D1127033

Bone Marrow Transplantation

The Jones and Bartlett Series in Nursing

Bone Marrow Transplantation

Principles, Practice, and Nursing Insights

Edited by

Marie Bakitas Whedon, RN, MSN, OCN
Hematology/Oncology
Clinical Nurse Specialist
Dartmouth-Hitchcock Medical Center
Hanover, NH

Jones and Bartlett Publishers
Boston

Editorial, Sales, and Customer Service Offices
Jones and Bartlett Publishers
20 Park Plaza
Boston, MA 02116

Library of Congress Cataloging-in-Publication Data

Bone marrow transplantation : principles, practice, and nursing
   insights / edited by Marie Bakitas Whedon.
      p. cm.
   Includes bibliographical references and index.
   ISBN 0-86720-440-0
   1. Bone marrow—Transplantation. 2. Bone marrow—Transplantation—
Nursing. I. Whedon, Marie Bakitas.
   [DNLM: 1. Bone Marrow Transplantation—adverse effects. 2. Bone
Marrow Transplantation—nursing. WH 380 B71192125]
RD123.5.B657 1991
617.4′4—dc20
DNLM/DLC
for Library of Congress   90-15614
                                                                   CIP

Printed in the United States of America
10 9 8 7 6 5 4 3 2 1

Contributors

Linda Z. Abramovitz, RN, MSN
Pediatric Bone Marrow Transplant
Clinical Nurse Specialist
The Medical Center at the University of
    California
San Francisco, California

Tim A. Ahles, PhD
Associate Professor
Behavioral Medicine Section
Department of Psychiatry
Dartmouth-Hitchcock Medical Center
Hanover, New Hampshire

Bruce Ballard, RN, BSN
Renal Care Coordinator
Fred Hutchinson Cancer Research Center
Seattle, Washington

Marilyn K. Bedell, RN, BSN, OCN
Nursing Director
Medical Hematology/Oncology
Dartmouth-Hitchcock Medical Center
Hanover, New Hampshire

Patricia Corcoran Buchsel, RN, BSN
Director of Nursing, Outpatient Department
Fred Hutchinson Cancer Research Center
Seattle, Washington

Kathryn Ann Caudell, RN, MN, OCN
Doctoral Candidate
University of Washington
Seattle, Washington

Dana Grossman, BA
Editor, *Dartmouth Medicine*
Dartmouth Medical School
Hanover, New Hampshire

Joleen Kelleher, RN, MS
Director of Nursing
Fred Hutchinson Cancer Research Center
Seattle, Washington

Lynna M. Lesko, MD, PhD
Assistant Attending Psychiatrist
Psychiatry Service
Department of Neurology
Memorial Sloan-Kettering Cancer Center
New York, New York

Deborah K. Meriney, RN, MN, OCN
Staff Nurse
Medical Hematology/Autologous Bone Marrow
    Transplant Unit
University of California at Los Angeles Medical
    Center
Los Angeles, California

Janet W. Nims, RN, BSN
Long-Term Follow-Up Consultant
Fred Hutchinson Cancer Research Center
Seattle, Washington

Jamie S. Ostroff, PhD
Research Fellow
Psychiatry Service
Department of Neurology
Memorial Sloan-Kettering Cancer Center
New York, New York

Peggy Plunkett Shedd, RN, MSN, CS
Psychiatric Liaison Clinical Nurse Specialist
Dartmouth-Hitchcock Medical Center
Hanover, New Hampshire

Karen S. Vanacek, RN, MSN
Clinical Nurse Specialist
Bone Marrow Transplant
Duke University Medical Center
Clinical Associate
Duke University
Durham, North Carolina

Pamela A. Weinberg, RN, BS
Director of Community Development
National Marrow Donor Program
St. Paul, Minnesota

Marie Bakitas Whedon, RN, MSN, OCN
Hematology/Oncology
Clinical Nurse Specialist
Dartmouth-Hitchcock Medical Center
Hanover, New Hampshire

Teresa J. Wikle, RN, BA, OCN
Nursing Supervisor
Bone Marrow Transplant Unit

Shands Hospital at the University of Florida
Gainesville, Florida

John R. Wingard, MD
Medical Director
Bone Marrow Transplant Outpatient Clinic
Associate Professor in Oncology
The Johns Hopkins Oncology Center
Baltimore, Maryland

To my husband, Jim, and my sons, Jimmy and Ryan,
whose love and support helped me to take the idea for this book
from dream to reality

Contents

Foreword

The early attempts (1956–1960) to carry out marrow grafts in human patients following high-dose chemo-radiotherapy were largely unsuccessful except for the occasional patient who had an identical twin to serve as donor (a syngeneic marrow graft). Allogeneic marrow transplants (a donor not genetically identical with the patient) were plagued by uncontrollable graft-versus-host disease. During the 1960s the development of better transfusion supportive care, better antibacterial antibiotics and, most important, definition of the human histocompatibility antigens set the stage for further investigation of allogeneic marrow transplantation. By 1967 my colleagues and I had been able to show that DLA-matched littermate dogs usually survived an allogeneic graft while DLA-mismatched littermates almost invariably died of complications related to graft-versus-host disease. These observations convinced us that it should be possible to identify an HLA-matched brother or sister of the patient in need of a bone marrow transplant.

During our early experiences with allogeneic and syngeneic marrow grafts we had recognized the difficulty in caring for these critically sick patients. In 1967 we wrote a program project grant application in order to establish a team of physicians, nurses, and laboratory technicians to carry out marrow grafts in a setting of optimal chance for success. The grant was funded in 1968, and we assembled a team of physicians and nurses who were then trained in the skills required for management of patients without bone marrow function. We carried out our first sibling transplant for a patient with advanced leukemia in March 1969.

Over the following years, we were able to show that some patients even with advanced refractory leukemia or aplastic anemia could be cured by an allograft from the matched sibling.

In recent years the list of diseases amenable to treatment involving marrow transplantation has expanded and results have improved, in part because of increasing skills and in part because of the ability to carry out transplants earlier in the course of the disease. More recently, the availability of large numbers of HLA-typed unrelated volunteer donors has made marrow grafting an option for some patients who do not have a family member donor.

Even so, there are many patients without a matched donor. These patients may be candidates for a graft with their own marrow, an autologous marrow graft. An autologous marrow graft after intensive chemotherapy and/or radiotherapy will almost always restore marrow function. The advantage of an autologous graft is that graft-versus-host disease is avoided. The disadvantage is that there may be tumor cells in the graft and this, along with the loss of the graft-versus-leukemia effect, may result in a greater relapse rate.

Marrow graft recipients almost always go through a period of critical illness because of their disease and the effort to treat it. Specialized problems include transfusion support and regimen related toxicity such as veno-occlusive disease of the liver, renal failure, pulmonary damage, and cardiac and central nervous system toxicity. The problems of graft-versus-host disease and opportunistic infections further complicate the care of these patients. Absolutely essential is a dedicated nursing team skilled in the critical care of such patients. Further, nurses play an important role in research protocols designed to improve the well-being and long-term survival of the patients. Nurses must keep up with the new and exciting developments in marrow transplantation including new anticancer agents and combinations of agents, new antibiotics and antiviral agents, the use of monoclonal antibodies, either alone or combined with a toxin or radioactive isotope, hematopoietic growth factors, biologic response modifiers and, perhaps soon, gene transfer therapy. Yet, with all these technical developments, nurses must not forget that they are in the best position to offer emotional and psychological support to the patient and family.

I have described our nursing team in Seattle as our "secret weapon" without which we could not have accomplished our goals.

E. DONNALL THOMAS, MD
Professor of Medicine Emeritus
University of Washington
School of Medicine
Member, Fred Hutchinson Cancer Research
    Center
1990 Nobel Laureate, Medicine/Physiology

Preface

It has been many years since the science and technology necessary to accomplish bone marrow transplants left the laboratory for the bedside; yet there is still much to learn. This presented a major challenge to the contributors of this book. Our charge was to integrate transplant science with the practical but complex daily informational needs of the clinician. Further, we were to intrigue the reader by supposing the future directions that the specialty would take and provide a nursing framework to guide that evolution.

As is the case with many textbook authors, my inspiration to produce this work was the wish that such a reference were available when I first entered the field. Like many other clinicians, I spent precious hours attempting to gather information from a variety of sources to grasp the nature of marrow transplantation. At the same time, I needed to provide care and counsel to patients and nurse colleagues and integrate physician and scientist's basic discoveries into the clinical setting. This text is designed to assist my colleagues who might otherwise struggle to develop a knowledge base and clinical expertise in the midst of chaos and crisis.

Although this text will be of primary interest to clinical hematology/oncology and transplant nurses, many sections will be of interest to others. These include health care providers who may refer patients for transplant, nursing and medical students or house staff, and hospital administrators contemplating the development of a transplant program.

Part I provides an overview of the scope of transplant in the treatment of adults and children: where we've been, where we're going, and general scientific concepts. Part II provides an in-depth analysis of the acute and long-term effects of the transplant procedure on each body system, including acute psychosocial effects. Common nursing diagnoses and nursing interventions for each disturbance are organized into plans of care (in Appendix A at the end of the book) which can be used to develop an individual patient's care or assist in the development of transplant-unit standards.

Part III considers the patient's transition to the world outside of the hospital and some additional post-transplant patient sequelae: psychosexual, psychosocial, and survivorship. Finally, Part IV addresses the important issues of the environment in which transplant occurs: the caregivers' responses and ethical issues, as well as physical and economical issues related to BMT programs. A patient's view concludes the book as a reminder of why we're doing this and to give a first-hand perspective on the positive and negative aspects of the procedure.

Bone marrow transplantation is still finding its place: standard therapy, investigational therapy, state-of-the-art treatment, or competing therapy. Indications for allogeneic transplants are becoming well-defined while indications for autologous transplantation are still being explored. The number of transplants performed annually and the number of teams performing these transplants is growing exponentially. Herein lies a major nursing challenge: many centers that were not designed or prepared to manage the specialized care needs of such a complex patient have begun to perform bone marrow transplants. Although little change in philosophy or environment need take place for an allogeneic transplant center to undertake autologous transplants, significant changes must occur in order for an oncology unit to provide this type of care. Therefore, a book such as this can assist nurses and other team members to quickly develop a sound knowledge base and an appreciation of the complexity of care needs for these patients.

There are references throughout the text to medical diagnoses, treatment, and care in order to give a complete picture of the spectrum of transplant nursing care. This information is not intended to prescribe or present a complete overview of physician's management of bone marrow transplant patients, but rather to emphasize the collaborative and integrated nature of providing care to this complex group of patients.

Transplantation technology changes daily and scientific discoveries increase the patient's hope for survival. Clearly discoveries will be made by the time this text is published that will make some of the content incomplete or outdated. Nevertheless, it is our hope that this reference will assist those who provide care every day to assure the success of this potentially curative procedure: the patients and their families, the nurses, the doctors, and all of the other team members.

Marie Bakitas Whedon

Acknowledgements

My sincere thanks to the many reviewers: Ted Ball, MD (Chapters 2 and 3), Cyndy King, RN (Chapter 3), Patricia Corcoran Buchsel, RN (Chapter 2), Fran Wiley, RN (Chapter 4), Bruce Davis, MD and Charles Bean BS, RPh (Chapter 6), Donald Ayers, MD (Chapter 11), Francine Lessard, RN (Chapter 11 and Nursing Care Plans), Diane Stearns, RN (Nursing Care Plans), and the cogent editorial assistance of Susan Scown.

To Ted Ball, MD, Gibbons Cornwell III, MD, Letha Mills, MD, Lamia Schwarz, Miriam Leach, and all of the rest of the members of the transplant team at Dartmouth-Hitchcock Medical Center for their support and ideas. A special thanks to all of the bone marrow transplant patients who motivated and inspired me by their efforts and dedication into believing that this book was important and to persist until it was complete. To Vincent Memoli, MD, for the helpful suggestions on Pathology illustrations.

To the staff nurses on the Medical Hematology/Oncology/ABMT unit and the nursing leadership (Marilyn Bedell, Amy Stansfield, Diane Stearns) at Mary Hitchcock Memorial Hospital who were always supportive and interested and who tolerated my brief absences during the critical times of manuscript development and review.

To the members of Nursing Administration of Mary Hitchcock Memorial Hospital who provided me with the time, resources, secretarial support (Barb Jarrell and Bev Cavanaugh), and emotional support necessary to complete this work while still maintaining my full-time status. To my clinical nurse specialist colleagues who supported and encouraged me throughout this arduouous process; especially Virginia Kilpack, RN, PhD, for her helpful suggestions on the use of nursing diagnoses in care plan development.

To Fred Pond, Tom Mead, Donna Jacob, Elaine Bent, and the other Dana Medical Library staff whose expert searching skills, computer education, and rapid attention to every detail assisted in the development of several chapters.

To Margaret Barton-Burke, RN, who ignited my spark from thinking to doing. To the wonderful people at Jones and Bartlett, particularly Jim Keating, Maureen Neumann, Rafael Millán and Clayton Jones who were always most helpful and encouraging.

Finally, in memory of my mother, Helen, and to my dad, Thomas H. Bakitas, who raised me to believe I could do anything I put my mind to.

Bone Marrow Transplantation

PART I

Bone Marrow Transplantation

Process and Indications

Chapter 1

Historical Perspectives and Future Directions

John R. Wingard

Introduction

The mythical figure of the chimera has often been used to symbolize the field of bone marrow transplantation (BMT). The **chimera** was a fire-spouting monster with a lion's head, a goat's body, and a serpent's tail. This creature was feared, killing many animals and people. The monster was eventually killed with the consent of the gods, hoping to free the earth of this scourge.

In the field of BMT, the term chimera was first used by Ford et al. in 1956 to describe animals lethally irradiated and then given bone marrow from another animal: this maneuver resulted in the recipient animal carrying a foreign hematopoietic system derived from the other animal. It is somewhat ironic that this name, which originally evoked fear and revulsion and represented a cruel perversion of nature, has come to evoke hope and concern and represents one of modern medicine's successful attempts to correct a number of nature's ailments afflicting human beings.

Evolution of BMT As a Treatment of Human Disease

Human bone marrow administration as a treatment for disease has been attempted sporadically since the late nineteenth century. Many of the early applications involved feeding or injecting bone marrow or spleen extracts into patients with a variety of ailments, such as several kinds of anemia, including the "anemia of rapid growth, overwork and underfeeding," leukemia, and chlorosis (Quine 1896). Sometimes, arsenic and iron were given adjunctively. While some benefits were ascribed to the bone marrow treatments, the reason for improvement was unclear, and these efforts now seem quaint and unscientific.

In the modern era, human bone marrow transplantation began in 1957, when French and Yugoslav physicians treated several laboratory workers who had been exposed to radiation during the Vinca nuclear reactor accident (Mathe et al. 1959). One patient received fetal spleen and liver cells but died from hemorrhage. Four patients were given allogenic bone marrow cells and all recovered marrow function. However, although there was some evidence of temporary engraftment, whether or not the bone marrow transplant offered any lasting benefit was uncertain (van Bekkum and de Vries 1967).

During the early years of human BMT, attention was directed to determining the source of bone marrow cells and methods of preserving the cells, achieving safe techniques for administering marrow intravenously to avoid pulmonary emboli, estimating the number of cells needed, and defining the types of illnesses to which BMT could be applied (Thomas et al. 1957; Thomas and Storb 1970).

In 1970, a review of the reported human bone marrow transplant experience indicated that approximately 200 transplants had been performed over the preceding decade (see Table 1.1) (Bortin 1970). The early results did not auger well. More than half of the patients had failed to engraft; three-fourths had died before being reported in the literature. There was evidence of chimerism in only a few of the cases in which there were markers of donor cells and only three chimeric patients were alive at the time of reporting. Of the patients with aplastic anemia treated by al-

logeneic marrow none engrafted, but five of seven patients given syngeneic bone marrow transplants recovered.

Because of this very disappointing early experience, the number of marrow transplants performed during the early 1960s declined (see Figure 1.1). Improvements in the results of BMT awaited developments in several ancillary fields: supportive care (especially transfusion support and antibiotics), histocompatibility testing, conditioning regimens, and control of graft-versus-host disease (GVHD). These developments are discussed below.

As a result of the advances in these related fields, a resurgence of interest in bone marrow transplantation took place in the late 1960s. At this time human tissue typing permitted intentionally matched marrow transplants, which were applied to the treatment of genetic immunodeficiency syndromes. These disorders are rare but have provided important biologic insights.

The wider application of BMT in the 1970s occurred initially in the therapy of severe aplastic anemia or acute leukemia where other treatment had failed. Improved results were reported in 1975 (Thomas et al. 1975) (see Figure 1.2). As supportive care of patients improved and more effective conditioning regimens were applied, six-month survival rates increased from less than 20% to greater than 70%.

Table 1.1.   Results of 203 Reported Human Bone Marrow Transplants

Disease	Number of patients	Number with no engraftment	Number with secondary disease	Number of allogeneic diseases
Aplastic anemia	73	66	5	0
Leukemia	84	33	32	3
Malignant disease	31	23	1	1
Immune deficiency	15	3	11	7
Total	203	125	49	11*

*Three alive at the time of this report.
M.M. Bortin, A compendium of reported human bone marrow transplants, *Transplantation* 9(6): 571–587, © Williams and Wilkins, 1970, with permission.

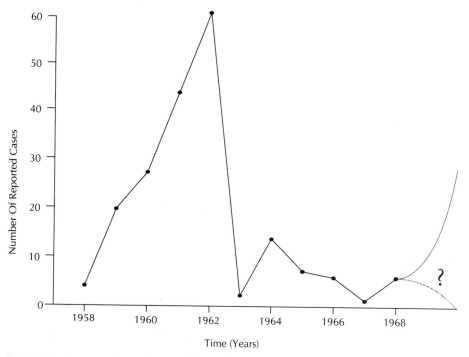

M.M. Bortin, A compendium of reported human bone marrow transplants, *Transplantation 9* (6): 571–587, © Williams and Wilkins, 1970, with permission.

Figure 1.1.   Reported Human Bone Marrow Transplants from 1958 to 1968

Since then, steady increases in interest have paralleled improved long-term outcomes and wider applications. By 1986, more than 200 bone marrow transplant centers (60% established since 1980) were performing almost 5,000 cases annually (Bortin et al. 1988) (see Figure 1.3).

An important advance that has evolved slowly over time is the development of criteria for performing BMT. It has become recognized that certain factors (both related and unrelated to the disease to be treated by BMT) must be considered in patient selection. Examples of factors unrelated to the disease to be treated that increase the risk of performing a BMT include advanced age of the patient, significantly impaired ventilatory function, abnormal hepatic function, and the presence of an active infection.

The status of the disease to be treated by BMT is an important determinant of the outcome for the patient. When BMT was performed in patients with acute leukemia in full relapse, long-term disease-free survival rates of approximately 15% were seen. In contrast, when BMT was attempted in patients in chemotherapy-induced remission, the mortality rate fell dramatically, due to both a lower relapse rate and a decreased rate of transplant-associated mortality. Similarly, it has become recognized that the earlier the transplant is performed in the course of the disease the better (rather than after multiple relapses or multiple courses of therapy): the risk of relapse is lower and the likelihood of toxicity from the conditioning regimen is less.

By adopting patient selection criteria one can minimize the risk of failure from toxicity. By performing the transplant at the appropriate time in the course of an individual's disease one can op-

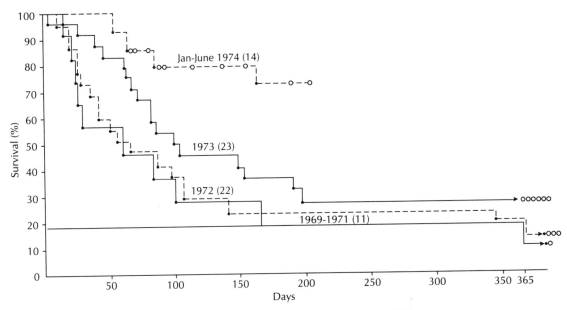

Reprinted by permission of the *New England Journal of Medicine Vol. 292*, p. 841, 1975.

Figure 1.2. Survival Curves in 70 Patients with Acute Leukemia Given a Marrow Graft from a Major-Histocompatibility-Complex-Matched Sibling (Open circles indicate living patients)

timize the likelihood of success in control of the underlying disease.

Conditioning Regimens

Some form of conditioning is necessary for BMT, except in certain rare situations where a monozygotic twin is used as a donor or where the recipient has a certain form of immunodeficiency and the donor is HLA-identical. From animal experiments, it was learned early on that there are several prerequisites for a conditioning regimen (Santos 1974). The conditioning regimen must first suppress the recipient immunity to prevent graft rejection. Secondly, it must create "space" for the donor marrow: not physical space, but rather an effect (still poorly understood) on the marrow microenvironment that permits the establishment and growth of hematopoietic progenitors. A third requirement for recipients trans-

planted for malignant disease is an antitumor effect, to eradicate residual tumor cells.

Total body irradiation (TBI), cyclophosphamide, or a combination of the two, were the first conditioning regimens used. Both agents possess all three properties desirable in conditioning agents.

Experiments in mammals (reviewed by van Bekkum and de Vries 1967) had demonstrated three types of syndromes after exposure to irradiation. Animals exposed to lethal TBI up to 1200 cGy die 8–14 days later from the effects of marrow aplasia (the so-called "hematopoietic syndrome"). Mice given 1200 to 12,000cGy die 4–5 days later due to the sequelae from gut damage (the gastrointestinal syndrome). Animals subjected to > 12,000cGy die hours to 1–2 days after exposure due to toxicity to the central nervous system (the cerebral syndrome). Infusions of syngeneic bone marrow will reverse the hematopoietic syndrome, but have no effect on the

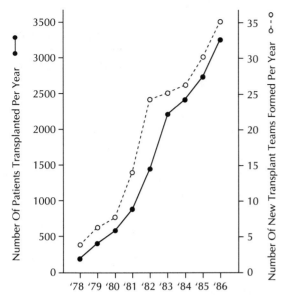

With permission. M.M. Bortin, Current status of BMT in humans: Report from the International Bone Marrow Transplant Registry. *Nat'l. Immun. Cell Regul. 7*: 339, © S. Karger A.G., Basel.

Figure 1.3. Annual Number of Patients Receiving Allogeneic Bone Marrow Transplants and Annual Number of New Tranplant Teams Formed 1978–1986

other two syndromes. In animals subjected to less than lethal irradiation, the frequency and persistence of engraftment after marrow transplant was found to be related to the TBI dose. In general, supralethal TBI doses were necessary for long lasting chimerism.

Aside from the extensive experience with TBI in animals, there were several other reasons TBI was a good choice as a preparative regimen. Irradiation was known to be effective in killing leukemic cells. It was able to bypass supposed sanctuary sites, such as the testes and central nervous system, to eliminate any occult contaminating tumor cells. One of its major organ toxicities, bone marrow, is not a concern when it is to be replaced by donor marrow. Initially, TBI doses of 800–1000cGy were given at a rate of 3–6cGy/min as

a single dose. This was successful in achieving engraftment, but was not very effective in eradicating leukemia.

Experience with cyclophosphamide in animals (Santos et al. 1970) similarly led to its use in man. The combination of cyclophosphamide plus total body irradiation (CyTBI) was introduced very early, and since has become the most commonly used conditioning regimen in the treatment of malignant disease. During the 1970s it was recognized that the risk for another major non-hematologic toxicity, interstitial pneumonitis, could be reduced by fractionation of the TBI, rather than administration in one dose (Meyers et al. 1983). Another regimen, busulfan plus cyclophosphamide (BuCy), was developed as an alternative preparative regimen to CyTBI. Busulfan has very little immunosuppressive potency, but has excellent antitumor and space-making properties. The combination regimen of BuCy has been shown to be at least as effective as CyTBI in the treatment of ANLL (Santos et al. 1983). In recent years it has also been found to be effective as a conditioning regimen for chronic myelogenous leukemia (CML), Hodgkin's Disease, non-Hodgkin's lymphoma, and beta-thalassemia.

Other agents have also been introduced into preparative regimens to try to improve the antitumor efficacy. One agent used increasingly is etoposide (VP16), which has excellent antitumor activity, as well as some immunosuppressive activity although not as much as cyclophosphamide (Gassmann et al. 1988). Caution must be exercised in allogeneic transplantation to avoid agents with little or no immunosuppressive properties, especially in situations where there is an increased risk of graft rejection, such as with a non-sibling donor, a mismatched donor, or a marrow graft manipulated ex vivo to remove T lymphocytes.

With autologous BMT, there is no such concern for graft rejection or the need for immunosuppression, and thus a panoply of preparative regimens have been and continue to be explored. The major objective is to develop combinations of drugs and/or radiotherapy with additive or synergistic antitumor activity and toxicities that do not overlap or where non-hematologic toxicities are minimal.

With respect to severe aplastic anemia there is no necessity for antitumor activity, but the risk of graft rejection is substantive, and immunosuppression of the host is the paramount consideration in choosing a conditioning regimen. In the first 66 patients transplanted with allogeneic marrow for aplastic anemia, none benefitted, and none demonstrated chimerism (Bortin 1970). This was due in large measure to the fact that none received vigorous immunosuppressive pretreatment. Santos developed the use of high-dose cyclophosphamide alone as a conditioning regimen for patients with aplastic anemia (Santos 1974). Today this continues to be the most commonly used preparative regimen for allogeneic BMT for aplastic anemia. For patients who had been sensitized to the donor, through blood transfusions or prior pregnancy (by exposure to fetal alloantigens), one of the major difficulties to overcome was graft rejection. It was learned that by increasing the immunosuppression in the conditioning regimen rejection could be reduced. Initially this was done by adding TBI to cyclophosphamide; the rejection rate decreased, however, there was no improvement in survival due to the sequelae of the irradiation toxicity. Subsequently, the use of cyclosporine or total lymphoid irradiation has provided better immunosuppression without the added mortality from toxicity.

Developments in Tissue Typing

Dausset (1954 and 1958) first presented evidence of leukoantigens in patients receiving multiple transfusions. Initially thought to be autoantibodies, they were later shown to be alloantibodies to antigens expressed on the leukocytes. Family studies showed the leukocyte antigens to be genetically determined. These antigens are the gene products of the HLA (or major histocompatibility) complex, which is a series of genes located on human chromosome 6. Although initially thought to be leukocyte specific, the HLA antigens subsequently were found to be broadly distributed tissue antigens. The HLA system plays a critical role in the cellular interactions that occur as part of immune reactions to viruses and other foreign antigens: viz., T lymphocytes only recognize foreign antigens when they are physically associated with HLA gene products. They have been recognized as important determinants of allograft rejection.

In 1964 Terasaki and McClelland introduced the microlymphocytotoxicity assay, which continues to be the major type of procedure to perform HLA typing. During the 1960s two serologically defined loci (the A and B loci) were identified, and in 1970 the C locus was defined. These now are grouped as Class I loci. The D region was initially assessed by the mixed lymphocyte reaction. It has subsequently been learned that there are several loci within the region, some of which can be defined serologically (such as DR and DQ). The D loci are grouped as Class II loci.

The dismal results of the initial human bone marrow transplantation experience were in large measure due to the lack of use of tissue typing in the selection of donors. In the compilation of early human BMT experience by Bortin (1970), matched donors (using the mixed leukocyte culture test) were used in only three cases, and all three lived, while only two of the 200 transplanted patients in which histocompatibility matching was not performed survived.

Beatty et al. (1985) has shown the importance of HLA identity between the host and the donor in determining the outcome of allogeneic BMT. As the number of HLA antigens not shared by both donor and recipient increases, the rate and severity of GVHD increase, the risk for delayed engraftment or nonengraftment increases, and the rate of survival decreases. Attempts to improve the potential success for transplantation using donors who are unrelated or who are only partially matched is in the developmental stages in the field of BMT, and the issues involved will be discussed in subsequent chapters.

Developments in Supportive Care

Blood Banking

The presence of different blood groups has been known since the early part of the twentieth century. Initially, the major ABO groups were defined in the first decade of this century, and in 1940 the Rh system was described. Subsequently, over 200 blood group systems have been discovered. Blood preservation and anticoagulation were also developed in the first half of the twentieth century. The first blood banks were organized in the 1930s, and during the 1940s blood transfusion was available in many American hospitals. The introduction of plastic equipment in the late 1940s facilitated wider applications of transfusion. Refrigeration, improved preservative solutions, automated equipment for separating and processing blood, and serologic testing for viruses all have led to improved utilization and safety of blood components.

The introduction in the 1960s of component therapy, in which whole blood could be divided into red cells, plasma, platelets, and other components, enabled the targeted use of blood products to replace specific needed elements and avoid unnecessary components. This led to improved safety and efficacy, and has enabled better utilization of donor supplies, since a larger number of therapeutic units are derived from each donation.

The advances of BMT have depended heavily on the availability of blood component support. In the early 1960s platelet transfusions were available only at some large hospitals with cancer treatment programs. The use of platelets has subsequently grown meteorically. For example, the American Red Cross Blood Services distributed 196,000 units in 1972, but more than three million units in 1986. This increase is attributable to the development of standardized criteria for the use of these products, the increasing use of aplasia-producing cytotoxic therapy in the treatment of malignant diseases, and improved technology with the advent of differential centrifugation increasing the availability of these products. In 1963, the relationship between the number of circulating platelets and the risk for hemorrhage was described (Gaydos et al. 1962). The incidence of spontaneous hemorrhage was found to not significantly increase until the count fell below 20,000/ul. The risk of hemorrhage also was shown to be reduced by transfusion (Freireich et al. 1963). Using these data, in many centers, the general practice has evolved to prophylactically transfuse patients at counts less than 15,000–20,000/ul in chemotherapy-treated patients. Platelets can be obtained either by concentration of pooled multiple donor components or by single-donor platelets obtained by plateletpheresis. Both techniques are used widely, but the latter is preferred as it exposes the patient to fewer different HLA antigens, reduces the chance for alloimmunization, and lessens the risk of exposure to infectious agents in the product.

Neutropenic patients were found to be at greater risk for infection, especially with neutrophil counts less than 500/ul. The initial attempts to correct neutropenia used transfusions from patients with chronic myelogenous leukemia (CML) with high circulating neutrophil counts. During the early 1970s the source of neutrophils shifted from CML patients to normal donors with a yield of only 10% of that used in early studies. One early technique used to obtain neutrophils was to obtain cells from donors by leukopheresis and pass the cells over nylon wool columns to which neutrophils selectively adhered. This provided an excellent yield, but some damage to the neutrophils impaired their functional capacity; most important, donors occasionally suffered potentially serious toxicities, such as activation of complement, and signs and symptoms of leukostasis. Accordingly, this technique was abandoned and the technique of flow centrifugation has become prominent with the use of an erythrocyte sedimenting agent, such as hydroxyethyl starch, to facilitate the separation. Sometimes, corticosteroids are also used to elevate the donor's neutrophil count and improve the yield. Generally, 1×10^9 to 1.5×10^{10} cells are obtained. Neutrophil transfusions have been shown to be efficacious in the treatment of bacterial sepsis. Trials where neutrophil transfusions are given prophylactically during neutropenia have generally shown a reduction in infections but no reduction in death. During the late 1970s, several BMT studies (Winston et al. 1980) demonstrated that the risk of death from infection by CMV, a virus that is transmitted via blood products, was significantly increased in BMT patients given neutrophil transfusions. Subsequently, the routine use of neutrophil transfusions has largely been abandoned in the management of the aplasia soon after BMT, due to the concern of exposure to CMV.

There are several unique challenges in the area of transfusion support in BMT. In the setting of profound immunosuppression present shortly after BMT, donor lymphocytes present in blood transfusions can transiently engraft and produce GVHD. Transfusions of all types of cellular blood products have been shown to cause GVHD. Therefore, all cellular blood products should be irradiated with 1500 to 3000cGy rads to eliminate the proliferative potential of lymphocytes.

As mentioned, CMV infection is a major cause of morbidity and death after BMT (Meyers et al. 1983). Seropositive patients can reactivate latent endogenous virus and, to date, there is no effective preventive strategy. However, seronegative patients can acquire the virus through the marrow graft (if the donor is seropositive) or through blood transfusions since the majority of adult Americans who constitute the donor pool are seropositive. One possible way to avoid acquisition of CMV is through the use of blood products screened to eliminate CMV-positive donors; this approach has been found to eliminate CMV

primary infection (Bowden et al. 1986). It is applicable to only the situation in which both donor and recipient are seronegative, however. Fortunately, the risk of CMV disease in such patients is low even without CMV screening (Wingard et al. 1990a), and the question of significance of the benefit remains unanswered. Also, the use of CMV-screened blood products in syngeneic and autologous BMT patients does not appear necessary, since studies have shown the risk of CMV disease to be low (Wingard et al. 1988a).

The genes controlling the major blood groups are located on chromosome 9, not chromosome 6 where the HLA complex resides. Thus, it is possible for a patient and donor to be HLA identical yet ABO mismatched. Since red cells make up a substantial part of the marrow product, techniques had to be developed to avoid major hemolytic transfusion reactions when the patients were infused. One early technique was intensive plasma exchange of the recipient to remove anti-A and/or anti-B isohemagglutinins. With the advent of cell separators, the most common technique now used is to differentially centrifuge the marrow product using hydroxyethyl starch to remove the donor erythrocytes, and resuspend the marrow in recipient-type erythrocytes (Braine et al. 1982). The recipient is also given copious fluids and monitored closely to minimize the hazard for an ABO-incompatible transfusion reaction.

Antimicrobial Therapy

As previously mentioned, life-threatening infection has been a major obstacle to advances in BMT (Winston et al. 1979). The most common cause of death in the early history of not only BMT, but also in the treatment of leukemia by chemotherapy (Hersh et al. 1965; Levine et al. 1974), was infection.

One of the first advances in this area was the recognition of the association between neutropenia and the risk for infection (Bodey et al. 1966). The incidence of any type of infection has been found to increase as the number of circulating neutrophils falls below 500/ul; the incidence of serious infection was noted to be particularly high at neutrophil counts below 100/ul. The duration of neutropenia also was found to be significantly correlated with the risk of infection. The major type of infection in neutropenia was due to enteric Gram-negative bacteria. During the second or third week of neutropenia, fungi, especially *Candida* and *Aspergillus*, emerged as important pathogens. In recent years, with the routine use of indwelling venous catheters, Gram-positive bacteria have become increasingly important pathogens during neutropenia.

An equally important advance in the control of infection was the recognition that fever during neutropenia was usually due to an infection, and that the use of empiric broad-spectrum antibiotics was much more effective in successfully treating the infection than waiting until the infection was documented by culture or some other diagnostic test. Initially, various combinations of a semisynthetic penicillin plus an aminoglycoside were used, but more recently, single-agent therapy with ceftazidime has been found to be effective (Pizzo et al. 1986).

A variety of antimicrobial agents have been used over the years to prevent infections. Combinations of nonabsorbable agents (such as orally administered vancomycin, gentamicin, and nystatin) and absorbable agents (such as trimethoprim-sulfamethoxazole) have been studied in multiple centers but have not been found to be consistently useful. In recent years the advent of the quinolone family of antibiotics has provided a group of agents that can be administered orally and have a wide antibacterial spectrum, including *Pseudomonas*. Norfloxacin, one member of this family, has been found to be an effective prophylaxis against Gram-negative bacterial infection in neutropenic patients treated for leukemia (Karp et al. 1987). With the emergence of Gram-positive bacterial pathogens, many of which are methicillin-resistant, some clinicians advocate the use of intravenous vancomycin prophylactically (Karp et al. 1986).

The most elaborate strategy to prevent infections is isolation of the patient in a laminar air flow (LAF) room along with the use of topical and oral antibiotics and sterile food. This has been shown to be effective but is very expensive. It also exacts an emotional toll on the patient because of the isolation from human contact. In addition, several studies showed no improvement in survival (Bodey 1984; Armstrong 1984). One study showed a reduced rate of GVHD in aplastic anemia patients transplanted in LAF (Storb et al. 1983). However, in the absence of a substantial benefit of LAF, and with its high cost, most BMT units do not use LAF. Moreover, with the introduction of a panoply of safe and effective antibiotics with a wide spectrum of activity, death from bacterial infections has diminished. Many BMT units use simple reverse isolation, with patients placed in single rooms, or in rooms equipped with high-efficiency particulate air (HEPA) filters.

As the control of bacterial infections has been refined, attention has increasingly turned to the more problematic fungal infections, which continue to be the most common cause of death from infection before engraftment. Because of the difficulty in early diagnosis and the poor success rate when therapy is delayed, efforts to prevent *Candida* infection have been numerous. Orally administered agents have not been consistently effective, in part, because of poor tolerance of oral medications after chemotherapy. Two strategies have been found to be effective. Amphotericin B given intravenously, started empirically 6–10 days after the start of the antibacterial empiric regimen in persistently febrile patients reduces fungal infections (Pizzo et al. 1982; EORTC 1989). Alternatively, intravenous miconazole given concomitantly with the empiric antibiotic regimen started at the first incidence of fever has also been found to be effective (Wingard et al. 1987a). Unfortunately, miconazole and the other members of the imidazole family of antifungal agents (such as ketoconazole), which are less toxic than amphotericin B, are not effective against *Aspergillus*. In the past, *Aspergillus* infections were uniformly fatal, despite the use of amphotericin B (Wingard et al. 1987b). In recent years, however, use of the CT scan to detect early distinctive pulmonary lesions, coupled with the use of early, high-dose amphotericin B has resulted in improved control rates (Kuhlman et al. 1987, Burch et al. 1987).

Over the years the major postengraftment infectious complication has been CMV pneumonitis; indeed, this has represented one of the most common causes of death after BMT. Until recently, there was no effective therapy. Thus, over the past decade, efforts have focused on prevention through the use of CMV-negative blood products, anti-CMV immunoglobulin, and high-dose acyclovir (reviewed in Wingard 1990b). However, even in the absence of such measures, the incidence of CMV pneumonia in some centers has decreased in recent years (Wingard et al. 1988b and 1990a), without any change in CMV infection rates. This appears to be largely related to the adoption of cyclosporine as anti-GVHD prophylaxis and to improved control of GVHD. More recently, several studies have shown the combination of ganciclovir plus intravenous immunoglobulin to be an effective therapy for CMV pneumonitis, with 50–70% survival rates (Reed et al. 1988). Ganciclovir prophylaxis is presently under study in several centers.

Nutritional Considerations

The gastrointestinal side effects of the chemoradiotherapy employed in the conditioning regimen include anorexia, nausea, vomiting, and diarrhea. Additionally, graft-versus-host disease and enteric viruses can cause severe, prolonged diarrhea. Up to half of BMT patients have enteritis severe enough to cause a protein losing eneropathy (Weisdorf et al. 1983). Mucositis often makes oral intake of fluid and nutrients difficult. In sum, nitrogen loss occurs as a result of reduced intake of nutrients, enteral loss in diarrhea, and the direct catabolic effect of the cytotoxic therapy, infection, graft-versus-host disease and corticosteroids, and immobilization.

Early in the history of BMT, when patients referred for BMT often had residual leukemia, malnutrition was frequently present. Animal studies demonstrated that hematopoietic recovery was compromised without adequate nutrition (Stuart and Sensenbrenner 1979). Thus, many BMT centers routinely used total parenteral nutritional (TPN) support to replete nutrition and ensure marrow engraftment. In recent years, the character of transplant patients has changed. Patients are mostly in remission at time of transplant and are well nourished. Thus, the goal has changed from nutritional repletion to maintenance. Many studies of well-nourished patients undergoing chemotherapy and radiotherapy have shown no benefits from total parenteral nutrition (Koretz 1984), while some have noted more rapid hematologic recovery (Hays et al. 1983). One randomized trial in BMT patients compared patients given TPN to those given maintenance IV fluids plus enteral feedings as tolerated (Weisdorf et al. 1987). Patients who received TPN had improved overall survival and disease-free survival rates. In contrast, another study in BMT patients compared TPN and an enteral feeding program in a randomized trial (Szeluga et al. 1987). The Weisdorf study began the trial during cytoreductive therapy; the Szeluga study started the nutritional program just before marrow infusion (after completion of the conditioning regimen). Both studies found that patients were unable to achieve maintenance nutritional status with an enteral feeding program. The Szeluga study, in contrast, found no long-term benefit in survival or disease-free survival. Szeluga and colleagues (1987) speculate that TPN may have potentiated the effects of the antineoplastic therapy rather than supported marrow recovery; thus, an effect would be seen when given during chemotherapy, but in the absence of a gross nutritional deficiency, TPN would not offer a benefit.

A survey of BMT centers in 1987 indicated that various methods were being used to provide oral nutritional support (Dezenhall et al. 1987). Sterile food was rarely used due to cost and poor patient acceptance. Most commonly used were either a reduced-bacterial diet or a house diet without fresh vegetables or fruit. Frequently, patients have prolonged poor oral intake after marrow engraftment. In the past this necessitated delays in hospital discharge. Now, with the availability of home IV therapy, many patients can still be discharged and continue to receive TPN without compromising their nutrition (Lenssen et al. 1983).

Nursing Care

As the field of bone marrow transplantation has evolved, so too has BMT nursing, which has become one of the most challenging of nursing specialties. Its roles have become more complex and have expanded enormously in recent years.

The traditional major concern of attending to the acute care needs of patients has become increasingly difficult. BMT patients are generally young, but span the age range from infancy to the middle years of life: thus, skill in managing pediatric, adolescent, and adult fields of nursing are prerequisites. BMT nurses are frequently called upon to provide the highly technical critical care services needed to manage the problems of nutritional support, electrolyte and fluid management, aplasia, sepsis, severe graft-versus-host disease, transfusion management, and vital organ failure (O'Quin and Moravec 1988). In recent years, the introduction of computerized information systems to the clinical setting have required mastery of automated data system skills. Within the Oncology Nursing Society (ONS) a special interest group (SIG) has developed, focusing soley on the concerns of BMT nurses. These concerns include efforts to develop national standards of BMT nursing care, especially with respect to management of mucositis, skin care, indwelling venous catheter care, and isolation procedures.

The role of nursing in patient and family education has also expanded. Patients and their families require orientation to the treatment modalities and to the specific objectives in the plan of care. Although many patients have been under the care of an oncology treatment team before referral, few have a good understanding of what is to be undertaken. Specific issues that require emphasis in patient orientation include: a prolonged hospitalization with some type of isolation, the attendant loss of control associated with the restrictions of being in a hospital environment, the unique problems of graft-versus-host disease, and the need for months of isolation from the general public even after recovery of marrow function, to avoid contagious illness until the slower recovery of cellular immunity occurs. Teaching self-care tasks, especially with respect to exercise, nutrition, and care of indwelling catheters, to encourage the patient to exercise as much control over his/her care, is very important. For patients newly referred to the transplant center, orientation to the inpatient and outpatient units is important to enable them to utilize optimally the hospital's resources.

A greater emphasis on the psychosocial needs of patients and families has also emerged (Haberman 1988). Nurses play an increasingly pivotal role in the recognition of patients' psychosocial needs and are called on to ensure that appropriate resources are directed to dealing with problems that arise. Patients who do not reside in the same community as the transplant center are especially in need of psychosocial resources since their network of family and friends is unable to be physically present during much of the BMT experience. Changes in family roles are universal concerns for patients and significant others. The primary nurse or case manager must be adept at utilizing the services of social workers, psychiatric liaison nurses, child life specialists, occupational therapists, etc.

Follow-up care is becoming increasingly important as there are more and more long-term survivors (Nims and Strom 1988). During the first year after transplant the patient and primary care team must be vigilant for the possible occurrence of chronic graft-versus-host disease, infections, obstructive airway disease, and recurrence (if transplanted for malignancy). Ovarian failure, which requires hormonal replacement, is a concern for adult women. Issues regarding sexuality are frequent concerns for both men and women. For children, growth and development must be monitored to detect pituitary, thyroid, or adrenal insufficiency. Reintegration into employment and former family social roles emerges as an increasingly important task for patients as the acute illness recedes into the background. Awareness of these "late" concerns, and assisting patients and families in dealing with these issues of survivorship have become important roles for nursing.

Developments in the Control of GVHD

Once techniques to ensure engraftment by adequate conditioning were developed, it became clear that GVHD was a major obstacle for allogeneic BMT. From animal studies it was recognized that GVHD was caused by donor T lymphocytes. It was learned that the frequency and severity of GVHD was dependent on the degree of HLA compatibility and the dose of lymphocytes. Although GVHD had harmful effects, being one of the major causes of death, it was found to also have beneficial effects, to be associated with an antileukemic effect (Weiden et al. 1979). Thus, the goal of prevention and treatment of GVHD was moderation of its severity without complete elimination.

Based on studies in dogs, methotrexate was employed as a prophylaxis against GVHD in some centers, and based on studies in rodents, cyclophosphamide was used in other centers. In recent years cyclosporine has been found to be an effective preventive measure and has been substituted as the preferred GVHD prophylaxis by many centers (Santos et al. 1987). Some centers employ a combination of methotrexate and cyclosporine.

High doses of corticosteroids have been the mainstay of treatment of GVHD over the years.

In cases of refractory GVHD, antithymocyte globulin (ATG) has sometimes been useful.

Another strategy investigated in the past decade is the removal of the T lymphocytes from the donor marrow. A variety of techniques have been used: anti-T cell monoclonal antibodies, corticosteroids, lectins, counterflow centrifugal elutriation. These have been shown to reduce GVHD in a variety of studies. Unfortunately, these techniques have also been associated with increased rates of relapse (Goldman et al. 1988), apparently eliminating the graft-versus-leukemia (GVL) effect seen with allogeneic BMT (Wingard 1990c).

For chronic GVHD, combination therapy with steroids plus azathioprine was the preferred treatment for many years (Sullivan 1983). Recently, a study comparing prednisone plus azathioprine versus prednisone showed prednisone alone to be as effective and to be associated with fewer infectious complications (Sullivan et al. 1988). Thalidomide has recently been shown to be active in the treatment of chronic GVHD and currently trials are investigating its role in the treatment of GVHD (Vogelsang et al. 1987).

Future Considerations

It is ironic that the initial steps in human BMT were taken in the wake of a nuclear reactor accident. Almost three decades later, in 1986, a nuclear reactor accident of significantly larger proportions with hundreds of individuals hospitalized in the Soviet Union led to the employment of marrow transplants once again to attempt to reverse the hematologic toxicity from accidental radiation exposure (Baranov et al. 1989). Of the 33 persons estimated to have received > 600 cGy, half had severe nonhematologic toxicity (mainly burns), which made survival unlikely. Thirteen received marrow transplants and one was given fetal liver because no histocompatible related donor was available. Of the marrow transplants, ten were from siblings (five HLA-identical, the remainder were one-haplotype identical). Although transient hematologic recovery occurred in most patients, there were only two long-term survivors. Most of the deaths were due to burns and other non-hematologic radiation injury. Thus, even today, nearly three decades later, we are reminded of the limitations of BMT and any other treatment modalities used to deal with radiation accidents, since the mortality related to the non-hematologic toxic effects of radiation, such as burns, gastrointestinal, pulmonary, or central nervous system injury, are not affected.

In the three decades of human bone marrow transplantation, enormous strides have occurred in the treatment of human disease. Currently, success rates in severe aplastic anemia exceed 70%, in acute nonlymphocytic leukemia in first remission 60%, in acute lymphoblastic leukemia in second remission 55%, in relapsed Hodgkin's or non-Hodgkin's lymphoma 55%, and chronic myelogenous leukemia 40–50%. There are a variety of other less common diseases in which success rates exceed 50%.

There remain a variety of limitations to the greater application of BMT, which require further improvements. The major causes of failure are graft-versus-host disease, immunodeficiency and infection, toxicities from the preparative regimen, and relapse. Further, only one-third of patients have an HLA-identical sibling to serve as a potential donor.

One strategy to address the problem of a lack of a compatible donor is the development of the National Bone Marrow Donor Registry. This will be addressed in a subsequent chapter. The use of related donors who are haplo-identical is another alternative, but remains limited as an option at present until better techniques are developed to control graft-versus-host disease.

With ex vivo purging of T cells from the donor graft, serious GVHD can be effectively prevented. Unfortunately, this and other measures successful in preventing GVHD have generally resulted in an increased relapse rate, by abrogation of the graft-versus-leukemia effect. There is some experimental evidence that the cell populations that mediate the GVL effect differ from the lymphocytes that mediate GVHD, although other data do not support this (reviewed in Wingard 1990c). In the future there will certainly be attempts to identify, characterize, and grow cells that mediate GVL and not GVHD. If successful, the marrow graft can be engineered to contain enriched populations of GVL cells while depleted of cells that mediate GVHD. Attempts to enrich the marrow with NK cells or LAK cells to enhance the anti-leukemic potential are also likely in the near future.

Another approach for adoptive immunotherapy may be to identify antigens enriched on tumor cells and, using cell culture techniques now available, to grow large numbers of T lymphocytes with desired specificity to be administered to the transplant recipient. Alternatively, administration of an antibody (perhaps linked with a cellular toxin or radio-isotope) specific for tumor antigens can be performed post-transplant. Such immunoadjuvant therapy would be expected to be most effective at a time of minimal residual disease, shortly after transplant.

The role of various biologic response modifiers in BMT will be more fully explored. Interferon is being studied for a possible antileukemic effect (Meyers et al. 1987). Erythropoietin may well reduce the need for red cell transfusion support. A variety of other growth factors, such as GM-CSF and G-CSF and IL-3, are being studied to determine their capacity to speed myeloid recovery without affecting the growth of any residual tumor cells. Quicker engraftment will result in both reduced morbidity and shorter hospitalizations.

An alternative way to avoid the limitations of GVHD and unavailability of a donor is with the use of autologous BMT. Results with autologous BMT have been improving in recent years, especially with lymphomas and acute nonlymphocytic leukemia (Santos et al. 1989). With the absence of GVHD, the early post-transplant mortality is lower than after allogeneic BMT. However, the relapse rate is generally substantially higher. This is due to the frequent contamination of the marrow graft with occult tumor cells and also to the absence of any GVL effect. Efforts to improve elimination of contaminating tumor cells are under development. Use of pharmacologic methods, such as 4-hydroperoxycyclophosphamide, monoclonal antibodies directed against tumor-associated antigens, immunoabsorption columns, and cell separation techniques are being studied.

Additionally, the deliberate creation of autologous GVHD is being investigated as a potential adjunctive to exert an immunotherapeutic effect. We have found that in man (as shown earlier in animals), autologous or syngeneic GVHD can be produced routinely after autologous GVHD when low-dose cyclosporine is administered (Jones et al. 1989). Cells that mediate this autologous GVHD are very similar to the cells that mediate chronic GVHD after allogeneic BMT; they are autoreactive against target cells that express Ia antigens (Hess and Fischer 1989). Ia antigens are expressed on lymphoma and nonlymphocytic leukemia cells. Thus, these effector cells may be capable of mediating an antileukemic effect, similar to that seen with chronic GVHD after allogeneic BMT (Weiden et al. 1981). Fortunately, autologous GVHD, unlike the acute GVHD after allogeneic BMT, is generally mild, and is easily controlled with either no therapy or a short course of corticosteroids. Studies are just beginning to purposely create autologous GVHD, with a goal of demonstrating an antitumor effect. If successful, the results of autologous BMT will exploit the benefits of the antileukemic effect of chronic GVHD without the harmful effects of acute GVHD with attendant immunodeficiency and risk for life-threatening infection.

One concern increasing in emphasis in recent years is the quality of life of survivors of various cancer treatments. This has been poorly studied as yet in BMT patients. Several small studies suggest that outcomes are similar to other types of cancer (Andrykowski et al. 1989a and b).

We have conducted a retrospective study of quality of life in 135 survivors of BMT (Wingard et al. 1990; Baker et al. 1988 and 1989; Curbow et al. 1989 and 1990). We have found that survivors reported both positive and negative changes in plans and activities, relationships, physical status, and existential concerns, but positive changes exceeded the negative changes, except in physical status. Seventy-nine percent reported the positives balanced with losses. Life satisfaction was rated favorably by most. Eighty-one percent reported their health to be good or excellent and 92% were able to perform normal activities with little or no difficulty. Seventy-eight percent were employed or in school. Twenty to thirty percent reported improved family relations, greater compassion, redirected life goals, and existential recovery, and 36% reported psychological gains after recovery from the transplant. While most appear to have been successful in reintegrating their life, some reported significant losses: 16% reported their health to be ill or bad, social function was limited "a good bit" in 9%, and 13% reported moderate to severe pain. These issues clearly need further prospective study. We are presently conducting such a study at Johns Hopkins, with a goal to examine stressors and patient resources as they change over time and interact in life satisfaction and psychological adjustment after BMT.

In summary, the historical developments of BMT have occurred because of the dedication and perseverance of specialists from many different fields. The advances in the biological sciences, supportive care, and nursing care have resulted in improved outcomes for BMT patients and patients undergoing other types of cancer therapy as well. These developments bode well for the future of BMT as an important treatment modality with expanding applications.

Acknowledgments: I am grateful for the helpful suggestions of Jane Shivnan, R.N. and Frances Phillips-Wingard, R.N., M.S.N.

References

Andrykowski, M.A., Henslee, P.J., and Farrall, M.G. 1989a. Physical and psychosocial functioning of adult survivors of allogeneic bone marrow transplantation. *B.M.T.* 4: 75–81.

Andrykowski, M.A., Henslee, P.J., and Barnett, R.L. 1989b. Longitudinal assessment of psychosocial functioning of adult survivors of allogeneic bone marrow transplantation. *B.M.T.* 4: 505–509.

Armstrong, D. 1984. Protected environments are discomforting and expensive and do not offer meaningful protection. *Am. J. Med.* 76: 685–689.

Baker, F., Curbow, B., and Wingard, J.R. 1988. Role retention and quality of life of bone marrow transplant survivors. *Social Science and Medicine,* In press 1990.

Baker, F. et al. 1989. Quality of life of cancer survivors after bone marrow transplantation. *The Society of Behavorial Medicine,* Abstract.

Baranov, A. et al. 1989. Bone marrow transplantation after the Chernobyl nuclear accident. *N. Engl. J. Med.* 321: 205–212.

Beatty, P.G. et al. 1985. Marrow transplantation from related donor other than HLA-identical siblings. *N. Engl. J. Med. 313:* 765–771.

Bodey, G.P. et al. 1966. Quantitative relationships between circulating leukocytes and infection in patients with acute leukemia. *Ann. Intern. Med.* 64: 328–340.

Bodey, G.P. 1984. Current status of prophylaxis of infection with protected environments. *Am. J. Med.* 76: 678–684.

Bortin, M.M. 1970. A compendium of reported human bone marrow transplants. *Transplantation 9:* 571–587.

Bortin, M.M., Horowitz, M.M., and Gale, R.P. 1988. Current status of bone marrow transplantation in humans: Report from the International Bone Marrow Transplant Registry. *Natl. Immun. Cell Regul.* 7: 334–350.

Bowden, R.A. et al. 1986. Cytomegalovirus immune globulin and seronegative blood products to prevent primary cytomegalovirus infection after marrow transplantation. *N. Engl. J. Med.* 314: 1006–1010.

Braine, H.G. et al. 1982. Bone marrow transplantation with major ABO blood group incompatibility using erythrocyte depletion of marrow prior to infusion. *Blood* 60: 420–425.

Burch, P.A. et al. 1987. Favorable outcome of invasive aspergillosis in patients with acute leukemia. *J. Clin. Oncol.* 5: 1985–1993.

Curbow, B. et al. 1989. Personal changes and psychological adjustment to an aggressive cancer treatment. *American Psychological Association,* Abstract.

Curbow, B. et al. 1990. Loss and recovery themes in survivors of bone marrow transplantation. *Eastern Psychological Association,* Abstract.

Dausset, J. 1954. Leukoagglutinins. IV. Leukoagglutinins and blood transfusions. *Vox Sang.* 4: 190.

Dausset, J. 1958. Iso-leuco-anticorps. *Acta Haematol.* (Basel) 20: 156–166.

Dezenhall, A. et al. 1987. Food and nutrition services in bone marrow transplant centers. *J. Am. Dietetic Assoc.* 87: 1351–1353.

EORTC International Antimicrobial Therapy Cooperative Group. 1989. Empiric antifungal therapy in febrile granulocytopenic patients. *Am. J. Med.* 86: 668–672.

Freireich, E.J. et al. 1963. Response to repeated platelet transfusions from the same donor. *Annu. Intern. Med.* 59: 277–287.

Gassmann, W. et al. 1988. Comparison of cyclophosphamide, cytarabine, and etoposide as immunosuppressive agents before allogeneic bone marrow transplantation. *Blood 72:* 1574–1579.

Gaydos, L.A., Freireich, E.J., and Mantel, N. 1962. The quantitative relation between platelet count and hemorrhage in patients with acute leukemia. *N. Engl. J. Med.* 266: 905–909.

Goldman, J.M. et al. 1988. Bone marrow transplantation for chronic myelogenous leukemia in chronic phase: Increased risk of relapse associated with T cell depletion. *Ann. Intern. Med.* 108: 806–814.

Haberman, M.R. 1988. Psychosocial aspects of bone marrow transplantation. *Seminars in Oncology Nursing* 4: 55–59.

Hays, D.M. et al. 1983. Effect of total parenteral nutrition on marrow recovery during induction therapy for acute nonlymphocytic leukemia in childhood. *Med. Pediatr. Oncol.* 11: 134–140.

Hersh, E.M. et al. 1965. Causes of death in acute leukemia. *JAMA* 193: 99–103.

Hess, A.D., and Fischer, A.D. 1989. Immune mechanisms in cyclosporine-induced syngeneic graft-versus-host disease. *Transplantation* 48: 895–900.

Jones, R.J. et al. 1989. Preliminary communication: Induction of graft-versus-host disease after autologous bone marrow transplantation. *Lancet* 1: 754–757.

Karp, J.E. et al. 1986. Empiric use of vancomycin during prolonged treatment-induced granulocytopenia: Randomized, double-blind, placebo-controlled clinical trial in patients with acute leukemia. *Am. J. Med.* 81: 237–242.

Karp, J.E. et al. 1987. Oral norfloxacin for prevention of gram-negative bacterial infections in patients with acute leukemia and granulocytopenia. *Ann. Intern. Med.* 106: 1–7.

Koretz, R.L. 1984. Parenteral nutrition: Is it oncologically logical? *J. Clin. Oncol.* 2: 534–538.

Kuhlman, J.E. et al. 1987. Invasive pulmonary aspergillosis in acute leukemia. *Chest* 92: 95–99.

Lenssen, P. et al. 1983. Parenteral nutrition in marrow transplant recipients after discharge from the hospital. *Exp. Hematol.* 11: 974–981.

Levine, A.S. et al. 1974. Hematologic malignancies and other marrow failure states: Progress in the management of complicating infections. *Semin. Hematol.* 11: 141–202.

Mathe, G. et al. 1959. Transfusions et greffes de moelle osseuse homologue chez les humains irradies á hautes dose accidentellement. *Rev. Fr. Etudes Clin. Biol.* 4: 238.

Meyers, J.D. et al. 1983. Biology of interstitial pneumonia after marrow transplantation. In Gale, R.P. (ed.) *Recent Advances in Bone Marrow Transplantation.* New York: Alan R. Liss, Inc., pp. 405–423.

Meyers, J.D. et al. 1987. Prophylactic use of human leukocyte interferon after allogeneic marrow transplantation. *Annu. Intern. Med.* 107: 809–816.

Nims, J.W., and Strom, S. 1988. Late complications of bone marrow transplant recipients: Nursing care issues. *Seminars in Oncology Nursing* 4: 47–54.

O'Quin, T., and Moravec, C. 1988. The critically ill bone marrow transplant patient. *Seminars in Oncology Nursing* 4: 25–30.

Pizzo, P.A. et al. 1982. Empiric antibiotic and antifungal therapy for cancer patients with prolonged fever and granulocytopenia. *Am. J. Med.* 72: 101–111.

Pizzo, P.A. et al. 1986. A randomized trial comparing ceftazidime alone with combination antibiotic therapy in cancer patients with fever and neutropenia. *N. Engl. J. Med.* 315: 552–558.

Quine, W.E. 1896. The remedial application of bone marrow. *JAMA* 26: 1012–1013.

Reed, E.C. et al. 1988. Treatment of cytomegalovirus pneumonia with ganciclovir and intravenous cytomegalovirus immunoglobulin in patients with bone marrow transplant. *Annu. Inter. Med.* 109: 783–788.

Santos, G.W. et al. 1970. Rationale for the use of cyclophosphamide as immunosuppression for marrow transplants in man. In Bertelli, A., and Monoco, A.P. (eds.) *International Symposium on Pharmacological Treatment in Organ and Tissue Transplantation.* Amsterdam: Experta Medical Foundation, p. 24.

Santos, G.W. 1974. Immunosuppression for clinical marrow transplantation. *Semin. Hematol.* 11: 341–351.

Santos, G.W. et al. 1983. Marrow transplantation for acute nonlymphocytic leukemia after treatment with busulfan and cyclophosphamide. *N. Engl. J. Med.* 309: 1347–1353.

Santos, G.W. et al. 1987. Cyclosporine plus methylprednisolone versus cyclophosphamide plus methylprednisolone as prophylaxis for graft-versus-host disease: A randomized, double-blind study in patients undergoing allogeneic marrow transplantation. *Clin. Transplantation* 1: 21–28.

Santos, G.W., Yeager A.M., and Jones, R.J. 1989. Autologous bone marrow transplantation. *Ann. Rev. Med.* 40: 99–112.

Storb, R. et al. 1983. Graft-versus-host disease and survival in patients with aplastic anemia treated by marrow grafts from HLA-identical siblings. Beneficial effect of a protective environment. *N. Engl. J. Med.* 308: 302–307.

Stuart, R.K., and Sensenbrenner, L.L. 1979. Adverse nutritional deprivation of transplanted hematopoietic cells. *Exp. Hematol.* 7: 435–442.

Sullivan, K.M. 1983. Graft-versus-host disease. In Blume, K.G., and Petz, L.D. (eds.) *Clinical Bone Marrow Transplantation.* New York: Churchill Livingston, pp. 91–130.

Sullivan, K.M. et al. 1988. Prednisone and azathioprine compared with prednisone and placebo for treatment of chronic graft-versus-host disease: Prognostic influence of prolonged thrombocytopenia after allogeneic marrow transplantation. *Blood* 72: 546–554.

Szeluga, D.J. et al. 1987. Nutritional support of bone marrow transplant recipients: A prospective, randomized clinical trial comparing total parenteral nutrition to an enteral feeding program. *Cancer Research* 47: 3309–3316.

Terasaki, P.I., and McClelland, J.D. 1964. Microdroplet assay of human serum cytotoxins. *Nature* 204: 998–1000.

Thomas, E.D. et al. 1957. Intravenous infusion of bone marrow in patients receiving radiation and chemotherapy. *N. Engl. J. Med.* 257: 491–496.

Thomas, E.D, and Storb, R. 1970. Techniques for human marrow grafting. *Blood* 36: 507–515.

Thomas, E.D. et al. 1975. Bone marrow transplantation. *N. Engl. J. Med.* 292: 832–843, 895–902.

van Bekkum, D.W., and de Vries, J.J. 1967. *Radiation Chimeras.* London: Logos.

Vogelsang, G.B. et al. 1987. Thalidomide therapy of chronic graft-versus-host disease. *Blood* 70: 1116.

Weiden, P.L., Flournoy, N., and Thomas, E.D. 1979. Antileukemic effect of graft-versus-host disease in human recipients of allogeneic marrow grafts. *N. Engl. J. Med.* 300: 1068–1073.

Weiden, P.L. et al. 1981. Antileukemic effect of chronic graft-versus-host disease. *Medical Intelligence* 304: 1529–1533.

Weisdorf, S.A. et al. 1983. Graft-versus-host disease of the intestine: A protein losing enteropathy characterized by fecal alpha-1-antitrypsin. *Gastroenterology* 85: 1076–1081.

Weisdorf, S.A. et al. 1987. Positive effect of prophylactic total parenteral nutrition on long-term outcome of bone marrow transplantation. *Transplantation* 43: 833–838.

Wingard, J.R. et al. 1987a. Prevention of fungal sepsis in patients with prolonged neutropenia: A randomized, double-blind, placebo-controlled trial of intravenous miconazole. *Am. J. Med.* 83: 1103–1110.

Wingard, J.R. et al. 1987b. Aspergillus infections in bone marrow transplant recipients. *Bone Marrow Transplantation* 2: 175–181.

Wingard, J.R. et al. 1988a. Cytomegalovirus infection after autologous bone marrow transplantation with comparison to infection after allogeneic bone marrow transplantation. *Blood* 71: 1432–1437.

Wingard, J.R. et al. 1988b. Interstitial pneumonitis after allogeneic bone marrow transplantation. Nine-year experience at a single institution. *Medicine* 67: 175–186.

Wingard, J.R. et al. 1990. Health, functional status, and employment of long-term survivors after bone marrow transplantation. *Ann. Intern. Med.* In press.

Wingard, J.R. et al. 1990a. Cytomegalovirus infections in patients treated by intensive cytoreductive therapy with marrow transplant. *Rev. Infect. Dis.* 12 (Suppl. 7): 805–810.

Wingard, J.R. 1990b. Advances in the management of infectious complications after bone marrow transplantation. *Bone Marrow Transplant.* In press.

Wingard, J.R., Burns, W.H., and Santos, G.W. 1990c. Bone marrow transplantation: A form of adoptive immunotherapy.

In Mitchell, M.D. (ed.) *The Biomodulation of Cancer.* Elmsford: Pergamon Press, Inc. In press.

Winston, D.J. et al. 1979. Infectious complications of human bone marrow transplantation. *Medicine* 58: 1–31.

Winston, D.J. et al. 1980. Cytomegalovirus infections associated with leukocyte transfusions. *Ann. Intern. Med.* 93: 671–675.

Chapter 2

Allogeneic Bone Marrow Transplantation: Clinical Indications, Treatment Process, and Outcomes

Marie Bakitas Whedon

Introduction

Bone marrow transplantation has been described as both intensive investigational therapy for end-stage disease and as standard curative treatment for malignant and nonmalignant conditions. Both descriptions are accurate, given the wide variety of bone marrow transplant types and clinical indications. While controversies in the literature persist regarding the use and place of bone marrow transplantation, thousands of transplants are performed annually at more than 250 centers worldwide (see Figure 2.1), for nearly one hundred different diseases. Nurses are on the frontline of caring for these complex patients and need to be knowledgable about and distinguish among the many uses, treatment processes, and prognoses to serve as patient advocates, educators, and expert clinicians.

The three major types of bone marrow transplant, **syngeneic**, **allogeneic**, and **autologous**, are

so named to indicate the source of "healthy" marrow that is obtained and then transplanted into the patient, for example, from an identical twin, from someone else, or from the patient himself. Syngeneic transplants, first attempted in the early 1960s to treat aplastic anemia, allowed investigators to learn that the hematopoietic system in man could be replaced by that of a genetically identical donor. However, when allogeneic transplantation was first attempted, patients developed a "secondary disease" (later called **graft-versus-host disease [GVHD]**) that interfered with **engraftment** and was often fatal. As more was learned about the need to match tissue types and condition or prepare the host to receive a bone marrow graft from a donor, greater success in preventing graft rejection was evident. Host immunosuppression allowed the new, healthy graft to "take" rather than attack a seemingly "foreign" host.

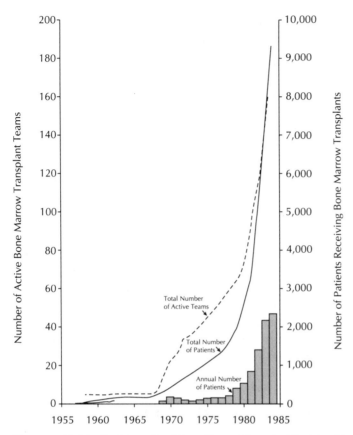

Figure provided by the International Bone Marrow Transplant Registry. *Directory of Bone Marrow Transplant Teams,* August 1988.

Figure 2.1. Vertical bars represent number of patients who received bone marrow transplants annually. Solid line indicates cumulative number of patients who received bone marrow transplants from 1958 through 1984. Dashed line represents number of active bone marrow transplant teams from 1958 through 1984.

Most reported cases of allogeneic bone marrow transplantion since the first successful cases in the late 1960s, involved transplants between siblings with identical bone marrow tissue types (**human leukocyte antigen [HLA]** matched-explained later). However, since only about one-third of eligible patients had identical sibling donors, other sources of marrow were sought. Discoveries in the field of immunology allowed the successful transplantation of marrow from HLA-matched unrelated donors and HLA-partially matched related and unrelated donors. Recently, locating HLA-matched unrelated donors for large numbers of patients has become potentially more feasible with the creation of bone marrow **donor registries** (see Chapter 5). Cadaver donors are another reported source of allogeneic marrow (Blazar et al. 1986; Mugishima et al. 1985), which in the future could potentially expand the donor pool.

Finally, investigators have developed a renewed interest in the use of the patient's own (autologous) marrow. High-dose drug regimens with hematologic toxicity as their primary limiting factor and the development of methods to remove disease from autologous marrow have shown promise against certain resistant cancers.

Given the above it is no wonder that bone marrow transplantation is one of the most challenging specialties to understand and in which to maintain expertise. Basic educational programs give little or no specialized formal education to nurses regarding transplantation, and they must often rely heavily on the transplant center for clinical and theoretical orientation to the field. Nurses in nontransplant settings might seek out continuing education programs or search through professional journals to develop a base of current knowledge.

This chapter provides an overview of the field and a framework for understanding bone marrow transplantation as a treatment modality, with a focus on allogeneic bone marrow transplantation. Subsequent chapters will look at the development of autologous marrow transplantation and the application of marrow transplantation to the pediatric population.

Clinical Indications

Tables 2.1 and 2.2 list the uses of allogeneic bone marrow transplantation for nonmalignant and malignant disorders. Each disease has been categorized according to whether the use of bone marrow transplantation as a treatment modality is most often considered as a standard or investigational therapy. The first successful allogeneic transplants were performed on patients with immunodeficiency diseases. This success and the prevalence of often fatal bone marrow malignancies quickly led to the conducting of clinical trials of bone marrow transplantation in these cancers. Today, most bone marrow transplant procedures are performed for malignancies, primarily leukemias, rather than for the more rare nonmalig-

Table 2.1. Nonmalignant Diseases Treated with Allogeneic Bone Marrow Transplantation

Acquired	Congenital
Aplastic anemia	Severe combined
Paroxysmal nocturnal	immunodeficiencies
hemoglobinuria*	(SCIDS)
Myelofibrosis	Mucopolysaccharidoses
Wiskott-Aldrich	Lipid storage diseases*
Syndrome	Osteopetrosis
Thalassemia*	
Chronic granulomatous	
disease*	

*Indicates diseases in which role of BMT is still under study.

nant indications (Bortin and Rimm 1986; Bortin and Rimm 1989).

The following discussion is an overview of some of the diseases for which an allogeneic transplant may be an option. Examples of major disease categories are presented. However, greater detail on the use of bone marrow transplant in childhood diseases appears in Chapter 4.

Congenital Disorders

Severe Combined Immunodeficiency Syndrome (SCIDS)

One of the most commonly transplanted congenital disorders is **severe combined immunodeficiency syndrome (SCIDS)**. This group of diseases

Table 2.2. Malignant Diseases Treated with Allogeneic Bone Marrow Transplantation

Acute myelogenous leukemia (AML)
Acute lymphocytic leukemia (ALL)
Chronic myelogenous leukemia (CML)
Preleukemia*
Hairy cell leukemia*
Non-Hodgkin's lymphoma
Burkitt's lymphoma*
Hodgkin's disease
Multiple myeloma*
Selected solid tumors*

*Indicates diseases in which the role of BMT is still under study.

can result from either an inborn error of lymphogenesis that is characterized by profound deficiencies in normal T, B, and plasma cell populations, or from inborn errors of metabolism as is the case with SCIDS due to adenosine deaminase (ADA) deficiency. The goal of transplanting normal marrow in this disease is primarily to reconstitute the lymphoproliferative branch of the immune system that is either defective or absent. Since patients are already immunosuppressed, there is usually no need for additional preparative (immunosuppressive) therapy prior to transplant, thus eliminating the toxicities of chemotherapy and **total body irradiation (TBI)**. Without treatment, most patients with SCIDS will die within a year, so marrow transplantation must be carried out early in the disease process. SCIDS patients transplanted with an HLA-identical donor have a 60% survival rate (Fonger 1987; Cowan 1985).

Aquired Disorders

Severe Aplastic Anemia

Severe aplastic anemia (SAA) is one of the most common nonmalignant marrow failure diseases successfully treated with bone marrow transplantation. Although patients are already immunosuppressed as a result of the disease, additional immunosuppressive agents (e.g., cyclophosphamide, antithymocyte globulin) may be administered to further prepare the patient. These agents are used pretransplant in the hope of ridding the patient of defective stem cell clones, which harbor immunologic abnormalities that potentially caused the disease. They are used post-transplant to prevent GVHD (Weisdorf 1990).

If bone marrow transplant is not anticipated and patients receive therapeutic red blood cell transfusions the rate of marrow graft rejection increases significantly, ranging as high as 30–60% (Deeg et al. 1988). This rejection appears to occur due to patient sensitization from these transfusions. Therefore transfusions should be avoided if transplant is anticipated. Transplant should especially be considered in younger aplastic anemia patients (under age 45), since the outcome of the

procedure is often successful. Older patients have an increased risk of transplant-related complications and an alternative treatment may be more appropriate. Some alternative treatments for older patients, as well as for those without an HLA-identical sibling donor, include immunosuppression with antithymocyte globulin (ATG) (Fairhead et al. 1983), cyclosporine, and/or monoclonal antibodies.

Hematologic Malignancies

Acute Lymphocytic Leukemia (ALL)

Although ALL was originally thought to be the disease most likely to benefit from bone marrow transplant, it currently appears that in most cases combination chemotherapy regimens are the treatment of choice. Most patients experience excellent survival and cure rates (approximately 60–70%) (Poplack and Reaman 1988). However, there are subgroups of patients with poor-risk ALL who may still be considered for transplant while in first remission. These groups include patients younger than 2 or older than 15, patients with high blast counts at diagnosis, mediastinal masses, and certain chromosomal abnormalities (Barrett et al. 1989, Bortin et al. 1988). Limiting cranial irradiation in prospective transplant candidates should be considered in order to reduce the complications of leukoencephalopathy, and impairments of growth and psychological functioning following the additive toxicities from the conditioning regimen for transplant.

In addition to patients with poor-risk ALL, allogeneic transplant is also considered for patients in a second complete remission and for some patients with advanced disease (Wingard et al. 1990). In these patients, recurrent leukemia following transplantation continues to be a serious problem (IBMTR 1990).

Acute Myelogenous Leukemia (AML)

Transplantation in AML was originally considered a salvage therapy for patients with end-stage disease (Bortin and Rimm 1989). However, as it was shown that this treatment could cure some patients with even far advanced disease, its use has grown and expanded to include patients in earlier stages of the disease (Gale et al. 1989). Now a well-established treatment concept, transplantation of patients with AML often occurs when the patient is in remission or early relapse, when the tumor burden is less and patient performance status is better. The outcome of transplantation does appear to be age-related, however, as many treatment teams have shown that younger patients, especially those under 25, have a significantly increased survival rate over those ages 25–50 (Santos 1989a). Leukemia relapse also appears to be reduced in patients who are transplanted in earlier stages of the disease (Gale et al. 1989). Despite favorable outcomes, whether allogeneic transplant in younger AML patients with a suitable HLA-matched donor is the treatment of choice is still controversial and subject to debate each time a clinical trial matures comparing this modality to chemotherapy alone (Santos 1989a).

Chronic Myelogenous Leukemia (CML)

HLA-matched donors should be sought in all patients with CML under 55 years of age, since transplantation provides the only hope for cure in these patients (Fefer and Thomas 1990; Deeg et al. 1988). For this group, the major issue is when in the disease process the transplant should be carried out; CML often has a long natural history and transplantation has significant morbidity and mortality (Fefer and Thomas 1990). CML patients have acheived cures when transplanted at any stage of disease, but the best results to date have occurred when patients were transplanted soon after diagnosis, while they were still in the chronic phase (Martin et al., 1988; Thomas et al. 1989). Prolonged treatment with busulfan, for patients who were later transplanted, seemed to worsen post-transplant pulmonary toxicity. Therefore, it may be recommended for potential transplant candidates to be treated with alpha interferon or hydroxyurea (Copelan 1989a; Copelan 1989b).

Other Malignancies/Second Transplants

Some patients with end-stage lymphomas and multiple myeloma have been successfully treated with allogeneic transplants (Sullivan 1989). Other malignancies have been treated with allogeneic transplantation in situations where an autologous transplant would have been an appropriate treatment option but the patient lacked an adequate bone marrow reserve, or the marrow was contaminated with disease. Prior intensive chemotherapy or irradiation can damage marrow so that adequate cell numbers are not available to reconstitute normal hematopoiesis, and in some diseases purging methods to remove residual disease may not be available. Patients with refractory Hodgkin's disease have been treated under these circumstances with limited success (Philip et al. 1989).

Allogeneic transplantation has been used as salvage therapy for non-Hodgkin's lymphoma patients who had relapsed after an autologous transplant and had HLA-identical siblings (Schouten et al. 1989). Although one patient died on day seven, the second patient was alive disease-free two years later.

Although the use of allogeneic transplant for certain diseases is well established, active investigation continues to reduce the morbidity and mortality associated with the procedure. Consequently, allogeneic transplantation of other diseases that are not cured with current treatments will certainly continue. Examples of expansion of this therapy are its recent use for treatment of lysosomal deficiency and storage diseases (van Bekkum 1989), and x and x-linked adrenoleukodystrophy, an inherited childhood genetic disease (Aubourg et al. 1990).

Radiation Injury

In April 1986, the nuclear reactor accident at Chernobyl heightened public and professional awareness to the use of bone marrow transplant for the treatment of radiation-induced injury (Baranov et al. 1989). "The First Consensus Development Conference on the Treatment of Radiation Injuries," held in May 1989, cited the following conclusions about the appropriateness of bone marrow transplantation as a potential treatment for this problem: bone marrow transplantation can help radiation victims, although the transplanted marrow need not completely replace the host marrow to be effective; bone marrow can simply provide cellular support to the victim while their own marrow has a chance to recover; bone marrow transplant should only be done on persons with no other fatal radiation-induced organ toxicity (Marx 1989).

Areas of controversy include how to identify which victims should undergo such a procedure, given the risks to both the patient and donor, and how quickly does the transplant need to be done to be effective. An alternative to marrow transplantation for some victims might be the use of marrow colony stimulating factors (Marx 1989). Clearly, everyone hopes that no future experiences require us to develop this modality of treatment for this purpose, although continued exploration of nuclear energy as a common household power source requires our understanding of the use of this treatment modality in the event of occupational exposure even in the absence of nuclear war (Cassel and Leaning 1989).

Unrelated Matched and Partially Matched Transplants

Many of the diseases discussed above have also been treated with allogeneic transplants, using marrow from HLA-matched unrelated volunteer donors and partially matched related or unrelated donors. In both cases there are greater risks of graft-versus-host disease and graft failure and hence poorer survival than with HLA-identical transplants (Kaminski 1989). However, for some patients who lack HLA-matched sibling donors and have diseases that are highly curable with transplant (e.g., CML and severe aplastic anemia),

the increased risk is considered acceptable since there are no better therapeutic alternatives.

Today the National Marrow Donor Registry Program (established in 1986) locates many HLA-matched unrelated donors, although other smaller donor registries still operate throughout the world. The national registry locates donors only for patients with diseases shown to be successfully treated with matched sibling donors. To date, hundreds of transplants with unrelated donors have occurred due to the registry's efforts, and the outcomes have been promising. (Greater detail about the program is provided in Chapter 5.)

When an HLA-matched sibling is not available, and there is a choice between an unrelated HLA-matched and partially matched related donor what choice should be made? Although a few studies have started to look at this question there is currently no clear answer. In an early study by Hows and colleagues (1986), a 50% survival rate was reported in 14 patients with histocompatible unrelated donors. The patients were being treated for severe aplastic anemia, Fanconi's anemia, and CML. This compares with a 19% survival rate (3 of 16 survived) in a similar group transplanted with HLA-mismatched marrow. Clearly, matched unrelated donors fared better in this series than did partially matched pairs. It was concluded that unrelated matched donors should be considered in certain situations (Hows et al. 1986). These results continue to be supported by Ash and colleagues (1990). However, since there are higher rates of complications and a lowered survival rate, indications for the use of partially matched donors is currently less clear (Ash et al. 1990).

Recently, Mackinnon et al. (1990) and McGlave et al. (1990) reported results from two studies of patients with CML treated with bone marrow from HLA-matched unrelated volunteer donors. They concluded that CML patients who lacked matched sibling donors should pursue this option although graft failure and a higher incidence of moderate to severe acute GVHD continued to be important complications to consider before undergoing the procedure.

Other Factors Influencing the Use of a Transplant

Many factors, in addition to the type of disease, must be considered when determining whether a bone marrow transplant is appropriate for a particular patient. Factors such as the stage of disease, patient age, availability of a histocompatible donor, concomitant medical conditions, and financial resources are among the most important.

In most cases it is not enough to know the types of diseases that are treated with bone marrow transplantion, but also the point in the course of a disease when a transplant should be considered. Will certain procedures or treatment decisions exclude a patient from eligibility for a transplant protocol or worsen his chances of surviving transplant? Such is the case with giving red blood cell transfusions to aplastic anemia patients prior to transplantation (Bortin et al. 1988). As stated earlier, patients are more likely to tolerate intensive therapy at earlier stages of disease. However, if a particular type of transplant has high treatment-related toxicities and the outcome is not well-defined, then only patients with advanced disease and few or no treatment options may be considered. Transplant in this type of situation is most often conducted within the setting of a clinical trial.

Age is an important factor in patient selection, since older patients experience an unacceptably high treatment-related mortality (Bortin et al. 1988). Major complications include interstitial pneumonitis, graft-versus-host disease, and infections. In many transplant centers an upper age limit is set (often somewhere between 50 and 60), after which patients will not be considered eligible. However, the age factor may become less important in the future as more tolerable conditioning regimens are developed. For instance, replacing total body irradiation (TBI), a major source of treatment-related toxicity, with the drug busulfan in a transplant protocol for older leukemia patients resulted in a similar survival rate and less toxicity, when compared to a similar but younger group (Copelan et al. 1989). This combination continues to be tested in a variety of malignant and nonmalignant diseases (Santos 1989).

Donor availability is becoming less and less of a problem with the growing network of donor registries and persons interested in becoming bone marrow donors (see Chapter 5). The continued development of tissue matching technology, immunosuppressive regimens to control or prevent GVHD, and other methods to reduce the morbity and mortality from unrelated transplants are all areas of intense investigation (Ash et al. 1990, Krensky et al. 1990). As mentioned earlier, results of allogeneic transplants with unrelated matched donors is very promising.

Concomitant medical conditions such as acquired immune deficiency syndrome (AIDS), major organ abnormalities or dysfunction such as pulmonary or cardiac damage from previous treatment and antibiotic allergies (i.e. allergy to amphotericin, commonly needed to treat fungal infections that can occur during post-transplant immunosuppression), and platelet refractoriness are but a few of the additional considerations in determining whether a patient will be eligible for transplant. Evaluation of these factors usually takes place at the time of consultation at a transplant center if an initial screening did not already rule out the patient from eligibility.

Finally, patient's financial resources are increasingly scrutinized when determining eligibility for transplantation, since reimbursement of the procedure costs by third party payors has become less predictable. Figures on the number of patients ineligible for transplant due to lack of financial resources have not been reported. These issues are discussed in detail in Chapter 17.

Treatment Process

Despite different clinical indications for allogeneic transplants, the basic treatment process is similar. Patients are evaluated for eligibility, a course of treatment is chosen, the disease is stabilized, a source of marrow is located, the patient's marrow is ablated, donor marrow is infused, and engraftment occurs. The following section describes each of these steps in detail including the nursing role.

Patient Evaluation and Eligibility

Deciding to undergo a procedure that is filled with hazards and life-threatening toxicities is difficult. The patient and family are often required to make this decision while under a great deal of stress. Often the best treatment option is uncertain and the patient and family must be active participants in the decision-making process. Exploring options for transplant can be time-consuming, frightening, and expensive whether or not the final decision is to actually have the procedure.

Nurses play a key role during the evaluation phase. The nurse in the referring center together with the physician can help the patient and family locate and secure consultations at appropriate transplant centers. They can provide general information on the overall treatment process and outcomes. Of critical importance is the role of helping the patient and family to develop questions and criteria on which to evaluate a prospective center and to aid them in assimilating information about one or more centers being considered after the initial consultation. The referring health care team is in a unique position—with the knowledge of the patient's medical, psychosocial, and emotional background—to assist the patient in choosing the most suitable option. This is especially true in situations where there is more than one treatment possibility or center that would be appropriate. Table 2.3 lists some potential questions and information that the patient might wish to consider when selecting a treatment modality and center. Although much of this would be covered in a typical informed consent process, the patient may not yet be at that stage when initially investigating several treatment centers or protocols.

In some diseases it is critical to identify potential transplant candidates early and seek im-

mediate consultation from a transplant center. This is especially true of patients with SCIDS and aplastic anemia, since pretransplant care may well affect transplant eligibility, efficacy, and outcome. As a practical matter it should be recognized that many centers can have significant waiting lists, relocating families will need to secure housing, and in general, funding sources must be secured and guaranteed before the patient will be accepted into the program.

Further delays are created by the need to undergo an extensive pretransplant evaluation, which includes an in-depth history and diagnostic testing. Table 2.4 describes some of the typical preevaluation information that may be required. Preevaluation testing requirements should be determined early in consultation with the specific transplant center since each program may have requirements for tests that may be done at the local institution while other tests may need to be performed at the transplant center. Considerable unnecessary expense can be avoided by not repeating tests that the transplant center requires be done there.

Disease Stabilization/Remission Induction

Occasionally patients are evaluated for transplantation prior to attaining a remission or stabilization of their disease. In this way they can be placed on waiting lists and avoid delay once their disease is at a point allowing them to enter a program. This is often a time of hope, anticipation, and worry for the patient and family as they consider the possibility of a future chance of cure while still in the uncertain phase of attaining a stable course or remission. Also, since some leukemia transplants may be done at the first sign of first or subsequent relapse—a relatively brief therapeutic window—prior investigation of transplant options will decrease the need for locating a program with undue haste.

During this phase the nurse is a key team member, serving as an important liaison between

Table 2.3.   Questions Patients/Families May Wish to Ask about the Prospective Transplant Facility

How many procedures like this have they done? or How many per year?
How long have they been doing bone marrow transplants?
Is the unit where I will be cared for just for transplant patients or are there other types of patients? Is the unit only for children or adults or is it mixed?
What type of specialized education do the nurses and others who care for me have?
What type of isolation procedures will I follow? Are there any visitor restrictions?
Can I visit the unit and meet the staff who will be responsible for my care?
What other centers perform the type of bone marrow transplant that I am eligible for?
What will this cost?
Will my insurance cover the costs? If not, what other payment sources are available?
What are major causes of morbidity and mortality from the procedure at this setting?
Who is the main physician(s) in charge of my care? Will I be cared for by interns and residents?
What support services are available for family? Can family stay in the hospital? In the area?
What type of financial support is available for non-hospitalization type expenses, e.g., living expenses, child care, phone calls, etc.
What are the acute and chronic effects of BMT?
What are the statistics of cure and relapse for my disease?
What are the effects to the marrow donor?
What if I don't have a matched donor, what are the alternatives?

the local facility and the transplant center in ensuring adequate exchange of information. Transplant center nurses also play an important role in developing and sharing patient teaching booklets, brochures, and communicating other vital information about the treatment facility and local area to prospective patients and families (Buchsel and Parchem 1988). Often a particular nurse at the transplant center will serve as a coordinator and will perform an initial evaluation and become an ongoing contact for potential candidates.

Donor Search

Once a patient is considered eligible for bone marrow transplant, a search for an appropriate donor ensues. Usually all family members are tested to determine histocompatibility with the patient. Depending on the disease, if no matches are found within the family unit then a bone marrow donor registry may be consulted to locate an unrelated HLA-matched donor. (This process is described in detail in Chapter 5.) Alternatively, an autologous transplant may be considered.

When an appropriate donor is located, extensive donor testing occurs.

Marrow Harvest

In general, bone marrow is technically one of the simplest forms of organ transplantation. Few if any adverse effects to the donor from the harvest procedure have been reported (Thomas 1987).

Bone marrow is harvested aseptically in the operating room (see Figure 2.2), while the donor is under general anesthesia. Multiple bone marrow aspirations are performed from the posterior and/or anterior iliac crests and occasionally from the sternum to remove bone marrow stem cells. The procedure can last from one to four hours (about 90 minutes is the average) depending on the number of bone marrow cells needed and the ease of aspiration from the donor. Far less difficulty in aspiration is expected in a normal healthy donor than in an autologous marrow aspiration from a person who has been heavily pretreated and may have hypocellular marrow or areas of fibrosis.

Table 2.4. Preevaluation of the Bone Marrow Transplant Candidate

Discussion with the patient, family and/or referring medical team (if referral is only tentative) of the
   transplantation procedure including rationale, risks/benefits, alternative treatment options
Complete medical history including:
   confirmation of diagnosis
   other medical/surgical problems
   previous treatment
   any difficulties with patient medical management during past treatment
   transfusion history
   infectious history
   allergies
   psychosocial assessment
Histocompatibility testing on patient and donors type all family members for syngeneic/allogeneic match
      mixed leukocyte culture (MLC) testing on patient and donor
Transfusion support planning
   determine allosensitization to blood components
   determine ABO match between patient and donor and plan management for ABO mismatch
Evaluation of major organ function
   Serum tests of renal, hepatic, hematopoietic, endocrine function
   Pulmonary and cardiac function tests
   Creatinine clearance
Tumor staging studies
   bone marrow aspirate and biopsy
   x-rays, computerized tomagraphy (CT) scans, magnetic resonance imaging (MRI) of sites of current/
      previous disease
   lumbar puncture and cerebrospinal fluid (CSF) cytology
Reproductive considerations
   sperm banking/ova storage

Adapted from Deeg et al. 1988. *A Guide to Bone Marrow Transplantation.* N.Y.: Springer-Verlag, p. 27.

Nucleated marrow cell counts are performed during the procedure to ensure adequate cell numbers for transplantation. Many centers consider an adequate number of cells for allogeneic transplant to be $1–8 \times 10^8$ cells per kilogram of body weight (Storb 1989). This equals only about 3–5% of the donor's viable bone marrow and is easily replaced by the donor within a couple of weeks. The total fluid volume from harvesting this amount of marrow stem cells is between 500 and 1000ml depending on the number of cells needed, which is determined by the size of the recipient. Additional marrow may be collected for reserve in circumstances where cell damage from manipulation may occur, i.e., if marrow is being frozen or treated. Several units of autologous blood may be collected preoperatively from the donor for use during the procedure, although the donor often tolerates the procedure well without needing additional blood component replacement once the procedure is complete. Occasionally red cells will be removed from the harvested marrow and will be returned back to the donor following the procedure.

A variety of methods are used for initially processing bone marrow in the operating suite. Filtering or straining is accomplished by running aspirated marrow through a separating device in order to remove bone fragments or other tissue particles (see Figure 2.3). Then the marrow is collected directly into a bag or poured into some other collection apparatus (see Figure 2.4) for further processing or infusion into the host (Thomas and Storb 1970). A similar method is to infuse

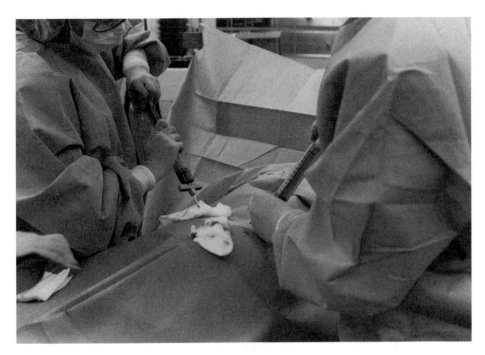

Figure 2.2. Bone marrow is harvested aseptically in the operating room while the donor is under general anesthesia.

the collected marrow directly into the infusion bag through sterile gauze that is lightly packed in a syringe. This method reportedly decreases the incidence of bacterial contamination of the marrow that may occur with multiple manipulations (Neudorf et al. 1989).

Postoperatively, the donor is stabilized in the recovery room and pressure dressings over the harvest sites are assessed for any unusual bleeding. The donor is then returned to floor care and may be discharged on the same or following day. Of note are recent reports of harvest procedures done in the outpatient setting as well as harvests performed using mild general analgesia and local anesthesia, or epidural anesthesia rather than general anesthesia (Brandwein et al. 1989; de Vries et al. 1989). In this era of cost containment and shortage of hospital beds, these trends are likely to continue and become standard procedure as long as donor safety and comfort can be maintained.

Donor complications are rare but can include complications from anesthesia, blood loss, and infection. Pain at the harvest sites is alleviated by mild analgesics like acetaminophen and/or oxycodone, and remaining mobile. The donor can usually resume limited activities within a day or so postoperatively and normal activities within a week or so. Other general donor considerations and issues are discussed in Chapter 5.

Marrow should be infused within three hours if it is not frozen for transport or processed further. Marrow may be frozen prior to infusion also when it is obtained from cadavers (Blazar et al. 1986) or from volunteer unrelated donors for future use. Cryopreservation of marrow, first established for use in autologous transplantation, has also been shown to reconstitute the host successfully in allogeneic transplantation (Lasky et al. 1989). Semiautomated methods for processing bone marrow on blood cell separators are also

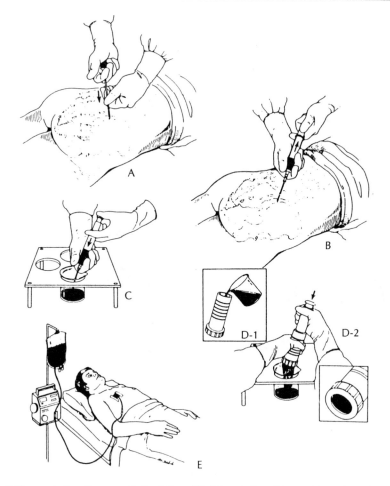

With permission, Corcoran-Buchsel, P. and Kelleher, J. Bone Marrow Transplantation. *Nursing Clinics of North America 24* (4): 918.

Figure 2.3.   Bone marrow is processed in the operating room.

being investigated, especially for use in autologous transplantation where smaller total volumes of marrow for storage are desirable (English et al. 1989). Additional considerations in the manipulation of bone marrow in autologous transplantation are discussed in Chapter 3.

Conditioning/Preparative Regimens

Conditioning, preparation, and **ablation** are all terms used to describe the process by which the host (patient) is made physiologically ready to receive the bone marrow graft. The purpose of conditioning is threefold: (1) to create "room" for the donor graft to "take"; (2) to immunosuppress the host to allow graft acceptance; and (3) to eliminate residual malignant disease in some instances (Deeg 1988).

Specific combinations of radiation and chemotherapy, in a variety of doses and schedules, are selected based on their mechanism of action and ability to accomplish these three goals. For instance, conditioning a patient with a nonmalignant disorder for transplant eliminates the need

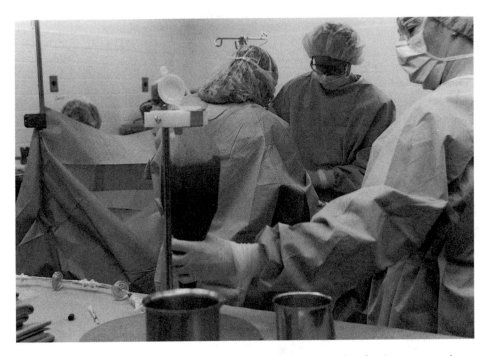

Figure 2.4. The marrow is collected directly into a bag for further processing.

to use agents with an antitumor effect. Likewise, conditioning a patient who is already severely immunosuppressed from an immunodeficiency disorder may obviate the need for further immunosuppression. A combination of ionizing radiation and cyclophosphamide is often chosen as a conditioning regimen that meets all three criteria. Inadequate conditioning can result in failure of engraftment, graft rejection, or relapse of the original disease (see chapter on hematopoietic complications).

In many protocols, conditioning days are referred to by negative numbers, like a countdown. The day of transplant is referred to as "day 0" and each day thereafter is given a positive number which is then indicative of the number of days that have transpired since the marrow infusion. Most post-transplant events are described in relation to this numbering system, e.g., the patient spiked a fever on day three but the first neutrophil

was not seen until day 14. Figure 2.5 shows a typical treatment schedule.

Since the goals of conditioning vary with the many different diseases currently being treated with allogeneic transplant, it is unlikely that a standard conditioning regimen will ever be determined to be useful for all allogeneic transplants. Furthermore, many different pharmaceuticals and biologicals (some of which are also used as conditioning agents) are being tested as lymphocyte purging agents for the donor marrow as well as for definitive therapy should GVHD occur.

The nurse must be well-versed in the purpose of the therapy as well as its actions and toxicities to effectively design appropriate nursing interventions to lessen or prevent complications of this therapy. Survival figures for all types of allogeneic transplant can be improved by decreasing or preventing the mortality caused by conditioning, an outcome partially affected by nursing care.

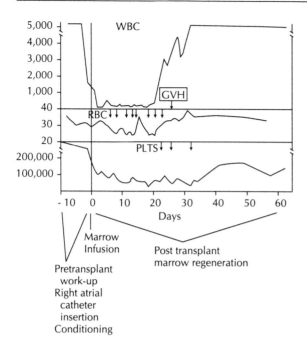

Figure 2.5. Stages of bone marrow transplantation. Uppermost graph indicates WBC counts, middle portion indicates hematocrit, lower portion indicates platelet count. Arrows indicate RBC and platelet transfusions.

Innovative dosage schedules, new drugs, and hence new side effects and toxicities will continue to present a challenge to nurses who administer these agents. Designing efficient and effective patient care regimens that prevent or lessen drug effects is an important nursing function. It is beyond the scope of this discussion to provide an in-depth analysis of each of the individual or combination drug regimen effects and related nursing interventions. However, it is hoped that reports, like two recent excellent reviews published in the nursing literature on busulfan (Rohaly 1989) and cyclosporine (Truog and Wozniak 1990), will continue to be developed to provide a foundation for nursing care. Such reports can also spark clinical nursing care trials to compare the effectiveness of various nursing interventions in minimizing or preventing drug side effects.

Immunosuppressive/Antineoplastic Drug Therapy

A brief summary of agents or methods that have been used in conditioning regimens for immu-nosuppressive or antineoplastic effects is presented here; some agents have a dual effect. Improvements in immunosuppressive therapies continue to be sought since many current methods cause serious toxicities or increase the incidence of disease relapse (Bearman et al. 1988).

Many of the antineoplastic drugs described here have already been studied to determine their maximal non-hematologic dose-limiting organ toxicity so that enhancement of antineoplastic effect is unlikely to occur simply by further escalating doses of these drugs. Rather, future advancements in antineoplastic therapy will occur most likely through the development of new drugs, new ways to protect the patient from non-hematologic organ effects in higher doses of currently effective drugs, or by developing synergistic combinations of current drug therapy.

Some of the more common agents and methods used for conditioning are listed here. The list and specific information about each drug is by no means exhaustive, and the nurse should refer to pharmacology texts or original study reports in the transplant literature for more complete information on all drugs currently in use or under investigation. (Additional drugs/methods used in autologous transplantation for conditioning, antineoplastic therapy, or marrow purging are described in Chapter 3.)

Antithymocyte Globulin (ATG).   Primarily immunosuppressive in its action, ATG has been used in combination with methotrexate and prednisone for GVHD prophylaxis (Weisdorf 1990). ATG has also been used as part of a marrow purging regimen and in the treatment of GVHD (Vogelsang et al. 1988). Inconsistent findings in clinical trials for all of the above stated uses makes it difficult to define a specific role for its use outside of further clinical trials.

Busulfan (Myleran).   Recently reviewed by Rohaly (1989), this oral agent is used for its antineoplastic effect and in combination with cyclophosphamide also appears to offer adequate immunosuppression to allow for successful allografting. Its use as a substitute for TBI in combination with many other chemotherapeutic agents is being actively investigated in both allogeneic and autologous transplantation for both malignant and nonmalignant diseases due to its reduced toxicity (Rohaly 1989). A variety of schedules and doses are used but most commonly reported is 2mg/kg in 16 divided doses, e.g., four times/day for four days. The major toxicities include acute nausea and vomiting during the period of administration, severe leukopenia, anemia, thrombocytopenia, pulmonary fibrosis ("busulfan lung"), and hyperurecemia. Less common effects include endocardial fibrosis, seizures, hyperpigmentation, alopecia, and cataracts (Rohaly 1989).

One unique nursing consideration specific to the use of this agent is management of the acute nausea and vomiting that can occur during oral administration, to enable the patient to tolerate the entire drug dose. Antiemetics, use of capsules to encase the significant number of tablets to be ingested for the typical transplant dose, and if necessary, placement of a nasogastric tube may be necessary to manage this problem.

Carmustine (BCNU).   Used primarily in combination with other agents for antineoplastic effects, carmustine was originally part of a regimen designed to substitute for TBI. Its current use is mostly in autologous transplantation in the treatment of lymphomas (see Chapter 3).

Cyclophosphamide (Cytoxan).   Used primarily for its immunosuppressive qualities in doses of 120–200mg/kg, it is a standard component of many conditioning regimens. Hemorrhagic cystitis and in higher doses (200mg/kg or greater) cardiomyopathy are the major toxicities. Hemorrhagic cystitis is easily prevented by vigorous hydration, diuresis, and/or continuous bladder irrigations. Maintaining the urine output at 100ml/ hour or greater by any of these methods during the infusion and for 6–8 hours following the completion of the infusion is a typical procedure followed by many transplant centers to prevent hematuria and subsequent bladder hemorrhage.

Cyclosporine (CyA).   Since it first became available and was tested in the 1970s, cyclosporine has become a mainstay of GVHD prevention. Exclusively immunosuppressive, it acts primarily against T lymphocytes by inhibiting the production of interleukin-2, which suppresses the proliferation and production of cytotoxic T cells while sparing suppressor T cell populations. It does not affect mature T cells. It is not effective if given once GVHD is already evident (Truog and Wozniak 1990). It is associated with little if any damage to hematopoietic/myelogenous tissues and has no anti-inflammatory properties. It is administered to the host following allogeneic transplant in a variety of schedules (e.g., in the adult 25mg/kg daily for 18 days beginning on the day of transplant; in the child 3mg/kg daily IV or 13mg/kg daily by mouth when the child can tolerate it) to prevent the development of GVHD. A recent survey of administration practices of cyclosporine demonstrated that many different schedules are frequently being used and that the schedule can interfere with providing the patient with other medications, transfusions, and nutritional support (Caudell and Adams 1990). The surveyors recommended cyclosporine administration as a piggyback through hyperalimentation as one possible solution.

Side effects associated with intravenous drug administration include paresthesias, palmar and solar pain, and peripheral or facial flushing, all of which have been reported to lessen when the infusion is slowed or cease when the drug is given orally (Truog and Wozniak 1990). Serum peak and trough drug levels have been done to monitor for appropriate dosing, although absolute therapeutic and toxic levels have not been determined. Toxicities include hypertension, nephrotoxicity, hepatoxicity, and central nervous system effects like ataxia and tremor (Truog and Wozniak 1990).

Cyclosporine has been tested in combination with a variety of other agents including methotrexate, prednisone, and ATG with promising results. Vogelsang and colleagues (1988) have recently conducted a comprehensive review of these studies and concluded that the incidence of acute GVHD was reduced when cyclosporine was used in combination with other agents.

Cytarabine (ARA C). Cytarabine has demonstrated a high antileukemic effect, but poor immunosuppressive qualities. In the rat model it was found to be inferior to cyclophosphamide in its prevention of graft rejection (Gassmann et al. 1988). It has been used in high and conventional doses in combination with cyclophosphamide and TBI for leukemias (Deeg 1988).

Etoposide (VP-16-213). Although this agent has significant antineoplastic properties, like cytarabine, it is a poor immunosuppressive agent. Even when used in combination with busulfan as a conditioning agent, in the rat model high rates of graft rejection occurred (Gassmann et al. 1988). Therefore, this agent has been used primarily in combination with other agents as mentioned above under cytarabine and in autologous transplant for its antineoplastic properties (Stadtmauer et al. 1989).

Methotrexate. Methotrexate was one of the earliest drugs used for prevention of GVHD and was considered the drug of choice before the introduction of cyclosporine. It has been used successfully alone, and in combination, and as a lymphocyte marrow purging agent. Another use in leukemia therapy has been in the treatment and prophylaxis of CNS leukemia. In contrast to cyclosporine, it is toxic to hematopoetic tissue.

T Lymphocyte-Depleted Donor Marrow. Removal of T cells from donor marrow is immunosuppressive in nature and is a specific therapy aimed at preventing acute GVHD. Mature T lymphocytes cause GVHD, so donor marrow is T cell depleted in vitro to decrease or eliminate these cells. Several ex vivo depletion methods (shown in Figures 2.6 and 2.7) have been used, including soybean agglutinin followed by rosetting with sheep erythrocytes and monoclonal antibodies specific to T lymphocytes in combination with complement or toxins (such as ricin) (McGlave 1985).

T cell depletion has reduced the incidence and severity of GVHD, but at the cost of increases in leukemia relapse and marrow failure. Thus, disease-free survival rates have stayed constant in diseases using this modality of GVHD prophylaxis (Santos 1989). Because some series of patients receiving T cell-depleted marrow have not experienced a higher than expected leukemia relapse rate, it has been postulated that the T cell depletion method may be a factor (Biggs et al. 1989).

Total Body Irradiation (TBI). Ionizing radiation is used, usually in the form of total body fractionated doses, to immunosuppress the host, "make space" for the donor marrow and for its antileukemic effect in hematologic malignancies (Vitale et al. 1989). Early marrow transplants were done almost exclusively with TBI and its

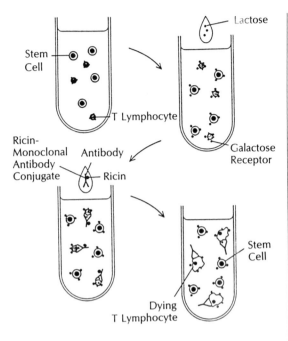

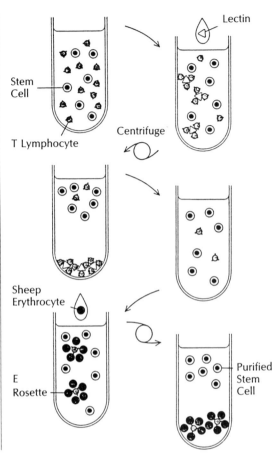

With permission, McGlave, P.B. 1985. The status of bone marrow transplantation. *Hospital Practice* 20 (11): 104.

Figure 2.6. One approach to stem-cell purification involves the use of monoclonal (anti-T lymphocyte) antibody-ricin conjugates, or immunotoxins. Ricin binds to nucleated cells via galactose receptors, pentrates cells, and inhibits protein synthesis. Ricin linked to anti-T lymphocyte monoclonal antibodies will bind selectively to T lymphocytes. The system is flooded with lactose to block ricin's native binding site (galactose) and thereby render it antibody specific. Dying T lymphocytes are infused along with the viable bone marrow stem cells.

With permission, McGlave, P.B. 1985. The status of bone marrow transplantation. *Hospital Practice* 20 (11): 105.

Figure 2.7. Ex vivo removal of T lymphocytes from donor marrow prior to transplantation may reduce risk of graft-versus-host disease. With double agglutination technique, lectin (soybean agglutinin) removes majority of thymocytes. Rosetting with sheep erythrocytes removes the rest, leaving a purified stem-cell population in marrow.

effects have been well studied in both animals and man (van Bekkum and De Vries 1967).

In addition to its beneficial (therapeutic) effects, TBI can also produce dose-dependent damage to the host. Evidence of this effect in man was first studied in victims of the unfortunate and tragic nuclear bomb explosions during World War

II and the nuclear power plant explosion at Chernobyl. Radiation injury in man results in three distinct syndromes (see Table 2.5): the bone marrow syndrome (500–1,000cGy), the gastrointes-

Table 2.5. Causes of Mortality After Total Body Irradiation

Syndrome	Bone marrow or Hematopoietic Syndrome	Gastrointestinal Syndrome	Central Nervous System
Dose of irradiation (cGy)	500–1000	1000–10,000	> 10,000
Day of death post-transplant	7–30	3–7	< 1
Cause of death	Bone marrow aplasia, hemorrhage, infection	Destruction of GI mucosa, fluid loss, electrolyte imbalance	Apnea, cardiac arrest
Protection from BMT	Yes	No	No

With permission, Petz and Blume (1983). *Clinical Bone Marrow Transplantation.* N.Y.: Churchill-Livingstone Publishers, Inc. p. 38.

tinal syndrome (1,000–10,000cGy), and the central nervous system syndrome (> 10,000cGy) (Petz and Blume 1983).

Radiation doses to adequately immunosuppress the host and create space within the marrow for the newly infused donor immune system are in the "bone marrow" range. Higher doses would cause irreversible host organ damage that would not be corrected simply by infusion of donor marrow. Although an ideal treatment to accomplish the aforementioned desired effects, ionizing radiation alone does not provide an adequate antileukemic effect and therefore other agents described above are necessary adjuncts when the disorder to be corrected by transplantation is leukemia.

Despite careful dosimetry, TBI, especially when used in combination with antineoplastic therapy, can result in serious or life-threatening toxicities. A variety of dosing and blocking techniques have been reported, which have attempted to reduce these toxicities particularly to the lungs, kidneys, lens, and liver (Lawton et al. 1989; Vitale et al. 1989; Labar et al. 1989). Employing these techniques might allow delivery of higher, more immunosuppressive radiation doses, which are most desirable in the setting of T cell-depleted or only partially matched donor marrow to increase the success of engraftment in these higher-risk procedures. Irradiating only the lymphatic system

(described later) is another variation on this idea under study.

Another approach to reducing TBI toxicity evident in some leukemia protocols is to substitute a chemotherapy agent and remove TBI from the conditioning program (Tutschka et al. 1989). That is, some programs have been designed using only chemotherapy. Kanfer and McCarthy (1989) critically analyzed studies that replaced TBI with a variety of agents, to compare the incidence and severity of toxicities, immunosuppressive effects to enable successful engraftment, and antileukemia efficacy. They found a favorable trend toward the efficacy of non-TBI containing regimens. Future investigations of this type are sure to be conducted to answer the question of the need for TBI in allogeneic transplant.

Regardless of dose, technique, or toxicity the patient's experience in undergoing the actual radiation treatment is often described as at best uncomfortable and at worst terrifying. Many radiation therapy departments were not originally designed to accommodate a total body approach and novel positioning and treatment schemes have been developed to fit the patient's total body in the treatment field. Patients may need to remain perfectly still in a curled or fetal position for 15–20 minutes per treatment—a significant feat for a nauseated, sedated patient. Special stands (Glasgow et al. 1989) or boxlike containers

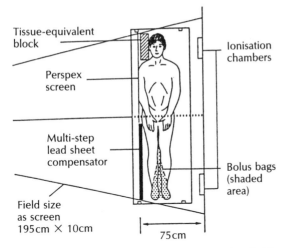

Tissue-equivalent block

Perspex screen

Multi-step lead sheet compensator

Field size as screen 195cm × 10cm

Ionisation chambers

Bolus bags (shaded area)

75cm

With permission, James, N.D. et al. 1989. Total lymphoid irradiation preceeding bone marrow transplantation for myeloid leukemia. *Clinical Radiology 40*: p. 196.

Figure 2.8. Details of the field set-up for TBI. Parallel opposed lateral fields. FSD 5m.

have been devised to assist patients to remain immobile and facilitate special positioning for the necessary extended periods of time (see Figure 2.8). It is no wonder that patients have described this apparatus as "the casket" or "torture chamber." Although the patient will not experience any sensations from the delivery of the radiation per se, some may become fearful of being "closed in" or experience muscle cramps and tremors from lying or sitting in the required contorted positions.

A visit to the radiation department to see the equipment and to develop a rapport with radiation technologists and nurses involved in delivery of treatments prior to the actual treatments can do much to ease the patient's fears and anxieties about these treatments. Other nursing interventions include administration of premedications for antiemesis or antianxiety and sedation if indicated. Also, coordination of premedication and other required patient care with the radiation therapy personnel to facilitate accurate timing of the treatment schedule is critical, as the actual

treatment involves much time and personnel in a typically busy department. The nurse must be particularly diplomatic and sensitive to the patient who, out of fear and dread of the treatment, has difficulty getting prepared to be transported to the department. Adequate preparation time must be built into the busy conditioning regimen days. Many a transplant nurse can share an anecdote about the patient who refused to leave the bathroom or needed to make an important phone call just when it was time to leave for his or her radiation treatment.

Total Lymphoid Irradiation (TLI).   TLI was first used to treat patients with Hodgkin's disease and later to prevent allograft rejection in renal transplant patients. This method of immunosuppression was first employed in bone marrow transplant in 1985 to decrease the incidence of graft failure in CML patients receiving T cell-depleted marrow from matched or partially matched donors (James et al. 1989). TLI has the potential benefit of contributing the desirable T cell immunosuppressive effects with potentially less host toxicity than is normally experienced with a total body approach. In transplant, TLI has been administered as a single dose (range 300–750cGy) or as twice-daily fractionated doses (1000–1200cGy total dose) (James et al. 1989; Deeg et al. 1988). It is also used in preparation for autologous transplantation in advanced or refractory Hodgkin's disease with reported success (Yahalom et al. 1989). Figure 2.9 illustrates one approach to delivery of TLI.

Infusion of Bone Marrow

Intravenous infusion of bone marrow has been established as the route of choice since the 1940s, although other routes including intraperitoneal, intrasplenic, and oral have been attempted. Marrow cells may be dripped in by short infusion or pushed centrally using a syringe. Institutions vary regarding policies allowing nurses or others to actually administer the marrow cells. In either case the staff, the patient, and the environment

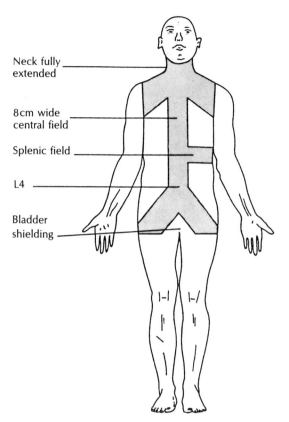

Neck fully extended

8cm wide central field

Splenic field

L4

Bladder shielding

With permission, James, N.D. et al. 1989. Total lymphoid irradiation preceeding bone marrow transplantation for myeloid leukemia. *Clinical Radiology 40*: p. 196.

Figure 2.9. Details of the field set-up for TLI. Parallel opposed fields two fractions/day with a 6h gap, FSD 120cm.

should be prepared to deal with the uncommon but potential reactions in the host resulting from the infused marrow. Ideally a one-to-one staffing ratio should be enacted during this time. Standing orders that can be instituted immediately for appropriate medications and other therapies will help to ensure that all health care team members are prepared for an emergency situation should it arise.

Emergency medications, such as diphenhydramine, epinephyrine, hydrocortisone, and neosynephrine may be ordered by the physician and should be readily available. Also, resuscitation equipment, oxygen, and saline should be nearby. Frequent or continuous monitoring of vital signs, constant observation, and asking the patient to report any untoward effects can detect any early signs of a reaction, thereby minimizing the need for extensive support.

Common signs of bone marrow infusion-related reactions are similar to those seen with other blood product infusions and can include shortness of breath, hypotension, chills, fever, chest pain, rash, hives, and nonspecific malaise. Treatment is symptomatic and may include slowing the rate of infusion, medications (described above), and temporary oxygen to relieve dyspnea. Although much preparation can occur on the transplant day (or day 0), many patients describe the reinfusion of marrow as anticlimatic given all the preparation they have already experienced.

Following infusion of marrow, the stem cells travel to marrow spaces, a process known as "homing," and within 7–14 days begin to reestablish normal bone marrow function. It appears that the marrow environment provides the proper stimulus for hematopoietic proliferation.

Immediate Post-Infusion Care

Once the patient is stabilized following the infusion, the tedious wait begins for marrow engraftment and return of normal bone marrow function and blood counts. This time is filled with potential for many life-threatening complications, which are discussed in detail in Part II of the text. A summary of the complications and the timing of their approximate appearance is shown in Figure 2.10.

Discharge Planning and Follow-up Care in the Community

Patients are discharged from the hospital when their granulocyte count reaches over 500mm³ and they are in otherwise stable medical condition. Early discharge can decrease chances of serious hospital-acquired infections, decrease costs, and

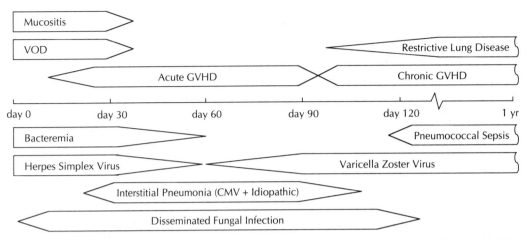

Source: Press O.W., Schaller R.T., Thomas E.D.: Complications of Organ Transplantation. New York, Marcel Dekker, 1987. Reprinted courtesy of Marcel Dekker, Inc.

Figure 2.10. Temporal Sequence of Major Complications After Allogeneic Bone Marrow Transplantation on Day 0

begin the lengthy process of rehabilitation and reacclimation to a "normal" life (Stream 1983). Depending on whether the transplant center is near the patient's home or whether the patient's home is near a medical center where appropriate intensive outpatient care and support can be provided often determines how long the patient must stay within the immediate area of the transplant center. Anticipating discharge and initiating planning during the early stages of transplant as well as soliciting the active involvement of the patient, family, and any outpatient services can do much to ensure a smooth and timely transition to the outpatient setting (Buchsel and Parchem 1988; Buchsel and Kelleher 1989).

After discharge, the nurses in the ambulatory care clinic play a vital role in patient assessment and social support. It is beneficial if outpatient nursing staff have had an opportunity to meet the patient before the first clinic visit so that they have an opportunity to establish a rapport and learn preferences in care routines from the inpatient nursing staff, patient, and family. Outpatient nursing staff will continue to be involved in assessing

patients for the appearance of chronic GVHD, as well as assisting in the acquisition of post-transplant follow-up care. (See Chapter 13 for a more detailed description of ambulatory nursing care considerations.)

Financial considerations may also play a role in the discharge of patients to intensive ambulatory care. In general, many oncology patients have been able to receive insurance reimbursement for much of the care they receive in an outpatient setting and home setting; bone marrow transplant patients are no exception. Insurance companies will often reimburse such outpatient and home services as intravenous antibiotics, hyperalimentation, blood product support, and other types of nursing and supportive care. "High-tech home care" is often an accurate description of the level of sophisticated outpatient care that many transplant patients continue to receive after discharge.

Many patients are so familiar with their care routines that they may play a vital role in orienting the health care team at their home medical center about the specifics of care that work for them.

Many centers have local temporary low-cost or free housing near the center, although the family may have already secured some living arrangements while the patient was in the hospital.

Long-Term Complications following Bone Marrow Transplant

Major long-term complications are discussed at the time of informed consent. However, patients will often focus their attention on the actual complications of the procedure and the immediate transplant phase. Most notable of the long-term complications include failure of the procedure to accomplish the desired result, i.e., cure the cancer or correct the disease, failure of the graft to function normally, relapse of the disease, and complications of graft-versus-host disease. Additionally, infertility, disorders of growth and development, cataracts, and even secondary cancers may occur (Buchsel 1986). Psychosocial function and return to normal lifestyle can take some time and adjustment. However, normal psychosocial and emotional functioning is more likely when physiologic complications are well managed or prevented. These complications are discussed in detail in Part III of the text.

Outcomes of Allogeneic Bone Marrow Transplantation

The danger of reporting generalizations of outcomes in a text such as this is that it soon becomes out of date. Also, when the results of many institutions and regimens are grouped, individual successes and shortcomings are diluted. Despite these problems, it is hoped that the generalized outcomes summarized here provide nurses with an understanding of the state of the art and trends that began the discoveries and investigations of the 1990s.

Outcomes of allogeneic transplants are illustrated in Figures 2.11–2.14 and discussed below.

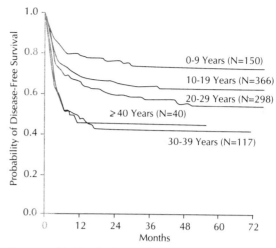

Figure provided by the International Bone Marrow Transplant Registry, 1990.

Figure 2.11. Actuarial Probabilty of Survival After BMT for Severe Aplastic Anemia According to Age at Transplant

The majority of the results were obtained from data compiled by the International Bone Marrow Transplant Registry (a voluntary organization of more than 190 transplant teams that collects and analyzes data on bone marrow transplants worldwide at a centralized statistical center) and other scientific publications as noted.

Nonmalignant Conditions

Severe Aplastic Anemia

Aplastic anemia is by far the most common nonmalignant disease treated with allogeneic bone marrow transplantation. For patients under age 40 with an HLA-identical sibling donor, it may be considered the treatment of choice (IBMTR 1990). Results of nearly a thousand such transplants worldwide summarized by Sullivan (1989) for the years 1972–88 demonstrate a 40–82% actuarial survival for patients treated with a variety of regimens (cyclophosphamide alone, cyclophosphamide + thoracoabdominal irradiation/total lymphoid irradiation; and cyclophosphamide and total body irradiation) at a variety of centers.

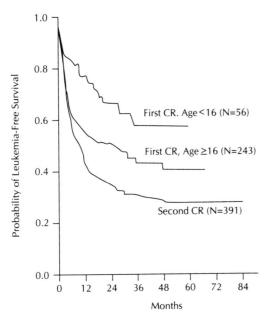

Figure provided by the International Bone Marrow Transplant Registry, 1990.

Figure 2.12. Actuarial probability of leukemia-free survival after bone marrow transplantation for acute lymphoblastic leukemia according to remission status and age at transplant.

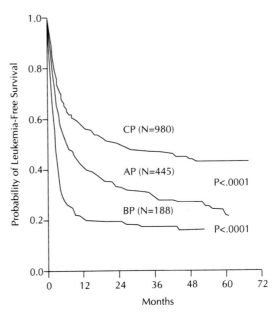

Figure provided by the International Bone Marrow Transplant Registry, 1990.

Figure 2.13. Actuarial probability of leukemia-free survival after bone marrow transplantation for chronic myelogenous leukemia according to disease phase at transplant (CP = chronic phase; AP = accelerated phase; BP = blast phase).

In general, survival is greatly improved in this disease when patients do not receive red blood cell transfusions prior to transplant.

Nonidentical donor transplants have been conducted in a much smaller group of aplastic anemia patients. In these patients there is greater morbidity and mortality from graft rejection and a survival rate (between 15–50%) significantly less than that observed with an HLA-identical sibling donor.

Hematologic Malignancies

The major cause of bone marrow transplant failure is death from treatment toxicity, unlike with chemotherapy, where treatment failure is predominantly from recurrent disease. If patients could be selected who would do well with chem-

otherapy, in situations where it is unclear which choice is best, some would argue that bone marrow transplant should not be attempted due to the high procedure-related toxicity. It is unknown whether the poor risk characteristics in chemotherapy and bone marrow transplant are the same. That is, is the factor causing a poor outcome in a patient treated with chemotherapy the same factor that will bode a poor outcome if bone marrow transplant is used (Barrett et al. 1989)?

Early transplants, before 1975, were done only on patients with advanced or refractory disease. However, even in this group of poor risk patients the long-term survival was 15%; a result that encouraged further investigations into the usefulness of transplant in earlier stages of disease.

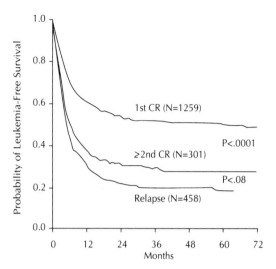

Figure provided by the International Bone Marrow Transplant Registry, 1990.

Figure 2.14. Actuarial probability of leukemia-free survival after bone marrow transplantation for acute myelogenous leukemia according to remission state at transplant.

Acute Lymphocytic Leukemia

There is considerable controversy surrounding the selection of appropriate candidates for transplantation (Kersey 1989), especially for patients in first remission as discussed earlier. The outcomes of more than a thousand patients reported by the International Bone Marrow Transplant Registry (IBMTR) conducted at 107 centers worldwide demonstrated an actuarial disease-free median survival for patients in first remission of 42% (±9%) and 26% (±6%) for patients in second remission. Overall survival was better for children (56%) than for adults (39%) (Barrett et al. 1989). Disease- and treatment-related variables explained differences in outcomes among these large heterogenous groups.

Acute Myelogenous Leukemia

Currently, patients with acute myelogenous leukemia can expect a 45–55% long-term disease-free survival if transplanted in first remission (Sul-

livan et al. 1989). Morbidity and mortality of transplantation even in HLA-identical donors and the ability of combination chemotherapy to cure a percentage of patients and induce a second remission in others still makes a clear choice for a "best treatment" between bone marrow transplant and postremission chemotherapy difficult and unclear (Tallman et al. 1989). Transplantation in subsequent remissions or in relapse results in actuarial survival range 20 to 30% (Sullivan et al. 1989), although ongoing improvements in conditioning and immunosuppressive regimens and supportive care may increase these figures in the near future.

Chronic Myelogenous Leukemia

Fifty to sixty percent of patients in the chronic phase of chronic myelogenous leukemia survive disease-free more than five years after HLA-identical matched allogeneic transplant. In patients transplanted during the blastic phase, survival drops to around 20%. In addition to disease status at the time of transplant (e.g., accelerated or blastic), other factors associated with poorer outcome include age greater than 35, occurrence of moderate to severe acute GVHD, and use of T cell-depleted donor marrow (Bortin et al. 1988).

Other Malignancies

Patients with lymphoma and multiple myeloma have also been treated with allogeneic transplantation and initial results have been encouraging (Sullivan et al. 1989).

General Considerations Regarding Outcomes— Discussion

Currently, whether bone marrow transplantation is or is not the treatment of choice for particular diseases, and at what stage of disease it should be considered is still a debate (Mayer 1988). While we await the design of such a large multi-

Table 2.6. Incidence and Types of Complications and Long-term Survival After Transplantation of Unmodified Marrow from HLA-Identical Siblings for Patients with Leukemia

Disease	Disease Phase	Disease-free Long-term Survival (%)	Relapse (%)	GVHD (%) Acute, Grade 2–4	Chronic	Interstitial Pneumonia (%)*	VOD (%)
ANL	1st CR	50	22 ⎫				
	2nd + CR	25	45 ⎬ 40–45	25–35	15–35	28	
	1st REL	34	31 ⎭				
ALL	1st CR	54	34 ⎫				
	2nd CR	35	45 ⎪				
	3rd CR	30	48 ⎬ 35	25	15	7	
	2nd + REL	18	75 ⎭				
CML	1st CP	58	17 ⎫				
	AP	30	45 ⎬ 45	35	22	25	
	BC	20	70 ⎭				

ANL, acute nonlymphoblastic leukemia; ALL, acute lymphoblastic leukemia; CML, chronic myelocytic leukemia; CR, complete remission; REL, relapse; CP, chronic phase; AP, accelerated phase; BC, blast crisis; GVHD, graft-versus-host disease; VOD, veno-occlusive disease of the liver; VZV, varicella-zoster virus.
*Includes both idiopathic and cytomegalovirus interstitial pneumonias.
†Includes cardiorenal failure, bleeding, encephalitis, leukoencephalopathy, adult respiratory distress syndrome.
‡% applies to patients given fractionated total body irradiation; % usually considerably higher with single-dose irradiation.
With permission, Storb, R. 1989. Bone marrow transplantation. In DeVita, V. et al. (eds.) *Cancer: Principles and Practice of Oncology*. Phil.: J.B. Lippincott, Co. pp. 2480–2481.

institutional, prospective, randomized trial comparing the "best" standard chemotherapy with the "best" transplant regimen, judgments still need to be made for the individual patient. The outcomes summarized here seem to suggest that bone marrow transplantation is an effective if not superior treatment in some instances. For some patients at certain disease stages, transplant can offer significant increases in long-term survival and cure when compared to other standard therapies.

This guarded optimism is further tempered by the fact that, unlike standard chemotherapy where treatment failures and death are most often due to recurrent, resistant disease—death from bone marrow transplant is often due to the toxicity of the treatment (see Table 2.6). It is a nursing challenge to assist patients and families who have to make choices to undergo significant pain and suffering to cope with the idea that cure is not guaranteed and that their treatment choice may in fact lead to death (from treatment toxicity) earlier than if they had chosen a different treatment or no further treatment.

If both chemotherapy and transplant have similar results it is likely that chemotherapy would

| Bacerial and Fungal Infections During First 3 Mos (%) | | | | Moderate | | | VZV | | Late |
Before Engraft-ment	After Engraft-ment	After 3 Months	Nephro-toxicity (%)	to Severe Mucositis (%)	Other† (%)	Graft Failure (%)	Infec-tions (%)	Cataracts (%)	Secondary Malignancies (%)
20	12	20	13	38	5	< 1	40	18‡	1–2

be the treatment of choice because it currently appears to be the less expensive option. Some claim that bone marrow transplant is less expensive when compared to particular chemotherapy regimens for leukemia (Watson et al. 1981). Others claim that although the initial transplant procedure is more expensive than a course of induction chemotherapy, it is in fact more cost-effective per additional year of life offered over a standard chemotherapy regimen outcome (Welch and Larson 1989). Chapter 18 analyzes the procedure costs in detail.

Treatment of Recurrent Disease

When a standard conditioning regimen of cyclophosphamide and total body irradiation is used to treat advanced leukemia a relapse rate of 40–70% has been reported (Sullivan 1989). When AML patients are transplanted in first and second complete remission, relapse rates are around 23% and 48%, respectively (IBMTR, 1990). Relapse caused by the donor cells is unlikely but has been reported (Boyd et al. 1982). More often, recurrent disease is due to residual disease in the host from an inadequate conditioning regimen. Salvage therapy at this point is not well-defined although both chemotherapy and second bone marrow transplant have been attempted (Wagner et al. 1989). Highly resistant disease favors the more intensive bone marrow transplant approach, but a thorough assessment of the patient's ability to tolerate the expected treatment-related toxicities should be performed. Improving the ability of conditioning regimens to eradicate disease without increasing mortality from regimen-related toxicities is an active area of transplant research (Sullivan 1989).

Patients need to be prepared physically and emotionally to once again undergo the rigors of this treatment. Emotionally, patients are devastated having failed the hope for cure with bone marrow transplant and having their disease behind them. Although relapse is included as one of the risks explained in the informed consent process it may never have been thought of again as the patient occupies his thoughts with hope and the idea of cure.

Summary

The scientific basis underlying allogeneic transplant has been presented to familiarize the new nurse or review for the expert clinician the complexities of the procedure and its outcomes. The nursing roles of patient advocate, care coordinator, educator, and expert clinician are vital to the success and function of the transplant team. The nurse needs to understand these general concepts in order to appreciate fully the potential scope of side effects and toxicities, and the depth and breadth of the patient experience in order to plan appropriate nursing interventions. Developing a knowledge base about the broad indications for this treatment modality, its potential risks and benefits, the treatment process, and outcomes are but a beginning step to providing expert care to this complex and challenging patient population.

There is an explosion of new knowledge in bone marrow transplant. Throughout this text it will be obvious that there are many areas in need of nursing research to determine the most effective nursing interventions to complement the medical treatment-related advances that continue to be made.

References

Ash, R.C. et al. 1990. Successful allogeneic transplantation of T cell-depleted bone marrow from closely HLA-matched unrelated donors. *N. Engl. J. Med. 322* (8): 487–494.

Aubourg, P. et al. 1990. Reversal of early neurologic and neuroradiologic manifestations of x-linked adrenoleukodystrophy by bone marrow transplantation. *N. Engl. J. Med. 322* (26): 1860–1866.

Baranov, A. et al. 1989. Bone marrow transplantation after the Chernobyl nuclear accident. *N. Engl. J. Med. 321* (4): 205–212.

Barrett, A.J. et al. 1989. Marrow transplantation for acute lymphoblastic leukemia: Factors affecting relapse and survival. *Blood 74* (2): 862–871.

Biggs, J.C. et al. 1989. Can morbidity and mortality of matched allogeneic marrow grafts be reduced? *Transplantation Proceedings 21* (1): 3058–3059.

Blazar, B.R. et al. 1986. Successful donor cell engraftment in a recipient of bone marrow from a cadaveric donor. *Blood 67* (6): 1655–1660.

Bortin, M.M., Horowitz, M.M., and Gale, R.P. 1988. Current status of bone marrow transplantation in humans: Report from the International Bone Marrow Transplant Registry. *Nat. Immun. Cell Growth Regul. 7:* 334–350.

Bortin, M.M., and Rimm, A.A. 1986. Increasing utilization of bone marrow transplantation. *Transplantation 42* (3): 229–234.

Bortin, M.M., and Rimm, A.A. 1989. Increasing utilization of bone marrow transplantation: II. Results of the 1985–1987 survey. *Transplantation 48* (3): 453–458.

Boyd, C.N., Ramberg R.C., and Thomas E.D. 1982. The incidence of recurrence of leukemia in donor cells after allogeneic bone marrow transplantation. *Leukemia Research 6:* 833–837.

Brandwein, J.M. et al. 1989. An evaluation of outpatient bone marrow harvesting. *J. Clin. Oncol. 7* (5): 648–650.

Buchsel, P.C. 1986. Long-term complications of allogeneic bone marrow transplantation: Nursing implications. *O.N.F. 13:* (6): 61–70.

Buchsel, P.C., and Parchem, C. 1988. Ambulatory care of the bone marrow transplant patient. *Seminars in Oncology Nursing 4* (1): 41–46.

Buchsel, P.C., and Kelleher, J. 1989. Bone marrow transplantation. *Nurs. Clin. North Am. 24* (4): 907–938.

Cassel, C.K., and Leaning, J. 1989. Chernobyl: Learning from experience. *N. Engl. J. Med. 321* (4): 254–255.

Caudell, K.A., and Adams, J. 1990. Cyclosporine administration practices on bone marrow tranplant units: A national survey. *O.N.F. 17*(4): 563–568.

Copelan, E.A. 1989a. Bone marrow transplantation without total body irradiation in patients aged 40 or older. *Transplantation 48* (1): 65–68.

Copelan, E.A. 1989b. Indications for marrow transplantation in chronic myelogenous leukemia (letter). *Blood 74* (8): 2771–2772.

Cowan, M. et al. 1985. Haplocompatible bone marrow transplantation for severe combined immunodeficiency disease using soybean agglutinin-negative, T-depleted marrow cells. *Journal of Clinical Immunology* 5 (6): 370–376.

Deeg, H.J., Klingemann, H.-G., and Phillips, G. L. 1988. *A Guide to Bone Marrow Transplantation.* New York: Springer-Verlag.

de Vries, E.G.E., Sleijfer D.T., and Mulder N.H. 1989. Outpatient bone marrow harvesting without general anesthesia. *J. Clin. Oncol.* 7 (9): 1367–1368.

English, D. et al. 1989. Semiautomated processing of bone marrow grafts for transplantation. *Transplantation* 29 (1): 12–16.

Fairhead, S.M. et al. 1983. Treatment of aplastic anaemia with antilymphocyte globulin. *British Journal of Hematology* 55: 7.

Fefer, A., and Thomas, E.D. 1990. Bone marrow transplantation for treatment of chronic myelogenous leukemia. In Devita, V.T., et al. (eds). 1990. *Important Advances in Oncology 1990.* Philadelphia: J.B. Lippincott Co, pp. 143–158.

Fonger, P. 1987. Nursing care of the child with severe combined immune deficiency. *Journal of Pediatric Nursing* 2 (6): 373–380.

Gale, R.T. et al. 1989. IBMTR analysis of bone marrow transplants in acute leukemia. *B.M.T.* 4 (suppl. 3): 83–84

Glasgow, G.P. et al. 1989. A total body irradiation stand for bone marrow transplant patients. *Int. J. Radiation Oncology Biol. Phys.* 16: 875–877.

Gassmann, W. et al. 1988. Comparison of cyclophosphamide, cytarabine, and etoposide as immunosuppressive agents before allogeneic bone marrow transplantation. *Blood* 72 (5): 1574–1579.

Hows, J.M. et al. 1986. Histocompatible unrelated volunteer donors compared with HLA nonidentical family donors in marrow transplantation for aplastic anemia and leukemia. *Blood* 68 (6): 1322–1328.

International Bone Marrow Transplant Registry (IBMTR). 1990. An overview of allogeneic bone marrow transplantation. *Directory of Bone Marrow Transplant Teams. 3rd ed.* Milwaukee, WI.

James, N.D. et al. 1989. Total lymphoid irradiation preceeding bone marrow transplantation for chronic myeloid leukemia. *Clinical Radiology* 40: 195–198.

Kaminski, E.R. 1989. How important is histocompatibility in bone marrow transplantation? *B.M.T.* 4: 439–444.

Kanfer, E.J., and McCarthy D.M. 1989. Cytoreductive preparation for bone marrow transplantation in leukemia: To irradiate or not? *British Journal of Haematology* 71: 447–450.

Kersey, J.H. 1989. The role of marrow transplantation in acute lymphoblastic leukemia. *J. Clin. Oncol.* 7 (11): 1589–1590.

Krensky, A.M. et al. 1990. T lymphocyte-antigen interactions in transplant rejection. *N. Engl. J. Med.* 322 (8): 510–517.

Labar, B. et al. 1989. Total body irradiation with or without lung shielding for allogeneic bone marrow transplantation. *B.M.T.* 4 (suppl. 1): 108.

Lasky, L.C. et al. 1989. Successful allogeneic cryopreserved marrow transplantation. *Transplantation* 29 (2): 182–184.

Lawton, C.A. et al. 1989. Technical modifications in hyperfractionated total body irradiation for T lymphocyte depleted bone marrow transplant. *Int. J. Radiation Oncology Biol. Phys.* 17 (2): 319–322.

McGlave, P.B. 1985. The status of bone marrow transplantation for leukemia. *Hospital Practice* 20 (11): 97–105, 108–110.

McGlave, P.B. et al. 1990. Therapy for chronic myelogenous leukemia with unrelated donor bone marrow transplantation: Results in 102 cases. *Blood* 75 (8): 1728–1732.

Mackinnon, S. et al. 1990. Bone marrow transplantation for chronic myeloid leukemia: The use of histocompatible unrelated volunteer donors. *Exp. Hematol.* 18: 421–425.

Martin, P.J. et al. 1988. HLA-identical marrow transplantation during accelerated-phase chronic myelogenous leukemia: Analysis of survival and remission duration. *Blood* 72 (6): 1978–1984.

Marx, J.L. 1989. Bone marrow transplants approved. *Science* 244: 768.

Mayer, R.J. 1988. Allogeneic transplantation versus intensive chemotherapy in first-remission acute leukemia: Is there a "best choice"? *J. Clin. Oncol.* 6 (4): 1532–1536.

Mugishima, H. et al. 1985. Bone marrow from cadaver donors for transplantation. *Blood* 65 (2): 392–396.

Neudorf, S. et al. 1989. A modified method for human bone marrow filtration prior to bone marrow transplantation. *B.M.T.* 4: 97–100.

Petz, L.D., and Blume, K.G. 1983. *Clinical Bone Marrow Transplantation.* New York: Churchill-Livingstone.

Phillips, G.L. et al. 1989. Allogeneic marrow transplantation for refractory Hodgkin's disease. *J. Clin. Oncol.* 7 (8): 1039–1045.

Poplack, D.G., and Reaman, G. 1988. Acute lymphoblastic leukemia in childhood. *Pediatr. Clin. North Am.* 35 (4): 903–931.

Rohaly, J. 1989. The use of busulfan therapy in bone marrow transplantation: A nursing overview. *Cancer Nursing* 12 (3): 144–152.

Santos, G. 1989a. Marrow transplantation in acute nonlymphocytic leukemia. *Blood* 74 (3): 901–908.

Santos, G. 1989b. Busulfan (Bu) and cyclophosphamide (CY) for marrow transplantation. *B.M.T.* 4 (suppl. 1): 236–239.

Schouten, H.C. et al. 1989. Allogeneic bone marrow transplantation in patients with lymphoma relapsing after autologous marrow transplantation. *B.M.T.* 4: 119–121.

Stadtmauer, E.A. et al. 1989. Etoposide in leukemia, lymphoma, and bone marrow transplantation. *Leukemia Research* 13 (8): 639–650.

Storb, R. 1989. Bone marrow transplantation. In Devita, V.J., et al. (eds). *Cancer: Principles and Practice of Oncology.* Philadelphia: J.B. Lippincott Co.: 2474–2489.

Stream, P. 1983. Functions of the outpatient clinic before and after marrow transplantation. *Nurs. Clin. North Am. 18* (3): 603–610.

Sullivan, K.M. 1989. Current status of bone marrow transplantation. *Transplantation Proceedings 21* (3, suppl. 1): 41–50.

Sullivan, K.M. et al. 1989. Long-term results of allogeneic bone marrow transplantation. *Transplantation Proceedings 21* (1): 2926–2928.

Tallman, M.S. et al. 1989. Analysis of prognostic factors for the outcome of marrow transplantation or further chemotherapy for patients with acute non-lymphocytic leukemia in first remission. *J. Clin. Oncol. 7* (3): 326–337.

Thomas, E.D. 1987. Bone marrow transplantation. *CA 37:* 291–301.

Thomas, E.D. et al. 1989. Indications for marrow transplantation in chronic myelogenous leukemia. *Blood 73:* 861.

Thomas, E.D., and Storb R. 1970. Technique for human marrow grafting. *Blood 36* (4): 507–515.

Thompson, H.W., and McCullough, J. 1986. Use of blood components containing red cells by donors of allogeneic bone marrow. *Transfusion 26:* (1): 98–100.

Truog, A.W., and Wozniak, S.P. 1990. Cyclosporine-A as prevention for graft-versus-host disease in pediatric patients undergoing bone marrow transplants. *O.N.F. 17* (1): 39–44.

Tutschka, J. et al. 1989. Replacing total body irradiation with busulfan as conditioning of patients with leukemia for allogeneic marrow transplantation. *Transplantation Proceedings 21* (1): 2952–2954.

van Bekkum, D.W., and De Vries, M.J. 1967. *Radiation Chimaeras.* London: Logos Press Ltd.

van Bekkum, D.W. 1989. From radiation chimeras to 1988. *B.M.T. 4* (suppl. 1): 216–221.

Vitale, V. et al. 1989. Total body irradiation: single dose, fractions, dose rate. *B.M.T. 4* (suppl. 1): 233–235.

Vogelsang, G.B. et al. 1988. Acute graft-versus-host disease: Clinical characteristics in the cyclosporine era. *Medicine 67* (3): 163–174.

Wagner, J.E. et al. 1989. Second BMT after leukemia relapse in 11 patients. *B.M.T. 4:* 115–118.

Watson, J.G. et al. 1981. Acute myeloid leukemia: Comparison of support required during initial induction of remission and marrow transplantation in first remission. *Lancet* Oct. 31: 957–959.

Weisdorf, D.J. 1990. Bone marrow transplantation: What you need to know. *Postgrad. Med. 87* (1): 91–101.

Welch, H.G., and Larson, E.B. 1989. Cost effectiveness of bone marrow transplantation in acute nonlymphocytic leukemia. *N. Engl. J. Med. 321* (12): 807–812.

Wingard, J.R. 1990. Allogeneic bone marrow transplantation for patients with high-risk acute lymphoblastic leukemia. *J. Clin. Oncol. 8* (5): 820–830.

Yahalom, J. et al. 1989. Total lymphoid irradiation, high-dose chemotherapy, and autologous bone marrow transplantation for chemotherapy-resistant Hodgkin's disease. *Int. J. Radiation Oncology Biol. Phys. 17* (5): 915–922.

Chapter 3

Autologous Bone Marrow Transplantation: Clinical Indications, Treatment Process, and Outcomes

Marie Bakitas Whedon

Introduction

Like many other medical therapies, modern autologous bone marrow transplantion, also called marrow support or "rescue," is actually a recycled idea. As described in Chapter 1, its use in the late 1950s as a rescue from "high dose" chemotherapy was met with only minimal enthusiasm since at that time patients seemed to recover from high-dose chemotherapy equally well without the infusion of autologous marrow. Today, most patients can be supported through the nadir caused by modern combination chemotherapy doses and recover without event, or with only mild toxicity. Thus, the need for autologous marrow infusion in these cases continues to be unnecessary.

However, the more recent trend of dose escalation has redefined high-dose chemotherapy. For today's patients, hematologic recovery would be significantly delayed or absent without reinfusion or rescue with autologous marrow. Hence

one reason for renewed enthusiasm concerning this treatment modality.

Unlike allogeneic transplant in which the replacement of the diseased organ is the treatment, reinfusion of autologous marrow for patients with solid tumors is a rescue from the treatment toxicity (i.e., prolonged pancytopenia). In many ways the purpose of reinfusion of autologous marrow today is just as it was historically envisioned—as a supportive care measure to ensure return of hematopoiesis after administration of high-dose chemotherapy and radiation therapy.

Another reason for renewed enthusiasm for autologous bone marrow transplant was alluded to in Chapter 2. About two-thirds of patients with hematologic malignancies who could potentially benefit from a bone marrow transplant lack an HLA-identical sibling donor and therefore an available source of disease-free marrow (Gale and Butturini 1989). In this case, alternative sources of marrow have been sought, including HLA-matched unrelated donors, partially matched related and unrelated donors (described in Chapter 2), and the patient's own marrow.

In the treatment of hematologic malignancies, the goal of autologous bone marrow transplant is often similar to that of allogeneic transplant, that is, to replace diseased marrow with healthy, normal marrow. The patient is "conditioned" in a fashion similar to the allogeneic patient (as described in Chapter 2). There may also be an additional step of ex vivo removal of malignant cells from the autologous marrow. This later step is accomplished by the use of marrow purging techniques (described later in this chapter) designed to eliminate malignant cells from the marrow while preserving adequate numbers of normal healthy stem cells. When these healthy stem cells are returned to the host, normal hematopoiesis results (Gee 1990).

An added benefit of autologous transplant has been the elimination of one of the most significant complications of allogeneic bone marrow transplant: graft-versus-host disease. Autologous marrow does not recognize the host as foreign and is generally accepted by the host with little or no acute or delayed immunologic consequences. Again, the goal of autologous transplant is quite similar to that of allogeneic bone marrow transplant treatment (i.e., replacing a damaged or diseased organ); the difference lies in the source of healthy marrow.

To this point, only the advantages of autologous transplant have been mentioned. However, there are some disadvantages to this approach. In hematologic malignancies the lack of a graft-versus-host effect seems to come at the cost of a lack of a **"graft-versus-leukemia"** effect and a proportional rise in the relapse of the disease (Gale and Butturini 1989). Also, since bone marrow is known to contain leukemic clones even when the patient is in remission, leukemic clones capable of causing disease relapse may be returned to the host at the time of marrow reinfusion (Gale and Butturini 1989). Despite the increasing popularity of marrow purging methods (Gross 1990), it is

not known whether these methods are necessary to prevent leukemia relapse (Burnett 1989), or if necessary, whether the current purging methods are capable of removing all clonogenic malignant cells (Gross 1990).

In the treatment of solid tumors there continues to be a lack of effective (curative) chemotherapy regimens. Consequently, recurrent disease after transplant is a significant problem (Appelbaum 1987). In those tumors where effective treatment regimens are available, for instance with lymphomas (Frei et al. 1989), methods to remove disease from the bone marrow may not yet be feasible (if marrow contamination by malignant cells has already occurred). However, purging methods to remove malignant disease from the marrow of patients with many solid tumors continues to be actively explored (Gross 1990).

As stated above, the purpose of reinfusing autologous bone marrow differs depending on the disease being treated. However, the broader intent of autologous bone marrow transplant as a treatment modality is cure. Whether in the clinical or investigational setting, autologous bone marrow transplantation is a highly toxic treatment. Therefore, many transplanters agree that the treatment must provide significant improvements in median survival over standard chemotherapy regimens to account for the increased morbidity, mortality, and costs (Frei et al. 1989). However autotransplant may be a preferred treatment option if the trends demonstrate comparable costs, acceptable treatment toxicity, and a potential shortened length of treatment. If the latter is true, which may be the case when one compares the length of intensification treatment for AML versus a single high-dose treatment and autotransplant, a reduced cost of treatment may be evidenced with autotransplant.

Recognizing the advantages and limitations of this relatively new and investigational treatment and its potential to cure previously fatal diseases, it is no wonder that there is an explosion of autologous bone marrow transplantation treatment programs being developed throughout the world. Hence, there is a proportional explosion in the need for expert nurses to provide sophisticated clinical care to these patients. The purpose of the following chapter is to set forth a framework from which current knowledge of this exciting treatment modality can be summarized for application by the nurse in the clinical setting.

Clinical Indications

In order for autologous bone marrow transplant to be effective (curative) the disease being treated needs to meet the following four criteria (Santos, 1985):

1. the malignancy is responsive to cytoreductive therapy,

2. the effective treatment has only marrow failure as its dose-limiting toxicity,

3. the procedure can be performed early in the disease when the tumor burden and drug resistance are minimal, and

4. the source of hematopoietic stem cells is free of tumor cells and clones.

These criteria can be satisfied by both hematologic and solid tumors. This in part explains the wide application and investigation of autologous bone marrow transplant for so many types of malignancies (see Tables 3.1 and 3.2). However, unlike allogeneic transplant, autologous transplant is exclusively applied to the treatment of malignant diseases.

As mentioned earlier, autologous bone marrow transplants are a rather heterogeneous group of procedures and it may be some time until all of the possible uses are determined and tested for superiority over current therapy. Their use in hematologic malignancies and solid tumors continues to be actively explored in clinical trials throughout the world (as shown in Figure 3.1). Although for unknown reasons the frequency with which the procedure is done for different cancers varies between the continents. For instance, in North America, autotransplant is most often done

Table 3.1. Solid Tumors Treated with Autologous Transplant

Breast
Lung (small cell and non-small cell)
Neuroblastoma
Testicular/Germ cell tumors
Ovarian
Colon
Melanoma
Sarcomas
Gliomas
*Renal cell
*Pancreatic
*Gastric

*Few cases reported.
Adapted from Cheson et al. 1989; Armitage and Gale 1989; Antman et al. 1986; and Souhami and Peters 1986.

for lymphomas, whereas leukemias are the diseases most frequently treated in this manner in Europe (Advisory Committee of the International Autologous Bone Marrow Transplant Registry 1989). Clinical indications for both hematologic and solid tumors are discussed below, describing areas of demonstrated usefulness, undetermined usefulness, and areas that have lacked success.

Hematologic Malignancies

Overview

Hematologic malignancies are among the most responsive to chemotherapy, making them a perfect choice for investigating a treatment modality that employs high-dose therapy. However, several difficulties can potentially interfere with the success of this treatment. First, all malignant clones

Table 3.2. Hematologic Malignancies Treated with Autologous Transplant

Acute myelogenous leukemia (AML)
Acute lymphocytic leukemia (ALL)
Chronic myelogenous leukemia (CML)
Hodgkin's and non-Hodgkin's lymphoma
Multiple myeloma

A.

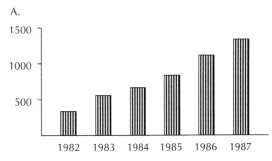

B.

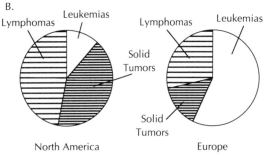

With permission, Advisory Committe of the International Autologous Bone Marrow Transplant Registry. 1989. Different Indications for ABMT in North America and Europe, *Lancet* (Aug. 5): p. 318.

Figure 3.1. A. Annual Number 1982–87; B. Indications for Autotransplants in Europe and North America

must be eliminated from the patient. This is a task potentially more difficult than in the allogeneic transplants, where there is a predicted benefit from a graft-versus-leukemia effect, which is lacking in autologous marrow transplants (Gale and Butturini 1989; Gorin 1986). Second, all malignant clones must be eliminated from the harvested marrow. Clearly, strategies must be designed to attack each of these problems. Some of these are mentioned below.

Infusion of autologous cells for the treatment of acute leukemias and chronic myelogenous leukemia (CML) was first reported in the late 1970s, and this experience was recently reviewed (Gorin 1986). In this early experience bone marrow stem cells were collected from patients while still in remission and were later infused to either support

patients during periods of neutropenia or, in the case of CML, to return patients to a chronic phase of the disease after ablative therapy for blast crisis (Goldman et al. 1981). Because most of these patients experienced a relapse of their disease, modifications in conditioning regimens and attempts to rid the marrow of malignant clones were undertaken (Gorin 1986).

Over the last decade, marrow purging techniques have expanded to include lymphomas (Hurd et al. 1988). Continued development and clinical trials that use various methods of autologous marrow purging continues in most hematologic malignancies. (See "Marrow Purging Techniques" later in this chapter for a more specific discussion of these techniques.)

In general, autologous transplantation for leukemia is usually considered when the patient lacks a histocompatible donor or is over age forty. In lymphomas, this has quickly become a treatment of choice for many patients. As results improve, the decreased toxicity of this treatment (as compared with allogeneic transplants), and the potential shorter duration of treatment compared with many conventional chemotherapy regimens might make this an even more attractive option.

Acute Myelogenous Leukemia (AML)

Transplantation is used in AML because although the majority of patients (50–80%) will achieve a chemotherapy-induced complete remission (CR) (Dicke et al. 1989), only 20–30% of these will continue to be in remission two years hence. Once relapse occurs, few if any will acheive a cure from subsequent chemotherapy (Appelbaum et al. 1989). Because of these statistics, other strategies have been sought to improve survival and effect cures in patients following the achievement of a first CR. Results from allogeneic transplant (summarized in Chapter 2) currently show some advantage over chemotherapy. Forty-five to fifty percent of patients are disease-free at three years compared to the above cited figures for chemotherapy (Appelbaum et al. 1989).

Autologous transplantation as a strategy for those patients lacking HLA-matched sibling donors has been used to improve the disease-free survival of patients with AML. It has been used in patients who have acheived a first remission as an intensification of first remission (Dicke et al. 1989; Gorin et al. 1990), at the time of first relapse (Meloni et al. 1985), and in second and subsequent remissions (Ball et al. 1990; Meloni et al. 1990; Yeager et al. 1986). The procedure toxicity is acceptable although the leukemia relapse rates have been high (Cheson et al. 1989). Because of the lack of randomized trials it is still unclear whether there is a need for marrow purging in AML (Gress 1990).

Acute Lymphoblastic Leukemia (ALL)

The role of autotransplant in ALL is even less certain than in AML, because even fewer patients have been treated with autologous transplant (Cheson et al. 1989). Most patients with ALL are children and most (60–70%) are cured by combination chemotherapy (Poplack and Reaman 1988). Because of this, few other treatment modalities have been used. Transplantation is often considered the next most reasonable option of choice (Kersey et al. 1987). Poor risk patients who lack an HLA-matched sibling donor and older patients are considered the most likely candidates for autologous transplant (Tura and Visani 1989; Sallan et al. 1989). Poor risk ALL patients are usually defined as those who have relapsed while on therapy, whose first remission was shorter than 18 months, those who present with a high white blood cell count or particular cytogenetic abnormalities, and adults (Tura and Visani 1989; Kersey et al. 1987).

Chronic Myelogenous Leukemia (CML)

Autologous transplant for CML has been attempted using bone marrow and blood-derived stem cells collected while the patient was in chronic phase and then returned to the patient after ablative therapy during blast crisis. The goal of the procedure was to return the patient to the more stable "chronic phase" (Marcus and Goldman 1986). A review of autologous transplant studies by Marcus and Goldman (1986) concluded that patients often achieved a second chronic phase of the disease, which was short-lived. After this they eventually returned to "blast crisis" from which they eventually died. More recently, autologous transplant has been combined with subsequent low dose interferon. Unfortunately, to date these results have been disappointing (Meloni et al. 1989b). Problems that still must be overcome for autotransplant in CML to be successful include: eradicating disease in the host and in the graft. Approaches to these problems continue to receive attention (Butturini et al. 1990).

Until then however, allogeneic transplant seems to be the only therapy offering a cure to CML patients, with the best results achieved when the patient is transplanted in chronic phase. Presently, it seems that in most situations autologous transplant is not an option for patients with CML (Deeg et al. 1988).

In summary, there are still many unanswered questions in determining the role of autologous transplantation in hematologic malignancies: What regimens are most effective to eliminate disease from the host? What are the best methods to eliminate disease from the autograft? When in the disease process should autologous transplantation be attempted? After acheiving a first remission? As a consolidation/intensification alternative? When a histocompatible donor is not available, should an autograft be recommended rather than an unrelated donor transplant in certain situations? How do patients decide?

Non-Hodgkin's and Hodgkin's Lymphomas

Non-Hodgkin's lymphoma is the disease for which most autologous transplants are currently performed (Advisory Committee of the International Autologous Bone Marrow Transplant Registry 1989). This is due to a high incidence of this disease in comparison to other cancers that are treatable with autotransplant. Additionally, lymphomas are very chemoradioresponsive and reinfusion of marrow contaminated with lymphoma cells does not seem to play a major role in disease recurrence (Armitage and Gale 1989; Sharp et al. 1989b). Autotransplantation currently appears to be the treatment of choice in some patients with intermediate and high grade non-Hodgkin's lymphomas, who are still responding to chemotherapy (Hurd et al. 1988) and have an acceptable performance status (Armitage and Gale 1989; Cheson et al. 1989). Although patient with advanced lymphoma have had long-term disease-free survivals (Gingrich et al. 1990), patients outcomes seem to be better in patients treated earlier in their disease (Philip et al. 1987). Consequently, it has been recommended that high dose therapy and autologous transplant be considered as frontline therapy, especially in selected poor prognosis lymphoma patients (Tura et al. 1986; Takvorian et al. 1987). Its use in lymphoma patients with low-grade histology is still being studied (Cheson et al. 1989).

The lower incidence and high cure rate with chemotherapy even in advanced disease (50% for patients with stage IV [Spinolo et al. 1989]) has resulted in fewer patients with Hodgkin's disease than other lymphomas being treated with autotransplant. It is usually considered as an option for patients who have relapsed while on therapy or for those with resistant disease in whom initial treatment fails (Gingrich et al. 1990; Armitage et al. 1989; Armitage and Gale 1989; Cheson et al. 1989; Jagannath et al. 1989; Gribben et al. 1989b). The use of autotransplant in Hodgkin's disease has been reviewed and reported to be most beneficial for patients with a good performance status, low tumor burden, and less than two prior treatment regimens (Ahmed 1990).

The promising outcome of autologous bone marrow transplants in lymphoma patients has prompted the use of high-dose treatment with the more recently developed method of periperal blood stem cell transplants (described later). Clinical trials using this method exist for patients who have been ineligible for traditional autolo-gous harvests due to a variety of bone marrow abnormalities (Kessinger et al. 1989a).

Solid Tumors

As stated earlier, for autologous bone marrow transplantation to be effective there must first be drugs available that have activity against a particular tumor and with hematologic effects as the only dose-limiting toxicity (Santos 1985). As drugs that show activity against resistant solid tumors continue to be developed, the usefulness of autologous bone marrow transplantation in solid tumors will continue to expand. Carboplatin (Shea et al. 1989) and ifosfamide are two examples of newer drugs being tested in dose escalation studies for usefulness in transplantation.

Table 3.1 lists some common cancers being treated with high dose chemoradiotherapy and autologous transplant. Results of clinical trials of autologous transplant in solid tumors are still maturing and at this point recommendations for diseases that will benefit from this therapy are premature. The diseases that presently seem to be the most responsive to this therapy include neuroblastoma and breast cancer (Cheson et al. 1989).

Identification of an Investigational Treatment Center

Many centers today are investigating and offering autologous bone marrow transplant for a variety of malignancies in children and adults. Development of new programs continues at a rapid rate. This growth can be appreciated when one considers that between 1986 and 1989 the number of centers worldwide reporting data to the International Autologous Bone Marrow Transplant Registry grew from 43 to 112 (Advisory Committee for the International Autologous Bone Marrow Transplant Registry 1986 and 1989). Additional centers not reporting to the International

Registry may have existed between those dates and others have been developed since then. Therefore, the number of centers in operation today is unknown and growth is difficult to predict.

This growth presents a potential challenge to the patient seeking such a procedure. The challenge first is knowing (discovering) whether a program is available for the disease, and second, evaluating the quality of the institution performing this procedure. The difficulty increases if the treatment being offered is still in the earliest stages of development in general, or in that institution in particular. Successful performance of high-dose therapy with transplantation requires a tremendous amount of coordination and an interdisciplinary team representing expertise in many different specialty areas (Kelleher and Jennings 1988; Frei et al. 1989; Gianni et al. 1989).

The patient approaching an unfamiliar institution that may offer him a "cure" can feel very threatened. It may be difficult to be assertive and ask the necessary questions to get enough information to fully evaluate the treatment and the institution. However, the patient must decide whether to pursue the treatment at that particular institution based on this information. The threatening nature of clinical trials to cancer patients in general has been well documented (Lesko et al. 1989). Because autologous transplants are available at many institutions for a wide variety of conditions, and mostly within the setting of a clinical trial, the above situation is currently a common one for many patients seeking this treatment.

The health care team of the referring institution can be instrumental in assisting the patient to get complete information and the team is obliged to be a patient advocate in this pursuit. Physicians can help by evaluating a prospective institution's treatment results, eligibility requirements, and any available publications in professional journals. The nursing role may include contacting nurses at the transplant center to inquire about how the patient can get through the system in addition to coaching the patient in asking pertinent questions and assisting the patient to formulate those questions in advance.

Depending on the transplant institution's protocol requirements, the patient should be assisted in gathering all pertinent records, specimens, and copies of diagnostic x-rays and scans. Occasionally the transplanting institution may need to repeat tests if actual specimen slides and x-rays do not accompany the patient and only reports of these tests are sent. The research protocol may require actual tissue or slides rather than reports of these tests.

Most centers have a program coordinator who can be contacted prior to an initial visit and consultation to assure that all necessary information is brought with the patient. All other arrangements and eligibility criteria must be critically analyzed by the referring team in advance (usually by phone). This will help to maximize the visit.

Patients can spend considerable time, effort, financial resources, and hope only to find out on evaluation at the transplant center that they have relapsed or are otherwise ineligible for a particular protocol due to a clinical finding that might have been recognized at the referring institution (e.g., inadequate blood counts to allow harvest, elevated liver function tests, etc.). This can occur even with a great deal of scrutiny and attention to detail because a patient with active disease can experience rapid changes in condition. However, it is frustrating to the transplant center, the patient, and the referring health care team when it occurs.

Treatment Process

Patient Evaluation and Eligibility

Patient evaluation methods for autologous transplants are similar to those described in Chapter 2. However, since the uses of autologous transplant are not yet fully defined, eligibility criteria may be broader and may allow patients in more advanced stages of disease to be treated than is the case with allogeneic transplant protocols. Patients older than typically accepted into allogeneic programs may be eligible. One reason for this is the absence of GVHD and other toxicities of allogeneic transplant, which make autologous procedures generally much better tolerated in the older patient.

Bone Marrow Harvest: Timing and Process

Although the basic harvest procedure is the same for autologous and allogeneic bone marrow transplants, some procedural and technical aspects differ. The point at which the marrow is harvested and reinfused also varies. For instance, most patients receiving autologous transplants will have been pretreated with chemotherapy and/or radiation therapy before transplant was even considered. This can affect the overall quality, cellularity, and ease of marrow harvest in contrast to a normal, healthy allogeneic marrow donor (Gee 1990).

In general, more total volume of marrow is harvested for autologous transplant procedures, especially if the marrow is to be treated or purged. Unknown effects of purging to the normal stem cells following these manipulations require a great deal of consideration and careful calculation of the amount of marrow to be harvested to ensure adequate hematopoiesis (Gee 1990). The physician generally anticipates a reduced cell count following the purging process and harvests more total cells than might normally be necessary to allow for adequate hematopoietic reconstitution. Occasionally harvests may need to be repeated or peripheral stem cell harvests may be necessary if postpurging cell counts are found to be inadequate. Inadequate harvests can result from marrow fibrosis in heavily pretreated patients, patients who received radiation to the pelvis, or possibly stem cell sensitivity to the agent used for marrow treatment (Williams et al. 1990). Prior to the ability to perform peripheral blood stem cell harvests, the inability to obtain adequate numbers

of nucleated cells and/or marrow contamination with malignant cells caused patients to be ineligible for an autologous transplant procedure (Williams et al. 1990). This may still be the case in institutions that do not routinely perform or lack the capacity to do peripheral harvests.

More recently, "double" transplants have been performed in which a single harvest is done to gather twice the required amount of marrow for repeated hematopoietic reconstitutions (Beaujean et al. 1989). A variation of this method calls for a repeated harvest and treatment after an initial high dose treatment and autologous marrow infusion (Gribben et al. 1989a).

Unlike allogeneic harvests, autologous marrow is rarely reinfused immediately. It may be processed and frozen for later use or processed, treated, and then frozen (cryopreserved). Dimethylsulfoxide (DMSO), a cryoprotective agent discovered in 1940, allow the safe freezing of bone marrow. After DMSO is added to the storage bag the marrow is frozen by a controlled-rate process usually at a rate of 1°C per minute until a temperature of -40 to $-50°C$ is reached. Variations of this method have been reported to result in successful engraftment (Allieri et al. 1989; Alessandrino et al. 1989).

Marrow frozen in this way can be stored for an undetermined amount of time. A recent survey of cryopreservation practices, in which 47 major transplant centers responded, showed that most centers (85%) tend to reinfuse greater than half of their cryopreserved marrows within a year with a maximal storage of three years at which point they may reharvest the patient if transplant is still being considered. However, 20% of the centers responding had successfully reinfused marrow that had been cryopreserved between 5–8 years (Areman et al. 1990).

It is not absolutely certain if increasing the number of infused stem cells above the amount needed to normally reconstitute the hematopoietic function provides any benefit in the quality or rapidity of return of hematopoiesis. However, trends in this practice have been reported (Rowley et al. 1989).

Peripheral Blood Stem Cell (PBSC) Harvests

Animal models have demonstrated that hematopoietic stem cells capable of reconstituting the bone marrow circulate in the peripheral blood. However, these cells are about 10–100 times more concentrated in the bone marrow than in the peripheral circulation. This explains the common use of the bone marrow as the site of stem cell harvest.

Both positive and negative results using only PBSCs for reconstituting the hematopoietic system of humans were reported between 1979–1984 (Hershko et al. 1979; Abrams et al. 1980; McCarthy and Goldman 1984). Consistent successful hematopoietic reconstitution of several patients with solid tumors and hematologic malignancies following ablative therapy began to be reported in 1986 (Kessinger et al. 1986; Reiffers et al. 1986). This has encouraged continued investigation of this method for use in selected patients. The early lack of success was thought to be due in part to the collection and reinfusion of a smaller than necessary dose of nucleated cells than is currently believed to be needed when this method of hematopoietic reconstitution is used (Juttner et al. 1988).

Transplantation by this method alone has resulted in both rapid and delayed hematopoietic recovery times (Juttner et al. 1990) when compared with the return of bone marrow function typical of traditional transplants. When PBSCs have been combined with bone marrow harvests rapid and complete hematopoietic recovery has been reported (Gianni et al. 1989). Clinical trials of this method of performing transplantation are continuing (Kessinger et al. 1989a and 1989b) and Table 3.3 lists some of the diseases for which PBSC transplants have been done. As successful clinical trials continue to be reported, more diseases are likely to be added.

Table 3.3. Malignant Diseases Treated with Peripheral Blood Stem Cell Transplantation

Acute nonlymphocytic leukemia
Acute lymphoblastic leukemia
Hodgkin's and non-Hodgkin's lymphomas
Breast cancer
Ovarian cancer
Small cell lung carcinoma
Neuroblastoma

Adapted from Lasky, 1989.

Peripheral blood stem cells (mononuclear cells) are obtained using an apheresis procedure on a cell separation (apheresis) device (e.g., Haemonetics Model 30 or V50, Haemonetics, Braintree, MA; or Fenwal CS-3000, Fenwall, Deerfield, IL). The patient is connected to the machine for a period of two to four hours while blood is automatically withdrawn, separated, and unneeded components (i.e., red blood cells, platelets, and plasma) are returned to the patient. This collection procedure is repeated as many times as necessary to obtain adequate numbers of mononuclear cells. An average number of eight collections is often reported over a span of days to weeks. After each individual collection, cells may be frozen with DMSO 10% or treated (purged) and then frozen.

Higher numbers of circulating peripheral stem cells and therefore higher yields of cells with pheresis procedures have been evidenced as a rebound effect during marrow regeneration following induction chemotherapy for leukemia. It is also believed that at this time there is probably less peripheral contamination with leukemia cells (Juttner et al. 1990). Use of this effect to the clinical advantage of leukemia patients and for other patients receiving myelosuppressive drugs is currently under study (Juttner et al. 1990). Additional mechanisms that can mobilize peripheral blood stem cells include: excercise, corticosteroids, repeated pheresis procedures, administration of colony stimulating factors (i.e. G-CSF, GM-CSF) (Juttner et al. 1990).

Only minor complications of circumoral tingling and lightheadedness, or coldness have been reported from this collection method. These effects are similar to those reported by patients who donate platelets or whole blood (Kessinger et al. 1989; Hubbard 1989).

One advantage of this procedure over a traditional bone marrow aspiration technique is that it eliminates the need for general anesthesia. More important, it enables patients who might otherwise be ineligible for transplant due to inadequate stem cell harvest an opportunity to receive this procedure (Williams et al. 1990). One indication for performing a peripheral harvest would be for a patient with a history of bone marrow involvement or current bone marrow metastases. This is because PBSCs may contain fewer malignant cells capable of causing disease than diseased marrow (Lasky 1989). Another indication would be patients with hypocellular marrow as might occur following pelvic irradiation (Juttner et al. 1988). Also, recently a case report of successful allogeneic transplantation using T cell-depleted PBSC in an 18-year-old ALL patient was reported (Kessinger et al. 1989b), indicating another potential clinical indication for this harvest method.

In situations where peripheral harvests are not purged it is not known if this procedure might also allow collection of undetectable circulating malignant cells capable of causing a relapse of the disease (Sharp et al. 1989). Purging methods for peripheral harvests are similar to those used for traditional bone marrow harvests (Lasky 1989), but often are more time-consuming. Each collection must be treated and frozen individually rather than in bulk as is done when marrow is harvested by traditional means. It seems logical that this additional manipulation puts the cells at greater risk for destruction or contamination by pathogens. However, this complication is as yet unreported.

It is unclear at this point whether peripheral blood stem cell collection will be more economically beneficial than traditional harvest procedures. For instance, one center estimated the cost to the patient of a typical pheresis collection procedure to be approximately $385 plus an additional charge of $250 for purging, for a total collection cost of $635 (Leach 1990). This procedure is often repeated 8–15 times depending on the yield from each collection, which averages out to a cost of $5,000–$9,500 to obtain an adequate amount of marrow for transplant. The same institution reports an average patient cost for a traditional harvest/monoclonal antibody purge for AML of $12,000 ($9,000 unpurged). At this point the expense of PBSC harvests, like many other cancer therapies perceived to be investigational by insurance companies (described in Chapter 17), may be more difficult to recover.

Marrow Purging Techniques

The major scientific basis for purging marrow is that malignant cells persist in the bone marrow in microscopic amounts even when patients are in remission (Sharp et al. 1989). The ability of these cells to cause relapse or recurrence of the original disease after high dose therapy is still subject to debate (Sharp et al. 1989a and 1989b; Armitage and Gale 1989a; Dicke and Spinolo 1989). Recurrence of chronic myelogenous leukemia following reinfusion of unpurged marrow in these patients (Goldman et al. 1981; Marcus and Goldman 1986; Butturini et al. 1990) demonstrates the ability of malignant cells to persist and repopulate the host, favoring a need for purging. Both positive results (Ball et al. 1990; Yeager et al. 1986; Rowley et al. 1989; Gorin et al. 1989) and limitations (Gale and Butturini 1989; Burnett 1989) of the benefits of purging continue to be reported.

Methods to detect minimal amounts of residual disease are not well established (Burnett 1989). Consequently, it is unclear which patients would obtain the potentially beneficial effects that purging might offer. The need for purging in acute leukemia patients in first remission is the most controversial. There does seem to be some benefit to patients in second and subsequent remissions

(Yeager et al. 1986; Tura and Visani 1989; Ball et al. 1990).

Some problems that have occurred with purging are profound aplasia and prolonged thrombocytopenia (Santos 1985) leading to the potential for higher infection rates and bleeding complications. Bacterial contamination of autologous marrow grafts has been reported to occur presumably due to ex vivo manipulation during purging and processing (Rowley et al. 1988). Although it occurred at the same rate as that of allogeneic harvests (17%) contaminants in addition to usual skin flora were more prevalant in autologous grafts. Since no major clinical effects could be attributed to the bacterial contamination in this study, Rowley and colleagues (1988) suggested that specific antibacterials did not need to be added to the graft. However, they suggested more attention be given to solving this problem considering the profound immunosuppression of the recipient.

A system to categorize the many different techniques used to eliminate marrow disease was proposed by Gross (1990), in the proceedings of the Second International Symposium on Bone Marrow Purging and Processing (1989), and is seen in Table 3.4. Purging methods are designed to take advantage of the structural, biological, and antigenic differences between normal and malignant cells. Theoretically, the more the malignant cell resembles a normal cell the more difficult it could be to design strategies to selectively eliminate it; hence a potential barrier to effective purging of some tumors. Furthermore, if different clones capable of causing disease coexist in the same host, use of only one purging method may be inadequate.

Negative stem cell selection methods are those which rid the marrow of malignant cells, by removal or destruction, presumably leaving normal cells behind. These methods are currently more prevalent. The first category, purging by cytotoxic methods that cause destruction of malignant cells, includes physical, pharmacologic, biophysical, and immunologic means (see Figure

Table 3.4. Negative Selection Purging Techniques Under Development for Removal of Malignant Cells from Marrow Grafts

Ex vivo purging by cytotoxic methods
Biophysical agents
   Photoradiation
   Radioisotopes
Pharmacologic agents
   Activated cyclophosphamides
     (e.g., 4-hydroperoxycyclophosphamide [4-HC])
   Cytosine arabinoside analogues
   Platinols
   Deoxycytidine
   Doxorubicin
   Etoposide (VP-16)
   Verapamil
   Glucocorticoids
   Alkyl-lysophospholipids
Immunologic agents
   Monoclonal antibodies with complement
   Monoclonal antibodies with ricin
   IL-2 leukocyte activated killer cells
   Alpha 2b interferon
Ex vivo purging by elimination
Immunomagnetic microspheres and monoclonal
   antibodies
Immunorosettes
Physical agents
   Counterflow elutriation
   Centrifugation
   Immunoabsorption

3.2). Sometimes multiple methods (for instance multiple monoclonal antibodies) may be used to reduce the chance of allowing resistent or different tumor clones to repopulate the host (Gross 1990).

The second category, purging by elimination of malignant cells from the graft, is accomplished by physically removing malignant cells. Examples of this category include the use of immunomagnetic manipulation of cells with magnetic beads (microspheres), immunorosettes, and physical agents.

Finally, although not officially recognized as a purging method, cryopreservation has been shown to adversely effect leukemia cell recovery

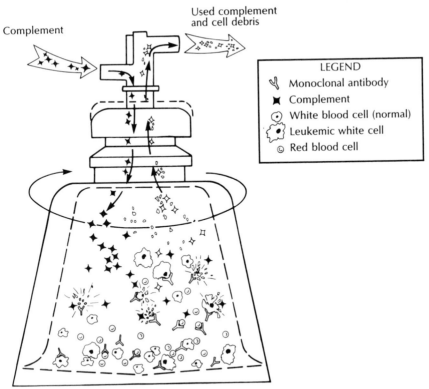

Illustrated by Joan Thompson, Dartmouth Medical School, Photography and Illustration.

Figure 3.2.   Monoclonal antibody treatment is started by mixing monoclonal antibodies, human serum albumin, DNAase, autologous or type-specific packed red cells, and 10 units/ml preservative-free heparin. The mixture is incubated with constant mixing at room temperature for 15 minutes.

over normal stem cells (Allieri et al. 1989; Alessandrino et al. 1989). Cryopreservation may play an unintended but beneficial role in injuring and reducing leukemia cells in autografts. It is possible that this advantageous effect may become systematically tested in future clinical trials.

In contrast to the above, positive stem cell selection methods are those that attempt to return to the host only cells known to be normal (Civin et al. 1990). These cells are first "immunologically" selected from the host and then grown in long-term cultures. One major advantage to this method is that it overcomes the difficulties of needing multiple purging methods to remove the heterogeneous malignant clones that often exist in a single tumor and theoretically may not be removed with a single agent or even combination of agents (Civin et al. 1990).

Despite the safety of the above methods it must be recognized that the success and quality of engraftment following purging may relate more to the amount of patient pretreatment and hence the marrow environment and have little to do with the purging agent or "purger" (Gee 1990).

Patient Conditioning/Antineoplastic Treatment

The goal of pretreatment in autologous transplantation is to treat and cure the cancer without the additional need to immunosuppress the patient. (The latter goal being of prime importance in allogeneic transplants to reduce or prevent host immune cells from attacking the "foreign" donor graft [GVHD] as described in Chapter 2). Although autologous bone marrow transplant allows for higher doses of chemotherapy and radiation therapy to be given, these higher doses are of no value unless they are able to cure the patient.

In solid tumors the pretransplant antineoplastic regimen is designed as a curative treatment since marrow reinfusion is only a rescue from the otherwise prolonged pancytopenia. In hematologic tumors there may be a double challenge; the treatment must eliminate the disease from the patient while another strategy may be employed to rid the potentially cancer-contaminated autologous marrow of malignant cells.

Many drugs have been employed in high doses against the variety of cancers being treated with this modality. It must be remembered that the drugs used must have only hematologic effects as their major dose-limiting toxicity. Table 3.5 lists some drugs that have been used or are being tested in the treatment of solid tumors. Chemotherapy texts or specific studies should be consulted for specific dosage regimens and side effects and toxicities for drugs not discussed in Chapter 2.

In transplant, greater, but reversible, nonfatal toxicities in other non-hematologic organs may be tolerated in an attempt to effect cure. Recognizing this, a toxicity grading scale, unique to transplant (described in Chapter 2), has been proposed that accounts for higher levels of organ toxicity than is typically used by many cooperative research groups to evaluate toxicity in nontransplant protocols (Appelbaum 1987; Bearman et al. 1988). The nurse is a key team member in recognizing and reporting new toxicities of these

Table 3.5. Commonly Used Antineoplastic Drugs Used as Single Agents or in Combinations in Solid Tumor Autologous Transplant

Alkylating agents
  Cyclophosphomide
  Ifosphomide
  Melphalan (L-Pam)
  Mechlorethamine hydrochloride (nitrogen mustard)
  Thiotepa
  4-Hydroperoxycyclophosphamide (4 HC)
  Busulfan
Alkylator-like agents
  Cisplatin
  Carboplatin
Nitrosoureas
  Carmustine (BCNU)
Antitumor antibiotics
  Bleomycin
  Doxorubicin
  Mitomycin C
Plant alkaloids
  Etoposide
  Vincristine
Antimetabolites
  5 Flurouracil
  Methotrexate
Acridinyl aisidide (M-AMSA)

Adapted from Cheson et al. 1989; Antman et al. 1986; Souhami and Peters 1986.

high doses of drugs and must be on the alert for unexpected toxicities as well. All of the possible long-term toxicities including secondary cancers have yet to be identified.

Radiation therapy is sometimes also used in autologous transplants for its antileukemic effect. The role of radiation in solid tumors is unknown but seems to be of benefit in some tumors such as multiple myeloma and lymphoma (Cheson et al. 1989; Gingrich et al. 1990).

Marrow Reinfusion

Frozen marrow is thawed quickly and brought to body temperature in a warm water bath, and reinfused immediately to guarantee the greatest cell viability. The preserving agent, DMSO, causes the patient to experience an immediate garlic taste, and since it is excreted by the lungs, this same odor is obvious in the immediate area of the patient's room. Some patients report a lessened taste if they suck on hard citrus candies or drink flavored beverages during and after the infusion. Taste and odor can persist for 12–24 hours following the infusion and may cause nausea, which is temporary and not very disturbing to most patients. Again, as mentioned in Chapter 2, agencies vary regarding their policies governing whether nurses may administer bone marrow cells. Regardless of who administers these cells, the nurse must be prepared to deal with potential adverse reactions.

Patients rarely experience any adverse effects during marrow reinfusion. One study of marrow reinfusion toxicity (Davis et al. 1990) in a sample of 70 patients identified only nausea and vomiting and headache in a group receiving a density gradient separated graft. In patients receiving buffy coat grafts, additional effects (listed in frequency of occurrence) included flushing, abdominal cramping, dyspnea and chest tightness, diarrhea, pulse and blood pressure changes, and increases in liver function tests. All patients had been hyperhydrated and premedicated with diphenhydramine, mannitol, and hydrocortisone. DMSO, cell damage or products of cell lysis, and large prehydration fluid load have all been implicated in causing these effects.

Single case reports of adverse effects during reinfusion have included anaphylaxis (Macy et al. 1989), adult respiratory distress syndrome (ARDS) (Roy et al. 1989), renal failure (Smith et al. 1987), and cardiopulmonary arrest (Vriesendorp et al. 1984).

Toxicity associated with reinfusion of peripheral blood stem cells has been reported in one study to include fluid overload, pulmonary edema, macroscopic hemaglobinuria, and temporary renal dysfunction (evidenced by a rise in the serum creatinine greater than 2mg/dl within 72 hours of the infusion) (Smith et al. 1989).

Immediate Post-Transfusion Care

Nursing care during the initial post-transfusion period includes careful monitoring of the patient's weight and fluid status as well as continued monitoring for fever or other signs that could indicate a potential transfusion reaction. The latter may be more common following transfusion of marrow treated with immunologic products. Residual foreign proteins and cellular debris can cause a hypersensitivity or anaphylactic response (Macy et al. 1989).

Except for GVHD many of the side effects and toxicities from autologous transplant are similar to those seen in allogeneic transplant and are described in Part II. Where differences exist they are mentioned within the appropriate chapter.

Toxicities unique to the antineoplastic regimens used in solid tumors transplants will continue to be discovered as new agents, higher doses, and new drug combinations are tested in order to develop curative therapies. These toxicities may differ significantly from those commonly seen in allogeneic transplant. Common toxicities experienced in the more standard autologous regimens are included in Part II of the text. Complete information on the wide spectrum of potential toxicities related to all of the specific chemotherapy or radiation regimens currently undergoing dose escalation in clinical trials is beyond the scope of this discussion. This information should be extrapolated from the experimental chemotherapy and radiotherapy literature.

Discharge Planning and Community Follow-Up

With increasing numbers of patients being treated with autologous transplant at specialized referral centers, community follow-up and knowledge of the unique needs of these patients upon discharge is of critical importance. As described in Chapters 2 and 14, a body of knowledge of long-term complications and rehabilitation considerations in bone marrow transplantation is just developing now that allogeneic transplantation approaches its third decade of existence. Increasing attention to cancer patient rehabilitation needs in general is causing a parallel development in rehabilitation programs specifically for cancer survivors (Frymark 1990). This effort is likely to include and benefit the long-term survivor of bone marrow transplant.

Long-term effects and complications of autotransplants are only beginning to be recognized. Many of the currently described/predicted complications have been extrapolated from allogeneic transplant literature (Nims and Strom 1988). This is a new and important area for nursing research as positive results of this treatment modality are reported. Once there is a better understanding of the adverse effects on long term survivors, then specific nursing interventions can be designed to help patients return to previous lifestyles or adapt to treatment-related limitations or disabilities. We owe much to our current, courageous patients who are the pioneers of this future knowledge.

Outcomes of Autologous Bone Marrow Transplant

Relapsed disease is the greatest cause of treatment failure in all the diseases described below. When patients relapse it is difficult to determine if the patient treatment was inadequate or if the marrow was contaminated with disease. As is the case with allogeneic patients whose relapsed leukemia can be determined to be of host origin we know that improvements in preparative regimens need to occur. Improvements in methods to remove disease from marrow were discussed earlier but the more fundamental question is whether marrow contamination with disease is a clinically important cause of disease relapse (Armitage and Gale 1989) and therefore outcome. The following discussion considers outcomes to date of the main diseases currently treated with autologous bone marrow transplant.

Hematologic Malignancies

Acute Myelogenous Leukemia (AML)

Reports of institutional trials (Yeager et al. 1986; Ball et al. 1990; Meloni et al. 1990; Gorin et al. 1990) and reviews have described the outcomes of different treatment programs using autologous transplantation in patients with AML in various stages of disease and compared these results with other therapies, i.e., allogeneic and conventional chemotherapy (Gorin et al. 1990; Burnett 1989; Cheson et al. 1989; Hurd 1987; Linch and Burnett 1986). The summarized results from these reviews demonstrate the following tentative conclusions:

1. relapse rates are comparable to those seen in syngeneic transplant (about 50%) a procedure which also lacks a possible graft-versus-leukemia effect,

2. disease-free survival rates are slightly lower (45–50%) than, but similar to, allogeneic transplant,

3. in some studies autologous transplant has better results than conventional chemotherapy,

4. autologous transplant with purged marrow may be superior to unpurged marrow transplant,

5. outcomes are better when patients are transplanted in earlier remissions, preferably first, rather than in later remissions,

6. patients with French-American-British (FAB) leukemia subtype M4 have a greater risk of relapse and do poorer than patients with other leukemia subtypes; patients with M3 subtype do slightly better, and

7. to date, patients with AML have had better outcomes from autologous transplant than patients with ALL.

Answers to the questions of when to harvest, when to transplant, whether to purge (and with what) still evade current researchers. However, these are the areas undergoing active study, so it is likely that in the near future the outcomes of these studies will hold the recommendations for tomorrow's patients with AML.

Acute Lymphoblastic Leukemia (ALL)

Far fewer patients have undergone autologous transplant for ALL versus AML due to the excellent outcomes achieved in children with both conventional chemotherapy (60–70%) (Poplack and Reaman 1988) and allogeneic transplant (Brochstein et al. 1987). Additionally, fewer adults are diagnosed with the disease.

Long-term survival after autologous transplant for ALL was reported to be uncommon for patients transplanted in relapse and better for patients transplanted in first or subsequent remissions. An overall complete response rate when all patients were combined from 16 different studies was 56% (Cheson et al. 1989). This is encouraging but certainly not a figure synonymous with cure. A recent study reported the following cure rates for autologous transplant in ALL:

1. 41% for standard-risk patients in first complete remission,

2. 17% for high-risk patients in first complete remission, and

3. 10% for patients in second complete remission at a 56-month follow up (Tura and Visani 1989).

In children with ALL who had relapsed or had refractory disease, an event-free survival ranged from 30–50% at five years depending on disease status at transplant (Sallan et al. 1989).

The most common cause of treatment failure following autologous transplant has been relapse (up to 70% reported) from residual disease in the patient (Prentice 1989; Sanders et al. 1989). This is also a common problem following allogeneic transplants especially in those poor risk/prognosis patients who do not develop GVHD (Kersey et al. 1987). It has been suggested that additional treatment following allo- or autotransplant directed at eliminating persistent minimal residual disease is an approach worth pursuing (Bostrom et al. 1990), rather than further manipulation of conditioning regimens.

Chronic Myelogenous Leukemia (CML)

As described earlier, most CML patients can be returned to a chronic phase of disease or even achieve a hematologic remission using intensive chemotherapy and autologous marrow collected during chronic phase. However, most patients experienced only a brief reprise before death from disease occurred (Cheson et al. 1989). New directions in the treatment of CML using interferon may influence a renewed interest in autologous transplant in this disease (Butturini et al. 1990).

Hodgkin's and Non-Hodgkin's Lymphomas

Hodgkin's and non-Hodgkin's lymphomas are among the diseases with the best long-term disease-free survival of all of the cancers treated with autologous transplant. In fact, autologous transplant has been used as first line therapy for some aggressive lymphomas (Tura et al. 1986).

The most significant predictor of long-term disease-free survival for non-Hodgkin's lymphoma has been response to chemotherapy before transplantation (Philip et al. 1987; Takvorian et al. 1987). Additionally, patients transplanted at earlier stages of the disease experience an improved long-term disease-free survival of about 70–80% compared with patients transplanted in more advanced stages (only about a 20% survival) (Armitage and Gale 1989a). Despite the decreased survival rates, patients with advanced stages of the disease have experienced cures with autologous transplant in situations where cures were rare or unlikely with conventional chemotherapy (Armitage and Gale 1989).

Consistent with the results found in the acute leukemias, Cheson and colleagues (1989) reported in a summary of all autologous transplants for non-Hodgkin's lymphoma that relapse of disease was the most common reason for treatment failure rather than drug-related toxicity or failure to respond to therapy.

The results from autologous treatment of Hodgkin's disease are based on more recent trials in fewer patients than have been treated for other lymphomas (Advisory Committee for the International Autologous Bone Marrow Transplant Registry, 1989). In a review summarizing the results of almost 200 patients treated by three different groups, complete response rates were near 50% with a long-term disease-free survival rate of 25–35% (Armitage et al. 1989). Toxic deaths approached 10% and relapse rates were 20–50%. Recommendations for future research based on these results included determining better selection criteria for patients, identification of the role of purging to reduce the relapse rate, and development of strategies to reduce treatment toxicities and mortality (Armitage et al. 1989).

Solid Tumors

As mentioned earlier, according to Frei and colleagues (1989), the goal for the use of autologous bone marrow transplant in solid tumors should be cure, not just minor improvements in relapse-free or overall survival. Although this laudable goal has yet to be achieved, the results of clinical trials have encouraged further development and refinement of this modality for the treatment of solid tumors both in the laboratory and the clinical setting.

Outcomes of the greater than one hundred clinical trials of autologous transplant in solid tumors to date have been extensively reviewed elsewhere (Cheson et al. 1989; Antman et al. 1986; Souhami and Peters 1986) and will not be repeated here. However, some general results and tentative conclusions from these reports are mentioned to give the nurse a general sense of the state of the art and potential future directions of autologous transplant for solid tumors.

Some guiding principles or keys to success that have evolved to improve the cure rates in solid tumors include: treating patients earlier in their disease when drug resistance may be less (Armitage and Gale 1989) or during stages of minimal disease, and use of combinations of agents that will more likely prove superior to single agents (Cheson et al. 1989). It is likely that different regimens will be needed for different tumor types (Cheson et al. 1989). Less certain are the optimal drugs, doses, and schedules that will im-

prove results with acceptable toxicities and the unknown advantage of repeated autologous transplant (so-called double autologous transplant).

To date, although response rates in many solid tumors have been high: 58% in breast (Antman and Gale 1988), 30% in gliomas, 50% in melanoma and colon cancer, and 60% for lung cancer, the responses are brief with patients eventually dying of refractory disease (Cheson et al. 1989). On the bright side, some patients with advanced disease historically refractory to standard therapy have experienced long-term survival (Cheson et al. 1989). As stated by Applebaum (1987), "though progress is slow and difficult, it seems reasonable . . . to keep hammering away" at solid tumors (with the use of autologous transplant).

Future Directions

The use of various biological response modifiers in conjunction with transplantation is one of the most exciting areas currently undergoing investigation. Although their ability to stimulate leukemia cells is not entirely known, these colony stimulating or hematopoietic growth factors (e.g., G-CSF, GM-CSF) are able to stimulate hematopoietic progenitors and speed the recovery of normal peripheral blood cell counts. Colony-stimulating factors may improve patient outcomes by reducing treatment toxicity from pancytopenia (Armitage and Gale 1989; Blazar et al. 1989) or in some situations may replace the need for marrow rescue. Administration of interleukin-2 may contribute to the secretion of cytokines, which have an antileukemic effect (Heslop et al. 1989). Finally, the addition of systemic antimyeloid antibodies to eliminate host or graft-related residual leukemia cells in vivo is under development (Ball personal communication, March 14, 1990).

Variations on the standard transplant procedure to improve outcomes are being investigated in a number of centers. Double sequential transplant is being tested to improve antileukemia efficacy in patients with AML (Meloni et al. 1989a; Gribben et al. 1989a) and in other solid tumors (Beaujean et al. 1989). Two patients with non-Hodgkin's lymphoma treated with autologous bone marrow transplant relapsed and were treated with allogeneic transplant (Schouten et al. 1989). The addition of peripheral blood stem cells to bone marrow derived cells (described earlier in this chapter) may continue to broaden the application of transplantation to more patients. Other novel interpretations of the ways to improve disease-free long-term survival are certainly on the horizon.

Strategies that have been proposed to reduce the current 50% relapse rate following autologous transplant for hematologic malignancies include: continuing development of purging techniques, and inducing GVHD in a controlled way to take advantage of the graft-versus-leukemia effect (Gale and Butturini 1989). It is also likely that clinical trials may be developed to combine autologous therapy with radiation, surgery, and biological response modifiers as adjuvant therapy.

A final pressing concern that can have an impact on many future developments in autologous transplant is whether insurance companies will continue to reimburse these procedures or develop a mechanism to standardize payment practices. This issue is addressed in detail in Chapter 17.

Summary

A great deal of progress has been made in individual diseases and the momentum is building as results from more and more patients are reported. However, autologous transplantation is still in its infancy. Over the next decade it is likely that there will be enough patients with a wide variety of diseases to begin to draw conclusions and further refine therapies. Nurses are at the forefront of these developments. Providing expert clinical care, observing and documenting the effects of new treatment methods, designing complemen-

tary clinical trials to test nursing interventions to have an impact on the high toxicity rate, educating, and acting as patient advocates, are but a few of the ways that nurses can make important contributions to the development of this exciting and promising treatment modality.

References

Abrams R.A. et al. 1980. Result of attempted hematopoietic reconstitution using isologous peripheral blood mononuclear cells: A case report. *Blood 56*: 516.

Advisory Committee of the International Autologous Bone Marrow Transplant Registry (ABMTR), 1986. Bone marrow autotransplants in man: Report of an international cooperative study. *Lancet (Oct 25)*: 960–962.

Advisory Committee of the International Autologous Bone Marrow Transplant Registry (ABMTR). 1989. Autologous bone marrow transplants: Different indications in Europe and North America. *Lancet (Aug 5)*: 317–38.

Ahmed, T. 1990. Autologous marrow transplantation for Hodgkin's disease current techniques and prospects. *Cancer Investigation 8* (1): 99–106.

Alessandrino, E.P. et al. 1989. Cryopreservation of marrow cells for ABMT. Is there any effect on the harvested leukaemic cells? *B.M.T. 4* (suppl. 4): 81–84.

Allieri, M.A. et al. 1989. Intrinsic leukemic progenitor cells' sensitivity to cryopreservation: Incidence for autologous bone marrow transplantation. In Dicke, K.A., et al. (eds.) *Autologous Bone Marrow Transplantation: Proceedings of the Fourth International Symposium 1989*. Houston: University of Texas, M.D. Anderson Cancer Center, pp. 35–39.

Antman, K. et al. 1986. High-dose chemotherapy with bone marrow support for solid tumors. In DeVita, V.T., Jr., et al. (eds.) *Important advances in oncology 1986*. Philadelphia: J.B. Lippincott Co., pp. 221–235.

Antman, K., and Gale, R.P. 1988. Advanced breast cancer: High-dose chemotherapy and bone marrow autotransplants. *Annu. Intern. Med. 108*: 570–574.

Appelbaum, F.R. 1987. Hammering away at solid tumors (editorial). *Cancer Treatment Reports 71* (2): 115–117.

Appelbaum, F.R. et al. 1989. Timing of bone marrow transplantation for adults with acute nonlymphocytic leukemia. In Dicke, K.A. et al. (eds.) *Autologous Bone Marrow Transplantation: Proceedings of the Fourth International Symposium 1989*. Houston: University of Texas, M.D. Anderson Cancer Center, pp. 21–26.

Areman, E.M. et al. 1990. Cryopreservation and storage of human bone marrow: A survey of current practices. In Gross, S., et al. (eds.) *Bone Marrow Purging and Processing*. NY: Alan R. Liss, Inc., pp. 523–529.

Armitage, J.O., and Gale, R.P. 1989. Bone marrow autotransplantation. *Am. J. Med. 86:* 203–206.

Armitage, J.O. et al. 1989. Bone marrow transplantation in the treatment of Hodgkin's lymphoma: Problems, remaining challenges, and future prospects. *Recent Results in Cancer Research 117:* 246–253.

Ball, E.D. et al. 1990. Autologous bone marrow transplantation for acute myeloid leukemia: Using monoclonal antibody-purged bone marrow. *Blood 75 (5):* 1199–1206.

Bearman, S.I. et al. 1988. Regimen-related toxicity in patients undergoing bone marrow transplantation. *J. Clin. Oncol. 6* (10): 1562–1568.

Beaujean, F. et al. 1989. Hemopoietic reconstitution after repeated autologous transplantation with mafosfamide-purged marrow. *B.M.T. 4 (5):* 537–541.

Blazar, B.R. et al. 1989. In vivo administration of recombinant human granulocyte/macrophage colony-stimulating factor in acute lymphoblastic leukemia patients receiving purged autografts. *Blood 73 (3):* 849–857.

Bostrom, B. et al. 1990. Bone marrow transplantation for advanced acute leukemia: A pilot study of high-energy total body irradiation, cyclophosphamide and continuous infusion etoposide. *B.M.T. 5:* 83–89.

Brochstein, J.A. et al. 1987. Allogeneic bone marrow transplantation after hyperfractionated total body irradiation and cyclophosphamide in children with acute leukemia. *N. Engl. J. Med. 317:* 1618–1624.

Burnett, A.K. 1989. Autologous BMT for AML without purging. *B.M.T. 4 (3):* 76–78.

Butturini, A. et al. 1990. Autotransplants in chronic myelogenous leukemia: Strategies and results. *Lancet 335* (May 26): 1255–1259.

Cheson, B.D. et al. 1989. Autologous bone marrow transplantation: Current status and future directions. *Annu. Int. Med. 110* (1): 51–65.

Civin, C.I. et al. 1990. Positive stem cell selection—Basic science . . . In Gross, S., et al. (eds.) *Bone Marrow Purging and Processing.* NY: Alan R. Liss, Inc., pp. 387–402.

Cogliano-Shutta, N.A., Broda, E.J., and Gress, J.S. 1985. Bone marrow transplantation: An overview and comparison of autologous, syngeneic, and allogeneic treatment modalities. *Nur. Clin. North Am. 20* (1): 49–66.

Davis, J. et al. 1990. Toxicity of autologous bone marrow graft infusion. In Gross, S., et al. (eds.) *Bone Marrow Purging and Processing.* NY: Alan R. Liss, Inc., pp. 531–540.

Deeg, H.J. et al. 1988. *A Guide to Bone Marrow Transplantation.* N.Y.: Springer-Verlag. p. 22.

Dicke, K.A. et al. 1989. Does high-dose intensification with autologous bone marrow rescue contribute to long-term disease-free survival in acute myelogenous leukemia in first remission? In Dicke, K.A. et al. (eds.) *Autologous Bone Marrow Transplantation: Proceedings of the Fourth International Symposium 1989.* Houston: University of Texas, M.D. Anderson Cancer Center, pp. 3–12.

Dicke, K.A., and Spinolo, J.A. 1989. High dose therapy and autologous bone marrow transplant (ABMT) in acute leukemia: Is purging necessary? *B.M.T. 4* (Suppl. 1): 184–186.

Frei III, E. et al. 1989. Bone marrow autotransplantation for solid tumors—Prospects. *J. Clin. Oncol. 7* (4): 515–526.

Frymark, S. 1990. Cancer rehabilitation in the outpatient setting. *Oncology Issues: The Journal of Cancer Program Management 5* (1): 12–17.

Gale, R.P., and Butturini, A. 1989. Autotransplants in leukaemia. *Lancet* (Aug 5): 315–317.

Gee, A.P. 1990. Bone marrow purging and processing: A review of ancillary effects. In Gross, S., et al. (eds.) *Bone Marrow Purging and Processing.* NY: Alan R. Liss, Inc., pp. 507–522.

Gianni, A.M. et al. 1989. Rapid and complete hemopoietic reconstitution following combined transplantation of autologous blood and bone marrow cells. A changing role for high-dose chemo radiotherapy? *Hematological Oncology 7:* 139–148.

Gingrich, R.D. et al. 1990. BVAC ablative chemotherapy followed by autologous bone marrow transplantation for patients with advanced lymphoma. *Blood 75* (12): 2276–2281.

Goldman, J.M. et al. 1981. Buffy coat autografts for patients with chronic granulocytic leukemia in transformation. *Blut 42:* 149.

Gorin, N.C. 1986. Autologous bone marrow transplantation in acute leukemia. *J.N.C.I. 76* (6): 1281–1287.

Gorin, N.C. et al. 1990. Autologous bone marrow transplantation for acute myelocytic leukemia in first remission: A European survey of the role of marrow purging. *Blood 75* (8): 1606–1614.

Gress, R.E. 1990. Purged autologous bone marrow transplantation in the treatment of acute leukemia. *Oncology 4* (8): 35–47.

Gribben, J.G. et al. 1989a. Double autologous bone marrow transplantation in acute myeloid leukaemia. *B.M.T. 4* (suppl. 1): 209–211.

Gribben, J.G. et al. 1989b. Successful treatment of refractory Hodgkin's disease by high-dose combination chemotherapy and autologous bone marrow transplantation. *Blood 73* (1): 340–344.

Gross, S. 1990. Perspectives in marrow purging. In Gross, S., et al. (eds.) *Bone Marrow Purging and Processing.* NY: Alan R. Liss, Inc., pp. xxix–xxxiv.

Hershko, C. et al. 1979. Cure of aplastic anemia in paroxysmal nocturnal haemoglobinuria by marrow transfusion from identical twin: Failure of peripheral-leucocyte transfusion to correct marrow aplasia. *Lancet 1 :* 945.

Heslop, H.E. et al. 1989. In vivo induction of gamma interferon and tumor necrosis factor by interleukin-2 infusion following intensive chemotherapy or autologous marrow transplantation. *Blood 74* (4): 1374–1380.

Hubbard, Susan. October 20, 1989. Personal communication.

Hurd, D. 1987. Allogeneic and autologous bone marrow transplantation for acute nonlymphocytic leukemia. *Seminars in Oncology* 14 (4): 407–415.

Hurd, D. et al. 1988. Autologous bone marrow transplantation in non-Hodgkin's lymphoma: Monoclonal antibodies plus complement for ex vivo marrow treatment. *Am. J. Med.* 85: 829–834.

Jagannath, S. et al. 1989. Prognostic factors for response and survival after high-dose cyclophosphamide, carmustine, and etoposide with autologous bone marrow transplantation for relapsed Hodgkin's disease. *J. Clin. Oncol.* 7 (2): 179–185.

Juttner, C.A. et al. 1988. Early lympho-haemopoietic recovery after autografting using peripheral blood stem cells in acute non-lymphoblastic leukaemia. *Transplant Proc.* 20: 40–43.

Juttner, C.A. et al. 1990. Peripheral blood stem cell selection, collection and autotransplantation. In Gross, S. et al. (eds.) *Bone Marrow Purging and Processing.* NY: Alan R. Liss, Inc., pp. 447–460.

Kelleher, J., and Jennings, M. 1988. Nursing management of a marrow transplant unit: A framework for practice. *Seminars in Oncology Nursing* 4 (1): 60–68.

Kersey, J.H. et al. 1987. Comparison of autologous and allogeneic bone marrow transplantation for treatment of high-risk refractory acute lymphoblastic leukemia. *N. Engl. J. Med.* 317 (8): 461–467.

Kessinger, A. et al. 1986. Reconstitution of human hematopoietic function with autologous cryopreserved circulating stem cells. *Exp. Hematol.* 14: 192–196.

Kessinger, A. et al. 1989a. High-dose therapy and autologous periperal blood stem cell transplantation for patients with lymphoma. *Blood* 74 (4): 1260–1265.

Kessinger, A. et al. 1989b. Allogeneic transplantation of blood-derived, T cell-depleted hemopoietic stem cells after myeloablative treatment in a patient with acute lymphoblastic leukemia. *B.M.T.* 4: 643–646.

Lasky, L.C. 1989. Hematopoietic reconstitution using progenitors recovered from blood. *Transfusion* 29 (6): 552–557.

Leach, Miram. Feb. 2, 1990. Personal communication.

Lesko, L.M. et al. 1989. Patients', parents', and oncologists' perceptions of informed consent for bone marrow transplantation. *Med. and Pediat. Oncol.* 17: 181–187.

Linch, D.C., and Burnett, A.K. 1986. Clinical studies of ABMT in acute myeloid leukaemia. *Clinics in Haematology* 15 (1): 167–186.

Macy, E. et al. 1989. Anaphylaxis to infusion of autologous bone marrow: An apparent reaction to self, mediated by IgE antibody to bovine serum albumin. *J. Allergy Clin. Immunol.* 83 (5): 871–875.

Marcus, R.E., and Goldman, J.M. 1986. Autografting in chronic granulocytic leukaemia. *Clinics in Haematology* 15 (1): 235–247.

McCarthy, D.M., and Goldman, J.M. 1984. Transfusion of circulating stem cells. *C.R.C. Crit. Rev. Clin. Lab. Sci.* 20 (1): 1–24.

Meloni G. et al. 1985. Cryopreserved autologous bone marrow infusion following high-dose chemotherapy in patients with acute myeloblastic leukemia in first relapse. *Leukemia Research* 9: 407–412.

Meloni, G. et al. 1989a. Acute myelogenous leukemia in first relapse treated with two consecutive autologous bone marrow transplantations: A pilot study. *Eur. J. Haematol.* 42: 441–444.

Meloni G. et al. 1989b. Autologous bone marrow or peripheral blood stem cell transplantation for patients with chronic myelogenous leukaemia in chronic phase. *B.M.T.* 4 (suppl. 4): 92–94.

Meloni, G. et al. 1990. BAVC regimen and autologous bone marrow transplantation in patients with acute myelogenous leukemia in second remission. *Blood* 75 (12): 2282–2285.

Nims, J., and Strom, S. 1988. Late complications of bone marrow transplant recipients: Nursing issues. *Seminars in Oncology Nursing* 4 (1): 47–54.

Philip, T. et al. 1987. High dose therapy in autologous bone marrow transplantation after failure of conventional chemotherapy in adults with intermediate grade or high grade non-Hodgkin's lymphoma. *N. Engl. J. Med.* 316: 1493–1498.

Poplack, D.G., and Reaman, G. 1988. Acute lymphoblastic leukemia in childhood. *Pediat. Clin. North Am.* 35 (4): 903–932.

Prentice, H.G. 1989. ABMT versus chemotherapy in high risk acute lymphoblastic leukemia. In Dicke, K.A., et al. (eds.) *Autologous Bone Marrow Transplantation: Proceedings of the Fourth International Symposium 1989* Houston: Univ. of Texas, M.D. Anderson Cancer Center, pp. 139–144.

Reiffers, J. et al. 1986. Successful autologous transplantation with peripheral blood hemopoietic cells in a patient with acute leukemia. *Exp. Hematol.* 14: 312–315.

Rowley, S.D. et al. 1988. Bacterial contamination of bone marrow grafts intended for autologous and allogeneic bone marrow transplantation: Incidence and clinical significance. *Transfusion* 28 (2): 109–112.

Rowley, S.D. et al. 1989. Efficacy of ex vivo purging for autologous bone marrow transplantation in the treatment of acute nonlymphoblastic leukemia. *Blood* 74 (1): 501–506.

Roy, V. et al. 1989. Adult respiratory syndrome following autologous bone marrow transfusion. *B.M.T.* 4: 711–712.

Sallan, S.E. et al. 1989. Autologous bone marrow transplantation for acute lymphoblastic leukemia. *J. Clin. Oncol.* 7 (11): 1594–1601.

Sanders, J.E. et al. 1989. Autologous marrow transplant experience for acute lymphoblastic leukemia. In Dicke, K.A., et al. (eds.) *Autologous Bone Marrow Transplantation: Proceedings of the Fourth International Symposium 1989.* Houston: Univ. of Texas, M.D. Anderson Cancer Center, pp. 155–160.

Santos, G.W. 1985. Overview of autologous bone marrow transplantation (ABMT). *Int. J. Cell Cloning* 3: 215–216.

Schouten, H.C. et al. 1989. Allogenic bone marrow transplantation in patients with lymphoma relapsing after autologous marrow transplantation. *B.M.T. 4* (1): 119–121.

Schryber, S., Lacasse, C. R., and Barton-Burke, M. 1987. Autologous bone marrow transplantation. *O.N.F. 14* (4): 74–80.

Sharp, J.G. et al. 1989a. Are occult tumor cells present in peripheral stem cell harvests of candidates for autologous transplantation? In Dicke, K.A., et al. (eds.) *Autologous Bone Marrow Transplantation: Proceedings of the Fourth International Symposium 1989*. Houston: University of Texas, M.D. Anderson Cancer Center, pp. 693–696.

Sharp, J.G. et al. 1989b. Recent progress in the detection of metastatic tumor in bone marrow by culture techniques. In Dicke, K.A., et al. (eds.) *Autologous Bone Marrow Transplantation: Proceedings of the Fourth International Symposium 1989*. Houston: University of Texas, M.D. Anderson Cancer Center, pp. 421–425.

Shea, T.C. et al. 1989. A phase I clinical and pharmacokinetic study of carboplatin and autologous bone marrow support. *J. Clin. Oncol. 7* (5): 651–661.

Smith, D.M. et al. 1987. Acute renal failure associated with autologous bone marrow transplantation. *B.M.T. 2*: 195–201.

Smith, D.M. et al. 1989. Peripheral blood stem cell collection and toxicity. In Dicke, K.A., et al. (eds.) *Autologous Bone Marrow Transplantation: Proceedings of the Fourth International Symposium 1989*. Houston: University of Texas, M.D. Anderson Cancer Center. pp. 697–701.

Souhami, R., and Peters, W. 1986. High dose chemotherapy in solid tumours in adults. *Clinics in Haematology 15* (1): 219–233.

Spinolo, J.A. et al. 1989. High-dose combination chemotherapy with cyclophosphamide, carmustine, etoposide, and autologous bone marrow transplantation in 60 patients with relapsed Hodgkin's disease: The M.D. Anderson Experience. *Recent Results in Cancer Research 117*: 233–238.

Takvorian, T. et al. 1987. Prolonged disease-free survival after autologous bone marrow transplantation in patients with non-Hodgkin's lymphomas with poor prognosis. *N. Engl. J. Med. 316*: 1499–1505.

Tura, S. et al. 1986. High dose therapy followed by autologous bone marrow transplantation (ABMT) in previously untreated non-Hodgkin's lymphoma. *Scand. J. Hematology 37*: 347.

Tura, S., and Visani, G. 1989. Long term survivors in adult acute lymphoblastic leukemia. *B.M.T. 4* (suppl. 1): 104–105.

Vriesendorp, R. et al. 1984. Effective high-dose chemotherapy with autologous bone marrow transplantation in resistant ovarian cancer. *Gyn. Oncol. 17*: 271–276.

Williams et al. 1990. Peripheral blood-derived stem cell collections for use in autologous transplantation after high dose chemotherapy: An alternative approach. In Gross, S. et al. (eds.) *Bone Marrow Purging and Processing*. NY: Alan R. Liss, Inc., pp. 461–469.

Yeager, A. et al. 1986. Autologous bone marrow transplantation in patients with acute nonlymphocytic leukemia: A phase II study of ex vivo marrow treatment with 4-hydroperoxycyclophosphamide. *N. Engl. J. Med. 315*: 141–147.

Chapter 4

Perspectives on Pediatric Bone Marrow Transplantation

Linda Z. Abramovitz

Introduction

Over the last several decades, bone marrow transplantation has become an accepted treatment modality for many diseases and disorders of childhood. Infants, children, and adolescents account for approximately one half of the transplants performed (Wiley and House 1988). Although there are many similarities between pediatric and adult bone marrow transplantation, several aspects of physical and psychosocial care differ. For this reason, a chapter has been devoted to the unique needs of the pediatric bone marrow transplant patient.

This chapter provides an overview of bone marrow transplant from a pediatric perspective. Major emphasis will be placed on the nursing management of the physiological and psychological needs of the child/family during the various phases of the transplant process.

Clinical Indications

Clinical indications for bone marrow transplantation in children include a wide range of diseases and disorders. Potential bone marrow transplant recipients include infants, children, and adolescents with congenital and acquired disorders as well as hematological malignancies and solid tumors (see Table 4.1).

Nonmalignant Disorders

The goal of transplanting a child with a hematological disease such as aplastic anemia, thalassemia, or Fanconi's anemia is to replace the defective or nonfunctioning marrow with normal stem cells that will differentiate into erythroid, myeloid, lymphoid, and megakarocytic cell lines. Thalassemia major is an inherited disorder which is characterized by abnormal hemoglobin synthe-

Table 4.1. Childhood Diseases Treated by Marrow Transplantation

Malignant	Nonmalignant
Acute lymphocytic leukemia (ALL)	Hematologic
	Aplastic anemia
Acute nonlymphocytic leukemia (ANLL)	Fanconi anemia
	Diamond-Blackfan syndrome
Chronic myelogenous leukemia (CML)	Thalassemia major
Neuroblastoma (Stage IV)	Genetic
	Osteopetrosis
Lymphoma	Mucopolysac-
Other solid tumors	charidoses
	Lesch-Nyhan syndrome
	Severe combined immunodeficiency (SCID)
	Wiskott-Aldrich syndrome

sis and red blood cell structure (Smith 1972). Children with the severest form of this congenital disease require chronic transfusions to prevent anemia and chelation therapy to minimize iron overload (Nuscher et al. 1984). In young children with thalassemia major, bone marrow transplantation is a promising treatment offering a 75% chance of disease-free survival at two years (Lucarelli 1990).

Aplastic anemia can be congenital or acquired and is characterized by a failure of the bone marrow to produce red blood cells, white blood cells, and platelets. This state of pancytopenia can be associated with high morbidity and mortality (Bayever 1984). As with adults, bone marrow transplantation is the treatment of choice in children with an HLA-matched sibling donor when compared to other approaches such as androgen therapy, antithymocyte globulin (ATG), and supportive care. Long-term survival based on transfusion status prior to the transplant is 83% (untransfused) and 65% (transfused), with an overall survival rate of 70% (Sanders et al. 1986a). There

are other rare congenital anemias, including Diamond-Blackfan syndrome and Fanconi's anemia, for which bone marrow transplantation has been used with varying degrees of success (O'Reilly et al. 1984).

In infants and children with congenital immunodeficiencies, the purpose of a bone marrow transplant is to restore normal lymphocyte function. Severe combined immunodeficiency (SCID) is characterized by the complete absence of cell-mediated (T cell) and antibody-mediated (B cell) immunity (Fonger 1987). The majority of cases are inherited either as an autosomal recessive disease or an X-linked disease. Adenosine deaminase (ADA) deficiency is seen in 50% of the patients with the autosomal recessive inheritance form of SCID.

Following birth, infants with immunodeficiency (SCID) have frequent bacterial, fungal, and viral infections. Clinical presentation typically includes recurrent infections, chronic diarrhea, otitis media, pneumonia, and oral thrush. Graft-versus-host disease (GVHD) due to maternal T lymphocytes that cross the placenta and enter the fetal circulation is a rare complication. Early diagnosis and treatment are critical to prevent life threatening infections. Even with the best supportive care, SCID is usually fatal within the first few years of life.

Bone marrow transplantation is the treatment of choice for an infant with SCID. The overall success of an allogeneic transplant from an HLA-matched sibling is 65% (Ammann and Hong 1980). In situations where there are no sibling donors, a parent's bone marrow can be processed to remove immunocompetent T lymphocytes. The success of transplantation using haplocompatible soybean lectin T cell-depleted marrow is 70% (Cowan et al. 1985).

Wiskott-Aldrich syndrome is an X-linked recessive immunodeficiency that is characterized by recurrent infections, eczema, and thrombocytopenia (Standen 1988). The underlying pathology of the syndrome involves a defect in the child's cellular immunity. Infants typically present within the first six months of life with petechiae or a significant bleeding episode. Similar to patients with severe combined immunodeficiency, these infants are susceptible to life-threatening opportunistic infections. Bone marrow transplant is recommended in cases where there is an HLA-matched sibling donor. Engraftment of both megakarocytes and lymphoid cells of donor origin offers a 90% cure rate (Parkman 1986b).

Children with inborn errors of metabolism are another group of patients that can benefit from a bone marrow transplant (O'Reilly et al. 1984). Derived from hematopoietic origin, tissue macrophages, including osteoclasts, Kupffer's cells, Langerhans cells, and alveolar macrophages are absent in some genetic diseases. Examples of inborn errors include osteopetrosis which is marked by abnormal osteoclast activity and Gaucher's disease where there is undegraded glucocerebroside in tissue macrophages. Disorders of mucopolysaccharide metabolism, such as Hurler's, Hunter's, Sanfilippo B, and Maroteaux-Lamy syndromes are also treated with bone marrow transplantation (Parkman 1986b). In these patients the goal of bone marrow transplantation is to restore normal hematopoietic cells and correct the metabolic defect.

As a child with mucopolysaccharidosis gets older, the central nervous system is affected. Once brain damage occurs it is not reversible. However, bone marrow transplantation may curtail further central nervous system involvement, if performed soon after diagnosis. There are still many unknowns regarding how these diseases affect the central nervous system and the impact of transplantation.

Malignant Disorders

Cancer is the most common cause of death by disease in children (Cancer Statistics 1990). Currently, 60–70% of children are cured of their malignancy (Odom 1989). The use of bone marrow transplantation as a treatment modality has made

a significant impact on long-term survival. Children with acute and chronic leukemias, lymphoma, neuroblastoma, and other solid malignancies have been successfully treated with bone marrow transplantation (Parkman 1986b). The aggressive conditioning regimen used prior to bone marrow transplantation is designed to destroy any residual malignant cells. The transplant itself is viewed as a "rescue" to restore normal hematopoietic and immunological function (Trigg 1988).

Leukemia is the most common childhood cancer, accounting for approximately one third of all malignancies seen in children (Neglia and Robison 1988). Acute lymphocytic leukemia (ALL) is the most common form of childhood leukemia and occurs in approximately 80% of the cases (Diamond and Matthay 1988). Acute nonlymphocytic leukemia (ANLL), most often seen in the adult population, accounts for another 20% of childhood leukemias (Kalwinsky et al. 1988). The chronic leukemias of both adult and juvenile forms are very rare in children, accounting for less than 5% of cases (Altman 1989).

The overall disease-free survival rate for children with newly diagnosed ALL is 60–70% (Coccia et al. 1988; Poplack and Reaman 1988; Wiley and Whalley 1983). In current practice, bone marrow transplantation is most often indicated for children with ALL who relapse, achieve a second remission, and have an HLA-identical sibling (Trigg 1988). Comparative clinical trials looking at conventional chemotherapy versus allogeneic bone marrow transplantation for patients in second remission have revealed that bone marrow transplantation offers a 30–40% disease-free survival rate compared to less than 10% with standard chemotherapy (Coccia et al. 1988). Another approach to patients without a matched sibling donor is to use an autologous monoclonal antibody-purged marrow; however, there is a significantly higher relapse rate in this group compared to allogeneic transplant (Ramsay 1989).

There is controversy surrounding the use of conventional chemotherapy versus bone marrow transplant in children with acute nonlymphocytic leukemia (Trigg 1988). Although there are intensive chemotherapy regimens that appear to be quite effective, bone marrow transplantation is still considered to be the treatment of choice in patients with a matched sibling donor (Dahl 1990). In first remission, children with ANLL who receive a bone marrow transplant from an HLA-matched sibling donor can have a 40–70% chance of long-term disease-free survival (Dahl 1990; Sanders et al. 1985). Further clinical studies are in progress to compare conventional chemotherapy with bone marrow transplantation (Trigg 1988). For patients without a matched sibling donor, autologous bone marrow purged with 4-hydroperoxycyclophosphamide (4-HC) or monoceonal antibodies has been shown to be quite successful in adult patients with ANLL in second and third remission (Yeager 1986; Ball et al. 1990). This treatment may hold promise for children in first remission with this disease.

The ideal donor for bone marrow transplantation is an HLA-matched sibling; although, parental haplocompatible transplants can be performed with T cell depletion of the marrow using a variety of methods including soybean lectin separation or a combination of monoclonal antibodies. The use of unrelated matched donors through the National Marrow Donor Program is yet another option. The risk of relapse while awaiting a suitable donor is a real problem, since the ideal time to perform the transplant is immediately after the child achieves a complete remission and the risk of relapse increases with time.

Chronic leukemia rarely occurs in childhood and much of what is known is derived from the adult population. Accounting for less than 5% of all leukemias seen in children, the adult (Philadelphia chromosome positive) and the juvenile form of chronic myelogenous leukemia (CML) are unfortunately not responsive to chemotherapy (Trigg 1988). Allogeneic bone marrow transplant offers a 60–75% long-term disease-free survival rate when the adult form of CML is transplanted in chronic phase (Trigg 1988).

Neuroblastoma is a childhood cancer that has been shown to respond to bone marrow transplantation. This tumor of the sympathetic nervous system accounts for 8% of pediatric malignancies and is staged based on size and metastases. Although the disease may rarely be seen in the adolescent and in adults, the median age at diagnosis is two years (Kushner and Cheung 1988). There are several prognostic factors that may be used to distinguish high risk patients, including serum neuron specific enolase (NSE) > 100ng/ml, serum ferritin >140 ng/ml, histopathology, and multiple N-*myc* oncogene copy number in primary tumor (Kushner and Cheung 1988). Children with Stage IV neuroblastoma and patients with Stage II or III with poor prognostic features may benefit from high-dose chemoradiotherapy followed by autologous bone marrow transplantation to cure their disease (Seeger et al. 1988). Without transplantation, these patients have a very poor outcome with long-term survival calculated at less than 10% (Seeger et al. 1988). An allogeneic transplant may be performed if there is an HLA-matched sibling; otherwise, marrow is harvested from the patient. The autologous marrow may then be treated to remove residual disease. One purging method uses anti-neuroblastoma monoclonal antibodies that are attached to magnetic beads. The treated marrow is then run through a series of magnets to remove any residual neuroblastoma cells prior to infusion (Seeger et al. 1988). Two-year disease-free survival for those children receiving an allogeneic or purged autologous bone marrow transplant is approximately 50% (Seeger et al. 1988).

Children with both Hodgkin's and non-Hodgkin's lymphoma have also achieved complete remissions and long-term disease-free survival following allogeneic or autologous bone marrow transplantation (Ramsay 1989). In addition, children with rhabdomyosarcoma, Ewing's sarcoma, brain tumors, retinoblastoma, Wilm's tumors, and other solid pediatric malignancies, have shown some benefit from a bone marrow transplant (Lenarsky and Feig 1983; Spitzer et al.

1984). These tumors are extremely chemosensitive and respond well to high doses of chemotherapy followed by an autologous marrow rescue (Pinkerton et al. 1986).

The disease, age of the patient, and type of transplant (allogeneic, autologous, unrelated) are variables that affect the outcome of the transplant. Although there are some similarities related to disease and type of transplant in both the pediatric and adult population, children appear to have better tolerance for the procedure and a better outcome than do older patients. The incidence of graft-versus-host disease is less in younger patients, as are the effects of chemotherapy and radiation on organ tissue (Shannon et al. 1987).

In summary, bone marrow transplantation is the treatment of choice for many immunological deficiency diseases of childhood and offers a reasonable chance of cure for several childhood cancers. Considered "experimental" or "investigational" in certain situations, overall, there is a postive outlook towards the application of bone marrow transplantation in the treatment of childhood diseases.

Issues During the Pretransplant Period

Decision Making/Informed Consent

The decision to proceed with a bone marrow transplant is never taken lightly. Both the bone marrow transplant team and the child/family must be comfortable with all aspects of the decision.

From the transplant team's perspective, a thorough evaluation of the child must be completed to ensure that the child is a good candidate for a bone marrow transplant. A variety of tests are performed to evaluate cardiac, pulmonary, neurological, hepatic, and renal function, as well as infectious disease status. Another important aspect of the bone marrow transplant team's evaluation is a detailed psychosocial history. A social worker or psychologist typically interviews the child/parents to gather information about family structure and dynamics, in order to evaluate their ability to deal with the stresses of a bone marrow transplant.

The health care team must provide detailed information about all aspects of the transplant. Informed consent can occur only when a parent or child is given adequate information upon which to make a decision (Davis and Aroskar 1983). There should be ample time for parents to discuss issues with members of the health care team and to have all of their questions and concerns addressed. Written information, and taping of family and informed consent conferences can be very helpful and should be available to all families. Copies of the consent forms for both the patient and the donor outlining risks and benefits should be given to the family to review before signing. Some transplant centers have a specific videotape that discusses all aspects of bone marrow transplantation including the decision to proceed.

It is important to provide concrete information that can be read, watched, or listened to several times and shared with other members of the family. Whenever possible, written materials should be in the patient's/parents' primary language. In addition, parents may be offered the name and phone number of another family whose child has gone through a transplant. The responsibility of the health care team at this point is to help the parents make as an informed decision as possible. Even with this knowledge, the ultimate choice of proceeding with a tranplant is never easy.

There are several elements that factor into the decision-making process. The level of stress, age of the parents, family constellation, cultural background, language, and religious/spiritul concerns can all affect how the information is given to a particular family and how it is processed. Young and uneducated parents may need more assistance and review of the information. Increased anxiety and stress surrounding the prospect of a bone marrow transplant often prevents families from hearing and comprehending much of what is discussed; therefore, members of the transplant team should reiterate the information several times. Language barriers must be overcome with exhaustive use of interpreters and other individuals who are knowledgeable about the patient/family culture. In many societies, the parents' view of Western medicine as well as the child's sex and position in the family are very important and can influence the family's decision.

Of great concern to most parents is not only the welfare of the patient but of a sibling donor (Wiley et al. 1984). While the risk of marrow donation is minimal; much attention is focused on protecting donors who are minors. A conflict of interest can arise when parents give informed consent for the recipient and donor who are both minors (Serota et al. 1981). General anesthesia, bleeding, infection, and postoperative pain are potential risks to the donor but to date, there have been no pediatric donor deaths reported (Bortin and Buckner 1983). In fact, pediatric donors tolerate the procedure extremely well and are often playing only hours after the harvest (Lenarsky and Feig 1983).

Parents want to be assured that the risks are kept at a minimum and frequently request such things as the availability of designated donor blood in case a transfusion is needed following the harvest. Some families prefer one sibling to be used instead of another. Most parents will proceed with the transplant by weighing the minimal risk to the donor against the great potential benefit to the recipient (Levine et al. 1975).

All pediatric donors must be adequately informed and prepared. In some states a guardian ad litem is appointed by the court to represent the interests of the pediatric donor (Levine et al. 1975). This guardian evaluates the donor and signs the consent forms on behalf of the child. In other states, a child advocate is appointed to protect the rights of a donor who is a minor (Serota et al. 1981).

If possible, both parents should be present during informational sessions and informed consent meetings to assure that they are hearing the same facts and are in agreement with the decision. Increasingly, the bone marrow transplant team must deal with nontraditional (divorce, single parent) families. In single parent situations, the parent with the custody of the child is responsible for making the final decision and signing the consent forms. If the other parent is involved with the child, an attempt should be made to meet with that parent and provide him/her with information about the transplant before the decision is made. In cases of joint custody or multiple parents due to remarriage, an effort is made to have a single consent conference with everyone present. Typically, bad feelings are put aside and the focus is on the best interest of the child. A visitation schedule should be discussed. The visitation schedule is important since it will provide the child with concrete expectations.

Depending on the child's age, he/she may or may not be involved in the transplant consent process. Infants, toddlers, and preschoolers do not have the ability to understand the implications of a bone marrow transplant. On the other hand, older school-age children and adolescents must be a part of the consent process. For a child who is intellectually seven years of age or older, assent (agreement to participate) must be obtained from the child according to guidelines established by the American Academy of Pediatrics (Fochtman et al. 1982). In addition to being a part of the informed consent and other family conferences, older pediatric patients should have the opportunity without the parent present to discuss any issues or ask questions that may be of concern. Most children want to protect their parents and may be uncomfortable talking in front of their parent about changes in body image, sexuality, and concerns about death. Direct and open dialogue must be encouraged between the child and parents and may need to be facilitated by members of the team.

During the decision-making process, the health care team may be forced to face ethical, moral, and legal dilemmas. For example, the parents must be able to provide adequate physical care for the child in the post-transplant period at home. Administering medications correctly, knowing who and when to call in case of emergency, and maintaining adequate isolation precautions until the child's immunity returns, are important aspects of care. In extreme situations, foster care may need to be considered during the medically vulnerable post-transplant period. Based on information gathered about a particular family, all concerns must be addressed prior to initiating a transplant. In difficult cases or if there is disagreement among team members, a medical ethicist/ethics committee can be consulted.

When presented with the alternatives of transplant or conventional therapy, parents may feel that there is no good choice. There is no right or wrong decision and most parents feel that they must go ahead with the transplant if there is a chance that their child may be cured. If a family elects to proceed with another form of conventional or investigational therapy rather than a bone marrow transplant, the bone marrow transplant team must ultimately support the family's final decision.

Despite the outcome of the transplant, parents must look back on this decision as the best decision they could have made based on all the information and facts available at that time. The nurse's role during this period of time is that of educator and supporter. Helping the family understand all aspects of the transplantation process and preparing the family for admission to the bone marrow transplant unit is of critical importance. Frequently the nurse feels a certain bonding with the family during this initial pretransplant phase. The opportunity to become acquainted with the child and family prior to admission into the hospital when possible assists the nurse in developing an individualized plan of care.

Preparation for Bone Marrow Transplant

Preparing the pediatric patient for all aspects of the transplantation process including pretransplant tests, catheter placement, bone marrow harvest (in the case of autologous transplant), isolation, treatment regimen, and side effects can be very challenging. The type of preparation will vary based on the child's age, previous experience, and intellectual capacities. Parental support is critical during the preparative phase. Along with the parent, the child life specialist, the nursing staff, and/or social worker are key team members in the task of preparing the child.

Preparation for the Transplant Workup

Although most of the pretransplant workup is noninvasive, it can be frightening and overwhelming for the child and the parent. Some of the tests may be familiar to the child and others may present a new experience. To decrease parental anxiety, all parents benefit from a thorough explanation of the test/procedure in both a written and visual format (Ronan and Caserza 1988). This provides parents with information to assist in the preparation of their child.

Preparation of the infant involves adequately preparing the parents and utilizing the parents to comfort the infant through the test or procedure. Infants may need to be sedated or restrained for some tests. Parents need to be forewarned if the child will need to be NPO prior to a test and if they will need to cope with a hungry baby. In this age group, emphasis is placed on the important role of the parent's presence and reassurance during the test.

Toddlers and preschool age children are best told about a procedure immediately prior to the test and tend to do best with a parent accompanying them (Petrillo and Sanger 1980). Fantasies are common at this age; therefore, simple explanations about the equipment or people in the room may help decrease anxiety. Most frequently, children want to know if it will hurt. If there will be no "owies," reassure the child. Not until the age of seven do most children have a sense of time; therefore, discussing the length of the test will not be useful. It is important to let the child know about his role in the test. Examples include holding perfectly still, taking a deep breath, or holding a piece of equipment. Making the test or examination into a game or letting the parent demonstrate first usually helps gain the cooperation of the child. Sometimes the procedure can first be demonstrated on a doll or stuffed animal.

Older children and adolescents usually will have more specific questions regarding the pretransplant test and procedures. They want to know how long it will take as well as the various details of the test/procedure. They may need to be reassured of their privacy. Even though an adolescent may not ask questions, the nurse should provide the information.

Preparation for Catheter Placement and/or Bone Marrow Harvest

Bone marrow harvest and/or catheter placement in a child requires general anesthesia. Many centers have a pre-op program to provide adequate preparation including hospital/unit tours, puppet and hospital play, which permits the child life worker/nurse to explain the procedure to the child in a nonthreatening environment (Bates and Broome 1986). The concept of body integrity is an issue in the preschool and school-age child. The use of Band-Aids and protection of body parts is an important aspect to include during this educational process. The child should know if there will be any pain or where the bandages will be when he/she awakes after the procedure.

The child usually has an opportunity to play with hospital equipment such as IV tubing or the anesthesia mask, hats, and masks wore by personnel in the operating rooms (see Figure 4.1). Children do best when reassured that they will not be left alone and that their parents will be there before and after the surgery. A favorite doll or stuffed animal provides additional security and can accompany them to the operating room.

Honesty is a good rule of thumb when working with any child. Distrust arises if the child is misled to or if information is hidden. The child needs to know enough information to be able to cope and adapt to the situation.

The nurse, along with other members of the transplant team (social worker, child life specialist, physician) must adequately address the informational needs of the older child and adolescent to prepare them for catheter placement and harvest. Information-seeking strategies used by this older age group help them to cope with their disease and treatments (Ohanian 1989). The older school-age child (older than seven years) and adolescent need to know information as far in advance as possible so they may make plans and ask questions. They frequently express concerns about the catheter and how it impacts on going to school, participating in activities, and changing their body image. Drawings can be useful to explain procedures. Age-appropriate play and/or discussions should be encouraged following any procedure to deal with feelings, misconceptions, and fears.

Preparation for Admission

Even though a younger child may not be present during the informed consent conference, the child must be prepared for admission into the transplant unit. The parent, child life worker, and nurse should show the child the transplant unit and patient room. Aspects of isolation, length of stay, daily routines such as baths, mouth care, physical examinations, dressing changes, and oral medications are discussed during the tour and again at other times prior to the hospitalization. Issues surrounding parent rooming-in and sibling visits should also be addressed. For instance, all children should be screened for recent exposure to chicken pox. Older children and adolescents who were a part of the informed consent process will benefit from a review prior to admission.

Patients want to know if a T.V., telephone, video games, computer, and toys can be brought into their room. The patient should plan to pack a suitcase and bring favorite toys, games, stuffed animals, clothes, and posters to decorate the room. If the bone marrow transplant is to be done in a laminar air flow environment, additional preparation is necessary.

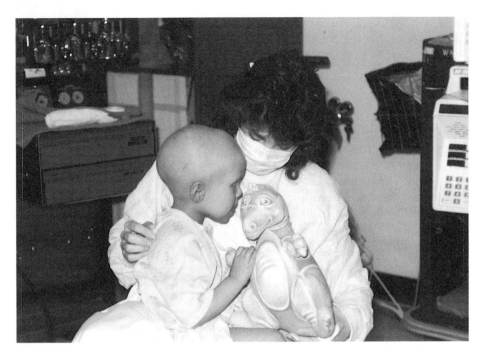

Figure 4.1. A favorite stuffed animal or doll provides additional security.

In addition to day-to-day care and the physical environment of the room, information regarding chemotherapy and/or radiation must be reviewed with the child. Although many children may have had prior chemotherapy or radiation, there are patients who have never received these therapies prior to the transplant. Parents and/or members of the transplant team must address side effects such as hair loss, nausea, vomiting, and mouth sores with the child. Details of the discussion will need to be tailored to the child's age. It is important for the child to understand that the transplant itself (infusion or reinfusion of the bone marrow) is not a painful procedure and only involves infusion of the marrow through the catheter, much like a blood transfusion. Some centers have developed patient education booklets that are tailored to the needs of both the child and his family (Almquist and Duchon 1986).

Aspects of care during the post-transplant period need to be reviewed. Children often want to know how long they will be in the hospital. The child under the age of seven typically does not comprehend the concept of time; therefore, a response using a number of weeks will not be helpful. The use of important dates, events, and holidays help mark the passing of time. A clock and a calendar where the days can be checked off are essential items for the room in children of all ages.

Preparation of the Family

The educational preparation of the parents is viewed as an ongoing process. Written materials such as booklets and handouts, as well as the informed consent process, help parents to learn about bone marrow transplantation. The National Institutes of Health organization has developed a handbook for parents of children with cancer, which contains excellent information about the disease, treatment, and resources available to families (NIH 1988). Like the child, parents must be prepared for all aspects of the transplant process. Many parents learn more than they really want to deal with or know. It is important for parents to understand their role during all phases of the transplant. Most parents want to be actively involved in their child's care. Parents can participate in daily activities such as catheter care, baths, mouth care, oral medication administration, diapers, and perineal care. The nursing staff can routinely negotiate and coordinate these activities on a daily basis with the parents. Parents need to know that "taking a break" or being less involved in their child's physical care is okay and will help maintain their strength during the long course of the hospitalization. In some situations, parents may increase their involvement to exert control and decrease their sense of helplessness.

Many parents have to deal with leaving their spouse and other children at home during the period of hospitalization. Whether the transplant center is around the block or thousands of miles away from home, parents must make arrangements regarding the care of their other children. Day care, carpooling, school, after school activities, and meals are daily routines that require planning and alternative arrangements. Preparation for many parents also involves taking off time from work. One parent may continue to work while the other spends the bulk of his/her time with the child in the hospital. The needs of the less visible parent are also important to consider, so that parent can can feel involved in the process even though far away.

Siblings must be included during the pre-transplant period as well as during other phases of the transplant process. They will need simple explanations of their brother or sister's disease, the bone marrow transplant, and hospitalization. Siblings frequently feel abandoned by their parents. Every family member must feel that they have an important role in the transplant; for some siblings, it is being the donor, for others it can be helping out at home. Parents should be encouraged to spend time with their other children and prearrange special activities.

The pediatric donor must be adequately prepared for all aspects of the donation experience. Most frequently, donors are healthy and have never been hospitalized. They need to know they will not "catch" what the brother or sister has, nor will they become sick. The sibling donor must be prepared for the surgical procedure. More detail about pediatric donors is included in Chapter 5.

In anticipation of the transplant, parents are encouraged to seek the assistance and support of family members, friends, and various community resources. Knowing that support is available often helps the parents to focus their attention on their child and the upcoming transplant.

Nursing Management of the Physiological Needs of the Child During the Transplant Process

Although the child undergoing a bone marrow transplant faces many of the same problems and complications as adults patients, there are aspects of care that are unique to pediatrics. Meeting the physiological needs of the child provides the bone marrow transplant nurse with a challenge. Those areas of care to be addressed include administration of chemotherapy, total body irradiation, fluid and electrolyte imbalances, skin care, myelosuppression, pain, and nutrition management.

Chemotherapy and Total Body Irradiation Administration Issues

The majority of preparative regimens utilize both chemotherapy and total body irradiation (TBI). Some conditioning regimens exclude radiation based on the patient's disease, type of transplant, and/or age. Examples of chemotherapeutic agents commonly used for immunosuppression and disease/marrow ablation include cyclophosphamide, cytosine arabinoside, busulfan, antithymocyte globulin, melphalan, and etoposide. The potential side effects and toxicities of these drugs when administered to children at high doses are similar to what is observed in the adult population. In general, children tend to tolerate the chemotherapy and radiation better than adults (Shannon et al. 1987).

Drug Dosing

There are several issues that are unique to children related to dosage, administration, and monitoring of chemotherapy. The dose of chemotherapy is based on the child's body surface (mg/m^2), weight (mg/kg), or age (Meeske and Ruccione 1987). In children less than two years or less than 12 kilograms, chemotherapy is usually calculated using the weight of the infant rather than the body surface area. At greater risk for chemotherapy-induced toxicities, the infant receives a reduced dose when dosing is adjusted in this manner (Meeske and Ruccione 1987). Unless the drug is routinely ordered in mg/kg, pediatric patients older than two years receive chemotherapy based on total body surface area. If intrathecal drugs are utilized, doses are based on the child's age and disease status (Bleyer 1988).

Drug Administration

Busulfan, a drug commonly used in the conditioning regimen, is commercially available as two milligram tablets and provides the nurse with a challenge in its administration to infants and young children who cannot swallow pills. Pharmacists can make an oral suspension of busulfan, however, it is highly recommended that the busulfan in its liquid form be given through a nasogastric tube to ensure that the entire dose is given. The patient should be NPO for an hour prior and post dose to permit adequate absorption. If the child does vomit in the one hour period post administration, some protocols suggest that the emesis be collected and readministered

through the nasogastric tube to ensure that the entire dose is given.

Hemorrhagic Cystitis

Most protocols include the use of cyclophosphamide (Cytoxan). Hemorrhagic cystitis is a potential side effect of the drug and requires careful nursing mangement. In a telephone survey of five pediatric bone marrow transplant units, all patients received increased hydration prior, during, and post cyclophosphamide administration. In addition to increased fluid hydration, continuous bladder irrigation was utilized in three of the five units surveyed (Bracken and Decuir-Whalley 1989). Intravenous hydration at twice the maintenance body fluid replacement requirements, along with normal saline boluses and diuretics adequately prevent hemorrhagic cystitis in most patients who do not receive bladder irrigations (Shannon et al. 1987).

If bladder irrigation is to be used, a straight bladder catheter (foley catheter) is adapted to create a three-way irrigating system, since three-way catheters are not available in pediatric sizes. To select the appropriate size catheter in the pediatric patient, the following guidelines will assist the nurse: infant (5 french), child < 4 years (8 french), child > 4 and < 10 years (10 or 12 french), and child > 10 years (14 french) (Bracken and Decuir-Whalley 1989). The child's bladder capacity, usual volume of urine output, and sensations experienced during instillation help determine the amount of bladder irrigant to be administered hourly. Neomycin GU irrigant is commonly added to saline irrigation bags, which is instilled and drained in 30-minute intervals until 24 hours after the last dose of cyclophosphamide (Bracken and Decuir-Whalley 1989). This procedure makes continuous bladder irrigation very time-consuming for the nurse. Nursing care of all patients receiving cyclophosphamide includes hourly monitoring of urine output, checking each void for specific gravity and microscopic blood as well as administering any antiemetics and diuretics (Nuscher et al. 1984). Recently, the concurrent intravenous administration of the drug mesna, a uroprotectant agent, has been tested to prevent hemorrhagic cystitis (Brugieres et al. 1989). Results to date have shown promise.

Nausea and Vomiting

Nausea and vomiting typically occur during and following the period of chemotherapy administration. Based on the child's weight, chlorpromazine (0.5mg/kg), metaclopramide (1–2mg/kg), diphenhydramine (0.5–1mg/kg), dexamethasone (4–8mg/m2), lorazepam (0.04mg/kg), and benzquinamide HCl (0.4mg/kg) are the more commonly used antiemetics in pediatrics. Several studies in the literature have revealed the efficacy of these antiemetic agents in children to control nausea and vomiting (Howrie 1986; Berg 1985). Diphenhydramine can be used in conjunction with phenothiazines and metoclopramide to prevent acute dystonic reactions (Clark 1989). In order to achieve an adequate antiemetic effect in some patients, combinations of medications are used as well as an around-the-clock schedule.

Due to vomiting and the sedative effects of antiemetics, nurses must be aware of the potential risk of aspiration in infants and younger children (Meeske and Ruccione 1987). Older children and adolescents frequently complain about the antiemetic making them feel "weird" and may refuse to let the nurse administer the medication. This situation can potentially lead to a conflict where the nurse is caught between the wishes of the patient and the parents. A scopalamine patch can be an effective solution in the older patient who objects to the intravenous medications. In some children, distraction, imagery, and relaxation techniques can be effective alternative or adjuvant approaches (Sauers et al. 1982).

Total Body Irradiation (TBI) Dosing

There are issues surrounding the use and administration of radiation therapy in children. Radiation is associated with numerous acute and chronic effects on many organs of the body; however, it is particularly toxic to a young child's developing central nervous system (Kramer and Moore 1989). Central nervous system complications following cranial or total body irradiation include leukoencephalopathy and a decrease in cognitive function (van der Wal et al. 1988).

In selecting a treatment protocol for a young child requiring bone marrow transplantation, the use of radiation must be carefully evaluated. If radiation is necessary only to ensure engraftment, it is common practice to shield the brain. Typically this technique is used for children with nonmalignant diseases; for instance an infant with severe combined immunodeficiency. In addition, blocks are made to shield the lungs from the effects of radiation. In patients with malignant diseases such as leukemia, the brain cannot be shielded because of the potential risk of failing to eradicate cells that may be harbored there. Chemotherapy agents such as cyclophosphamide and busulfan may be used instead of radiation therapy as a conditioning regimen (Yeager 1986).

Sedation for TBI

A challenge facing the bone marrow transplant team is the administration of radiation to infants and young children who cannot remain still during the treatment. A variety of approaches have been used to accurately deliver the radiation therapy. The infant or small child can be physically restrainted with a papoose board. This method should be avoided if at all possible since most children do not like being tied down and parents usually become upset seeing their child restrained and crying.

Sedation is an effective alternative that prevents the child from moving during the treatment. Administered intravenously, various combinations of medications can be used safely including narcotics (morphine), benzodiazepines (midazolam), and barbituates (pentobarbital) to provide adequate sedation. The child must be monitored very closely for signs of respiratory depression.

Emergency equipment and naloxone should be readily available.

Sedating an infant or child can be difficult since some children have paradoxic reactions and become agitated with these medications. Others may require higher doses than routinely administered, raising the concern about overdosing. The length of time spent in an already busy radiation oncology department is markedly prolonged if the patient is not easily sedated. It is not only stressful for the nurse and health care team but also anxiety-provoking for parents who feel helpless and are unable to comfort their child.

In the pediatric oncology setting, general anesthesia has been safely used for patients requiring painful procedures such as bone marrow aspirates and biopsies (Perin and Frase 1985). This approach has been applied successfully to infants and children who are receiving radiation treatments. The advantages of general anesthesia are that the treatments are smoother and quicker, the anxiety of the nurse, other team members, and parents is lessened, and the child is awake immediately following the treatment. However, the amount of coordination and cooperation required among the various departments is enormous.

If general anesthesia is selected the patient must be NPO for about six hours prior to the radiation. The anesthesiologist administers an inhaled anesthetic (halothane, nitrous oxide) through a facemask and passes a small flexible nasal tube once the child is asleep (Fisher et al. 1985). The anesthetic agent continues to be administered via this tube throughout the rest of the procedure. Turning the child midway through the treatment is done carefully so that the taped nasal tube does not fall out. Continuous monitoring of the patient's respirations and oxygen saturation occur during the treatment via the camera/TV. The anesthesia and the radiation treatment are usually tolerated without incident.

Depending on the total amount of radiation and the dose rate, the length of radiation takes anywhere from 20 minutes to 45 minutes to deliver. To decrease toxicity, radiation may be given in several fractions over several days. Even though heavy sedation is not used for older children and adolescents, these patients frequently find the treatment difficult. Most patients are anxious because this is their first experience with radiation. A mild sedative such as lorazepam can be helpful. The patient may also be premedicated with an antiemetic to lessen the amount of nausea and vomiting experienced. Being alone in the room can be very scary. Watching stuffed animals, playing tapes, having a story read by a parent or staff member, and singing or counting help decrease the feeling of loneliness as well as help pass the time. The older patient often selects favorite music on a tape player in the room.

Alteration in Fluid and Electrolyte Balance

There are numerous causes for the fluid and electrolyte imbalances in children receiving a bone marrow transplant. The preparative regimen contributes to many potential complications including tumor lysis syndrome in those patients with a significant tumor burden, the syndrome of inappropriate antidiuretic hormone (SIADH) and fluid overload in children receiving cyclophosphamide or melphalan, and hypomagnesemia associated with cisplatin administration. Careful monitoring of electrolytes and fluids is essential. Hourly input and output, frequent weights (QD or BID), and blood draws to evaluate electrolyte status are a part of the nursing care.

In children who require hydration, intravenous fluids are usually started at twice the maintenance level, and urine output is maintained at 3ml/kg/hour or greater. Refer to Table 4.2 for guidelines in determining a child's daily maintenance fluid needs and electrolyte requirements (Waskerwitz 1984). The nurse must assess the child for signs and symptoms of fluid overload including edema, sudden weight gain, and a bulging fontanelle in infants. Elevated blood pressure, tachycardia, and rales may provide additional

Table 4.2. Guideline for Determining Child's Daily Maintenance Fluid Needs

Daily Maintenance Fluids for Children

100cc/kg—for the first 10kg of child's weight
+ 50cc/kg—for the next 10kg of child's weight
+ 20cc/kg—for each kg in excess of 20kg
-Or-
2 liters/m²/day

Waskerwitz, 1984.

clues. If a child is taking fluids orally, hourly fluid intake is based on both intravenous and oral fluids. The nurse will need to adjust intravenous fluids accordingly, to avoid fluid overloaded.

There are times during the transplant when the child should be well hydrated and other times when keeping the patient below their fluid maintenance requirement is indicated. Fluid reductions are often necessary during and after radiation when patients tend to "third space" fluid, secondary to tissue trauma. In pediatrics, all intravenous fluids and medications are delivered by an infusion pump to ensure accuracy. When the child is fluid restricted, concentrating antibiotics and minimizing the amount of flush solution before and after medications by altering the infusion delivery system helps decrease unneccessary fluid intake.

In an overzealous attempt to manage the fluids, children can quickly become dehydrated. Due to a greater need for fluids relative to body size, infants and younger children are more prone to water and electrolyte imbalances usually with a rapid onset and a slower response to treatment (Whaley and Wong 1983).

Hypokalemia may be the result of nausea and vomiting, diarrhea, and the effect of chemotherapy, diuretics, and amphotericin. Potassium should be added to the child's total parenteral nutrition or maintenance fluids to keep the child's potassium level within normal limits. To prevent an accidental overdose, solutions containing supplemental potassuim should not be used to flush medications. It may be necessary to infuse an intravenous potassium bolus to promptly adjust the serum level. The child may need to be placed on a cardiac monitor and careful calculation made of the potassium dose to ensure safe delivery. In addition to potassium, patients may require magnesium, calcium, and phosphorus replacement, which also demand careful administration and monitoring.

Alteration in Nutritional Status

Much attention is paid to the nutritional needs of a child. High-dose chemotherapy and radiation can induce nausea and vomiting, anorexia, diarrhea, mucousitis, alteration in taste, and salivation (Cunningham 1983). These sequelae in turn may preclude adequate oral intake and thus significantly alter the nutritional status of the child.

For those children who can maintain an oral intake, changes in the gastrointestinal mucosa may affect the body's ability to adequately absorb nutrients (Weisdorf et al. 1984). Malabsorption can also be caused by graft-versus-host disease. Infections and fevers will increase caloric requirements.

Prior to admission to the transplant unit, a nutritionist should perform a thorough assessment of the child's nutritional status. In addition, the nurse should obtain a brief diet history about food intake patterns, food preferences (special formulas or diet), feeding schedule and amounts, and use of special nipples, bottles, or cups. High chairs and infant seats can be brought in from home and used to make meal times a more familiar experience.

Most commonly, children stop eating during the pretransplant conditioning therapy due to the nausea and vomiting. In the post-transplant period, nausea and vomiting continue to be problems. Additionally, the complication of mucousitis makes eating painful. It is important to keep in mind that medication such as narcotics, antibiotics, and cyclosporine can all have an impact on the child's nutritional status (Aker 1983). To meet the child's caloric needs, total parenteral

Table 4.3. Daily Caloric and Protein
Requirements

	Calories Required Kcal/kg	Protein Required gram of protein/kg
Infant/Toddler	90–110	2.5
Child	65–90	2
Adolescent	40–60	1.5–1.8

nutrition (TPN) is frequently initiated early in the transplant process.

In anticipation of requiring TPN and multiple intravenous drugs, the pediatric patient usually enters the transplant unit with two single lumen right atrial silastic catheters or a multiple lumen catheter. Often one lumen is designated for nutritional support and the other is used for other medications, fluids, and blood products. To avoid complicating the fluid and electrolyte management of the child, TPN is often started following the last day of chemotherapy.

Adequate nutritional support for the pediatric bone marrow transplant patient is necessary to prevent weight loss, and maintain muscle mass and adipose tissue reserve. The ultimate goal is to promote and support normal growth and development of the child, although this may not be feasible during the early post-transplant period due to the demands that the transplant places on the body. Refer to Table 4.3 for daily caloric and protein requirements for the pediatric patient based on age groups. These caloric and protein requirements are based on the age of the patient but also should be adjusted according to the child's level of activity, baseline nutritional status, and daily condition of the child during the transplant period.

The dextrose in the TPN should be concentrated to minimize fluid volume since most patients receive multiple intravenous antibiotics and blood transfusions. The concentration of dextrose may be increased up to 35% to provide the calories in as little fluid as possible. Intravenous fat emulsion (20%) is used to provide the balance of requirements in a calorically dense vehicle as well as to prevent deficiency of essential fatty acids. Nursing care of the child receiving TPN involves monitoring daily weights, accurate hourly intake and output, and blood draws to monitor serum electrolytes, BUN, creatinine, glucose, triglycerides, and liver function values, as well as urine testing to check glucose and ketones.

Enteral feedings are an option for infants and children who do not take enough calories orally and have an intact gastrointestinal tract. Nasogastric feedings via a small, flexible tube (6 or 8 french) may be administered over 12 hours at night while the patient is encouraged to eat during the day. Continuous nasogastric tube feeding may be necessary for patients who are unable to take enough calories during the day. A clinical study comparing TPN and enteral feedings revealed several advantages to the latter method for nutritional support in those patients who could tolerate oral feeds. These included decreased catheter complications, less need for diuretics, fewer problems with hyperglycemia, and reduced cost (Szeluga et al. 1987). However, nasogastric tubes are contraindicated when the mucosa is friable or the platelet count is low.

Patients who receive a relatively mild conditioning therapy that excludes radiation may continue to eat and drink throughout the entire hospitalization. Infant formula may require modification because of a temporary lactose intolerance and/or need to increase the caloric and nutrient density of the formula. Meeting the nutritional demands of the pediatric patient is very time-consuming for the nurse. Infants rely solely on adults to be fed, and a young child needs a considerable amount of assistance and encouragement at meal time.

Eating can become a tremendous control issue for the child, nurse, and parent. Placing too much emphasis on food is inappropriate during the acute period post-transplant when there are numerous complications facing the child. As discharge approaches however, eating does resurface as an issue that frequently causes much anxiety for both the parents and the child. Total parenteral nutrition is tapered and then stopped in hopes that the child will start eating and drinking. Once the isolation is modified, parents are encouraged to bring favorite foods from home and eat with their child. Most children do best when offered small and frequent servings of foods they enjoy.

Older children can keep track of the foods they eat and drink by maintaining a diary at their bedside. In planning for discharge, both the patient and parent must be told how much oral intake is satisfactory. Most children understand fluid volumes by the number of glasses they must drink within a specified period of time. Creativity on the nurse's part can help entice a child to eat and drink.

If the patient is ready for discharge and is not taking in adequate oral nutrition, nocturnal enteral feedings or total parenteral nutrition may need to be continued at home. In addition to learning how to set up a pump and administer the formula, parents are taught nasogastric insertion. In those patients who receive total parenteral nutrition, parents easily learn how to use very sophisticated IV pumps. Patients are generally referred to a local home infusion company that will supply the equipment and support services needed in the home.

Alteration in Skin Integrity

Several factors have been identified that place pediatric bone marrow transplant patients at high risk for skin breakdown (McConn 1987; Abramovitz and Baache 1988). This list includes the type of chemotherapy, the dose rate/dose of radiation, the age and diagnosis of the patient, the use of diapers, the presence of graft-versus-host disease, diarrhea, immobility, and malnutrition. The immunocompromised state of a child post chemotherapy and radiation, as well as potentially compromised nutritional state, interferes with adequate wound healing if skin breakdown exists.

Nursing care of the patient is aimed at prevention of skin breakdown and aggressive management of skin problems that are unavoidable. The nurse must do a thorough skin assessment daily in order to quickly diagnose skin problems and inititate a treatment plan. As with the adult patient, this can frequently be accomplished at bathtime.

Chemotherapeutic agents have been associated with toxic effects of the skin. The amount and dose rate of the radiation also plays a significant role in skin problems. Children who receive craniospinal radiation or abdominal radiation prior to their conditioning regimen are at risk for developing an additive local effect on the skin which can subsequently lead to redness and breakdown.

The diagnosis of the child that comes to transplant can help predict the susceptibility to skin breakdown. For example, an infant with severe combined immunodeficiency frequently presents with diarrhea, predisposing the patient to perineal breakdown. Children who receive a bone marrow transplant for neuroblastoma receive intensive chemotherapy/radiation, which often leads to breakdown around the catheter dressing, skin folds, and perineal areas.

Infants and young children who wear diapers are most susceptible to perineal breakdown. Urine and stool that remain in contact with the skin can result in excoriation. Patients who receive chemotherapy excrete metabolites in their urine which can act as an irritant to the skin unless immediately removed. Diarrhea caused by the use of non-absorbable antibiotics as well as from the side effects of chemotherapy and radiation can increase the likelihood of skin breakdown both in patients with diapers and without. Intense hydration and uncontrollable diarrhea may cause incontinence in children who were previously potty trained.

The nurse, parent, or child must follow meticulous perineal care in order to prevent breakdown from occurring. For infants and children in diapers, the diaper should be changed as soon as it is soiled. This is often an impossible task due to the frequency of episodes of diarrhea and the increased urine output caused by increased hydration. For all patients, cleanse the perineal area well after each stool. This can be done with an antimicrobial solution (diluted chlorhexadine or povidone iodine in sterile water). For infants a very dilute solution is made up or soapy water is used. The patient's skin should be cleaned with the solution, rinsed with water and then patted dry with sterile gauze. Finally, a thin layer of polysporin and nystatin ointment is applied to the perineal area. A variety of ointment combinations can be used to reduce infection and serve as a barrier to protect the skin.

Other approaches can be utilized for those children who fall into a high-risk category or for those patients who show evidence of impending perineal breakdown. Cloth diapers, which are less harsh to the skin, can be used to line disposable diapers. Also warm water sitz baths several times a day for periods of ten minutes can be effective. Leaving the perineal area open to air at times during the day may be of some assistance. Heat lamps or blow dryers are contraindicated. Areas of breakdown should not be rubbed. A syringe with a soft catheter tip can be used to squirt the area clean. Mineral oil works well to easily remove stool and residual ointments.

The nurse should employ an ointment that provides a stronger barrier for patients at high risk for skin breakdown or children who show evidence of excoriation. Combinations of Desitin®, stomahesive powder, and nystatin powder mixed as a balm and applied liberally to the perineal area protects the skin from stool and urine. Orabase® has also been used successfully. It provides a moist environment for reepithelization to occur and also functions as a skin barrier. Although some reepithelization of open lesions may occur, healing is usually delayed until the patient shows evidence of granulocyte recovery.

A bath is given to the child daily using water and an antimicrobial solution such as chlorhexidine or povidone iodine. These solutions should be avoided in infants less than six months since they can be systemically absorbed or cause skin irritation. Therefore a mild soap (Neutrogena®) should be substituted at bathtime. Mineral oil or other lubricants can be added to the bath water to moisturize the skin.

Children are also susceptible to the development of pressure ulcers of varying degrees during periods of immobility or extended bedrest. Inflatable and water bed mattresses as well as special air beds with HEPA filter attachments are available to reduce interface pressure. Similar devices are also available for cribs.

Care of the right atrial silastic catheter exit site presents a challenge to the nurse. In general, children dislike having tape removed from their skin. This is particularly true following chemotherapy and radiation since their skin is more sensitive and susceptible to tearing. Protective skin gel provides a film barrier and can be applied to areas where tape is in contact with the skin. Also, products such as Duoderm® and skin barrier can be placed on irritated areas to prevent direct contact of tape on the skin. Instead the nurse tapes directly onto the barrier which can remain in place for several days. Band-net® vests can be used to avoid tape. The area around the catheter exit site can easily become irritated. Povidone iodine is used to cleanse the skin; however, it should be removed with warm normal saline or sterile water before applying the dressing to prevent irritation and dryness. Skin care remains an active area of nursing research.

Alteration in Protective Mechanisms

The care of a myelosuppressed pediatric patient and an adult bone marrow transplant patient does not differ greatly. The focus of nursing care is to minimize infection through maintaining strict isolation. Personal hygiene such as bathing, oral and perineal care, and right atrial silastic catheter care are typical institution-specific nursing policies and procedures designed to reduce exposure to bend colonization of harmful pathogens.

Young children need supervision in order to comply with established isolation policies. For example, picking toys up from the "dirty" floor or playing with the nurse's hair or earrings would be unacceptable according to many institutions' isolation guidelines. Pediatric patients from infancy through the school-age years require complete or partial assistance in carrying out many aspects of care including bathing, perineal care, and mouth care. Parental involvement for these activities as well as performing catheter dressing changes is encouraged.

Transfusions are often necessary during the aplastic period and are administered according to physician and institution guidelines. Although this can vary, the patient is usually transfused for a hemoglobin between 7–10g/dl unless symptomatic and with a platelet count below 20,000 mm³ or higher if the child is actively bleeding (Buchanan 1989). Packed red blood cells (PRBCs) are ordered at 10ml/kg to raise the hemoglobin by 2.5–3g/dl (Buchanan 1989). For a small child, quad packs (75ml) may be ordered to minimize the amount of blood wastage. Platelets are ordered as individual random units or as a pediatric or adult platelet pheresis pack. An adult or full pheresis pack contains approximately six to eight units of platelets from a single donor, which can be split into two pedi-pheresis units (3–4 units apiece). As a general rule, one unit is required for every 6kg to increase the platelet count (Buchanan 1989). Therefore a 20kg patient would be transfused with three single random units of platelets or a pedi-pheresis unit.

Anemia may cause the child to feel weak and tired. Periods of rest such as naps or passive activities may be necessary to prevent exhaustion. Maintaining a safe environment for a child with thrombocytopenia is important. For an active toddler or preschooler, padding bed rails, removing all sharp objects, and supervising play can decrease accidents. Nosebleeds can be a real problem in children. Most children do not like pressure held on their nose in order to stop the bleeding. In addition, scabbed areas are often "picked" leading to recurrent episodes of epistaxis. Constant verbal reminders or cotton mittens may be helpful.

Based on their transfusion history, some patients may require premedication prior to blood product administration. Of particular concern in children is the amount of fluid the child will receive with any blood product transfusion. The administration of a diuretic (furosemide) in the middle or at the end of a transfusion may be indicated in those patients in which fluid overload is an issue. The use of normal saline to prime and flush the line is avoided in pediatric patients to minimize the total amount of fluid. Also, platelets can be "spun" or "dried" to decrease the total volume, allowing only the platelet concentrate to be given. Other special considerations include the use of irradiated blood products in all bone marrow transplant patients and the use of CMV antibody-negative blood products in those patients who are CMV antibody-negative and have a CMV antibody-negative donor. (These issues are discussed in Chapter 6.)

Alteration in Comfort

Both acute and chronic pain may be experienced by a child who is receiving a bone marrow transplant. Pain occurs with invasive procedures such as bone marrow aspiration/biopsy, blood draws, skin, liver, and other biopsies or as a result of chemotherapy and radiation-induced side effects such as mouth ulcerations and skin breakdown. Anxiety, age, fear, and parental attitudes are factors that can affect the child's perception of pain (Wofford 1985).

The McCaffery definition, that "pain is whatever the experiencing person says it is and exists whenever he says it does," also applies to children (McCaffery 1984). However, not all children can let the nurse know that they are experiencing pain. Even if a child admits to pain, the amount, location, and other describing features can be difficult to elicit. Restlessness, inconsolable crying, changes in vital signs, lack of interest in eating or playing, and inability to sleep are signs that can alert the nurse that an infant or young child is in pain (Whaley and Wong 1983). In all age groups, but especially in patients who cannot talk, the parent's assessment and changes in the child's body language and behavior can alert the nurse that something is wrong. Both subjective and objective data are used to assess a child's level of pain (Wofford 1985). On the other hand, the lack of pain expression does not mean the child is not in pain since both physiological and psychological adaption does occur (McCaffery 1984).

Assessing pain in children requires the use of tools and language that is familiar to the child (Beyer and Wells 1989). The child frequently uses the word "owie" or "boo-boo" or "hurt" to describe pain; therefore, the nurse should phrase pain questions using these terms. The location of pain can often be determined by having the child point to the area on his body or use a body outline and color in the spot that hurts (Eland and Anderson 1977). For the school-age child, asking them to assign their pain a number on a scale 0–10 (10 being the worst) will help the nurse assess the amount of pain the child is experiencing. This scale can also be used to evaluate the effectiveness of pain medications. Several other Likert-type tools are available as are drawings and pictures to assist the nurse in her assessment of the child's pain (Wofford 1985). One example is the Oucher scale, which uses photographs of faces to evaluate a child's level of comfort (Beyer and Wells 1989). The older child and adolescent usually can describe the amount, type, duration, and location of the pain.

There are several misconceptions regarding pain management in children. Infants and children do experience as much pain as adults. Health care providers often have fears concerning addiction and respiratory depression in pediatric patients, which can result in the undertreatment of the pain. These issues need to be addressed in order for the child to get adequate pain relief.

Based on body weight and age, acetaminophen is the most common non-narcotic analgesic used in children. Given for mild discomfort, this drug can be administered only in its oral form since medications given per rectum are discouraged in neutropenic patients. However, oral medications may be difficult to administer to a child who does not want to take anything orally due to severe oral ulcers and or nausea/vomiting.

Morphine is the drug of choice in relieving pain in the child undergoing a bone marrow transplant. For effective continuous pain relief and in an attempt to avoid multiple intravenous line breaks, a morphine drip can be initiated. A continuous morphine drip is started at 0.04mg/kg/hour and titrated by the patient's response (Benitz and Tatro 1988). Intermittent boluses may be indicated during painful treatments such as mouth care. A PCA (patient control analgesia) pump has been used successfully in children as young as six years of age to allow them to control the dosing of the medication.

Noninvasive techniques in pain control used alone or in conjunction with medications are distraction, relaxation, and cutaneous stimulation (McCaffery 1980). Some children respond favorably to hypnosis and guided imagery (Zeltzer et al. 1989). Distractions with play, television, and video games may help the child get his mind off the pain.

Alteration in Body Image

There are several aspects of bone marrow transplantation that cause changes in body image. Most oncology patients who come to transplant have experienced hair loss; however, the side effect of alopecia in particular is often emotionally traumatic for those children and adolescents who have never received chemotherapy prior to the transplant. Parents of infants and young children are often bothered by the thought of their child losing his hair. Open discussion prior to admission to the transplant unit can help both the parents and child plan for the event. Many children want their hair cut short, buy baseball caps and scarfs, and rarely, a wig. Talking with other children and parents can be helpful.

Children who require either steroids or cyclosporine must deal with the undesirable side effects of these drugs, including fluid retention, weight gain,and excess facial and body hair. Both the patient and the parents need to be reassured that the unwanted side effects disappear when the medication is stopped. School-age children and adolescents have the most difficulty coping with changes in body image.

Nursing Management of the Psychological Needs of the Child during the Transplant Process

To meet the psychosocial needs of a pediatric patient receiving a bone marrow transplant, the nurse must first have a basic understanding of normal growth and development. In addition, the nurse must be able to provide care using a family-centered approach that views the child and the other members of the family as a unit. The main concern of the pediatric nurse who applies this philosophy of care is the welfare of both the child and his family (Whaley and Wong 1983).

In providing care to a child with a life-threatening disease, three elements need to exist if the health care team is to utilize a family-centered approach: open honest communication between the child, parents, and all team members; involvement of patient/familiy in care; and ongoing education (Waechter et al. 1985). Examples of family-centered care in the bone marrow tranplant setting include sibling visitation, parental participation in physical care, and involvement in decision making including the consent/assent process.

Any model of nursing care delivery can work (e.g., primary nursing, case management) if the underlying philosophy of care is family-centered. A family-centered focus of care can be incorporated into either a pediatric or combined pediatric/adult bone marrow transplant unit. In a unit with a mix of both adult and pediatric patients, supplies, equipment, and care by the physicians and support staff must be attuned to the special needs of the child. Patients who are referred from a children's hospital frequently have a difficult time adjusting to the ''adult'' environment found in a unit with both adults and children.

In a study looking at attitudes of pediatric nurses who care for bone marrow transplant patients, nurses viewed the care provided to these children to be demanding; however, it was not depressing. Open communication, a family-centered care approach and involvement in the informed consent process were identified by the nurses as important factors in providing care to these children and their families (Abramovitz 1987).

Developmental Issues

As previously stated, the nurse must have knowledge regarding normal growth and development across the age spectrum since children who require bone marrow transplant range from newborns to teenagers. Frequently observed problems of children undergoing bone marrow transplantation include anxiety, fear of death, anger, regression, dependence, and lack of cooperation with many aspects of care (Gardner et al. 1977). An understanding of major developmental milestones and charactics of each age group (infant, toddler, preschool, school age, and adolescent) will assist in directing nursing care and other interventions related to the child's experience of the bone marrow transplant and hospitalization (see Table 4.4).

Infant

According to Erickson (1963), acquiring a sense of basic trust is characteristic of the infant. The development of this trust hinges on meeting physical needs, maintaining a safe environment, and positive parent/infant interactions. The infant's need to suck is extremely important during this oral phase of development providing both comfort and gratification (Lewandowski 1984). The in-

Table 4.4. Guidelines for Working with Pediatric Bone Marrow Transplant Patients

Age/Dev. Stage	Major Concerns	Interventions
Infant (0–1 yr.) Trust vs. mistrust Sensorimotor	Separation anxiety Fear of strangers	Encourage parent participation in day-to-day care (feeding, diapering, holding, comforting, bathing) Provide consistent nurses and caretakers and routines Elicit info. from parents about preferred methods of dealing with their child Decorate crib with mobile, stuffed animal, mirror Provide age-appropriate toys, music box, rattle
Toddler (1–3 yr.) Autonomy vs. shame and doubt Preoperational	Separation anxiety Loss of control	Encourage parent participation in day-to-day care Limit separation from parents as much as possible, always reassure the child that the parent will return Establish as much routine and rituals in the child's day-to-day care as possible Plan for consistent nursing and other caretakers Provide a safe environment Keep potty chair in room although child may be using diapers Explain all procedures to the child in simple language, allow time to play with any medical equipment Bring favorite blanket, stuffed animals, etc. from home to make the environment feel more secure Keep family pictures at bedside Provide play area in room with toy box if possible Provide appropriate toys and books Provide high chair or table for mealtime
Preschool (3–6 yrs.) Initiative vs. guilt	Body injury Fear of the unknown Loss of control	Encourage parent participation in care Carefully choose words so they are not misinterpreted Prepare child in advance for procedures Use Band-Aids and medical play around invasive procedures Establish routines for care as well as visiting schedule Provide activities: story telling, books and other age-appropriate games and toys
School age (6–12 yrs.) Industry vs. inferiority Concrete operations	Bodily harm Loss of control Death Negative feelings about self	Encourage the child to actively participate in his care Maintain parent involvement Provide tutor service Provide activities: schoolwork, books, video games, arts and crafts, cards, exercise bike
Adolescent (12–18 yrs.) Identity vs. identity diffusion Formal operations	Altered body image Lack of privacy Decreased independence Feeling different from peers	Encourage active self participation in care Maintain privacy Encourage friends to visit or call Be available to answer questions Provide activities: schoolwork, listening to music, reading, T.V., video games, computer Decorate room with posters of favorite musicians or athletes

Sources of reference: Wiley and House 1988; Lewandowski 1984; Waechter and Wong 1983.

tellectual development of an infant is characterized by Piaget as the sensorimotor stage of development (Stone and Church 1973).

Several aspects of normal development are disrupted when an infant is hospitalized for a bone marrow transplant. The infant's established patterns of eating and sleeping are interrupted by nursing and medical care. Side effects experienced from the chemotherapy and radiation affect the infant's desire to eat and need to suck. Although the parents remain active in the care of their baby, unfamiliar caretakers may not be as sensitive to responding to the subtle needs of the child (Whaley and Wong 1983).

In providing care to the infant, the nurse should encourage the parents to remain extremely involved in their child's day-to-day care including feeding, holding, diapering, bathing, and comforting. The nurse should elicit specific information from the parents regarding preferred methods of feeding, holding, and comforting as well as interpretation of the infant's cry and other behaviors. This information should become a part of the nursing care plan and be implemented accordingly. Minimizing the numbers of caretakers is important to the patient but also helps the parents develop trust in a small group of staff nurses.

Toddler

Autonomy is the single most accurate term to describe a toddler's stage of emotional and psychosocial development (Erickson 1963). Ranging between one and three years of age, a toddler's world centers around the child's ability to control their body and their environment. Mastering new motor skills and gaining control over bladder and bowel function are important aspects of a toddler's development (Whaley and Wong 1983). Asserting independence is seen in such behavior as temper tantrums, saying ''no,'' and refusing to eat at mealtime. If the toddler is unable to gain control and mastery, the child may experience negative feelings of doubt and shame (Erickson 1963). Despite becoming more independent, separation from parents continues to be very difficult for the child.

Toddlerhood is a period of time when the child makes enormous gains in intellectual development. According to Piaget, the child between the ages of one and two is in the final stages of the sensorimotor development (Stone and Church 1973). During this period of time the toddler begins to differentiate himself from others and displays egocentric thinking, understands simple cause and effect relationships, and develops some memory (Petrillo and Sanger 1980). Magical thinking and ritualistic behaviors are also seen during this period of development. After two years of age the toddler enters the preoperational phase of cognitive development characterized by an increase in language skills, a belief in animism and transductive reasoning (Lewandowski 1984). A child's belief that his doll is alive is a typical animistic manifestation. Associating all health care professionals who wear white lab coats with a painful procedure is an example of a toddler's transductive reasoning.

Hospitalization can be a terrifying experience for a toddler. The unfamiliar environment and a lack of routine are extremely hard on a toddler. Egocentric thinking by the toddler may cause the child to think that the hospitalization was a direct result of bad behavior or thoughts (Lewandowski 1984). In addition, concerns of abandonment and punishment exist when the child is separated from his parents. Mastery over bowel and bladder control may be completely disrupted due to the medical treatments imposed on the child such as fluid hydration, diuretics, and gut sterilizing medication.

The child's anxiety can best be minimized by limiting separation from his parents (Lewandowski 1984). Liberal visiting hours or rooming in is routine practice in many bone marrow transplant units. Consistency in day-to-day activities such as medications, baths, catheter, and mouth care can help reestablish some routines and ritual behaviors into the child's life. Incorporating some rituals and familiar items from home such as bedtime stories, naptime, favorite blankets, and stuffed animals help to provide some security. Pictures of family members decorating the bedside and a tape made by the parents can be reassuring when the parents are not physically present. Ideally, a small group of nurses who can develop a trusting relationship with the child can minimize the variety of schedules and personalities the child needs to deal with on a daily basis (Lewandowski 1984). Having a small core group of nurses also decreases the parent's anxiety level.

The nurse must provide a safe environment for the active toddler. High top cribs and side rails in the up position will prevent the child from falling out of bed. Play out of bed should be supervised to avoid accidental dislodging of the venous access catheter or hitting the head. Potty chairs should be near the bedside of those children who are in the process of being toilet trained or who have already mastered this control, although most patients revert back to diapers.

All procedures, no matter how painless or simple, should be explained to the child. Most toddlers do best when able to see and play with the equipment in advance. Both the nurse and the child life specialist can be of great assistance in preparing the child. Athough not always feasible in a transplant environment, procedures should not be performed in the safety of the child's bed or room. If possible allow the child to sit in the parents lap during the procedure or be near the child's face to provide comfort.

Despite all of these efforts to minimize the emotional trauma associated with hospitalization for transplantation, many children regress in some previously learned skills. Both staff and parents need to be reassured that this is normal in response to the stresses the child is experiencing. On the other hand, acquisition of new skills can occur during the transplant period if appropriate stimulation and activities are made available. Parents, nurses, the child life specialist, and physical therapist all can assist in promoting normal growth and development.

Preschooler

Erickson defines the psychosocial stage of a child between the ages of three and six as a period of gaining a sense of initiative (Erickson 1963). Dur-

ing this stage the child continues to develop motor and verbal skills along with exploration and a new mastery of the physical and social environment (Petrillo and Sanger 1980) Although parents and family remain central figures in the child's life, friends become extremely important. Preschoolers can tolerate brief separation from their parents and are more accepting of strangers. During these preschool years the child learns right from wrong, obeys simple rules, and can comprehend rewards and punishments (Lewandowski 1984). Guilt and disappointment may surface if the child's ability to complete a task or skill is obstructed.

The preschooler's state of intellectual development is preoperational or preconceptual (Stone and Church 1973). During this intuitive stage, preschoolers question everything, wanting to know "why" even though there may not be any explanation (Lewandowski 1984). As egocentric and magical thinking continues, the child may not be able to distinguish reality from fantasy. It is common for a child to have imaginary friends.

In dealing with children of this age group honesty is extremely important. Preparation for any procedures must be done in advance and reiterated just prior to and during each step of the procedure itself. This will greatly decrease the child's level of anxiety and will facilitate his cooperation (Lewandowski 1984). Explanations must be kept simple and include what the child will see, hear, smell, and taste. Play using dolls, stuffed animals, puppets, drawings, and other toys will help make the explanation more concrete (Waechter et al. 1985).

Fears of body injury and mutilation are real concerns for the preschooler facing numerous nursing and medical treatments. The nurse and other members of the health care team must be sensitive to these fears and provide sources of comfort such as Band-Aids® (Lewandowski 1984). Since children often mishear or misinterpret what is really meant, the words used to describe a treatment need careful selection.

The day-to-day care in the transplant unit may become extremely trying for the child.

Regression may be used as a coping strategy by the child to deal with several aspects of hospitalization (Lewandowski 1984). In order to regain some aspects of control, the patient should be given a choice whenever possible. For example, ask "do you want to take your bath before or after the cartoon?" or "what do you want to drink when you take your medicines?" Stickers and other rewards such as watching a favorite video can be used to help a child comply with unpleasant aspects of care such as mouthwashes and medication administration.

School-age

A sense of industry is the phase of psychosocial development that marks the school-age period (Erickson 1963). Children between the ages of six and twelve take pride in their accomplishments and new responsibilities as they strive for increased independence (Lewandowski 1984). Feelings of inadequacy and inferiority may arise if the child fails, thus resulting in poor self-esteem. Peer relationships and acceptance are extremely important to the school-age child.

Since school is the major focus of a child's day-to-day life, various aspects of school can be incorporated into daily activities while the child is hospitalized for the transplant. Parents should be encouraged to obtain schoolwork assignments from the child's teacher. Many transplant centers have a teacher on the staff to help the child with their schoolwork. Fever, nausea and vomiting, sedation, and other treatments may interfere with the child's ability to concentrate. Ideally, sessions with the teacher should be planned on a daily basis around the condition of the patient, although schoolwork may be a good distraction from routine medical care and feeling poorly.

Parents should ask the child's hometown teachers to have classmates send cards, pictures, and letters to the hospital. In addition to lifting the child's spirits they can be used to decorate the room. Contact by phone, letter, videotape, or recorded messages with a few close friends can help connect the child to the outside world. Since most children are miles from their home, visiting may not be an option. In addition, some units will not allow visitation by children under the age of twelve years.

The period of preconcrete operations is the beginning of logical thought for the school age child. As a part of this phase of cognitive development, the child gains the ability to reason deductively, understands the concept of time, and comprehends other viewpoints in addition to his own (Lewandowski 1984). As the child learns to read and write, the desire to learn new things increases.

The school-age child is very aware of his surroundings and will be quite attuned to things that happen to him while in the transplant unit. Depending on where the isolation room is situated, the child might be sensitive to the other children in the unit (Lewandowski 1984). In addition, the school-age child to a large degree understands his prognosis, potential complications of treatment, and the meaning of death (Lewandowski 1984). The nurse and the health care team must be cognizant of what is said or being overheard by the child.

The older school-age child views rules as flexible; therefore, he or she will attempt to bargain and manipulate the nurse, other members of the transplant team, and his parents into not doing certain aspects of care. Even though magical thinking is much less prevalent in the school-age child, certain rituals continue to play an important role. The school-age child is not very knowledgeable about his body parts and function; therefore, all procedures need to be fully explained including location and function of the organs that may be affected since fears regarding bodily injury and harm exist. Advance preparation using body outlines can help inform the child about the procedure. Striving for independence, the school-age child may be upset by the lack of privacy, unfamiliar people, and the barrage of stimuli that occurs with hospitalization. The patient should be given choices in scheduling care as well as periods of undisturbed time.

Adolescence

The period of adolescence covers a wide spectrum of years ranging from 12 to 18. There are several developmental tasks that adolescents are dealing with, including gaining a sense of identity and autonomy, coping with changes in body image, and developing a sexual identity (Erickson 1963). The behavior of an adolescent is erratic while going through this period of physiological and psychological change. As the adolescent strives for independence, the teenager tends to spend more time away from home and his parents while intensifying relationships with his peer group. Conflicts between the adolescent and his parents may arise as the teenager asserts himself.

According to Piaget, the adolescent is in the final stage of cognitive development, formal operations (Waechter et al. 1985). The ability to think abstractly and to look toward the future are characteristic of this stage. The adolescent is capable of understanding his disease, treatment, and prognosis and must be included in deciding and planning his care. The teenager must be part of the informed consent process and must agree to undergo a bone marrow transplant.

The actual hospitalization for an adolescent is an extremely stressful experience. The loss of control, separation from his peer group, and changes in body image are major threats to the adolescent (Lewandowski 1984). The fear of dying, isolation, limited activities, and a "special" diet all add to the adolescent's vulnerability. In direct conflict with the process of differentiation that adolescents undergo, hospitalization for a bone marrow transplant is associated with close and constant parental support. To support the adolescent, the nurse should encourage the teenager to be an active participant in his care. Although the adolescent's goal is to be independent, he may regress in order to cope and become very demanding on his parents and the staff. Even with this behavior, the staff should encourage the patient to do as much for himself as possible to build self-esteem and return a sense of control.

Every attempt should be made to maintain privacy. The patient at this age is quite concerned about who will examine him or her. Teenagers frequently want to have their curtains pulled the entire time they are in the transplant unit. The lengthy period of isolation is difficult for a teenager. The room is extremely small and they can easily get bored. Teenagers should be encouraged to decorate their room with favorite posters and bring in other things from home. Working on school projects, watching television or videos, listening to music, using the computer, and talking on the telephone are activities that help to pass the time.

Depending on the distance from the patient's hometown, friends may visit. Adolescents may not want their friends to see them because of the hair loss, fluid retention, and other changes in body image. Frequently, the teenager will make close attachments to a few nurses or members of the transplant team and may open up and discuss feelings and concerns that the he cannot share with his parents. Sterility and doubts about the adequacy of body image may be difficult for the adolescent to discuss.

View of Death

In all cultures, children are valued and seen as society's hopes, dreams, and future (Bandman and Bandman 1985). The idea of losing a child is overwhelming. Bone marrow transplantation forces a family to deal with issues involving both the quality of life and death.

A child's view of death varies with age and reflects the level of cognitive and psychosocial development (Waechter et al. 1985) (see Table 4.5). Infants and toddlers do not have the cognitive abilities to understand the concept of death (Waechter et al. 1985). Toddlers will pick up on parents' and other care givers' feelings and anxieties and will tend to cling. Issues that arise when a young child is dying revolve around decreasing any pain and discomfort experienced as well as minimizing parent-infant separation.

Table 4.5. Child Development: Death and Grief

Stages	Frequently Observed	How Parent Can Help	Beliefs About Death
Sensorimotor (0–2 years)	Anxiety and fear of being left alone Picks up on feelings and emotions of the parents and staff	Minimize parent-infant separation	
Symbolic Imagery (2–5 years)	Acts out, relieves anxiety by acting out fantasy (vs. talking) Feels at fault, guilty Fears being left alone Regresses to earlier stages, needs Does not understand sadness around him	Allow child to pay respects as he chooses Help child come to terms with own feelings (anger, sorrow, etc.); help come to terms with finality Assure child IT'S NOT HIS FAULT: child did not cause it to happen Give ample reassurance and consistency; assure he will be cared for Inform school	Death not seen as final Death temporary—like sleep; reversing—will go away, come back—like a journey "It may be my fault"
Concrete (6–9 years)	Child wants to know many facts Becomes expert re: disease Death no longer denied, but is seen as something that happens to others	Answer questions directly, honestly Provide information Respect "need to know" (information gives child some form of control) "Memory book" may help Inform school, teachers	Great understanding because of life experiences Death may be in form of person or spirit
Cognitive (10+ years)	Peer relationships important Conflicts between peer-adult standards Perceives irreversibility of death for first time Emotions may be withheld or expressed	Be available, supportive Help with "good-byes" as child indicates need Help alleviate guilt, if it exists	Perceives irreversiblity of death Perceives OWN mortality
Adolescent (12+ years)	Peer relationships vs. family ties, loyalties School performance reflects stress Girls: promiscuity may be a way of seeking affirmation, love Boys: fear of crying, expressing feelings	"I'm here if you need me" Recognize adolescent's need to work through independently	Full recognition of own mortality/omnipotence Attitudes about death similar to adults

Developed by Bonnie Sibley, M.A.

The child under the age of five views death as a temporary and reversible condition (Waechter et al. 1985). Magical and egocentric thinking may lead a preschooler to believe his bad thoughts caused this to happen to him and now he is being punished (Lewandowski 1984). Discussions with a child about death in this age group should be based on the child's previous experience with death (pets, relatives) and his cognitive development (Waechter et al. 1985). When questioned "am I going to die?," the nurse should explore what the child means by "die." Letting a child know that everyone dies someday and that it will not hurt would be an appropriate response. Frequently parents want some guidance in dealing with their child's questions about death and others want to completely avoid the topic. There are several books in children's literature that deal with sadness and hope that can be read to the child (Waechter et al. 1985). These stories provide an avenue for the child to bring up concerns and feelings.

The greatest period of change in the concept of death is between the ages of six and twelve. School-age children are aware of the severity of their illness and that they could die (Waechter et al. 1985). Children at this age are very interested in the morbid details of the dying process and want to know exactly what happens to the body. For the adolescent the concept of personal death is difficult to accept. Denial is commonly observed since death does not fit into the personal plans and future of the adolescent.

Parents and children during their stay in the bone marrow transplant unit must deal with the issue of death, not only with themselves but with others around them. Due to a very long hospitalization, the child/parents are very much aware of the death of another child in the unit. Fear, anxiety, and guilt are the feelings expressed by patients who experience another child's death while in the transplant unit (Patenaude and Rappeport 1982).

Psychological and Emotional Issues for Parents and Siblings

In order to provide adequate support to family members throughout the transplant process, background information should be obtained prior to admission. Areas to be addressed include other children at home, financial and work status, support systems, and significant religious and cultural practices. It is also important to determine the functional position or the role of the BMT patient in the family and the degree of emotional interaction among family members. How the family has coped and adapted to previous crises in their lives is important as bone marrow transplantation will stress the entire family system. Many families are geographically separated from their homes, leaving behind their support systems at a time when they are most vulnerable (Patenaude 1979).

Families vary in their ability to express and tolerate intense or difficult feelings. If openly expressed feelings are not tolerated, this may lead to various forms of acting-out behaviors during the bone marrow transplantation process. This information is extremely useful to the entire team and serves as a basis for interactions and interventions.

As the child moves through the transplant process, parents frequently experience an array of emotions. This emotional roller coaster usually starts with a sigh of relief as the child enters the transplant unit; however, this quickly changes to second thoughts, and fear of death, as well as guilt feelings as they watch their child become sicker from the chemotherapy and radiation (Waechter et al. 1985). Feelings of helplessness and loss of control are often expressed.

Anger is another common reaction to the transplant process. Some parents blame themselves for having a sick child; others blame the sick child. Many parents and older patients become angry at members of the health care team for not making the treatment a more pleasant process or promising a cure. As the transplant progresses, parents often feel increasingly anxious about the disruption in their lives and the financial consequences. Anger must be seen as a normal reaction to this unusually stressful situation. It is important for the entire family to understand that anger toward themselves and their situation is often projected onto others close to them. Thus, the nurse can frequently be the target of their anger and frustration. Consistent nursing care as well as direct and open communication is critical during this period. Helping parents cope with day-to-day crises and mobilizing support systems are other interventions that the nurse can offer. Support groups are available at some transplant centers and are another way family members and significant others can discuss issues. There are numerous community resources that are available to parents and can provide a source of support.

Most parents tend to cope with the stress of transplant by spending an enormous amount of time in the isolation room with their child (Gardner et al. 1977). This causes a great disruption of the family and guilt feelings that parents cannot meet the needs of the other children at home. Although difficult, parents must find the time to spend with their other children, who have their own concerns and fears.

A bone marrow transplant involves everyone in the family. As parents try to cope with the demands of a critically ill child, they are stretched emotionally, physically, and financially. Healthy children in the family can feel neglected and resentful of the transplant patient. Kramer (1984), in her study regarding the impact of cancer on healthy siblings, identified three main sources of stress: emotional realignment, separation, and ill child's therapeutic regimen. Sibling responses included increased sibling rivalry, anger, frustration, rejection, and confusion, as well as several other emotions (see Table 4.6). These feelings can be eased by encouraging parents to provide the healthy siblings with a full explanation about bone marrow transplantation in words they can understand (see Table 4.7). Updating siblings on the

patient's progress is extremely critical and can be done weekly or as often as needed through informal family meetings or telephone calls. A family support group where healthy children gain practical knowledge and talk out negative emotions can be helpful.

The sibling who is a bone marrow transplant donor is a special person. Because the sick child is the central figure, an extra effort must be made to discuss the medical issues as well as feelings of being a donor. It is not unusual for donors of all ages to feel "left out" and unappreciated. When discussing these feelings with the sibling donor, the parent and nurse must emphasize his key role in the transplant process. On the other hand, the sibling donor should not be made to feel guilty if the transplant does not have a positive outcome. The child life staff at many bone marrow transplant centers is able to work with the donor and the other siblings.

Life After Bone Marrow Transplant

A rise in the child's total white blood cell count and absolute neutrophil count is often accompanied by a sigh of relief. Unless other complications prevail, engraftment marks the point of discontinuing isolation. The focus of attention turns toward preparing the child and the parents to go home.

Prior to discharge an enormous amount of information is reviewed with the child/family. Parents must understand isolation and dietary restrictions, housekeeping guidelines as well as the purpose for the medications the child will receive at home (Nuscher et al. 1984). Knowing who to call to report signs and symptoms of infections and other potential transplant complications (e.g., rash, diarrhea, etc.) is critical. Parents must be given the clear message throughout the discharge process that it is alright to call with their

Table 4.6. Childhood Cancer in the Family: Negative Impact on Healthy Siblings

Sources of Stress	Negative Consequences	Emotional Responses
Emotional realignment	Emotional deprivation Decreased parental tolerance Increased parental expectations	Increased sibling rivalry Anger, frustration Rejection Guilt
Separation	Lack of information Decreased family involvement Insufficient social support	Loneliness, isolation Sadness Confusion Anxiety
Ill child's therapeutic regimen	Witnessing ill child's physical and personality changes Witnessing ill child's anxiety and pain Adjusting to changes in family's usual routines	Embarrassment Anger, frustration Guilt Fear, anxiety

Kramer, R. 1984

questions and concerns following discharge from the hospital.

The amount of information given to families as well as the fear of leaving the protected environment of the hospital can be overwhelming. Discharge information must be available in a written format (booklet, handout) and serve as a handy reference once the child is at home. Discharge information handouts should include isolation and dietary restrictions, medications and side effects, list of common problems and complications, important phone numbers, and the follow-up plan.

The amount of teaching a family requires will vary based on their previous experience as well as their level of anxiety. Anxious parents will need the information repeated several times. Both parents as well as other family members or friends directly involved in the child's care are encouraged to attend the teaching sessions. Parents must be able to provide physical care to the child and are taught how to care for their child's catheter and safely administer medications. If the child is unable to take enough calories, the parents are taught nasogastric tube feedings or how to administer total parenteral nutrition via a pump. Most parents learn these skills without much difficulty.

Ideally, a referral to a public health nurse or a home-care agency should be made for every child discharged after bone marrow transplant. Most families report that having a nurse come to the home immediately following discharge helped validate the teaching done at the hospital and decrease their level of anxiety. The bone marrow transplant nurse is responsible for relaying information and educating the nurse(s) at the referring hospital as well as the nurse in the home setting.

The younger child may become distressed over the change in isolation routine and fear they will get sick after they leave the bone marrow transplant room. A simple explanation of germs and teaching about good hygiene will often allay fears. Older children and adolescents are usually upset by the isolation restriction of avoiding crowds, which can include school, movie theaters, and shopping centers. A home tutor should be set up as part of the discharge planning process. Discussions should focus on activities the child can participate in until further immune recovery.

The bone marrow transplant patient often suffers a loss of ego strength and needs special encouragement in the post-transplant period. Advice to parents includes: (1) suggest the child pursue a hobby or a special talent, (2) encourage the child to keep a daily journal, (3) involve an

Table 4.7. Working with Healthy Siblings: Nursing Interventions

Intervention Areas	Specific Suggestions
Initial family assessment	Inquire about well children at home
	Where will they be staying during the transplant?
	Have they been told about the diagnosis as well as information about the BMT?
	Do the parents need assistance or guidance in talking with their well children?
	What were the siblings' reactions, questions, and concerns?
	Provide parents with anticipatory counseling regarding healthy siblings' role in the illness experience, their unique concerns and responses
	Elicit parents perceptions of how you may be helpful
Sibling involvement	Encourage siblings to be involved in the care of the ill child in the hospital and home
	Encourage phone calls, letter writing, and picture exchanges during periods of separation
	Encourage both sibling and patient to send drawings and other artwork to one another
	Keep pictures of siblings and other family members at the bedside and vice versa
Education support	Encourage inclusion of siblings at the initial family conference
	Arrange for follow-up teaching sessions in the hospital or outpatient clinic at convenient times for the siblings
	Employ age-based teaching strategies including use of dolls, puppets, and hospital equipment
Emotional support	Encourage parents to call siblings frequently and give them updates while the ill child is hospitalized
	Develop a sibling support group or network if feasible
Family communication	Encourage honest and open family counseling
	Counsel parents that sibling communication should be age-appropriate
	Reassure family that it is OK to show their emotions
	Encourage parents to explore the meanings behind siblings' questions and statements
	Remind families that communication needs to be an ongoing process

Adapted from Kramer, R. 1984.

outside friend who can bring news about school activities, (4) keep the school informed about the child's health, (5) provide a desk area for home tutoring or school work, and (6) if available, ask the library van to stop at your home.

Once home, many parents tend to be overprotective and may feel they need to limit the child's activities and become overly concerned with the degree of cleanliness and isolation. Other concerns and problems parents face post-discharge include poor appetite, reestablishing a daily routine, and setting limits with their child and other siblings in the home. The nurse and other members of the transplant team should discuss these issues prior to discharge and provide anticipatory guidance.

Follow-up care varies from institution to institution; however, this usually involves weekly or monthly clinic visits for the first six months and then less frequently.

Long-Term Effects

The amount of information known about the late complications of bone marrow transplantation has increased as more children become long-term survivors. Most late effects can be anticipated; therefore, early recognition and interventions are critical. Even with close monitoring, complications post-transplant can cause significant morbidity and mortality (van der Wal et al. 1988).

In the post-transplant period many complications affect both children and adults. Infections and restrictive lung disease, cataracts, chronic graft-versus-host disease, secondary malignancies and relapse occur in both patient populations (Buchsel 1986). Of particular concern in children are the late effects involving growth and development and endocrine function. Age, previous treatment, and transplant conditioning regimen can all have an impact on the severity and degree of late complications observed in children (van der Wal et al. 1988).

In general, the more toxic the conditioning regimen, the greater the likelihood of long-term sequelae (Buchsel 1986). Children who received chemotherapy alone have fewer long-term complications than children who received both chemotherapy and TBI. In pediatric patients treated with chemotherapy alone, no effect on normal growth and development was observed (Buchsel 1986). There were no adverse effects on gonadal function in prepubertal children who received only chemotherapy. Although there is a slow return of normal menses following bone marrow transplant in postpubescent girls, normal pregnancies can occur (Sanders et al. 1988). Males when transplanted after puberty have been able to father children (Buchsel and Kelleher 1989).

When chemotherapy and radiation were used in the conditioning regimen, infertility was observed in both prepubertal and postpubertal patients (Sanders et al. 1986b). Primary ovarian failure, failure to develop secondary sexual characteristics, and delayed onset of puberty are of particular concern in prepubertal girls and boys who received TBI (Buchsel 1986). Hormone therapy may be instituted to facilitate the achievement of normal secondary sex characteristics in these children (Nims and Strom 1988). See Chapter 14 for more details on fertility concerns.

In children receiving both chemotherapy and radiation, hypothyroidism is observed in 39% of patients (Sanders 1986b). In patients diagnosed with hypothyroidism, thyroid supplementation should be initiated (Sanders 1986b). Affecting the growth centers of the vertebral bodies of the spine, radiation causes spinal shortening (Ruccione and Weinberg 1989). Growth hormone deficiency was noted in some children; however, all children had a decrease in their height velocity with a reduction in sitting height (Sanders 1986b). With growth hormone now readily available, children who are candidates should receive growth hormone therapy.

Rapid brain development occurs during early childhood making a child's central nervous system vulnerable to insult and injury (Kramer and Moore 1989). Studies have revealed that children treated with cranial radiation and intrathecal therapy have lower IQ scores and lower measurements of academic achievement, conceptual reasoning, visuo-spacial processing and math-related abilities (Kramer and Moore 1989). Many children who receive a bone marrow transplant have had previous central nervous system treatment and will have further injury when conditioned with radiation. Very careful monitoring for learning disabilities must be incorporated into the child's follow-up care.

Starting from the time of the initial informed consent, both parents and older children express concerns about the long-term complications of bone marrow transplantation. Ongoing monitoring, education, and emotional support should be provided in order to assist the patient and his family to deal with these potential effects.

In both the pediatric and adult literature, little is written about the long-term psychological effects of bone marrow transplantation (Buchsel 1986). Many of the studies reported have looked primarily at the concerns and needs of long-term survivors of childhood cancer. Mild psychiatric problems were reported in approximately 59% of long-term survivors, which is greater than that reported in "healthy" children (Hymovich and Roehnert 1989). In one study, parents of survivors of childhood cancer were concerned about the risk of relapse, ability of the child to marry and have children, emotional development, and communication among family members including siblings (Wallace et al. 1987). Other areas of concern that have been reported in the literature and need further research based on childhood survivors of bone marrow transplantaion include self-concept and body image, life-style, employment and insurance, and marriage and family (Hymovich and Roehnert 1989).

Bone marrow transplantation offers hope and a chance of cure for many children. As more children are being cured, attention must continue to focus on minimizing acute complications and long-term effects of treatment. The field of bone marrow transplantation is growing in both medical and nursing knowledge. Nurses have played an important role in the success of bone marrow transplantation with their involvement in day-to-day care as well as research. The pediatric nurse is continually being challenged to meet the physical and emotional needs of the child and his family. Cure is the goal, but the ultimate reward is to restore a child who will lead a long, healthy, and rich life (Wiley and House 1988).

References

Abramovitz, L. 1987. Nurses' attitudes in caring for the pediatric bone marrow transplant patient. *Journal of the Association of Pediatric Oncology Nurses* 4 (1&2): 39.

Abramovitz, L., and Baache, B. 1988. Management of skin care complications in pediatric bone marrow transplant patients: A nursing challenge. *Journal of the Association of Pediatric Oncology Nurses* 5 (1): 37.

Aker, S. 1983. Nutritional assessment in the marrow transplant patient. *Nutritional Support Services* 3 (10): 22–26.

Almquist, G., and Duchon, D. 1986. Pediatric bone marrow transplantation: Developing a patient education booklet. *Journal of the Association of Pediatric Oncology Nurses* 3 (1): 13–18.

Altman, A. 1989. Chronic leukemias of childhood. In Pizzo, P., and Polack, D. (eds.) *Principles and practice of pediatric oncology*. Philadelphia: J.B. Lippincott Company, pp. 383–396.

Ammann, A., and Hong, R. 1980. Disorders of the T cell system. In Stielm, E., and Fulginiti, V. (eds.) *Immunologic disorders in infants and children. 2nd ed.* Philadelphia: W.B. Saunders Company, pp. 257–315.

Ball, E.D. et al. 1990. Autologous bone marrow transplantation for acute myeloid leukemia using monoclonal antibody-purged marrow. *Blood* 75 (5): 1199–1206.

Bandman, E., and Bandman, B. 1985. *Nursing ethics in the lifespan.* Norwalk, Conn.: Appleton-Century-Crofts.

Bates, T., and Broome, M. 1986. Preparation of children for hospitalization and surgery: A review of the literature. *Journal of Pediatric Nursing* 1 (4): 230–239.

Bayever, E. et al. 1984. Comparison between bone marrow transplantation and antithymocyte globulin in the treatment of young patients with severe aplastic anemia. *J. Pediatr.* 105 (6): 920–925.

Benitz, W., and Tatro, D. 1988. *The pediatric drug handbook. 2nd ed.* Chicago: Year Book Medical Publishers, Inc.

Berg, S. 1985. Dexamethasone's new use in cancer treatment. *Journal of the Association of Pediatric Oncology Nurses* 2 (2): 46–48.

Beyer, J., and Wells, N. 1989. The assessment of children in pain. *Pediat. Clin. North Am.* 36 (4): 837–854.

Bleyer, A. 1988. Central nervous system leukemia. *Pediatr. Clin. North Am.* 35 (4): 789–819.

Bortin, M., and Buckner, C.1983. Major complication of marrow harvesting for transplantation. *Exp. Hematol.* 11 (10): 916–921.

Bracken, J., and Decuir-Whalley, S. 1989. Continuous bladder irrigation for children receiving high-dose cyclophosphamide before bone marrow transplantation. *Journal of Pediatric Oncology Nursing* 6 (3): 105–107.

Brugieres et al. 1989. Hemorrhagic cystitis following high-dose chemotherapy and bone marrow transplantation in children with malignancies: Incidence, clinical course, and outcome. *J. Clin. Oncol.* 7 (2): 192–199.

Buchanan, G. 1989. Hematological supportive care. In Pizzo, P. and Polack, D. (eds.) *Principles and Practice of Pediatric Oncology.* Philadephia: J.B. Lippincott Company, pp. 823–836.

Buchsel, P. 1986. Long-term complications of allogeneic bone marrow transplantation: Nursing implications. *Oncology Nursing Forum.* 13 (6): 61–70.

Buchsel, P., and Kelleher, J. 1989. Bone marrow transplantation. *Nurs. Clin. North Am.* 24 (4): 907–938.

Cancer Statistics. 1990. *C.A.* American Cancer Society, pp. 14.

Clark, R. et al. 1989. Antiemetic therapy: Management of chemotherapy-induced nausea and vomiting. *Seminars in Oncology Nursing* 5 (2): 53–57.

Coccia, P. et al. 1988. High-dose cytosine arabinoside and fractionated total body irradiation: An improved preparative regimen for bone marrow transplantation of children with acute lymphoblastic leukemia in remission. *Blood* 4 (April): 888–893.

Cowan, M. et al. 1985. Haplocompatible bone marrow transplantation for severe combined immunodeficiency disease using soybean agglutinin-negative, T-depleted marrow cells. *J. Clin. Immunol.* 5 (6): 370–376.

Cunningham, B. 1983. Nutritional considerations during marrow transplantation. *Nurs. Clin. North Am.* 18 (3): 585–595.

Dahl, G. 1990. Allogeneic bone marrow transplantation in a program of intensive sequential chemotherapy for children and young adults with acute nonlymphocytic leukemia in first remission. *J. Clin. Oncol.* 8 (2): 295–303.

Davis, A., and Aroskar, M. 1983. *Ethical Dilemmas and Nursing Practice.* Norwalk, Conn.: Appleton-Century-Crofts.

Diamond, C., and Matthay, K. 1988. Childhood acute lymphocytic leukemia. *Pediatric Annals* 17 (3): 156–170.

Eland, J., and Anderson, T. 1977. The experience of pain in children. In Jacox, A. (ed.) *Pain: A Sourcebook for Nurses and Other Health Professionals.* Boston: Little, Brown and Company, pp. 453–473.

Erickson, E. 1963. *Childhood and Society.* 2nd ed.: WW Norton and Company, Inc.

Fisher, D. et al. 1985. Comparison of enflurane, halothane and isoflurane for diagnostic and therapeutic procedures in children with malignancies. *Anesthesiology* 63 (6): 647–650.

Fochtman, D. et al. 1982. The treatment of cancer in children. In Fochtman, D. and Foley, G. (eds.) *Nursing Care of the Child with Cancer.* Boston: Little Brown and Company, pp. 177–232.

Fonger, P. 1987. Nursing care of the child with severe combined immune deficiency. *Journal of Pediatric Nursing* 2 (6): 373–380.

Gardner, G. et al. 1977. Psychological issues in bone marrow transplantation. *Pediatrics* 60 (suppl.): 625–631.

Howrie, D. 1986. Metoclopramide as an antiemetic agent in pediatric oncology patients. *Drug Intelligence and Clinical Pharmacy* 20: 122–124.

Hymovich, D., and Roehnert, J. 1989. Psychological consequences of childhood cancer. *Seminars in Oncology Nursing* 5 (1): 56–62.

Kalwinsky, D. et al. 1988. Biology and therapy of childhood acute nonlymphocytic leukemia. *Pediatric Annals* 17 (3): 172–191.

Kramer, J., and Moore, I. 1989. Late effects of cancer therapy on the central nervous system. *Seminars in Oncology Nursing* 5 (1): 22–28.

Kramer, R. 1984. Living with childhood cancer: Impact on healthy siblings. *Oncology Nursing Forum* 11 (1): 44–51.

Kushner, B., and Cheung, N. 1988. Neuroblastoma. *Pediatric Annals* 17 (4): 269–284.

Lenarsky, C., and Feig, S. 1983. Bone marrow transplantation for children with cancer. *Pediatric Annals* 12 (6): 428–435.

Levine, M. et al. 1975. The medical ethics of bone marrow transplantation in childhood. *J. Pediatr.* 86 (1): 145–150.

Lewandowski, L. 1984. Psychological aspects of pediatric critical care. In Hazinski, F. (ed.) *Nursing Care of the Critically Ill Child.* St. Louis: The C.V. Mosby Company, pp. 12–62.

Lucarelli, G. 1990. Bone marrow transplantation in patients with thalassemia. *N. Engl. J. Med.* 312 (7): 417–421.

McCaffery, M. 1980. Relieving pain with noninvasive techniques. *Nursing '80* (December): 55–57.

McCaffery, M. 1984. Pain assessment and relief in children with cancer. *Journal of the Association of Pediatric Oncology Nurses* 1 (4): 9.

McConn, R. 1987. Skin changes following bone marrow transplantation. *Cancer Nursing* 10 (2): 82–84.

Meeske, K., and Ruccione, K. 1987. Cancer chemotherapy in children: Nursing issues and approaches. *Seminars in Oncology Nursing* 3 (2): 118–127.

National Institutes of Health. 1988. *Young People with Cancer: A Handbook for Parents.* NIH Publication No. 88-2378.

Neglia, J., and Robison, L. 1988. Epidemiology of childhood acute leukemias. *Pediatr. Clin. North Am.* 35 (4): 675–692.

Nims, J., and Strom, S. 1988. Late complications of bone marrow transplant recipients: Nursing care issues. *Seminars in Oncology Nursing* 4 (1): 47–54.

Nuscher, R. et al. 1984. Bone marrow transplantion: A lifesaving option. *Am. J. Nurs.* 764–772.

Ochs, J., and Mulhern, R. 1988. Late effects of antileukemia treatment. *Pediatr. Clin. North Am.* 35 (4): 815–833.

Odom, L. 1989. New directions in childhood cancer therapy. *Journal of the Association of Pediatric Oncology Nurse* 6 (2): 18–19.

Ohanian, N. 1989. Informational needs of children and adolescents with cancer. *Journal of the Association of Pediatric Oncology Nursing* 6 (3): 94–97.

O'Reilly, R. et al. 1984. Marrow transplantation for congenital disorders. *Seminars in Hematology* 21 (3): 188–221.

Parkman, R. 1986a. Current status of bone marrow transplantation in pediatric oncology. *Cancer* 58: 569–572.

Parkman, R. 1986b. The application of bone marrow transplantation to the treatment of genetic diseases. *Science* 232: 1373–1378.

Patenaude, A. et al. 1979. Psychological costs of bone marrow transplantation in children. *American Journal of Orthopsychiatry* 49 (3): 409–421.

Patenaude, A., and Rappeport, J. 1982. Surviving bone marrow transplantation: The patient in the other bed. *Annu. of Intern. Med.* 97: 915–918.

Petrillo, M., and Sanger, S. 1980. *Emotional Care of the Hospitalized Child.* 2nd ed. Philadelphia: J.B. Lippincott Company.

Perin, G., and Frase, D. 1985. Development of a program using general anesthesia for invasive procedures in a pediatric outpatient setting. *Journal of the Association of Pediatric Oncology Nurses* 3 (4): 8–10.

Pinkerton, R. et al. 1986. Autologous bone marrow transplantation in paediatric solid tumors. *Clinics in Haematology* 15 (1): 187–202.

Poplack, D., and Reaman, D. 1988 Acute lymphoblastic leukemia in childhood. *Pediatr. Clin. North Am.* 35 (4): 903–932.

Ramsay, N. 1989. Bone marrow transplantation in pediatric oncology. In Pizzo, P. and Polack, P. (eds.) *Principles and Practice of Pediatric Oncology.* Philadelphia: J.B. Lippincott Company, pp. 971–990.

Roesser, K. 1988. Bone marrow transplantation. *California Nursing Review* 10 (1): 14–43.

Rohaly, J. 1989. The use of busulfan therapy in bone marrow transplantation: A nursing overview. *Cancer Nursing* 12 (3): 144–152.

Ronan, J., and Caserza, C. 1988. Development of an educational handbook: Preparing the pediatric patient and family for pre-bone marrow transplant procedures and consults. *Journal of the Association Pediatric Oncology Nurses* 5 (1): 29.

Ruccione, K., and Weinberg, K. 1989. Late effects in multiple body systems. *Seminars in Oncology Nursing* 5 (1): 4–13.

Sanders, J. et al. 1985. Marrow transplantation for children in first remission of acute lymphocytic leukemia. *Blood* 66 (2): 460–462.

Sanders, J. et al. 1986a. Bone marrow transplantation experience for children with aplastic anemia. *Pediatrics* 77 (2): 179–186.

Sanders, J. et al. 1986b. Growth and development following marrow transplantation for leukemia. *Blood* 68 (5): 1129–1135.

Sanders, J. et al. 1988. Ovarian function following marrow transplantation for aplastic anemia or leukemia. *J. Clin. Oncol.* 6 (5): 813–818.

Sauers, S. et al. 1982. The challenges of physical care. In Fochtman, D., and Foley, G. (eds.) *Nursing Care of the Child with Cancer.* Boston: Little, Brown and Company.

Seeger, R. et al. 1988. Bone marrow transplantation for poor prognosis neuroblastoma. *Advances in Neuroblastoma Research.* 2: 203–213.

Serota, F. et al. 1981. Role of a child advocate in the selection of donors for pediatric bone marrow transplantation. *J. Pediatr.* 98 (5): 847–850.

Shannon, K. et al. 1987. Pediatric bone marrow transplantation: Intensive care management. *Journal of Intensive Care Medicine* 2: 328–344.

Smith, C. 1972. *Blood Diseases of Infancy and Childhood.* 3rd ed. St. Louis: C.V. Mosby Company.

Spitzer, G. et al. 1984. High dose chemotherapy with autologous bone marrow transplantation. *Cancer* 54: 1216–1225.

Standen, G. 1988. Wiskott-Aldrich syndrome: New perspectives in pathogenesis and management. *Journal of the Royal College of Physicians of London* 22 (2): 80–83.

Stone, L., and Church, J. 1973. *Childhood and Adolescence.* 3rd ed. New York: Random House.

Szeluga, D. et al. 1987. Nutritional support of bone marrow transplant recipients: A prospective, randomized clinical trial comparing total parenteral nutrition to an enteral feeding program. *Cancer Research* 47: 3309–3316.

Trigg, M. 1988. Bone marrow transplantation for treatment of leukemia in children. *Pediatr. Clin. North Am.* 35 (4): 933–948.

van der Wal, R., Nims, J., and Davies, B. 1988. Bone marrow transplantation in children: Nursing management of late effects. *Cancer Nursing* 11 (3): 132–143.

Waechter, E. et al. 1985. *Nursing Care of Children.* 10th ed. Philadelphia: J.B. Lippincott Company.

Wallace, M. et al. 1987. Parents of long-term survivors of childhood cancer: A preliminary survey to characterize concerns and needs. *Oncology Nursing Forum* 14 (3): 3943.

Waskerwitz, M. 1984. Special nursing care for children receiving chemotherapy *Journal of the Association of Pediatric Oncology Nurses* 1 (1): 1625.

Weisdorf, S. et al. 1984. Total parenteral nutrition in bone marrow transplantation: A clinical evaluation. *Journal of Pediatric Gastroenterlogy and Nutrition* 3 (1): 95–100.

Whaley, L., and Wong, D. 1983. *Nursing Care of Infants and Children.* 2nd ed. St. Louis: C.V. Mosby Company.

Wiley, F., and House, K. 1988. Bone marrow transplant in children. *Seminars in Oncology Nursing* 4 (1): 31–40.

Wiley, F., and Whalley, S. 1983. Allogeneic bone marrow transplantation for children with acute leukemia. *Oncology Nursing Forum* 10 (3): 49–53.

Wiley, F., Lindamood, M., and Pfefferbaum-Levine, 1984. Donor-patient relationship in pediatric bone marrow transplantation. *Journal of the Association of Pediatric Oncology Nurses* 1 (3): 8–14.

Wofford, L. 1985. Pain in children with cancer: An assessment. *Journal of the Association of Pediatric Oncology Nurses 2* (2): 34–37.

Yeager, A. 1986. Autologous bone marrow transplantation in patients with acute non-lymphocytic leukemia, using ex vivo marrow treatment with 4-hydroperoxycyclophosphamide. *N. Engl. J. Med. 315* (3): 141–147.

Zeltzer, L. et al. 1989. The management of pain associated with pediatric procedures. *Pediatr. Clin. North Am. 36* (4): 941–964.

Chapter 5

The Human Leukocyte Antigen (HLA) System, the Search for a Matching Donor, National Marrow Donor Program Development, and Marrow Donor Issues

Pamela A. Weinberg

When I was diagnosed with leukemia it was like a death sentence. It was a special shock because I had never been sick in my life. My brother and sister were tested, but neither of them matched me. I was able to find a donor through the National Marrow Donor Program, and had my transplant last spring. Now each day and every little thing has taken on special meaning for me.

Unrelated Marrow Transplant Recipient

When patients are referred for marrow transplant, some of the first questions that must be answered are: "What is the patient's tissue type?" and "Can a matching donor be located?" Patients and families in the already stressful situation of a life-threatening disease may feel overwhelmed by the need to absorb new information and respond to questions and situations that are completely unfamiliar to them. The additional burden of the vocabulary of the tissue typing world and the uncertainty of finding a donor can add significant stress to patients and their families. Nurses who have a clear understanding of the HLA system and the mechanism by which a donor is identified, can be very helpful in both explaining and guiding the family through a difficult process. This chapter will attempt to provide a basic understanding of the human leukocyte antigen (HLA) system and provide some general information on donor identification that can be useful in instructing and assisting patients and families.

The Human Leukocyte Antigen System

In order to understand the mechanism of the HLA system and its role in marrow transplantation, it is necessary to understand antigen-antibody reactions as they occur elsewhere in the body. It is sufficient to conceptualize these reactions as cells with markers—antigens—on their surfaces that fit, or "recognize," only similar antigens on other cell surfaces. If cells enter the system that have significantly different antigens on their surfaces, the existing or host system will mount an immune response, creating antibodies to coat or destroy the foreign antigens as well as their carrier cells.

There are two histocompatibility systems in the human body: the ABO system, and the HLA system. The ABO system refers to antigens found on the red blood cells and is familiar to most of us through information we have learned regarding blood donor compatibility. For instance, a person with type A blood is so called because of the presence of A antigens on his/her red blood cells. Figure 5.1 will remind nurses of the basics of the immune response as mounted by the ABO system. Similarly, the HLA system refers to a series of antigens found on white blood cells (leukocytes) and most other body cells. The HLA system is the dominant histocompatibility system and most important in marrow transplantation. The HLA system is highly varied—polymorphic—containing more than 90 unique antigens (as opposed to the two—A and B—defined in the ABO system). Because of this variation, and the presence of these antigens throughout the body, the human leukocyte antigens can be considered the "fingerprint" of each individual's body. The human leukocyte antigens are capable of mounting immune reactions similar to the ABO antigen response. Because the human leukocyte antigens are found throughout the body they are a major component of the body's immune system. Marrow is the only source of new blood cells in the adult human including erythrocytes, leukocytes, and platelets as well as lymphocytes, the key cells of the immune system.

Marrow is also the source for hematopoietic stem cells, the progenitor cells for all blood and lymphoid cells, and is thus the *source* for the human immune system. It is easiest to conceptualize the marrow, this rich source of leukocytes and lymphocytes, as a sort of sentinel system for the body. The leukocytes migrate throughout the system constantly identifying what is "self" and what is "not self" according to the antigens found on the cells within the body.

This can easily be described to patients in terms of what happens when a splinter enters the body. As the "marrow sentinels" (leukocytes) patrol the body and identify cells as either self or not self, they may encounter the invading splinter. Not recognizing the antigens found on the cells of the splinter, the sentinels define the splinter as not self. By a complex series of reactions, the body then mounts an immune response to rid its system of the invader, the splinter, and thus restore the equilibrium of all cells being identified as self.

Patients and families can better understand the importance of a perfectly matched marrow transplant when told that if healthy, immunologically competent marrow is transplanted into the patient's system, the new marrow will set about its old function of determining what is self or not self. If the donor marrow is insufficiently matched to the recipient's body, the donor marrow will not recognize the recipient's body as self and will begin to mount an immune response to the patient's body just as effectively as it would have done toward a splinter in its original or "home" body. This immune response of the graft directed against the antigens of the recipient is known as graft-versus-host disease, a complication that can be just as deadly as the patient's original disease.

The HLA system was first described by a single antigen, "Mac," in 1965. Subsequently, Mac was found to be a system of several closely linked genes. Mac is now known to be equivalent to A2, an antigen of the HLA-A locus. The HLA system

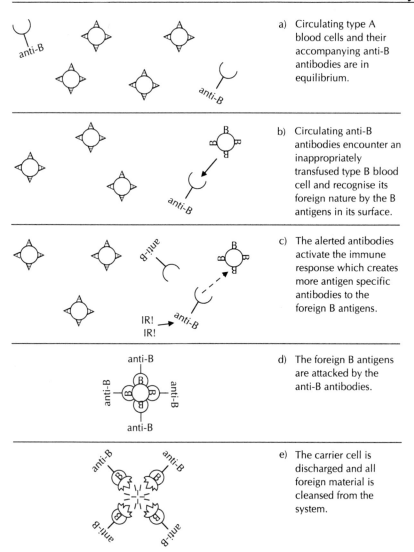

a) Circulating type A blood cells and their accompanying anti-B antibodies are in equilibrium.

b) Circulating anti-B antibodies encounter an inappropriately transfused type B blood cell and recognise its foreign nature by the B antigens in its surface.

c) The alerted antibodies activate the immune response which creates more antigen specific antibodies to the foreign B antigens.

d) The foreign B antigens are attacked by the anti-B antibodies.

e) The carrier cell is discharged and all foreign material is cleansed from the system.

Figure 5.1. Immune Response in the ABO Rh Histocompatibility System

is now known to include multiple loci including at least six antigen groups: HLA-A, B, C, DR, DQ, and DP, containing a total of more than 90 antigens. (Bruning, van Leeuwan, and van Rood 1975) Table 5.1 shows a complete list of the currently defined antigens. Antigens in the A, B, and C loci are referred to as Class I antigens, while the DR, DQ, and DP antigens are referred to as Class II antigens. By using increasingly fine typing methods, antigens once defined as a single specific antigen—specificities—have been found to be several different antigens or "splits." Referring again to Table 5.1, the originally defined broad antigen is shown in parenthesis following the split antigen. For example, note that antigens A23 and A24 are splits of A9. This means that an antigen originally defined as A9, was later found to actually be two antigens, A23 and A24. It is im-

Table 5.1. Acceptable Antigen Specificities

A	B (Private)	DR (Beta 1)
A1	B5	DR1
A2	B7	DR2
A3	B8	DR3
A9	B12	DR4
A10	B13	DR5
Aw19	B14	DRw6
A23(9)	B15	DR7
A24(9)	B16	DRw8
A25(10)	B17	DR9
A26(10)	B18	DRw10
A28	B21	DRw11(5)
A29(w19)	Bw22	DRw12(5)
A30(w19)	B27	DRw13(w6)
A31(w19)	B35	DRw14(w6)
A32(w19)	B37	DRw15(2)
Aw33(w19)	B38(16)	DRw16(2)
Aw34(10)	B39(16)	DRw17(3)
Aw36	B40	DRw18(3)
Aw43	Bw41	DR"BR"
Aw66(10)	Bw42	DR"5X6"
Aw68(28)	B44(12)	DR"5X8"
Aw69(28)	B45(12)	DRX
Aw74(w19)	Bw46	
AX	Bw47	
	B49(21)	
	Bw50(21)	
	B51(5)	
	Bw52(5)	
	Bw53	
	Bw54(w22)	
	Bw55(w22)	
	Bw56(w22)	
	Bw57(17)	
	Bw58(17)	Bw70
	Bw59	Bw71(w70)
	Bw60(w40)	Bw72(w70)
	Bw61(w40)	Bw73
	Bw62(15)	Bw75(15)
	Bw63(15)	Bw76(15)
	Bw64(14)	Bw76(15)
	Bw65(14)	Bw77(15)
	Bw67	BX

Table 5.2. Crossreactive Antigen Groups

A Locus
1. A1   A3   A11 A36
2. A9   A23 A24
3. A10 A25 A26 A34 A66 A43
4. A19 A29 A30 A31 A32 A33 A74
5. A2   A28 A68 A69

B Locus
1. B5   B18 B35 B51 B52 B53 B70 B71 B72
2. B12 B21 B44 B45 B49 B50
3. B14 B64 B65
4. B8   B59
5. B15 B17 B46 B57 B58 B62 B63 B70 B71 B72
   B75 B76 B77
6. B16 B38 B39 B67
7. B37
8. B7   B27 B42 B73
9. B7   B22 B54 B55 B56 B67
10. B7   B40 B41 B48 B60 B61
11. B13 B47

tigens in the original broad group as nonself. Many antigens, however, even those that do not come from the same parent group, may have some degree of compatibility with each other and are therefore classified as "crossreactive." Table 5.2 shows currently defined crossreactive groups. The ability to transplant marrow from a donor to a recipient successfully is always based on the degree of compatibility between the donor marrow and the recipient marrow. The varying antigeneity (strength) of the patient's and donor's antigens and the crossreactive nature of those antigens will either mitigate for or against the success of the transplant.

Definitions of HLA antigens are established periodically by a special HLA nomenclature committee of the World Health Organization (WHO). The WHO Nomenclature Committee usually bases its decisions on data presented by International HLA Workshops, which meet every three to five years to report results of collaborative study. The updated nomenclature then becomes the standard for national histocompatibility organizations. In the United States, the American

portant to define all possible splits when tissue typing patients, as splits are discreet antigens and may in many circumstances recognize other an-

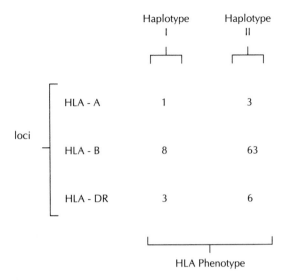

Figure 5.2. An Example of an HLA Phenotype

Society of Histocompatibility and Immunogenetics (ASHI) is such a national organization. Its functions include disseminating information about accepted antigens, setting standards for histocompatibility laboratories, and contributing to the research leading to further understanding of the HLA system.

Of particular importance in marrow transplantation is the inheritance mechanism of the human leukocyte antigens. The observed HLA antigens in a specific individual are called his or her HLA **phenotype** (see Figure 5.2). The phenotype consists of two sets of antigens; one set is inherited from the mother, and one set is inherited from the father. Each set is referred to as a **haplotype**, and one can be said to inherit one haplotype from one's father and one haplotype from one's mother. The genes that encode HLA antigens are clustered together in a region known as the HLA system on the short arm of the sixth chromosome. Referring to Figure 5.3 you can easily follow the inheritance of haplotypes from father and mother to offspring. It becomes readily apparent that there is a 25% chance that any two

siblings in a given family will match each other at both haplotypes.

With so many antigens in each of the human leukocyte antigen loci, the number of possible combinations that could form a given phenotype is over 26 million. Fortunately for the world of marrow transplantation, antigens form common linkages and are passed to the offspring in haplotype clusters. This kind of preferential association is referred to as positive linkage disequilibrium. The actual genetic makeup leading to the expression of the phenotype is known as the **genotype**. Genotypes are only definable by family study, and therefore what is most commonly discussed is the observed phenotype and component haplotypes of the HLA makeup of an individual.

Human leukocyte antigens can be typed by a variety of methods. Most common is the serological method of typing. This is quite similar to the typing method used in the ABO red blood system, in that it requires antisera. These are sera that have the ability to express antibodies to specific antigens. Antisera specific to certain antigens are placed in tiny wells in a tissue typing tray (see Figure 5.4). Lymphocytes from the individual to be typed are placed in each of the wells and after preparation and incubation the reaction is "read." Lymphocytes that are killed by the antisera obviously carry the antigen to which that antiserum is specific. Each of the human leukocyte antigens can be typed in this way.

Oligonucleotide and DNA probes are newer forms of typing and have several advantages and a few disadvantages. Oligonucleotide and DNA probes are used to detect differences in the nucleic acid sequences of the genes encoding HLA antigens. Since these sequences are unique to each specific antigen, the typing can be very exact. The technique breaks down the antigens into their molecular components. The resulting mixture is separated by molecular weight and forms an observable pattern that is specific to each antigen. The advantages of this system are that it requires very little blood or serum to perform the tests and that it is very accurate. DNA typing with

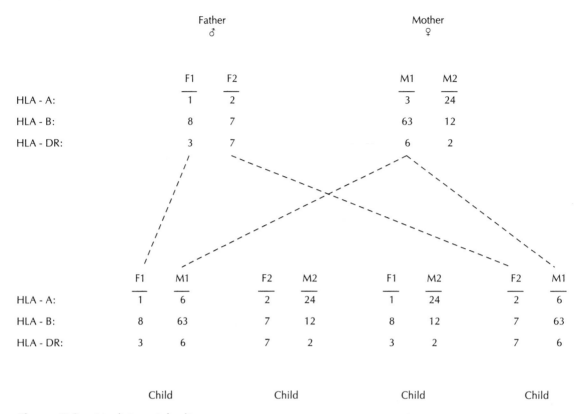

Figure 5.3.   Haplotype Inheritance

oligonucleotide probes is a new development, and the availability of reagents and technology is still very limited. Currently, the dominant mode of HLA typing continues to be serological.

The Search for a Matching Donor

A clear understanding of the basics of antigen inheritance and donor selection are important if the nurse is to assist the family in understanding the dynamics of finding a donor.

In seeking a donor for a patient, the HLA-A, -B, and -DR antigens are examined and a donor will be sought who matches the patient at all three loci (six antigens). Certainly the first source for a donor that will be explored is the immediate family. As mentioned earlier, there is a 25% chance that any two siblings in a given family will match. A patient lucky enough to have an identical twin may be a candidate for what is called a syngeneic transplant. In this case, there is complete genetic identity at all histocompatibility loci (see Figure 5.5). A patient who does not have a twin donor, but has a matching donor in the family may be a candidate for an allogeneic transplant.

Patients who do not find a marrow donor within their immediate family may face a desperate search for a donor. Many avenues of search are open to them, but all involve dedication of energy, time, intellect, and finance that most families will find overwhelmingly burdensome. The

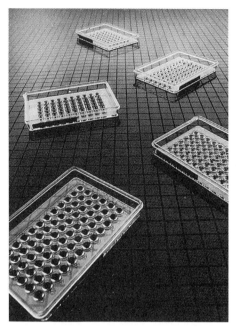

Source: One Lambda, Inc.

Figure 5.4. HLA Typing Tray

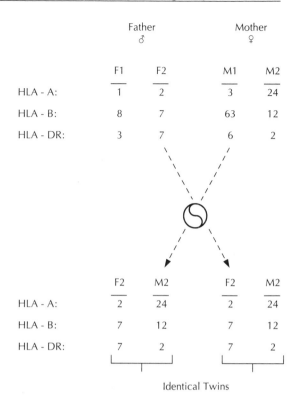

	Father ♂		Mother ♀	
	F1	F2	M1	M2
HLA - A:	1	2	3	24
HLA - B:	8	7	63	12
HLA - DR:	3	7	6	2

	F2	M2	F2	M2
HLA - A:	2	24	2	24
HLA - B:	7	12	7	12
HLA - DR:	7	2	7	2

Identical Twins

Figure 5.5. Haplotype Inheritance for Identical Twins

assistance of a knowledgeable histocompatibility specialist within the marrow transplant program can be invaluable to these families as they decide on their options in pursuing a donor.

A family histocompatibility study done at the time of referral for marrow transplant will give an indication of the source of antigens found within the patient's own HLA system (see Figure 5.6). Patients with a single very rare antigen and five common antigens may be well advised to pursue an extended family search for a matching donor. As can be observed in Figure 5.6, the patient has a single rare antigen in one haplotype, which is not shared by the other members of his sibling group. The use of the family study shows that the source of this antigen is on the mother's side of the family and gives clear direction for pursuing an extended family search through the mother's side. An examination of uncles, aunts, and cousins on the mother's side of the family may dis-

close an individual carrying the single rare antigen and also harboring the other more common antigens passed through to the patient by the mother and the father.

Failing to find a suitably matched donor within the immediate or extended family, patients must search for a donor within the unrelated population. It is worthwhile at this point to discuss the racial distribution of HLA antigens as this can be a significant factor in directing an unrelated donor search.

Patients and families can be helped to understand this concept by describing the inheritance of human leukocyte antigens in terms of inheritance of other more familiar features. It is generally recognized that two redheaded parents

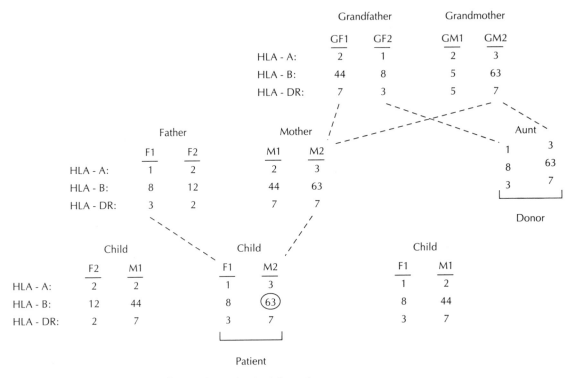

Figure 5.6. Family HLA Chart—Genealogical Search

will often have a redheaded child and similarly, two dark-skinned parents will usually have a dark-skinned child. We inherit our HLA-type in much the same way that we inherit our hair color, skin color, and other physical features. Thus, the most logical source for a matching marrow donor is within one's own family and secondarily, within one's own ethnic group.

Figure 5.7 shows genetic distances as described by the Third Histocompatibility Workshop and Conference held in Saporo, Japan, in the summer of 1986. The greater the genetic distance, the more disparate the group antigens. This international workshop focused specifically on the inheritance of HLA-types in ethnic groups. It was shown clearly that certain antigens follow ethnic groups in their migration paths around the world and that those antigens will only be found within that ethnic group. Many antigens, however, are classified as "pan-ethnic" and will be found with some frequency in all ethnic groups (Wakisaka et al. 1986).

The ethno-specific antigens are of particular interest when searching for a matching donor for a patient. Table 5.3 shows the HLA-A, -B, and -DR loci with their relative frequency in various ethnic groups. The HLA-type shown in Figure 5.8 is that of an African-American patient. Careful scrutiny of this HLA type shows that four of the six antigens of interest are pan-ethnic antigens, and two of the antigens, one at the A and one at the B locus, are most commonly found in the African-American population. This patient will be well advised to pursue a search within the African-American community in hopes of finding a similar donor who has inherited the specific African-

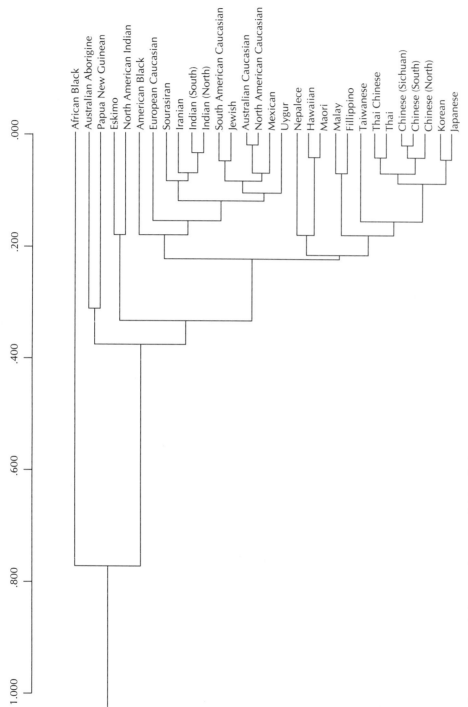

Figure 5.7. Phylogenetic Tree of 30 Ethnic Groups Constructed by UPG Method

Table 5.3. HLA Frequencies by Ethnic Group

HLA-A	C	N	O	HLA-B	C	N	O	HLA-DR	C	N	O
A1	27.0	6.5	1.0	B5	15.5	4.6	36.4	DR1	15.4	9.6	12.1
A2	45.7	27.3	43.2	B7	17.3	17.0	11.4	DR2	25.2	28.5	36.0
A3	23.0	14.2	1.1	B8	16.1	5.8	0.2	DR3	21.0	31.6	3.2
A9	29.3	26.1	59.6	B12	24.2	21.4	12.8	DR4	21.1	9.6	41.4
A10	11.0	8.2	18.8	B13	5.5	1.4	4.0	DR5	19.5	24.8	4.3
A11	11.8	1.1	17.2	B14	6.8	8.0	0.2	DRw6	2.5	6.5	5.3
A23	4.6	20.4	1.1	B15	11.3	2.5	17.1	DR7	23.5	18.6	1.0
A24	16.7	5.7	58.8	B16	9.3	3.6	6.1	DRw8	5.4	10.8	12.6
A25	3.8	0.8	0.1	B17	8.7	28.0	1.7	DRw9	2.4	5.3	23.0
A26	7.2	7.4	18.7	B18	10.8	7.7	0.0	DRw10	1.3	3.7	1.2
A28	8.3	16.6	1.1	B21	7.0	6.3	0.6				
A29	7.6	12.3	0.4	Bw22	5.5	1.6	22.1				
A30	4.8	28.3	0.3	B27	7.6	3.0	0.8				
A31	5.6	4.4	15.3	B35	17.5	12.1	14.1				
A32	8.3	3.0	0.1	B37	3.1	0.8	1.1				
Aw33	3.3	9.0	13.1	B38	5.3	0.0	0.4				
Aw34	1.0	12.5	1.9	B39	4.0	3.6	5.7				
Aw36	0.7	3.3	0.5	B40	10.8	3.5	29.5				
Aw43	0.1	1.9	0.0	Bw41	2.5	2.5	0.7				
				Bw42	0.6	14.8	1.2				
				B44	22.6	13.7	12.5				
				B45	2.0	7.7	0.3				
				Bw46	0.8	—	—				
				Bw47	1.1	0.3	0.4				
				Bw48	4.5	2.2	4.6				
				B49	2.5	4.9	0.6				
				Bw50	12.6	1.4	0.0				
				B51	2.9	2.7	15.9				
				Bw52	1.5	1.9	20.5				
				Bw53	0.0	12.6	0.2				
				Bw54	4.4	0.0	14.1				
				Bw55	1.1	1.6	5.8				
				Bw56	6.5	0.0	2.2				
				Bw57	2.2	7.7	0.0				
				Bw58	0.9	20.3	1.7				
				Bw59	7.9	1.6	4.2				
				Bw60	2.9	2.7	12.7				
				Bw61	10.1	0.8	16.8				
				Bw62	1.2	1.9	16.7				
				Bw63		0.8	0.4				

C-Caucasian, N-Negro, O-Oriental
Source: Histocompatibility Testing, 1980.

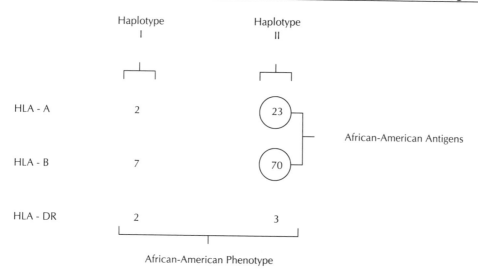

Figure 5.8. Example of an African-American Phenotype

American antigens in conjunction with the pan-ethnic antigens.

Similar patterns of inheritance are seen in other ethnic groups. In fact, whenever a human population settles in a geographic area and remains fairly isolated over a long period of time, specific antigens will become prevalent in that population. Studies have shown that antigen frequencies differ from one province to another in France (Ohayon and Cambon-Thomsen 1986), and HLA-types seem to differ significantly between varying Native American tribes in North America. It is also interesting that the prevalence of certain antigens can track the historical migration paths of nomadic peoples. B48 is found commonly in peoples along the migration path of the mammoth hunters, and A1 and A3 are found in China along those pathways travelled by Genghis Kahn (Wakisaka et al. 1986).

The search for a distantly related or unrelated donor either through a genealogical study or through recruitment of donors within an ethnic group can be a frustrating and overwhelming task for any patient or family. The obvious solution to the problem is the development of a large, ethn-ically diverse, unrelated donor registry. Such a registry could provide marrow donors for many patients in need of marrow transplant who lack a suitably matched sibling donor. The next section of this chapter will deal specifically with the development of such a registry and the projected use and growth of such a service in the future of marrow transplantation.

National Marrow Donor Program Development

The first unrelated donor marrow transplant took place December 3, 1973, at Memorial Sloan-Kettering Cancer Center in New York City (O'Reilly et al. 1977). The patient, a five-month-old boy with severe combined immunodeficiency, was transplanted not once, but seven times, from the same unrelated donor. This donor had been identified in a search through the HLA-typed blood donor file of the Blood Bank at Rigshopitalet in Copenhagen, Denmark. The series of seven transplants was spread over a 23-month period. Each successive transplant was performed to improve or correct the patient's physical condition. After the seventh transplant on November 7, 1975, engraftment was achieved and hematologic function rapidly became normal. The patient was discharged from the hospital on April 4, 1976, and returned home.

In the mid 1970s, pools of HLA-typed individuals began to be developed in laboratories and blood banks around the United States. Aggressive transplant centers made use of these local files to find an occasional unrelated donor for a patient in need of marrow transplant who had no matching donor within his or her own family. Because of the lack of availability of large numbers of HLA-typed individuals, the continued impression that marrow transplantation in general was quite risky, and the completely experimental nature of unrelated transplants, little attention was paid to the possibility of widespread unrelated transplants. In the late 1970s more attention was given to the possibility of unrelated transplants, but lack of available donors continued to be a problem, and few unrelated transplants were done.

In 1979, a normally inconspicuous event occurred that ultimately had tremendous importance in the field of unrelated transplants. A nine-year-old girl by the name of Laura Graves was diagnosed with acute leukemia in her hometown of Fort Collins, Colorado. After diagnosis and workup by local physicians, the entire family was HLA-typed to determine if a suitable donor could be found within the sibling group. Unfortunately, no suitably matched donor was found among the other three children. The family was referred to the Fred Hutchinson Cancer Research Center for ongoing treatment of the child's disease. Facing the lack of any suitably matched family donor, the family requested the staff at the Fred Hutchinson Cancer Research Center to search all possible pools of typed donors to find an unrelated donor for their daughter. Bearing in mind that the chance of finding an unrelated donor in the general population is very remote, it was astounding that an unrelated donor was located within the

laboratory staff at the cancer center itself. The donor located was a perfect six-antigen match for Laura Graves. Laura received her transplant, the donor marrow engrafted without complication, she suffered no graft-versus-host disease, and after 100 days Laura went home with her family as an apparently healthy child. The unfortunate ending to this story is that Laura's disease relapsed about a year later and she died from recurrent leukemia two years after the transplant. The initial success of this unrelated transplant and the perseverance of the Graves family, however, gave a clear message to many other patients and families: If a donor could be located, not just a donor within one's own family, but an unrelated donor, these patients could be offered new hope for life and health. Many families, facing the lack of an available family donor, returned to their homes and began to recruit, or invite participation, from friends and neighbors into local, family-operated donor registries.

It should require little effort to imagine the very frustrating and fragmented system that began to develop in the United States. Transplant centers searching for an unrelated donor for one of their patients might recall that one of their patients had gone home (ostensibly to die) and had reported recruiting local residents and having tissue typings done. Assertive transplant physicians might call this family and ask if a donor could be found for the current patient within their small local file. In the process of this inquiry, the transplanter might be referred to other families that had done similar recruitment. Additionally, inquiries might be forwarded to blood banks around the country that had HLA-typed their platelet donors. The search activity was very fragmented, tremendously time-consuming, and usually unsuccessful. Most of the patients who were the subjects of these searches died without ever finding an unrelated donor.

Laura's pioneering experience and the hope that she was given by her unrelated donor were not forgotten. Dr. Robert Graves, Laura's father, maintained contact with other patients, families, and physicians. In 1985, Dr. Graves contacted some of these physicians and families, and suggested that they make a mutual plea to the United States government to underwrite the costs of establishing a national marrow donor program. This group of physicians and concerned families were successful in gaining an audience with several members of Congress. They were able to show that if donors could be located quickly, and marrow transplants could be performed early in the disease process, the patient outcomes would improve dramatically. Their persistent efforts in contacting and lobbying members of Congress to support such a national marrow donor program were successful, and in July of 1986 the United States government awarded a contract for the establishment of the National Marrow Donor Program (originally called the National Bone Marrow Donor Registry) through the Department of Naval Research to a collaborative group consisting of representatives of the American Association of Blood Banks, the American Red Cross, and the Council of Community Blood Centers. Projections made at that time indicated that a file of 100,000 donors would provide a matched unrelated donor for between 40 and 75% of the patients in need of bone marrow transplant (Beatty et al. 1988), and that approximately 6,000 patients a year might make use of such a registry in the long run (Gale 1986). Figure 5.9 shows the structure of the program that was designed to fulfill the contract. This program was set up to perform three contract tasks: develop a large, centrally organized registry of unrelated potential marrow donors; develop a system to coordinate activities of donor centers and transplant centers in order to facilitate unrelated marrow transplants; and perform ongoing research on unrelated marrow transplantation, donor motivation and outcomes, and histocompatibility issues.

Program development from July 1986 to September 1987 involved many tasks:

1. Development and operational staff were hired.

2. Computer systems were designed to manage search activities.

3. It was acknowledged that transplant centers should be invited to participate in the program, but it was also acknowledged that it would be important in the long run to have adequate criteria for screening centers with the essential expertise to perform unrelated transplants with a reasonable probability of success. A team of transplanters was recruited from around the United States. They met in the fall of 1986 to establish criteria for participating transplant centers (see Table 5.4). Once these criteria were defined, letters were sent to transplant centers all over the United States inviting them to submit applications for participation.

4. The terms of the contract had required the development of a large, centrally organized registry of HLA-typed potential marrow donors. There were, however, very limited funds available for establishment of the program. It was therefore necessary to focus donor recruitment on those locations that already had large numbers of HLA-typed individuals. This led to a program focus on blood banks and their HLA-typed apheresis or platelet donor populations. Once again, the program administration recognized that it would be absolutely necessary in the long run to have membership criteria for participating donor centers. Blood bank physicians conferred on this issue and developed a set of criteria that was incorporated into the standards of the program (see Table 5.5). As these criteria were developed, invitations and information about the developing program were sent to blood centers across the United States inviting their participation.

5. Collection centers were defined as a third category of participating member centers. Many of the donor centers (blood centers) around the United States that had agreed to participate and recruit potential marrow donors from among their HLA-typed apheresis populations were not located in towns that had an active transplant program. It was therefore necessary to find local physicians and surgeons skilled enough and willing

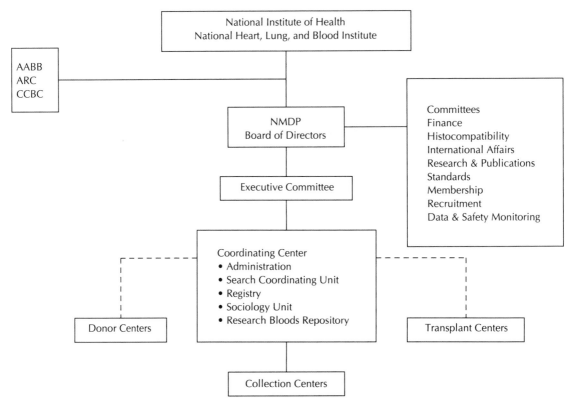

AABB – American Association of Blood Banks; ARC – American Red Cross; CCBC – Council of Community Blood Centers; NMDP – National Marrow Donor Program

Figure 5.9. National Marrow Donor Program Organizational Chart

to perform marrow collections on donors managed through those donor centers. It was acknowledged by all participants in the program that the greatest risk to the donor lay in the actual collection of the marrow, and it was therefore felt to be absolutely necessary that the collection centers recruited into the program be of high quality and meet stringent criteria. Once again criteria were established for collection centers and these were made part of the program standards (Table 5.6).

6. As transplant centers, collection centers, and donor centers began to apply for membership with the program, the second stage of activities began as well. This consisted of actual recruitment

of donors for participation in the program. Early attempts at marrow donor recruitment in localized blood centers had involved a multiple-step process of mailing out information in increasing detail and assessing the ongoing interest of donors. While this was a cumbersome process at best, many local donor centers had been very effective and successful in recruiting from among their apheresis platelet population in this fashion, with some centers having an overall consent rate as high as 70% (McCullough et al. 1988). No matter what the technique used at individual donor centers, the overall emphasis of the program focused on providing complete information so that donors could make a truly informed consent

Table 5.4. Transplant Center Participation Criteria

1. Centers must have performed at least ten allogeneic transplants per year during the previous 24 months and at least 30 in the previous five years.
2. A dedicated transplant team must have been in place for a minimum of two years.
3. Documentation of experience:
   There should be published or documented experience with marrow transplantation. Centers must submit a completed "Marrow Transplant History" form at the time of application documenting all allogeneic transplants for the previous five years.
4. The center director must have had two years experience in an NMDP-accredited transplant center or in a center recognized by publications in peer-reviewed journals to be capable and experienced. One of these years may be a period of training, but at least the previous year must be one in which the director had primary responsibility for the management of transplant recipients.
5. Designated nursing unit for marrow transplantation.
   This involves a nursing unit with specialized personnel and established procedures.
6. Patient care facility with proper air handling system to prevent nosocomial infections due to microbial material disseminated from central heating/cooling systems.
7. Protocols approved by local IRB:
   Local IRB approval is the minimal level of protocol review for participation in the program. Transplant centers submit protocols for transplantation using unrelated donors and copies of the IRB approval.
8. Adequate support by an HLA laboratory:
   There must be documented evidence of a willingness to participate and the laboratory must be accredited by the American Society of Histocompatibility and Immunogenetics.
9. Adequate blood bank support:
   A blood bank should agree to provide adequate blood component support and, where necessary, CMV testing. Irradiated blood products must be available.
10. Documented evidence that radiation therapy support is available if needed.
11. Compliance with patient outcome reporting policies established by the program, including completion of all required forms.
12. The Chief Financial Officer or Hospital Administrator must review the application and sign the Participation Agreement acknowledging financial responsibility for services rendered.
13. MCI electronic mail.
    All centers are required to participate in the MCI electronic mail network which links transplant centers with the National Coordinating Center. All search results are reported through this mechanism.
14. MLC data will be collected prospectively, and results will be analyzed as part of the research projects on extended histocompatibility testing coordinated through the National Marrow Donor Program.
15. The maximum degree of mismatch that will be allowed in any transplant facilitated by the National Marrow Donor Program will be a five-to-six antigen match.

to participate. Unfortunately, during the first year of donor recruitment, it became apparent that success rates across the United States would not be nearly as successful as they had been in some of the localized centers. Even after multiple contacts with apheresis platelet populations, the overall consent rate hovered at around 30%, yielding a participating donor pool of about 8,000 donors when the program began operation.

Program development had progressed sufficiently by September of 1987 that staff felt ready to begin accepting search requests. The first search request was accepted on September 1, 1987. As of that date there were 49 participating

Table 5.5. Donor Center Criteria

1. Center must have access to the following accredited facilities:
   a) Blood bank for collection of autologous blood units.
   b) Blood bank laboratory for infectious disease markers and CBC as defined by the standards.
   c) Blood typing laboratory.
   d) HLA typing laboratory for MLA-A, HLA-B typing newly recruited donors.
2. Center must have an HLA-typed apheresis file of at least 250 donors or be able to show community support for funding the HLA typing of at least 250 new marrow donors.
3. Center must have access to an IBM-compatible personal computer.
4. Center must be willing to designate a coordinator and time for that coordinator to work with the program.
5. Center must be willing to participate in MCI electronic mail communication network.
6. Center must be willing to have all requested HLA-DR typing performed at center contract laboratories.
7. Center must have a donor advocate identified and must offer this as an option to all donors.
8. Center must establish a cooperative relationship with a collection center.
9. Center must be willing to use and complete NMDP standard data forms.
10. Center must be willing to merge donor data on a routine basis with the NMDP Central Data File (Registry).
11. Center must have qualified medical director for their local program.
12. Center must carry liability insurance; suggested amount is $2,000,000.

donor centers, ten participating transplant centers, and 8,000 donors registered in the file. The first months were slow, as transplant centers became aware of the availability of the resource. Only one or two searches were received each month.

On November 25 of 1987, a search request was received at the National Marrow Donor Program offices in St. Paul, Minnesota, for a six-year-old girl with acute leukemia. The child was terribly ill, having been admitted to the hospital in relapse. The entire staff felt a tremendous sense of urgency. The search was run rapidly and a six-antigen match was identified that same day. The donor center nearest the donor was contacted and preparations began immediately for collection and transport of the marrow. The workup moved ahead swiftly, and on December 15 of 1987, marrow was collected from a donor in Milwaukee, Wisconsin, and flown through a raging blizzard to the Fred Hutchinson Cancer Research Center in Seattle, Washington, where it was transfused into the patient. The marrow engrafted, the child recovered, and was sent home several months later. This was the first transplant facilitated by the National Marrow Donor Program, and it began the escalation of activity and the long string of transplants that continues to grow.

It is useful, particularly for the practicing nurse clinician, to have some awareness of the progression of activities required in a donor search. Families will often inquire about the progress of their search and be confused and concerned over the time that is required to move through the process and actually deliver marrow to the bedside.

Participating transplant centers with the program may submit searches on behalf of their patients. The initial search, if received at the National Marrow Donor Program offices by noon, is run overnight, and the results (a list of potential marrow donors in decreasing order of compatibility [see Figure 5.10]) (NMDP 1989) are sent over the electronic network to the transplant center, where they appear on a computer screen at that center the next morning. Transplant centers can review the search results with the patient, family, and referring physician and decide

Table 5.6. Collection Center Criteria

Collection center criteria have been adopted by the Board of Directors of the NMDP to assure donor safety. Standards have also been established, many of which address the collection, storage, processing, labeling, and transportation of bone marrow collections facilitated by the NMDP. All collection centers participating in the NMDP must meet these criteria and must agree to comply with the standards of the NMDP.

1. The hospital must have an experienced bone marrow team that collects bone marrow on a regular basis.
   a) The bone marrow collection physician must have performed at least ten prior aspirations of bone marrow for transplantation. He or she must have done at least four collections in the last one year.
   b) The collection team must have a designated responsible physician who must agree along with the anesthesiologist that the donor is acceptable for the procedure. He or she must make certain that the donor has one or more autologous red cell units available prior to the marrow collection.
2. Hospital must provide a wide range of emergency and intensive care services.
   a) Marrow collection hospital must be accredited by the Joint Commission for Hospital Accreditation.
   b) Hospital must provide a surgical operating room and must have a medical intensive care unit.
   c) Collection center hospital must agree to have anesthesia supervised by a licensed, board certified anesthesiologist.
3. Hospital must have a staff which is experienced in handling bone marrow.
   a) Collection, storage and labeling of marrow must comply with standards of the NMDP.
   b) In the event of a medical emergency that requires homologous blood transfusion, collection center hospital must have irradiated blood products available for the donor.
4. Collection team must have a designated liaison with the donor center and NMDP staff.
5. Collection center liaison must complete the data collection forms in a timely manner.

whether any of the potential donors are sufficiently well matched to be of interest for the patient.

Transplant centers may then request that more extensive tissue typing be done on selected donors. The entire file of the National Marrow Donor Program is HLA-A and -B typed, but at the time of this writing only about 40% of the file is completely typed for HLA-A, -B, and -DR. Consequently, the second step in most search processes is to request HLA-DR typing on selected donors who are matched at the A and B loci. Requests for such HLA-DR typing are submitted by the transplant center to the National Marrow Donor Program offices. These requests are transmitted via the electronic network to the appropriate donor centers where selected donors are managed. Local donor centers call in selected donors, collect blood specimens, and forward those

blood specimens to national contract laboratories. These laboratories complete the HLA-DR typing and forward that typing information over the electronic network to the National Marrow Donor Program offices where it is automatically incorporated into the central computer system. Updated information thus appears on an almost daily basis on the computer screens at the transplant centers, so that they are kept constantly up-to-date on the status of their searches in progress.

As HLA-DR typings are reported to the transplant centers, the transplant centers may identify one or more donors who are sufficiently matched at all three loci to request mixed lymphocyte cultures (MLCs) for their patients. Once again the request from the transplant center is submitted to the National Marrow Donor Program and a subsequent request is forwarded to the appropriate donor center over the electronic network. Donor

NATIONAL MARROW DONOR PROGRAM
FORM 110A, PRELIMINARY SEARCH RESULTS
TRANSPLANT CENTER: 508   DATE OF RERORT: 01/04/90

Recipient: Smith, John   Search: 3
NMDP ID: 902-616-2   Date of Search: 01/04/90
Local ID: 999999999   Diagnosis: CML
HLA: A2   A3   B7   B35   DR1   DR4   Age: 40

Line No.	Donor Ref. No.	M Grd	A G E	S E X	ABO RH	C M V	A	B	B4,6	DRB1	DRB3/4	DQ	L A B
1	00-3609-5	111	41	M	A+	+	A2 ,3	B7 ,35		DR1 ,4		DQ1 ,3	
2	00-4040-2	111	40	M	A+	−	A2 ,3	B7 ,35		DR1 ,4		DQ1 ,3	
3	01-9563-6	111	52	M	AB+	I	A2 ,3	B7 ,35	B6	DR1 ,4	DR53	DQ5 ,7	
4	04-5490-0	111	43	M	A−		A2, 3	B7 ,35	B6	DR1 ,4	DR53	DQ1 ,3	
5	00-6172-1	211	35	F	B+		A2 ,11	B7 ,35		DR1 ,4	DR53	DQ1 ,3	1
6	00-9045-6	211	24	M	A+		A2 ,11	B7 ,35	B6	DR1 ,4	DR53	DQ5 ,7	3
7	01-0029-7	211	34	F	O+	−	A2 ,11	B7 ,35	B6	DR1 ,4	DR53	DQ1 ,3	2
8	01-6606-6	211	43	F	AB+		A2 ,11	B7 ,35	B4,6	DR1 ,4	DR53	DQ5 ,8	3
9	02-9676-4	211	27	M	B+		A2 ,11	B7 ,35	B6,6	DR1 ,4	DR53	DQ1 ,3	
10	03-1554-9	211	44	F			A2 ,11	B7 ,35	B6	DR1 ,4	DR53	DQ1 ,3	

Figure 5.10.   Sample Form 110A

centers call in their selected donors, collect the blood specimens, and forward these by Federal Express to the requesting transplant center for preparation and completion of the MLC. Many transplant centers do not actually use the MLC as a determinant in donor selection, but in order to complete the ongoing research on the effectiveness of the MLC as a predictor of marrow transplant outcome, transplant centers are required to report all MLC data to the NMDP data registry.

Once a donor has been identified as a compatible or acceptable match for a given patient, the transplant center notifies the National Marrow Donor Program, which, in turn, notifies the selected donor's managing donor center. Donors then move into the workup phase of the search.

The first step of the workup phase is a donor information session. Donors are asked to come into the local donor center with a significant other and meet with members of the local donor center

staff including the medical director and coordinator. Donors are offered the opportunity to view a film depicting marrow transplantation and collection, are offered an opportunity to discuss the disease and prognosis of their particular patient with the medical director, and have an opportunity to ask questions about the collection process and the risks to their own health. Once the information session is complete, donors are asked to go home and carefully consider their decision to proceed with the process. Donors are asked to call the center in a day or two after they have had a chance to think it over, and are reassured that they have every right to decline further participation at that point. Donors are further cautioned that they should make a good decision at this point, since a decision to not participate later in the process may endanger the recipient's life.

The second step in the donor workup process is the donor physical exam. In order to protect the rights and confidentiality of the donor, a third-party physical exam is scheduled with a physician in the community who is completely uninvolved with marrow transplant. This physical exam is meant to assure that the donor is physically capable of withstanding the rigors of the marrow collection process. It includes chest x-ray, EKG, complete blood work, and pulmonary function tests.

Donors who consent to participate after the information session and who pass the physical exam are ready to be scheduled for marrow collection. The managing donor center in the donor's local community works with the transplant center and collection center to coordinate the activities involved in moving toward collection and transplant of the marrow. Patients at this point will undergo a rigorous preparation for the marrow transplant, and it is absolutely necessary that the collection be scheduled to coincide with "D-Day" for the patient. It is often a source of frustration and puzzlement to the transplant centers that it can be difficult to schedule these collections, but it is important to bear in mind that donors have lives and constraints of their own. Often a donor will wish to wait until after some sort of holiday or family event, or will wish to get through some transient family illness before agreeing to participate. Transplant centers have the option of communicating to the donor center a particular urgency in completing a transplant, and donor centers and donors are amenable to meeting the needs of transplant centers and patients whenever possible.

A couple of weeks prior to the actual marrow collection, the donor is seen by the marrow collection physician at the collection center and by the anesthesiologist who once again verifies that the donor is an acceptable candidate for marrow collection. On the date of the marrow collection itself, the donor enters the hospital (usually in the early morning hours) and is taken to the operating room where he or she receives either general or spinal anesthesia (donors are offered this option at most centers, with approximately 50% choosing each mode of anesthesia). The donor is placed on his or her stomach and the marrow is removed through large needles inserted into the back of the pelvic bone. The marrow is filtered as it is collected and placed in a standard blood bag for transport.

Representatives from the local donor center or collection center then transport the marrow to the transplant center as rapidly as possible. Standards of the National Marrow Donor Program indicate that marrow should be transported and transfused within 24 hours of collection. Within the continental United States, this is certainly not a problem, but as the program has stretched and expanded around the world, it has become an increasing concern that marrow be transported quickly. Fortunately, in this age of expanding technology and shortened distances, it is now possible to transport and deliver marrow within 24 hours of collection to almost any location on the globe. The entire process from initial computer search to delivery of the marrow at the bedside takes an average of 120 days.

An important component of the National Marrow Donor Program standards and practice is the maintenance of donor and recipient confidentiality. Prior to establishment of the National Marrow Donor Program, there were instances of donor and recipient harassment (Caplan 1983) which led to concern over the protection of the identities of these individuals. It is therefore the policy of the National Marrow Donor Program that donors and recipients not know each other's identity before transplant and are only allowed to communicate in writing using first names for the first months after transplant. During this period, all communications are screened by coordinators at transplant centers and donor centers to assure protection of the donor's and the recipient's identities. If, after this period, both the donor and the recipient are persistent in their desire to communicate directly or even meet, the standards of the program do permit direct communication. Interestingly enough, surprisingly few patients and their donors actually continue communication beyond the first few months after transplant.

Another particularly interesting aspect of the marrow donor program is its research into donor motivation. Ongoing research is an integral part of the program and a particular emphasis has been placed on the motivation and life outcomes of donors. Extensive questionnaires have been developed to review donor motivation both before and after the transplant and personal telephone interviews are conducted as well. It is expected that results of this research will be published soon (Simmons).

An ongoing concern of the National Marrow Donor Program is donor physical safety. Most of the standards of the program are set up to protect the safety of the donor in his/her management at the donor center and in his/her care at the collection center, and to assure that, once donors have given a marrow donation, their marrow will be used at a center where patients have a reasonably good prognosis. It is always important to be able to reflect to donors the statistical outcomes of previous marrow transplants and to accurately outline for them the risks that they undergo in agreeing to become a marrow donor. Previously published data indicate that very few marrow donation procedures result in any adverse effect for the donor (Bortin et al. 1983), and that all adverse outcomes have been resolved without sequellae. Within the first 250 marrow donations facilitated through the National Marrow Donor Program there were approximately 20 donor safety incidents (usually involving local infection or unusual pain, and some involving anesthesia reactions including epidural leaks and allergic hypotensive episodes). Similar to the earlier reported data, all of these donor physical incidents have been resolved without sequellae and, on follow-up questioning, nearly 100% of these donors report their desire to participate in marrow donation a second time if possible (NMDP 1989).

Since the opening of the program in September, 1987, tremendous strides have been made within the National Marrow Donor Program and the availability of unrelated donors for transplant has increased enormously. From those first days with a donor file of only 8,000 and only ten domestic participating transplant centers, the program has grown to a registry of over 200,000 donors with over 35 transplant centers in the United States and around the world participating in both transplants and ongoing research (see Figures 5.11, 5.12, and 5.13). The Program transferred from the Office of Naval Research to the National Heart, Lung, and Blood Institute in May of 1989, but internal structure, tasks, and goals remained unchanged.

Recall, if you will, the initial contract tasks that were assigned to the National Marrow Donor Program as it began its activities in July of 1986:

1. Develop a large centrally organized registry of potential marrow donors.

2. Develop a system to coordinate activities of donor centers and transplant centers in order to facilitate unrelated marrow transplants.

3. Perform ongoing research on unrelated marrow transplantation, donor motivation outcomes, and histocompatibility.

It is obvious from the growth of the file that donor recruitment has grown far beyond the initial involvement of a few thousand apheresis platelet donors. Since December of 1988, donor recruitment has expanded out of the blood centers into the general community and special emphasis has been placed on recruitment within ethnic minority groups. Donor recruitment continues at a pace of about 5,000 new donors per month. As new HLA types are added to the file each month, new potential donors are identified for patients in need of marrow transplant. As the file has grown, the number of transplants per month has increased as well, and, as of the date of this writing, over 20 transplants per month are being facilitated through the National Marrow Donor Program. This is an interesting contrast to the total number of 250 unrelated transplants that had been done worldwide as of 1987 (I.B.M.T.R. 1987). The international development of the program is also of importance in the growth of the file and the increasing numbers of potential donors available. Donor registries have been devel-

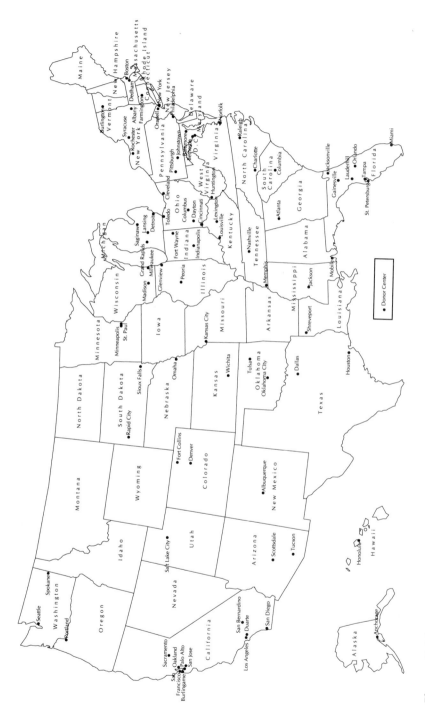

Figure 5.11. NMDP Domestic Donor Centers

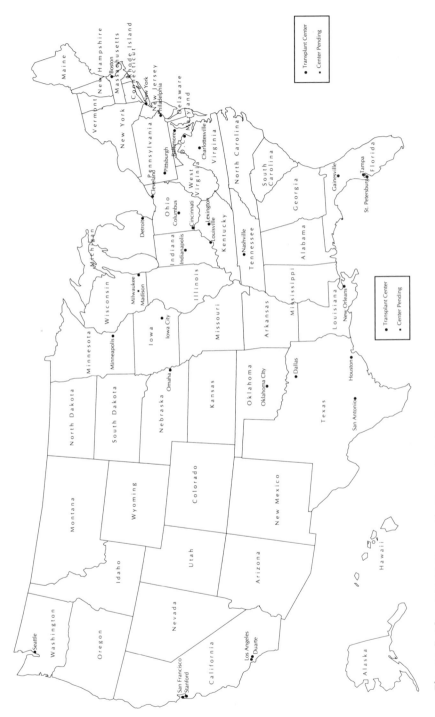

Figure 5.12. NMDP Domestic Transplant Centers

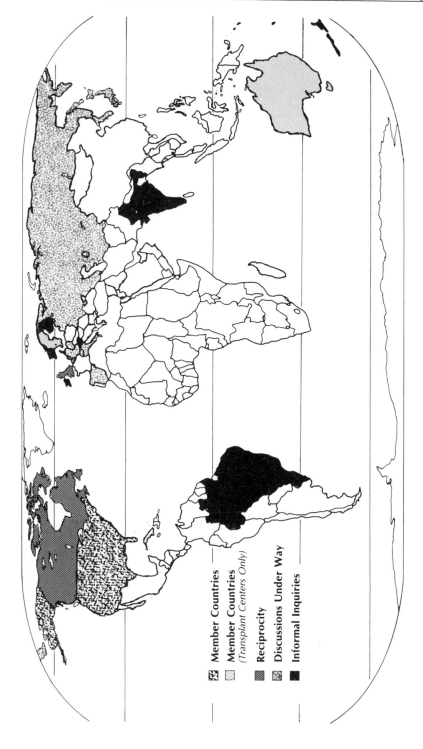

Figure 5.13.   National Marrow Program: Global Hope

oped in many countries around the world. Through the efforts of concerned hematologists and transplanters, the National Marrow Donor Program has begun to link the national registries together in a single computerized network that stretches around the world. The development of a large, ethnically diverse unrelated donor registry continues to be the central goal of the program. This has become particularly important as histocompatibility experts have determined that early projections of file effectiveness (40–70% with a file of 100,000) were overly optimistic. It is now felt that a worldwide, racially diverse file is of absolute necessity if significant numbers of patients are to be served.

The second contract task was facilitating searches. The first two years of program development saw an increase in the speed of performing searches and a broadening of the network of transplant centers and donor centers participating in such search requests. Of particular importance in facilitating searches is public and medical education. It is widely acknowledged that if there is to be a successful transplant and enough time to perform an adequate search, patients must be referred early in their disease process. It is therefore absolutely necessary that referring medical oncologists and clinicians have adequate information about access to the National Marrow Donor Program so that patients can be referred in a timely fashion. The National Marrow Donor Program has taken on an extensive public and medical education program to keep referring physicians abreast of the improved prognoses of patients undergoing marrow transplant, and make them aware of the methods of access to the file. It is a goal of the program that search speed will increase and that the program will continue to broaden its horizons. While the fastest search and delivery of marrow that has ever occurred has been approximately 14 days, the average time from search initiation to delivery of the marrow at the bedside remains at about 120 days. Patients who are in the chronic phase of chronic myelogenous leukemia may have sufficient discretionary

time to wait out a long search, but patients with aplastic anemia or other acute, time-limited diseases require a much faster search process. It is therefore an ongoing goal of the National Marrow Donor Program to increase the speed of the search process.

The third task originally designated under the terms of the contract was to perform ongoing research in the areas of marrow transplantation, donor motivation, and histocompatibility. Early in this chapter some of the work in donor motivation studies was discussed. It is important to note that an active Research and Publications Committee of the program designs and implements ongoing research studies. Currently underway are a matched control study for CML, a study of transplanted versus untransplanted patients to determine life outcomes and efficacy of transplant, and a donor physical safety study aimed at analyzing the physical impact of marrow donation on unrelated donors. Of particular and ongoing importance is the development of the Research Blood Repository. Prior to each transplant a blood specimen from the patient and one from the donor are shipped to the repository housed at the Irwin Memorial Blood Bank in San Francisco, California. One hundred days after transplant, an additional blood specimen is collected from the patient and is also shipped to the Irwin facility. Under development at this time are cell lines from each of these blood specimens which will be made available for ongoing research and will be an unprecedented source of cells for research into histocompatibility and clinical correlation studies.

The use of unrelated donors has increased tremendously over the past years. As the size of national registries increases and interaction between national registries improves, access to unrelated donors may make unrelated donor marrow transplantation even more prevalent than related donor transplantation. Many transplant centers around the United States are increasing their numbers of beds and their capabilities for performing transplants in order to meet this increasing need. Continued attention to the confidentiality and safety of donors and to the careful development of standards and research will further improve both the efficacy of the transplants and the opportunities for transplant.

Marrow Donor Issues

Many donor issues have been mentioned previously in this chapter, but for the nurse interacting with sibling donors or dealing with patients receiving marrow from unrelated donors, more information may be helpful.

Confidentiality

Whether the donor comes from within the family or is unrelated, confidentiality is an issue. Confidentiality for unrelated donors is well-protected by the National Marrow Donor Program. Confidentiality for related donors is quite vulnerable. In their desperate search for a donor, parents may not consider that a child may not want to donate for his brother or sister. Interesting ethical questions of parental control and self-determination are at issue here. The sensitive practitioner will shield family typings carefully until matching family members have had a chance to privately indicate their willingness to proceed.

Safety and Informed Consent

Safety issues were discussed earlier in this chapter. It is important to remember that donors are engaging in a potentially life-threatening ordeal. Donors, both related and unrelated, deserve clear, realistic explanations of the collection process and what can be expected physically. Providing adequate information for the donor to make a truly informed consent is the responsibility of those physicians and nurses preparing the donor for collection.

Unrelated Donor Process

The patient process in searching for an unrelated donor was described extensively earlier in this chapter. The perspective of the donor may be somewhat different and is worth describing.

Initial Recruitment

Potential donors may initially become interested in participating because they hear of the plight of a specific patient in their community (usually a child). The donor attends a "recruitment drive," views a film on the need for marrow donors, is given a brochure to read, fills out demographic forms, and signs a consent. The potential donor then has one or two tubes of blood drawn so that his/her HLA typing can be performed. The potential donor's information is sent to the National Marrow Donor Program computer, and it may be quite some time (if ever) before the donor hears anything further.

HLA-DR Typing

Most potential donors, when called to give a specimen for HLA-DR typing, are delighted. They are finally a possible match for a patient! After the blood draw, these potential donors will often call local donor center coordinators every day until they find out if their HLA-DR type matches that of the patient. About 5% of potential donors will choose to withdraw from the process at this point. Hurtful as it may be to the patient waiting for a donor, it is important to remember that donors do have the right to decline and may have legitimate reasons for so doing (illness in the family, etc.).

Mixed Lymphocyte Culture

Potential donors whose HLA-A, -B, and -DR typing matches the patient may be asked to give a second blood specimen for the MLC. Potential donors who get this far are usually very excited. Once again, these individuals will probably call their local coordinator every day or so to find out if a final decision has been made. Transplant centers that delay in setting up MLCs or reporting results should keep in mind how anxious these potential donors may be and how much we all depend on their willing participation.

Workup

Once a decision has been made to use a particular donor, the information session and physical exam are a final screening. Very few (less then 1%) of all potential donors decline to participate beyond this point. Of particular importance at this point is the significant other or donor advocate. All donors (related as well as unrelated) deserve a special confidant or attendant to listen, reflect concerns, and provide support.

Collection and Follow-up

The wait between workup and collection can be one of the most difficult times for a potential donor. These individuals realize that another person's life depends on theirs and they may become almost obsessed with not endangering their health or safety during this time. Many potential donors have been known to cancel Christmas holiday plans, family vacations, and business trips, in order to keep themselves available for "their patient." Transplant centers that anticipate long delays between workup and collection can help the potential donor by being very clear about the time frames.

Potential donors entering the hospital for collection of marrow may be entering a hospital for the first time. Staff dealing with these donors should keep in mind that even though this individual is well (and may be housed on a floor with very sick patients), he/she may have many questions and some trepidation. These people are giving selflessly and they deserve our kindness and admiration. Donors occasionally report hospital staff making comments like "I can't imagine why you would want to do this!" This is not helpful.

Donors should have been informed about the aftereffects of marrow collection and anesthesia (sore throat, low back pain, headache, etc.) but they may need reminding and support from floor staff. Most donors report that the actual pain at the collection site disappears within seven to ten days, but all donors should be reminded to report immediately any fever, excessive pain, drainage at the collection site, or persistent headache.

Finally, and not least important, is that all donors, related and unrelated, be thanked for what they have done. Often patients and families are so intensely caught up in sustaining life that writing thank-you notes is beyond consideration. A note from the transplant coordinator or primary care nurse can make a big difference. Donors usually like to hear how their recipient fared and want to be notified when marrow engrafts, when the patient goes home, or if the patient dies. It is simplest to say that without donors there are no transplants. We all need to maintain our awareness of donor needs and try to support and reinforce these individuals.

> I gave for a nine year old boy in Seattle. It's had a ripple effect in my life. The boy, his family, and I will never be the same again.
> —Unrelated Marrow Donor

References

Beatty, P. et al. 1988. Probability of finding HLA matched unrelated marrow donors. *Transplantation 45*: 714–718.

Bortin, M.M. et al. 1983. Major complications of marrow harvesting for transplantation. *Experimental Hematology 11* (10): 916–921.

Bruning, J.W., van Leeuwan, A., and van Rood, J. 1975. Leukocyte antigens. *Histocompatibility Testing 1975.* p. 275.

Caplan, A. 1983. Case study: Mrs. X and the bone marrow transplant. *Hastings Center Report 13* (3): 17–19.

Gale, R. 1986. Potential utilization of a national HLA-typed donor pool for bone marrow transplantation. *Transplantation 42* (1): 54–57

International Bone Marrow Transplant Registry. 1987. Milwaukee, WI.

McCullough, J. et al. 1988. Effectiveness of a regional bone marrow donor program. *JAMA 259* (22): 3286–3289.

National Marrow Donor Program. 1989. St. Paul, MN.

Ohayon, E., and Cambon-Thomsen, A. 1986. *Human Population Genetics.* Vol. 142. Inserm, Paris.

O'Reilly, R.J. et al. 1977. Reconstitution in severe combined immunodeficiency by transplantation of marrow from an unrelated donor. *N. Engl. J. Med.* 297: 1311–1218.

Simmons, R. Work in progress. University of Pittsburgh, Department of Sociology, Pittsburgh, PA.

Wakisaka, A. et al. 1986. Anthropological study using HLA antigen frequencies as a genetic marker. *HLA in Asia-Oceania.* Proceedings of the Third Asia-Oceania Histocompatibility Workshop and Conference, Sapporo, Japan, pp. 197–211.

PART II

Complications of Bone Marrow Transplant

Chapter 6

Hematopoietic Complications

Kathryn A. Caudell and Marie Bakitas Whedon

Introduction

One of the most critical complications of bone marrow transplantation is pancytopenia, resulting from the chemotherapy and/or total body irradiation employed in the conditioning regimens. Pancytopenia from BMT differs from the bone marrow suppression of other standard cancer therapies in that it is more profound and prolonged (Wingard 1990; Lum 1990; Atkinson 1990). Until the donor (or autologous) bone marrow begins to engraft, approximately two to three weeks after infusion, the patient is predisposed to potentially fatal neutropenic infections, thrombocytopenic hemorrhages (Phillips 1988), and anemia.

Due to the seriousness and complexity of pancytopenia, it is critical that the nurse understand the phenomena in its entirety, including the causative agents, the pathophysiological processes, the clinical manifestations, and the medical and nursing management. In this area of transplant care in particular, astute nursing assessment, early detection, and prompt intervention are able to reduce patient morbidity (Peters 1990; Oniboni 1990) and possibly mortality. This chapter provides a brief overview of normal hematopoiesis, followed by discussions of leukopenia, anemia, thrombocytopenia, and graft failure.

Normal Hematopoiesis

The blood-forming organs consist of the bone marrow, spleen, and liver. The cellular elements of the blood are produced in the bone marrow beginning at approximately the twentieth week of fetal life. In the fetus, hematopoiesis begins in the yolk sac and fetal liver, and also occurs in the spleen, lymph nodes, thymus, and in almost every bone. Hematopoietic activity takes place throughout an individual's life in the flat bones, which include the sternum, ribs, skull, pelvic and shoulder girdles, vertebrae, and innominates. In adulthood, marrow capable of hematopoiesis in the shaft of the long bones gradually diminishes and hematopoietic marrow is limited to the distal ends. Eventually, the inactive bone marrow is replaced by fatty tissue. However, inactive bone marrow may become active if there is a demand for an increased number of blood cells.

Bone Marrow

Several different cells are produced in the bone marrow. A pluripotent stem cell has the ability to differentiate into erythrocytic, granulocytic, monocytic, lymphocytic, or thrombocytic cell lines. In contrast, unipotential or committed stem cells are those that differentiate into one cell line and require a humoral poietin, a growth factor, to stimulate further differentiation. For instance, granulopoietin is needed specifically for the unipotential cells committed to the granulocyte, monocyte, and macrophage cell line (see Figure 6.1).

Spleen

The spleen contains lymphoid and reticuloendothelial cells and has many functions. Not only is it actively involved in antibody synthesis, the spleen has the ability to destroy old or imperfect red blood cells (RBCs) by phagocytosis, remove particles from intact RBCs without injuring them, serve as a storage area for platelets, remove worn out RBCs and platelets from the circulation, act as a mechanical filter trapping antigens, particularly of bacterial origin, and prepare antigens for phagocytic activity.

Liver

The liver produces many of the substances that are required in the coagulation process such as fibrinogen, prothrombin, accelerator globulin, and factors VII, IX, and X. If the demand for RBC production is accelerated or abnormal, the liver can participate in erythropoiesis (Griffin 1986).

White Blood Cells

In the human, the normal white blood cell count ranges from 4,000 to 11,000 cells per microliter. (See Table 6.1 for normal values for all blood cells.) The granulocytes comprise 50% to 70% of the total white blood cell population and are made up of neutrophils, basophils, and eosinophils. Lymphocytes and monocytes are also white blood cells and together with the granulocytes provide a powerful defense against a variety of antigens such as tumors, viruses, bacteria, and parasites (Ganong 1985). Characteristics and functions of various white blood cells are explained below.

Basophils

The basophils, comprising 0.5% to 2% of the total white blood cell count, release histamine during allergic reactions. In addition, they are essential in the prevention of clot formation due to their high content of heparin. Basophils are increased during asthmatic episodes, inflammatory bowel disease, chronic inflammation and in some carcinomas (Goodman 1987; Griffin 1986).

Eosinophils

Eosinophils comprise 1 to 4% of the total white cells and are involved in inactivating mediators released from mast cells during allergic reactions and attacking some parasites. The eosinophil count is elevated during allergic reactions, drug reactions (codeine and penicillin), parasitic infections (helminth, *Schistosoma* and *Trichinella*), skin diseases (exfoliative dermatitis), neoplasms (lung cancer and Hodgkin's disease), and infections (tuberculosis and leprosy) (Goodman 1987; Griffin 1986).

Neutrophils

Neutrophils, the most numerous of the granulocytes, have the ability to seek out, ingest, and destroy the majority of foreign invaders. This process involves a series of steps in which the neutrophils (1) adhere to the endothelium, (2) emigrate to extravascular regions and migrate specifically toward substances for ingestion (chemotaxis), (3) recognize and attach to membrane surfaces, (4) phagocytize, (5) degranulate, and (6) oxidize particles (Goldstein 1987). Slightly immature neutrophils, called "bands" or "stabs," comprise approximately 3% of the total

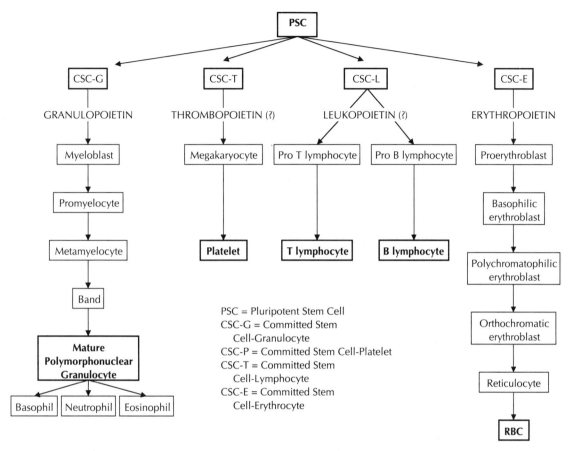

Figure 6.1.   Diagram of Cellular Development

Adapted from J.P. Griffin, 1986. Physiology of the hematopoietic system. In J.P. Griffin (Ed.). *Hematology and Immunology. Concepts for Nursing.* Appleton-Century-Crofts: Norwalk, 20.

white blood cell population. During periods of acute localized infections, such as appendicitis, the number of bands will increase. This increase in the circulating number of less mature neutrophils is commonly described as a "shift to the left." The increase in the band count is often proportional to the severity of the infection. The neutrophils are produced in the bone marrow and eventually migrate to tissues and body cavities via the blood stream. Neutrophil levels increase during periods of inflammation, with invasive tumors, and myeloproliferative disorders (Griffin 1986).

Monocytes/Macrophages

The mobile components of the reticuloendothelial system are the monocytes and the macrophages. Monocytes are immature macrophages that are produced in the bone marrow and migrate to tissues or body cavities. They differentiate into (1) free macrophages that have the ability to travel from the circulatory system through the endothelial membranes to ingest trapped particles, or (2) fixed macrophages or histiocytes that are found in the spleen, lymph nodes, bone marrow, capillaries of the liver, adrenal glands, pituitary,

Table 6.1. Normal Values for the Cellular Elements in Human Blood

	Cells/L (average)	Approximate Normal Range	Percentage of Total White Cells
Total WBC	9000	4000–11,000	***
Granulocytes			
Neutrophils	5400	3000–6000	50–70
Eosinophils	275	150–300	1–4
Basophils	35	0–100	0.4
Lymphocytes	2750	1500–4000	20–40
Monocytes	540	300–600	2–8
Erythrocytes			
Females	4.8×10^6	***	***
Males	5.4×10^6	***	***
Platelets	300,000	200,000–500,000	***

Reproduced with permission from W.F. Ganong, 1985. *Review of Medical Physiology Twelfth Edition*, Lange Medical Publications: Los Altos, p. 423.

lung, and the endothelial cells of the blood vessels (Griffin 1986).

The macrophages play a role in both the nonspecific immune system (through phagocytosis) and in the specific immune system (through their role in cellular immunity). Macrophages that have enveloped and processed an antigen come in contact with or "present" the antigen to the T lymphocyte enabling it to proliferate and specifically attack the antigen that was presented (Goodman 1987). Monocyte levels increase during chronic infections and recovery from infections, liver disease, and in neutropenia (Griffin 1986).

Lymphocytes

The lymphocytes comprise approximately 20% to 35% of the white blood cell population. The majority of lymphocytes are formed in the lymph nodes, thymus, and spleen from stem cells that have originated in the bone marrow. They are also distributed to the liver and intestines. Mature lymphocytes differentiate into cells that can express cell-mediated immune responses (T lymphocytes) or humoral immune responses (immunoglobulin-producing B lymphocytes). T lymphocytes

undergo differentiation in the thymus gland whereas the B lymphocytes are thought to undergo their differentiation in the bone marrow.

Plasma Cells

B lymphocytes have the ability to differentiate into antibody-producing plasma cells after they have been stimulated by an antigen. For this reason, the B lymphocytes are thought to be plasma cell precursors (Griffin 1986). The antigen binds to the appropriate B lymphocyte as it enters the body. It initiates division of the B lymphocyte and produces a clone that also binds to the antigen. T lymphocytes, specifically the helper lymphocytes, facilitate this process, whereas the suppressor T lymphocytes inhibit it (Goodman 1987).

Erythrocytes

Erythrocytes, or red blood cells (RBCs), contain hemoglobin, which carries oxygen from the lungs to all body tissues. They also remove carbon dioxide from the tissues for excretion by the lungs, and serve as a major buffer system for the body to assist in the maintenance of acid-base homeostasis (Guyton 1986; Griffin 1986). Normal quantities of red blood cells, the hemoglobin concentration in the blood (Hgb), and concentration of RBCs in the blood as measured by the hematocrit are listed in Table 6.1. The normal range for the quantity of RBCs in an individual varies and is effected by age, sex, and the altitude at which one lives (Guyton 1986).

The control and stimulus of RBC production in the bone marrow results from the humoral stimulus of the RBC growth factor, erythropoietin. Erythropoietin production is influenced by tissue oxygen tension and stimulates erythroblast formation from progenitors. The stages of RBC development from early progenitor (proerythroblast) to mature RBC are illustated in Figure 6.1.

Reticulocytes are immature red blood cells at their final stage of maturation, and normally constitute about 0.2 to 2% of the total circulating RBC peripheral blood count (Griffin 1986). Once released from the bone marrow, reticulocytes circulate for about 24 hours before maturing into RBCs. Hemoglobin synthesis ceases after the reticulocyte matures into a functional RBC. Reticulocytes are a constant source of replenishment for the approximately 1% of senescent RBCs that die and are removed from the circulation daily (Griffin 1986). Reticulocytes are absent during bone marrow aplasia but are considered an early indicator of bone marrow regeneration.

Megakaryocytes

Platelets, the circulating cell fragments of the mature bone-marrow-derived megakaryocytes, play a major role in normal hemostasis and coagulation. They are produced in response to a humoral stimulator, thrombopoietin (Figure 6.1) and once released into the circulation survive for about 7–14 days (Griffin 1986). Large quantities of platelets in the circulation, spleen, and to a lesser extent other organs, and constant production of platelets in the bone marrow ensures replacement of the approximately 15% that are consumed in normal daily intravascular coagulation (Griffin 1986).

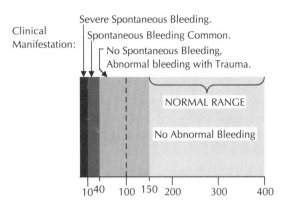

Figure 6.2. Bleeding Tendencies in Relationship to Platelet Count

Changes in bleeding tendencies related to decreased quantities of circulating platelets are illustrated in Figure 6.2. Minor decreases in quantity affect the normal function of the platelets in maintaining and repairing the normal "wear and tear" caused by blood flow and trauma to the vascular endothelium. This produces the clinical manifestation of pinpoint hemorrhages known as petechae. Major reductions in quantity can result in spontaneous and fatal hemorrhages. Qualitative defects in platelet function can also result in bleeding abnormalities even when the quantity is within the normal range (Griffin 1986).

Immunity

Immunity is defined as insusceptibility, or the status or quality of being immune. The two major components of the immune system are natural (nonspecifc) and acquired (specific) defenses.

Natural Nonspecific Defenses

The natural defenses are nonspecific, that is, they occur independently without prior contact with immunogens. These defenses usually are present at birth and grow or mature over the lifetime of the organism. The natural nonspecific immune defenses include inflammation, intact skin and mucosa, adequately functioning pyrogens that elevate body temperature and subsequently inhibit bacterial action, an acidic body pH that is not conducive to viral or bacterial growth, adequate amounts of normally functioning interferon, genetic integrity, phagocytosis, and preformed antibodies received from the mother (Griffin 1986).

Inflammation and Phagocytosis

It is important to briefly mention the process of inflammation since during neutropenia the clinical manifestations commonly observed during inflammation are absent or inconspicuous. This will be discussed in more detail later in the chapter.

Inflammation is a sequence of events involving white blood cell activity and vascular responses, which employ numerous substances from a variety of sources. Inflammation can occur in response to trauma or invasion by pathogens. When tissue injury occurs, damaged tissues release large quantities of histamine, bradydidnin, serotonin, and other substances into the immediate vicinity. These substances cause increased local blood flow and increased permeability of the vascular system. This, in turn, allows a large amount of fluid and protein, including fibrinogen, to pass from the vascular system into the extracellular area, which results in local edema. Fibrinogen, when in contact with the tissue exudates, results in clot formation. When pathogens are present this enclosed area is then invaded by macrophages and neutrophils. The inflamed tissues also release chemical substances that migrate to the bone marrow causing a dilation of the venous sinusoids of the bone marrow and a subsequent release of more neutrophils and other WBCs into the circulation. These cells, in addition to macrophages, permeate the inflamed area and, through a combination of efforts, begin to lyse the walls of bacteria (Griffin 1986).

The redness and warmth frequently seen in inflammation is a result of the increased amount of blood and compromised blood flow in the af-

fected area. The congestion and exudation produce swelling in the area. Pain, which commonly accompanies inflammation, is caused by pressure on or stretching of the nerve endings (nociceptors) during the process of swelling, and local changes in osmotic pressure and pH (Stedman 1982).

Acquired Specific Host Defenses

Cellular Immunity

The T lymphocytes are the cells responsible for cellular immunity. Antigens located on the surfaces of viruses, cells of another individual, or tumor cells activate the T lymphocytes when they come in contact with them. The T lymphocytes enlarge, divide, and release lymphokines, substances that assist the attack on the foreign protein. Some activated T lymphocytes also lyse foreign cells and are called cytotoxic or killer T lymphocytes.

The T lymphocyte system is responsible for the rejection of transplanted tissue. T lymphocytes recognize the histocompatibility antigens, those antigens found on circulating human leukocytes (HLA) that distinguish self from nonself. In the case of bone marrow transplantation, the viable graft (donor) T lymphocytes are the cells thought to be primarily responsible for graft-versus-host disease. Several treatment approaches have been employed to inhibit or prevent tissue rejection associated with graft T lymphocytes. The first involves destroying the T lymphocytes by killing all of the rapidly dividing cells with agents such as azathioprine. However, this method makes the patient susceptible to developing potentially fatal infections and cancer. The second approach employs glucocorticoids, which destroy T lymphocytes by unknown mechanisms. Glucocorticoids have many adverse side effects such as osteoporosis and Cushing's syndrome. The third technique utilizes antibodies against the T lymphocytes, such as antithymocyte globulin (ATG). The fourth approach involves treatment with cyclosporine, a fungus extract that does not affect B lymphocytes but prevents activated T lymphocytes from dividing (Ganong 1985). Finally, depletion of T lymphocytes in donor marrow in vitro has been accomplished by a variety of means. (See Chapter 7 for an expanded discussion of the above phenomenon.)

Humoral Immunity

Immunity achieved from circulating antibodies is called humoral immunity. B lymphocytes contain surface receptors for specific antigens. When the B lymphocyte comes in contact with a specific antigen, it divides and forms daughter cells that are subsequently transformed into plasma cells (or antibody factories), which secrete large amounts of antibodies into the circulatory system. These antibodies are also called immunoglobulins (Ig).

The B lymphocyte-plasma cell system produces five general types of immunoglobulin antibodies. They are IgG, IgA, IgM, IgD, and IgE. IgM is the first immunoglobulin formed. It undergoes maturation and eventually produces IgG. IgM whose function it is to fix complement, makes up approximately 10% of the total immunoglobulins. It is a prominent immunoglobulin in early immune responses to most antigens and also dominant in the natural blood group antibody. IgG accounts for 75% of the total immunoglobulins and is active against most bacteria, some parasites, viruses, and fungi. It is the only immunoglobulin that can cross the placenta in humans and it is responsible for protecting newborns in their first few months of life.

IgA is found predominantly in body secretions. Secretory IgA provides the primary defense against localized infections and is abundant in saliva, tears, bronchial secretions, nasal mucosa, prostatic fluid, vaginal secretions, and mucous secretions of the small intestine. It is postulated that due to the large amount of IgA found in membrane secretions, its primary function is to prevent antigen entry rather than to cause antigen destruction.

IgD makes up 0.2% of the total serum immunoglobulins. It is the predominant immunoglobulin on the surface of B lymphocytes; however, its primary function has not been determined. IgE accounts for the smallest amount of immunoglobulins; approximately 0.004% of the total amount. It binds efficiently to mast cells. Once exposed to and combined with allergens, IgE causes the release of chemical mediators from mast cells that produce the typical wheal and flare skin reactions seen on allergic individuals who have come in contact with the allergen (Goodman 1987).

Leukopenia

Virtually all bone marrow transplant patients experience severe immunosuppression lasting several months after transplantation. Profound neutropenia, usually defined as less than 500 neutrophils/microliter, commonly lasts for two to four weeks after the conditioning or antineoplastic regimen. After this time, it becomes evident that engraftment has occurred as the first neutrophils appear and steadily increase in number. Peripheral white blood cells reach normal quantities over a period of several weeks. However, completely normal immune function often does not return until months or years after transplantation (Engelhard et al. 1986; Lum 1990; Atkinson 1990).

Several investigators have determined that varying deficiencies of the immune system are observed in the different phases of the marrow transplantation procedure (Lum 1990; Atkinson 1990; Wingard 1990; Bowden and Meyers 1985; Lum 1987; Saral 1985; Young 1984). For instance, in the pretransplant phase, patients with relapsed acute leukemia or aplastic anemia begin the transplant procedure with compromised immune function due to their disease process (Phillips 1988), whereas patients in remission may have no evidence of immune dysfunction. Posttransplant as pancytopenia resolves, normal phagocytic function returns although continued cellular immune dysfunction may persist, especially in patients who develop GVHD. Humoral immune dysfunction can persist for up to a year post-transplant.

In an uncomplicated transplant, the recovery of the immune system is a gradual process. Several host and treatment-related factors have been found to influence the severity of hematopoietic toxicity experienced by an individual. Host factors include the age, nutritional status, renal and hepatic function, bone marrow infiltration by tumor, previous chemotherapy or radiotherapy, the proliferative state of the bone marrow, and the presence of infection. Older patients experience more severe hematopoietic toxicities than younger patients because of a decreased cellularity or smaller total marrow mass. Patients who are malnourished prior to therapy will have a decreased tolerance for chemotherapy and have a more severe myelosuppression (Marsh 1985). The latter can be a problem in patients who received chemotherapy preharvest (Visani et al. 1990) and in chemically purged and stored autologous marrow.

Treatment-related factors can also affect the rate of hematopoietic recovery. These include the conditioning regimen, GVHD, and the number of colony-forming unit cells (CFU-C) infused (Spitzer et al. 1980). Busulfan, which is sometimes used as an alternative to TBI, has less immunosuppressive activity. ATG, which is used to treat or prevent GVHD, delays the recovery of the humoral response to adequately phagocytize bacterial antigens. Infections themselves, like cytomegalovirus (CMV), can also inhibit immune function (Pizzo 1989). Immune recovery, as measured by the return of normal helper-to-suppressor ratios, skin test responses, and granulocyte chemotaxis, can be delayed post-transplant (Lum 1990).

Many antineoplastic agents used in the conditioning regimens cause hematologic toxicities. These toxicities result from the drugs' ability to interfere with the normal cell cycle functions (Griffin 1986), by decreasing the absorption of necessary cellular nutrients, by inhibiting the ac-

tion of required enzymes, or by other as yet unknown mechanisms.

Many conditioning regimens contain high doses of alkylating agents such as cyclophosphamide. This category of drugs produces cross-linking or complete breakage in the strands of DNA, which affects all the phases of the cell cycle and virtually all bone marrow cells. Cytarabine, an antimetabolite also used in many regimens, inhibits or blocks the synthesis of purine or pyrimidine components that subsequently affect DNA synthesis. The action of antimetabolites occurs during the entire cell cycle but they are particularly effective during the S-phase when DNA synthesis takes place (Lubran 1989). All of these effects interfere with or interrupt normal granulopoiesis.

The effect of drugs on granulocytes in the circulatory system is to alter either the function of the mature cell or the absolute number of circulating cells in the blood. Cell number may be influenced by decreased or inadequate production by the bone marrow, increased peripheral destruction, or by changes in the ratio of circulating cells.

Total body irradiation (TBI), a common component of most conditioning regimens, ablates immune function, residual normal bone marrow, and residual malignant cells (Slavin et al. 1983). Most patients who receive total body irradiation in combination with high doses of cyclophosphamide experience profound immune dysfunction for at least four months after transplantation (Noel et al. 1978). Phagocytic function is decreased including chemotaxis, phagocytosis, and the killing of intracellular microbes by neutrophils and pulmonary macrophages (Clark et al. 1976; Winston et al. 1982). Cellular immunity is affected as evidenced by a reversed helper/suppressor ratio mainly due to a reduction in helper cell numbers. Lymphocyte responses to various mitogens are reduced. Responses to skin test recall antigens such as *Candida* and mumps can be diminished for as long as four years after transplantation (Noel et al. 1978; Witherspoon et al.

1982). In contrast, natural killer cell function usually recovers within the first few months (Livnat et al. 1980; Lum 1990).

Dysfunctional humoral immunity in recipients despite normal numbers of B cells and normal immunoglobulin concentrations is due, perhaps, to a decreased antibody production. It has also been found that pretransplant concentrations of humoral antibodies to tetanus, diptheria, and polio are markedly reduced after the conditioning regimen. Complement concentrations, however, usually remain normal (Noel et al. 1978; Lum 1990).

In the allogeneic patient, hematopoietic reconstitution occasionally combines donor and recipient hematopoietic cells (often referred to as a mixed chimerism state). This situation occurs because the preparative regimen did not totally ablate the patient's marrow function; therefore, recipient hematopoiesis persists. This phenomenon can result in rejection of the donor marrow or occasionally the recipient marrow becomes tolerant of the donor cells and donor and recipient cells cohabitate (Roy 1990).

In autologous transplantation, marrow purging techniques can sometimes interfere with hematopoietic function, thereby prolonging the neutropenic period beyond what is considered a normal recovery phase in the allogeneic recipient (Wingard 1990). Although this does not generally change the patterns of infection during the first month post-transplant (described in the next section), beyond that time the autologous patient is often at higher risk for superinfections with antibiotic resistant pathogens (Wingard 1990).

Infections

The most frequently occurring complication of immunosuppression is infection. An infection exists when the body or part of the body is invaded by a pathogenic agent that multiplies (colonizes) and produces detrimental or injurious effects to the body. An opportunistic infection is one that

Table 6.2 Pathogenic Organisms

1. Infections resulting from cellular defects
   a) fungi: *Candida, Aspergillus*
   b) protozoa: *Pneumocystis carinii, Toxoplasma*
   c) virus: herpes simplex, varicella-zoster, cytomegalovirus
2. Infections resulting from humoral defects pyogenic organisms: *Streptococcus pneumoniae*
3. Infections resulting from phagocyte disorders low virulence local bacteria: Staph aureas, *Pseudomonas, Escherichia coli*

is usually the consequence of defective functioning of the normal immune system. It is caused by microorganisms that lack virulent infection-producing properties, unless a defect or group of defects is present in the host's immune system.

Infections caused by specific organisms can usually be linked to specific defects in immune function (see Table 6.2). For example, infections resulting from humoral defects are usually produced by the pyrogenic organisms such as *Streptococcus pneumoniae*. Phagocyte disorders, on the other hand, facilitate infestation of low virulence bacteria that usually remain localized such as Staph aureas, *Pseudomonas*, and *Escherichia coli*. Infections resulting from cellular defects include fungi (*Candida* and *Aspergillus*), protozoa (*Pneumocystis carinii* and *Toxoplasma*), and viruses (herpes simplex, varicella-zoster, and cytomegalovirus) (Atkinson 1990).

The type, severity, and frequency of these infections depends on a variety of host and treatment factors that are often related. Host factors include the underlying disease, presence of host endogenous flora, and presence of pretreatment infections. For example, patients who have aplastic anemia are at an increased risk after transplantation, more so than solid tumor patients because of the relatively high incidence of engraftment failure with concurrent prolonged neutropenia. Patients with Hodgkin's and non-Hodgkin's lymphomas have underlying defects in cellular immunity, and are therefore more susceptible to certain pathogens. Patients who have preexisting infections prior to transplantation are at a high risk of increased morbidity and, perhaps, mortality, unless those infections are eradicated before immunosuppression ensues. For this reason, most transplant centers attempt to treat and eradicate the infection before beginning the conditioning regimen. In some cases, infections may persist despite antibiotic therapy until the patient has achieved an immunologic recovery. Another host factor, the patient's normal endogenous flora, is a major source of infection in BMT recipients during the period of neutropenia. Patients can be colonized with undetectable amounts of such harmful pathogens as *Candida, Aspergillus,* and *Pseudomonas* (Drutz et al. 1985). Latent viral infections often are reactivated after transplantation. Exogenous or treatment-related factors also play a role in the nature of infections manifest in the BMT patient. For instance, different transplant centers are innoculated with different flora and these can vary over time (Pizzo 1989). *Aspergillus* is a major cause of nosocomial infection in some centers, but not in others. Pathogens endogenous to certain geographical areas, such as *coccidioidomycosis,* also present risks to BMT patients as well as other immunosuppressed patients.

The types of infections also vary with the different phases of treatment (see Table 6.3). During the first month, profound neutropenia, defined as neutrophil counts less than 100 cells per μL, causes BMT patients to be extremely susceptible to bacteremias, fungemias, and other types of disseminated infection (Lum 1990; Atkinson 1990). Viral reactivation is also likely during this period. Most pathogens at this time are from the patient's own flora, while some may have been recently acquired during the transplant hospitalization. For example a common skin inhabitant, the Gram-positive cocci, *Staphylococcus epidermidis,* frequently causes infections in BMT patients by gaining entry through the break in the skin barrier from a central venous catheter (Buckner et al. 1983; Meyers and Atkinson 1983). Also, the

Table 6.3. Spectrum of Infections After Marrow Transplantation

First Month (Preengraftment)
• Gram-negative bacteria
• Gram-positive bacteria
• Fungi
• Herpes simplex virus

Second and Third Months (Early postengraftment)
• Cytomegalovirus
• Fungi
• Gram-positive bacteria
• *Pneumocystis carinii*

After Three Months (Late postengraftment)
• Encapsulated bacteria
• Varicella zoster virus
• *Pneumocystic carinni*

Source: Wingard 1990, with permission.

longer the patient experiences neutropenia, the higher the incidence of disseminated fungal infections. *Candida,* particularly *Candida albicans,* and *Aspergillus* are the most common (Milliken and Powles 1990). *Histoplasma, Coccidioides, Mucor,* and *Trichosporon* have all been observed (Meyers and Atkinson 1983). This knowledge serves as the basis for the selection of the types of empiric antimicrobial therapy frequently initiated before results of cultures are known.

During the period immediately after transplantation, when the most severe neutropenia occurs ($< 0.1 \times 10^9$/liter), the oral and intestinal mucosa is often disrupted as well, due to the conditioning regimen. This, in turn, predisposes the patient to gastrointestinal tract infections, particularly those caused by typical bowel flora. In this phase, gastrointestinal mucosa disruption and the presence of indwelling central venous catheters are thought to be of primary importance for the development of infection.

Decreased numbers of neutrophils during the period of profound neutropenia produce minimal or atypical clinical signs of infection. For this reason, localized sites of infection may produce pain and mild erythema, but not swelling or abscess

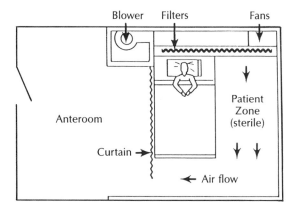

Blower   Filters   Fans

Anteroom

Patient
Zone
(sterile)

Curtain →

← Air flow

Figure 6.3. Laminar Air Flow Unit

formation. Fever normally accompanies infection. In the neutropenic BMT patient, fever may be nonspecific and result from the disease process, medications, or in conjunction with blood transfusions. The lungs, perirectal area, integument, mouth, and sinuses are the most common sites of local infection; however, any site may be involved.

Because an infection in a profoundly neutropenic patient can be fatal, many approaches have been utilized to prevent nosocomial infections in BMT recipients. Techniques to protect the patient's immediate environment include laminar air flow rooms (Lindgren 1983) (Figure 6.3), high efficiency particulate air (HEPA) filtration, and reverse or protective isolation. The latter consists of isolating the patient in a standard private room, requiring staff to wear masks, and use good hand-washing procedures. Oral nonabsorbable broad spectrum antibiotics including vancomycin, polymyxen, and nystatin have been administered to suppress endogenous flora alone or in conjunction with the above approaches (Pizzo 1989; Wade and Schimpff 1988). Placing the patients on sterile or low microbial diets and sterile water may be helpful in reducing the incidence of infection, although a controlled study investigating the use of sterile food has not been done (Engelhard et al. 1986). A recent report comparing the incidence of GVHD and infections in a pediatric population

revealed no significant differences between patients treated with nonabsorbable antibiotics in a laminar air flow environment and patients receiving standard reverse isolation procedures (Ogden et al. 1990). This same finding was reported in autologous transplant patients when these two methods were compared (Pizzo 1989).

Due to the serious and often life-threatening nature of infections in severely immunosuppressed patients, febrile episodes are treated as emergencies and immediate treatment with systemic broad-spectrum antibiotics is begun as soon as possible. Empiric, broad-spectrum antibiotic therapy often includes two or three antibiotics to provide coverage for the varehy of potential pathogens that may be involved in causing the fever. Examples of antibiotic combinations are a semisynthetic penicillin and an aminoglycoside or a third-generation cephalosporine and a broad spectrum agent such as Imipenem. Some physicians prefer to include vancomycin as specific antistaphylococcal prophylaxis because infections related to indwelling intravenous catheters are so common. On the other hand, other clinicians prefer not to add vancomycin until a *Staphylococcus epidermidis* infection is confirmed because of the expense of the drug and the lesser virulence and treatability of the organism (Rubin et al. 1988).

Broad spectrum antibiotic therapy is usually continued until the neutrophil count exceeds 0.5 × 10⁹/liter. If patients continue to be febrile after three or more days, a systemic antifungal agent such as amphotericin B, even in the absence of positive fungal cultures, may be added. Deep fungal infections are difficult to diagnose and must be treated vigorously early in their course to prevent mortality (Milliken and Powels 1990). Use of amphotericin B without positive cultures, however, is controversial. Initiation of that therapy must not be done without considering resistant bacterial infections, drug fevers, or indwelling central venous line infections as other causative agents.

When the neutrophil count recovers at approximately 30 days after transplantation, most bacterial and fungal infections will resolve. However, severe humoral and cellular immune dysfunction persists, maintaining host vulnerability to fungal and viral infections (Wingard 1990). Most of the critical infections experienced from day 30 to day 100 post-transplantation occur in patients with GVHD. These infections frequently involve the lungs and may be due to the additive pulmonary toxic effects of total body irradiation, antineoplastic agents, and/or a general impairment of mucociliary action (Phillips 1988). (See Chapter 8 for a full discussion of pulmonary complications.)

Pneumocystis carinii, a protozoa that causes interstitial pneumonia, used to be the most common protozoal pathogen seen in BMT patients. Prior to the advent of sulfamethoxazole-trimethoprim (SMZ-TMP, co-trimoxazole, Bactrim, or Septra), 6% of allogeneic BMT patients developed the highly fatal *P. carinii* pneumonia. Currently, transplant centers administer oral or intravenous SMZ-TMP (SMZ 25–50mg/kg/day, TMP 5–10mg/kg/day) two to three times daily prophylactically for up to 14 days prior to transplant and two days/week from day 30 through 150 after transplantation to prevent *P. carinii* (Engelhard et al. 1986). The delay in initiating SM2-TMP prophylaxis post-engraftment is primarily due to the fact that this drug can interfere with marrow engraftment (Pizzo 1989).

Cytomegalovirus (CMV), a ubiquitous virus that is a member of the herpes family, causes asymptomatic infections in the majority of individuals of the world population, but serious, potentially fatal infections in immunosuppressed patients. It has been isolated from saliva, tears, urine, breast milk, blood, semen, and cervical secretions. After inoculation, the virus usually establishes a latent infection. In the immunosuppressed BMT patient, the infection may result from reactivation of the latent virus or from exogenous acquisition of the virus by either blood product therapy or infected organ or bone marrow. The result of CMV in the BMT patient may range from an asymptomatic seroconversion to life-threatening dissemination. CMV, primarily CMV pneumonia, is the most common cause of death by infection in the BMT patient population and has a mortality rate of approximately 90% (Ford and Eisenberg 1990). In addition, CMV infection has also been found to inhibit immunologic recovery after BMT (Pizzo 1989). Incidence of CMV in autologous transplants is far less than that experienced by allogeneic patients (Wingard 1990).

The use of seronegative blood products is being employed in transplant centers in an effort to reduce the incidence of CMV infections in seronegative BMT patients (Mackinnon et al. 1988). Currently there is no data to support the hypothesis that immunosuppressed seropositive patients benefit from the use of seronegative blood products (Mackinnon et al. 1988). Unfortunately, the availability of CMV seronegative blood products and bone marrow is limited due to the widespread prevalence of the virus (Pomeroy and Englund 1987). Intravenous immune globulin and immune plasma may reduce the risk of CMV in seronegative patients. However, immune globulin therapy for the treatment of active CMV infections has not been found to be effective. Several investigations have utilized an active immunization with the Towne CMV strain. Data from these studies revealed that the vaccine did not decrease the incidence of CMV infection, but it did lessen the severity of the symptoms experienced (Balfour et al. 1984; Plotkin et al. 1984).

Ganciclovir (DHPG) is a new acyclovir derivative currently being investigated by several transplant centers for CMV prophylaxis (Ford and Eisenberg 1990). Fourteen of 18 immunosuppressed patients with virologically confirmed CMV infections exhibited clearing of CMV from all cultured sites. However, relapse of CMV infections was frequent when the drug therapy was stopped and those patients with CMV pneumonia did not respond well. Although neutropenia is a major side effect of ganciclovir, it has the most promising anti-CMV activity of antiviral drugs studied thus far (Pomeroy and Englund 1987; Ford and Eisenberg 1990).

Reactivation of oral or genital herpes simplex infections is common. These infections may present with similar clinical manifestations to that of therapy-induced mucousitis. Some transplant centers recommend administering systemic acyclovir prophylaxis to all patients who are seropositive for herpes simplex (Wingard 1990). Other centers administer acyclovir only to those patients who develop diagnosed herpetic lesions.

Topical antifungal agents such as nystatin, clotrimazole, ketoconazole, or miconazole may be helpful in preventing oropharyngeal candidiasis (Epstein 1990). Some clinicians recommend administering low-dose amphotericin B (20mg/day) for those who develop severe mucosal candidiasis (Phillips 1988).

Other infections frequently observed during this time period are Gram-positive bacterial or fungal sinusitis, cutaneous infections or indwelling CVC infections. Infections from unusual parasites such as *Toxoplasma* may be seen, although the incidence is rare.

Patients who live 100 days after transplantation and are free of GVHD are at less of a risk for many types of infection (Atkinson 1990). Some degree of immunosuppression still exists, however, in the form of specific antibody production and T cell abnormalities. The infections that do occur, therefore, are caused mainly by specific bacterial and viral organisms.

Bacterial infections, particularly those caused by encapsulated organisms such as *Streptococcus pneumoniae* and *Hemophilus influenzae*, are commonly seen in patients with chronic GVHD. If these infections occur, oral antibiotics such as SMZ-TMP or penicillin have been found to be helpful.

Viral infections are also common. Herpes zoster infections are the most frequently experienced viral infections observed during the late transplant period in both allogeneic and autologous patients (Schuchter et al. 1989). However, these infections are more frequently associated in patients with chronic GVHD (Deeg et al. 1988). Systemic acyclovir (500mg/m^2 intravenously every eight hours) is recommended for all cases of multidermatome or disseminated zoster (Phillips 1988).

Anemia

The bone marrow aplasia created by the conditioning regimens creates a reduction in the production and supply of red blood cells. This can result in a potential reduction in adequate tissue oxygenation. Altered hemoglobin and hematocrit levels offer another measurement of the adequacy of body/tissue oxygenation. Clinical manifestations of a reduced erythrocyte count include fatigue, pallor, and occasionally shortness of breath. All symptoms easily resolve with replacement of red blood cells by irradiated packed red blood cell transfusions.

About seven to ten days after marrow ablative chemoradiotherapy and donor or autologous marrow infusion, circulating nucleated red cells will be evident in buffy coat preparations (Burakoff et al. 1983). Circulating reticulocytes, however, often are not evident until about two to three weeks after marrow infusion. An average of 15 units of irradiated packed red cells were administered post-allogeneic transplant for a variety of diseases to maintain the hematocrit between 25 and 30% (Petz 1989). Prolonged red cell aplasia and increased transfusion requirements found in ABO-incompatible allogeneic transplants are discussed later in the chapter.

A variety of techniques including red cell antigen phenotyping and cytogenetic analysis have been used to distinguish between a host or donor source for erythrocyte repopulation following allogeneic BMT (Bar et al. 1989). This determination can be a useful measure of engraftment of donor marrow versus continued host RBC production. The latter is usually indicative of inadequate conditioning, which may also result in disease relapse. Return of normal erythropoiesis is generally first evidenced by the appearance of reticulocytes in the circulation (Griffin 1986).

The reticulocyte maturation index (RMI), another measurement of engraftment in autologous transplants, has been used to study erythropoiesis and has shown promise of detecting marrow engraftment potentially earlier than the reticulocyte or neutrophil count. The RMI is a proportional measurement of reticulocyte maturity determined by the content of reticulocyte RNA using flow cytometric reticulocyte quantification with thiazole orange. In one report, it was the earliest sign of bone marrow engraftment in the majority of patients studied (Davis et al. 1989).

Thrombocytopenia and Bleeding

The megakaryocyte is the last cell to arrive in the myeloid engraftment process; and then only after erythropoiesis is clearly established (Burakoff et al. 1983). Although most allogeneic patients are not platelet transfusion dependent beyond the first two weeks following bone marrow infusion (Osterwalder et al. 1988), normal platelet counts are usually not evident until one to three months and often later (Korbling et al. 1989; Wulff et al. 1983).

Factors related to delayed platelet engraftment (independence from platelet transfusions) include patients with GVHD (First et al. 1985; Anasetti et al. 1989a) and cyclosporine prophylaxis (Bensinger et al. 1989). Patients who are treated with autologous marrow for leukemia (Cahn et al. 1986; Beelen 1989) and some of those who received pharmacologically purged marrow (Korbling et al. 1989; Yeager et al. 1986) or monoclonal antibody-purged marrow (Ball et al. 1990) experienced delays in the return of platelet counts when compared to the allogeneic patient. In the Cahn study (1986), although platelet recovery was delayed compared with the typical platelet recovery time for allogeneic patients, there was no significant difference in hematopoietic recovery when the purged (monoclonal antibody and complement and mafosfamide [ASTA-Z]) and nonpurged groups were compared. Platelet recovery following solid tumor high-dose therapy and nonpurged autologous marrow transplant demonstrated a more rapid platelet recovery than was evident in patients with autologous transplantation for leukemia (Mulder et al. 1989).

Mechanisms of delayed platelet engraftment or prolonged thrombocytopenia are probably multifactoral and include platelet autoantibodies (Anasetti et al. 1989a), host-versus-graft antibodies (Panzer et al. 1988), viral infections (Cahn et al. 1989), GVHD (First et al. 1985; Anasetti et al. 1989a; Bensinger et al. 1989), and possibly the purging agent, cryopreservation techniques (Rowley et al. 1989), or CFU-GM content of the infused marrow (Ball et al. 1990; Rowley et al. 1987).

A factor under study to predict platelet recovery is megakaryocyte colony stimulating activity (MK-CSA) in the serum of patients during BMT (Fauser et al. 1988; de Alarcon et al. 1988). Levels appear to be biphasic and peak just after the beginning of the preparative regimen and again during the second week after bone marrow infusion, corresponding to the beginning of hematopoietic recovery (de Alarcon et al. 1988). Patients who failed to engraft did not show a spike during the second week, prompting the investigators to conclude that this spike was a physiologic response to marrow ablation and was associated with successful marrow engraftment (de Alarcon et al. 1988).

Thrombocytopenia can be transient or prolonged; however, persistent and prolonged thrombocytopenia can indicate a worse overall prognosis (First et al. 1985; de Alarcon et al. 1988). Despite occasional prolonged thrombocytopenia, mortality from bleeding complications in the general bone marrow transplant population is uncommon, probably due in large part to improvements in providing platelet transfusion support (see transfusion support described in the next section).

Graft Failure

Graft failure, a rare but potential complication following infusion of HLA-identical, partially matched allogeneic donor, or autologous marrow, can occur (is defined as) as complete absence of engraftment or as seemingly initial normal hematopoiesis with later decreasing blood counts and absence of normal hematopoiesis. As mentioned earlier, the appearance of peripherally circulating graft-generated blood cells (usually beginning with nucleated red cells) can be seen as early as seven to ten days following bone marrow stem cell infusion. However, since there is such a wide variation in time until complete myeloid regeneration has been observed (Burakoff et al. 1983), a diagnosis of graft failure may not be made until many weeks after the infusion. Additionally, graft failure may result even after apparent initial signs of engraftment (Deeg et al. 1988).

Graft failure in the allogeneic transplant patient is estimated to occur in less than 1% of patients receiving an HLA-identical sibling donor transplant (Storb 1989). With the more recent use of histoincompatible marrow grafts, a failure rate of 5–25% has been reported (Storb, 1989; Deeg 1988); with the likelihood of failure increasing with the degree of incompatibility (Anasetti et al. 1989b). Patients with aplastic anemia who have received blood transfusions prior to transplant demonstrated a 30–60% graft rejection rate compared with a 5% rejection rate in untransfused patients (Deeg 1988). The mechanism is thought to be sensitization of the recipient to minor histocompatibility antigens shared by the transfusion and marrow donor, or the persistence of host-derived cytotoxic T lymphocytes or natural killer cells (Barge et al. 1989). The practice of using family members for blood transfusions prior to allogeneic transplant for leukemia, however, does not seem to increase the rate of graft failure in this population (Ho et al. 1987).

In the allogeneic patient, graft rejection and subsequent failure is thought to result from marrow rejection by host T cells not eliminated during conditioning by a different mechanism from that seen in GVHD (Storb 1989; Voogt et al. 1990) or possibly from manipulation of allogeneic marrow during T cell depletion procedures employed to reduce the occurence of GVHD. In T cell-depleted donor marrow there is a reduced incidence of GVHD, but the immunosuppressive effect of the donor marrow is also lost, allowing the remaining host immune function to potentially reject the graft (Patterson et al. 1985; Voogt et al. 1990).

In the autologous transplant, the causes of graft failure are thought to be primarily related to infusion of inadequate numbers of stem cells to allow hematopoietic reconstitution, damage of the stem cells during in vitro manipulation (i.e., purging) (Deeg et al. 1988) and cryopreservation (Rowley et al. 1989), or the inability of the marrow environment to support (accept) marrow cells (defective soil) (Gee 1990). More recently, it has been proposed in heavily pretreated autologous marrow patients that although adequate cell numbers have been harvested and reinfused, inadequate engraftment or absence of engraftment has resulted due to some qualitative defect of the stem cells, possibly caused by the heavy pretreatment (Gee 1990; Visani et al. 1990). If this is the responsible mechanism, once again the question of when to harvest becomes an important one.

Death due to infection and hemorrhage that occurs due to prolonged pancytopenia may mask underlying graft failure as the cause. Therefore, the incidence of this complication is not well characterized. The incidence of marrow failure following the more recent practice of infusion of peripheral blood stem cells is even less well characterized.

Mortality rates with graft failure are extremely high and treatment is generally supportive. The idea of graft failure is devastating to the patient, family, donor (if allogeneic), and staff, and a feeling of despair and helplessness can permeate the team who are often only able to stand by and watch the inevitable deterioration of the patient. Treatments at this point include attempts at immunosuppression if the belief is that lack of engraftment is not graft failure but an immune phenomenon, discontinuation of drugs known to interfere with bone marrow function (e.g., trimethoprim-sulfamethoxazole [Bactrim]) (Storb 1989), searching for an allogeneic donor, marrow stimulation with colony-stimulating factors, or infusion of reserve marrow (if available). Autologous transplant centers have inconsistent policies regarding whether a "back-up" or reserve marrow is routinely collected. It is more likely when newer in vitro treatment (purging) methods are being employed; in that situation, an untreated back-up marrow may be stored. However, it is often difficult to obtain adequate marrow from many heavily pretreated autologous patients to ensure adequate cell numbers to accomplish a single reconstitution.

Management of the Patient with Pancytopenia

Immunosuppression

The nursing care of the immunosuppressed BMT patient is complex and multifaceted. When caring for a BMT patient, it is important to understand the dysfunctional components of their immune system, the resulting infections commonly observed during the different phases of transplantation, and the clinical manifestations of infections in neutropenic patients. This knowledge will facilitate adequate and thorough assessment of the patient and early detection of potential sepsis. It is also critical that the BMT nurse know the signs, symptoms, and pathophysiology of endotoxic shock caused by Gram-negative bacilli; the nurse should act immediately if such signs occur. These include chills, fever or hypothermia, prostration, tachycardia and tachypnea, hypotension, peripheral cyanosis, cold and clammy extremities, oliguria, and a decreased level of consciousness (Ketchel and Rodriguez 1978).

Nursing interventions are first aimed at preventing nosocomial or exogenously acquired infections. Patients are maintained in a total protective isolation environment or a private room to prevent or minimize the acquisition of exogenous pathogens while neutrophil counts are below 0.5 $\times$ 10^9/liter. As mentioned earlier, the use of laminar air flow rooms for this purpose is controversial in that data from some studies investigating protective isolation compared with standard hospital care did not reveal statistically significant differences in the overall incidence of infection, the length of time to the onset of infection, or the number of days with fever (Golden 1979; Neuseef and Maki 1981; Ogden et al. 1990).

One of the most important procedures in preventing the transmission of infections is *meticulous* handwashing. The use of antimicrobial soap, water, and friction are sufficient to remove most organisms. Some investigators have found that antiseptic agents produce excessively dry skin resulting in dermatitis and cracked skin, which can then harbor pathogens that are not easily removed, thus decreasing the efficacy of bacterial removal by handwashing. Others have found that bar and liquid soaps are an excellent medium for bacterial growth and, therefore, these products should be used with caution. Dehydrated soap flakes or liquid soaps that contain a bacteriostatic agent are potential alternatives (Steere and Mallison 1975; Wessler 1982).

Integumentary or mucosal interruptions allow various organisms to become pathogens and produce infection. These interruptions can be intentional as in bone marrow biopsies or venipuncture, or a consequence of therapy such as chemotherapy and total body irradiation. Avoidance of unnecessary enemas, venipunctures, bladder catheterizations, and finger sticks will help reduce damage to the body barriers. Stringent oral, perineal, and skin care may also reduce interruptions in skin integrity (Halliburton 1986).

Many transplant centers place their immunosuppressed BMT patients on low bacterial or sterile diets in an attempt to further reduce the incidence of exogenous acquired infections (Aker and Cheney 1983). *Escherichia coli, Klebsiella pneumoniae,* and *Pseudomonas aeruginosa* have been found on raw vegetable salads and fresh fruits (Remington and Schimpff 1981). Inadequate data exist to determine whether a low microbial diet can provide protection from infection equal to that of a sterile diet regardless of the environment the patient is in (Buckner et al. 1979; Clift et al. 1979; Kurrle et al. 1980). Some studies suggest that sterile food is not required for gut sterilization if oral nonabsorbable antibiotics are administered (Preisler et al. 1970; Levine et al. 1973; Siegel et al. 1971; Schimpff et al. 1975; Aker and Cheney 1983). Selective decontamination, gut sterilization, and special diets are considered in greater detail in Chapter 9.

Perineal abscesses are a frequent occurrence in immunosuppressed BMT patients. They are difficult to detect early in their course due to the minimal inflammatory response commonly seen in neutropenia. The patient, therefore, needs to maintain normal bowel function to reduce the incidence of pathogenic invasion into the altered gastrointestinal mucosa. Low bulk diets are recommended because they reduce total stool volume and reduce the total bacterial load that comes in contact with the anal orifice. Stool softeners may also be given to prevent constipation, which may result in further trauma to the intestinal mucosa (Schimpff et al. 1975; Brandt 1984). Sitz baths with antimicrobial irrigating solutions such as povidone iodine or chlorhexadrine can reduce the bacterial count and trauma from tissue paper cleansing of the anal orifice especially for patients with perirectal irritation from diarrhea. Avoidance of rectal temperatures, suppositories, enemas, or manipulations is recommended (Brandt 1984).

Most BMT patients have multiple lumen indwelling central venous catheters (CVC) during their hospitalization. An increase in the use of these catheters has been implicated in the rising rate of Gram-positive infections in cancer patients (Pizzo 1989). A prospective study of the use of

Hickman right atrial catheters in a BMT population noted a 44% infectious complication associated with these catheters (Viz et al. 1990). Meticulous care should be given when changing IV tubing, solutions, and administering medications. CVC sites should be inspected daily and assessed for erythema, skin breakdown, stitch abscess, drainage, swelling, and pain. However, drainage and swelling will be rare in severely immunosuppressed patients. It is recommended that bottles and IV solution sets be changed every 24 hours (Brandt 1984). A variety of protocols exist for CVC dressing changing procedures and frequency (Oncology Nursing Society 1989). Data is lacking to indicate which procedure is most effective to reduce the incidence of site or catheter-related systemic infections. In one prospective, randomized study comparing the use of transparent and gauze dressings, transparent dressings were found to be associated with increased rates of insertion site colonization, local catheter-related infection, and systemic catheter-related sepsis (Conly et al. 1989). Catheter care is a fertile area for nursing research.

Occasionally patients may require peripheral IV access especially if the CVC has been removed or does not provide adequate access for the tremendous IV medication, fluid, and blood product demands. Nosocomial staphylococcal septicemia due to intravenous needles has also been observed in immunosuppressed patients. A study by Band and Maki (1980) examining infection rates of peripheral IV sites revealed that all septicemias occurred in patients who had peripheral IV placements in the same site for more than 72 hours. Therefore, it is recommended that peripheral IV sites be changed every 48 to 72 hours if possible. Conversely, frequent peripheral IV site changes produce greater alterations in the integument and may place the patient at a higher risk for developing infections at a greater number of sites. Therefore nursing judgement should be used to determine a risk/benefit analysis for the individual patient.

As with all neutropenic patients, assessments should include: (1) frequent monitoring of vital signs, (2) inspection of all integumentary areas particularly the perineal area and those prone to dampness such as the axillae, beneath the breasts, and under fat folds, (3) inspection of oral mucosa, (4) auscultation of lungs every four to six hours to monitor the patient for changes in respiratory function, and (5) monitoring for changes in genitourinary function such as frequency, dysuria, cloudy urine, and hematuria. Application of an antifungal powder is recommended for areas prone to dampness to prevent fungal colonization.

Any sign of infection in an immunosuppressed BMT patient should be treated as a medical emergency. The nurse should notify the physician immediately, and anticipate a combination of further diagnostic assessments and prompt therapeutic interventions. Fever work-up cultures include blood cultures, both peripheral and through the CVC, urine, throat, sputum, and any draining wounds cultures. A chest x-ray is often ordered. Broad spectrum antibiotic therapy will often be initiated immediately after obtaining cultures. Antibiotic therapy is administered on a prescribed, around-the-clock basis to maintain effective serum levels. When possible, blood therapy should be administered in between antibiotics to reduce the chance of lowering serum antibiotic levels. Although controversial, some transplant centers obtain bacterial and viral surveillance cultures of the nose, oral cavity, throat, axillae, and/or perianal area, stool, and urine ranging from twice weekly to biweekly (Brandt 1984; Pizzo 1989).

After transplantation, patients vary in their ability to mount adequate antibody responses to antigens. Therefore, immunizations are not generally recommended during the first year after transplantation. Patients should, however, undergo immune function tests at approximately one year post-transplant to see if they can initiate a response at that time. Depending on the results of these tests, an immunization schedule may then be recommended (Lum et al. 1986; Lum 1990).

Pneumovax, attenuated Salk polio, influenza, diphtheria, pertussis, and tetanus toxoid are the booster vaccines usually recommended. Two to four weeks after patients receive their initial vaccinations, titers should be drawn to measure their response. If the titer levels are low, the primary series should be repeated (Lum 1987).

Individuals who have been exposed to varicella or herpes zoster should receive varicella zoster immune globulin (VZIG). Vesicles can appear from one to seven days after the initial exposure. The VZIG is most effective when administered within 96 hours after exposure and the effectiveness lasts for three weeks. After this time, if the patient comes in contact with chicken pox, another VZIG vaccination is necessary (Nims and Strom 1988).

It is important that BMT patients avoid individuals receiving live-virus vaccines during the first year post-transplant (Lum 1990). The Salk parenteral vaccine is recommended for family members who require a polio vaccination. Also, individuals who experience chronic GVHD that persists after the first year post-transplant should continue to avoid persons who have received live-virus vaccinations (Lum et al. 1986).

Blood Product Support

The ability to support the BMT patient post-transplant with RBCs and platelets is critical to the success of the transplant and has been the subject of many reviews (Osterwalder et al. 1988; Erickson 1990; Petz 1989; Brand et al. 1984; McCullough et al. 1984; Storb and Weiden 1981). Maintaining an adequate hemoglobin, hematocrit, and platelet count in the acute phase post-transplant is necessary for patient comfort and safety and provides a nursing challenge. Red cell and platelet support may have been required before BMT as a result of the underlying disease, and after the transplant due to the bone marrow suppressive (pancytopenia) effects of chemo and/or radiation therapy. Therefore, the duration of support may last as little as two to three weeks or continue as long as many months depending on the success (rapidity with which BM function returns) of bone marrow engraftment post-transplantation. Depending on the type of transplant, and the resulting severity and duration of marrow hypoplasia, a wide range in the number of transfusions required has been reported (Petz 1989; McCullough et al. 1984).

Most transplant center protocols advise RBC transfusion to keep the hematocrit at a minimum of 25–30%. In general, the majority of RBC transfusions are administered within the first four weeks following transplant, although it may be 6–12 weeks before erythropoiesis is adequate to maintain the hematocrit at this level. Blood loss can result from hemorrhage and excessive laboratory blood draws (up to 150ml/wk) during the acute phase.

Additionally, prolonged red blood cell support is routinely required for a longer period of time for BMT patients with major ABO incompatibility than when donor and recipient are ABO compatible (Wulff et al. 1983; Petz 1989; Gmur et al. 1990). The immunohematologic consequences of such transplants are summarized in Table 6.4. Removal of antibodies from the patient and removal of red cells from the donor product are two measures designed to overcome these problems (Petz 1989).

Viable lymphocytes (cells still capable of division) present in all cellular transfusion products, including stored RBCs, are thought to be capable of triggering GVHD. This rejection reaction of the graft against seemingly "foreign" host tissues can occur in both allogeneic (Petz 1989) and autologous patients (Postmus et al. 1988). Although GVHD can occur in HLA-matched sibling allogenic BMT recipients, and more frequently with lesser degrees of matches, using irradiated blood products can avert GVHD produced by blood product transfusions (Anderson and Weinstein 1990). The usual radiation dosage recommended is between 1.5 and 3.0Gy (1500–3000cGy) of gamma radiation (Petz 1989). The irradiation of blood products usually takes place in the radiation

Table 6.4. Immunohematologic Consequences of ABO-Incompatible Bone Marrow Transplants

Minor ABO incompatibility
  Anticipated problems
    Graft-versus-host disease
    Immune hemolysis at the time of infusion of the donor marrow caused by anti-A and anti-B in the plasma of the marrow product
  Unanticipated problem
    Immune hemolysis of delayed onset caused by red cell antibodies produced by the donor marrow
Major ABO incompatibility
  Anticipated problems
    Failure of stem cell engraftment
    Delay in onset of hematopoiesis, especially erythropoiesis
    Acute hemolysis at the time of infusion of the donor marrow
    Delayed onset of hemolysis associated with persistence of anti-A and/or anti-B after transplantation
    Hemolysis of infused red cells of donor type
    Hemolysis of red cells produced by the engrafted marrow
  Unanticipated problem
    Mixed hematopoietic chimerism

Source: Petz 1987, with permission.

therapy department just prior to transfusion, and takes about three minutes (McCullough et al. 1984). Occasionally, several units may be irradiated if a patient requires regular transfusions or is actively hemorrhaging. Some BMT centers have dedicated small irradiation equipment for this sole purpose. Since the other cellular functional components of irradiated blood products are not affected by this dose of radiation, these units of blood may be used for other appropriately crossmatched patients should the BMT patient for whom they were irradiated no longer need transfusion support.

Administration of irradiated blood products begins during the conditioning phase and is continued post-transplant. The length of time to continue irradiation of blood products post-transplant is a source of controversy. It currently seems logical to continue irradiation during the period of immunosuppression. However, this period of time is not well defined and may extend for years, especially for patients experiencing GVHD (see Chapter 7). This issue may present a discharge problem to some transfusion-dependent patients returning to a facility unfamiliar with transplant, since not all blood centers (banks) have the capacity to irradiate blood products (Messerschmidt et al. 1981).

Platelet transfusions are required by most transplant recipients for at least two to three weeks after marrow infusion. Most transplant centers typically maintain the platelet count above $20 \times 10^9/l$. Various platelet products including random donor, single donor apheresis products, HLA-matched, and more recently autologous products (Mulder et al. 1989) have been used to get the best response for the individual patient. These products are often used in the order described above, advancing towards a more specific product when the patient fails to achieve a satisfactory one-hour post-platelet increment (Erickson 1990). Currently, the benefit of this practice has not been supported by a prospective trial (Messerschmidt et al. 1988).

The presence of fever, bleeding, infection, and alloimmunization will all affect the survival of platelets being infused (Erickson 1990). Leukocyte removal filters, and premedication with acetaminophen and diphenhydramine may also help to reduce adverse reactions to platelet transfusions.

Other special considerations in blood product support include the use of CMV seronegative blood products (discussed earlier), which has reduced the incidence of this potentially fatal infection in seronegative allogeneic transplant patients. However, it has not had an impact on the autologous patient who generally experiences a much lower incidence of this infection (Mackinnon et al. 1988). Also, several cases of acquired immunodeficiency syndrome (AIDS) have been reported in patients who received blood products from infected donors (Atkinson et al. 1987), although with current blood screening this problem is unlikely in transplant centers today.

Future Directions

Shortening the duration and severity of pancytopenia following bone marrow transplantation is a major goal to reduce the morbidity and mortality of this common complication. Recent basic research efforts have identified a group of hematopoietic growth factors. These growth factors may revolutionize the treatments employed in hematology/oncology settings, as they provide opportunities for historically untreatable diseases to be amenable to medical treatment. Reduced infection-related morbidity is but one result, enabling high-dose chemotherapeutic and/or radiotherapeutic regimens to be used to treat a variety of neoplastic and myelodysplastic diseases. The growth factors being investigated include granulocyte-macrophage colony stimulating factor (GM-CSF), granulocyte colony stimulating factor (G-CSF), macrophage colony stimulating factor (M-CSF), and interleukin-3 or multicolony stimulating factor (Andreeff and Welte 1989).

GM-CSF and G-CSF have been found to induce cell cycle changes in suspension cultures of primary human myeloid leukemias (Murohashi et al. 1988; Andreeff et al. 1988; Tafuri et al. 1988). Not only did both growth factors increase the number of cells in the S-phase of the cell cycle, they also recruited cells from G_0 into G_1. These data demonstrated marked recruitment of leukemic cells into the cell cycle, which theoretically should make them more sensitive to the action of cell cycle specific drugs.

GM-CSF has also shown promising results in increasing neutrophils, eosinophils, and monocytes in a variety of immunosuppressed patients with subsequent reduction in clinical manifestations of infection. Vadhan-Raj and colleagues

(1987) administered GM-CSF by continuous infusion for two weeks to patients with aplastic anemia. The total WBC counts increased from 1.6 times to tenfold, with increases occurring primarily in the neutrophils. Brandt et al. (1988) administered GM-CSF to autologous BMT patients and noticed an accelerated granulocyte recovery and reduced toxicity. Groopman et al. (1987) administered GM-CSF to patients with AIDS and neutropenia. A dose-related increase in normally functioning circulating neutrophils, eosinophils, and monocytes was demonstrated in addition to an increased killing of HIV-infected lymphocytes. Side effects reported from various studies include low-grade fever, myalgia, phlebitis, flushing (Groopman 1987), pulmonary sequestration (Peters 1988), a decrease in serum cholesterol, and Sweet syndrome (Andreef and Welte 1989).

Clinical studies investigating the effect of GM-CSF and G-CSF are demonstrating exciting results in the recovery of normal hematopoiesis in leukemia patients after chemotherapy and in patients with a variety of neoplastic diseases after autologous bone marrow transplantation. Soon the use of growth factors may become a standard component of chemotherapy protocols in an attempt to alleviate some deleterious effects of chemotherapy-induced immunosuppression (Burdach et al. 1988).

The use of a combination of bone marrow-derived and peripherally derived stem cells also has been attempted to offset the immediate and long-term bone marrow suppressive effects of high-dose chemoradiotherapy used in transplant. The hypothesis is that bone marrow and peripheral stem cells potentially differ in function. The bone marrow cells are known to provide a lifelong supply of numbers and types of cells, while the properties of peripherally derived stem cells are still being investigated. It appears that following the peripheral stem cell infusion there is a quicker production and/or appearance of normal myeloid cells in the circulation (Gianni et al. 1989). This was demonstrated in the aforementioned study where myeloid recovery (greater than 500 granulocytes/L) occurred by day 13 following the combined bone marrow and peripheral stem cell graft, in constrast to the bone-marrow-only derived group, which did not show a median recovery until day 17.

Finally, as many of the most critical infections occur in patients with severe GVHD, decreasing the incidence and controlling the severity of GVHD can reduce the morbidity and mortality associated infections in this group. (See Chapter 7 on future directions for a complete discussion of these research efforts.)

Continued medical efforts will attempt to reduce the period preceding myeloid recovery. Future nursing research needs to be directed at determining the most effective nursing interventions that will protect the patient from harmful effects during the period of pancytopenia.

Summary

Due to defects in nonspecific and specific (humoral and cellular) immune function resulting from chemotherapy and total body irradiation utilized in conditioning regimens, a wide variety of bacterial, fungal, viral, and protozoal infections occur in patients undergoing bone marrow transplantation. Although often less severe, reduced platelet and red cell counts can also lead to significant morbidity and mortality. Because of current information on immunosuppression and immune recovery, many of these infections are predictable. Reductions in infection-related mortality are occurring due to improvement in diagnosis, antibiotic therapies, and thorough nursing and medical assessments. Reversal of the effects of anemia and thrombocytopenia through appropriate blood product support is an important nursing function in preventing adverse effects from these complications.

References

Aker, S.N., and Cheney, C.L. 1983. The use of sterile and low microbial diets in ultraisolation environments. *Journal of Parenteral and Enteral Nutrition* 7 (4): 390–397.

Anasetti, C. et al. 1989a. Graft-versus-host disease is associated with autoimmune-like thrombocytopenia. *Blood 73* (4): 1054–1058.

Anasetti, C. et al. 1989b. Effect of HLA compatibility on engraftment of bone marrow transplants in patients with leukemia or lymphoma. *N. Engl. J. Med. 320* (4): 197–204.

Anderson, K.C., and Weinstein, H.J. 1990. Tranfusion-associated graft-versus-host disease. *N. Engl. J. Med. 323* (5): 315–321.

Andreeff, M. et al. 1988. Cytokine modulation of leukemia cell proliferation and differentiation. *Cytometry* (suppl 2).

Andreeff, M., and Welte, K. 1989. Hematopoietic colony-stimulating factors. *Seminars in Oncology 16* (3): 211–229.

Atkinson, K. 1990. Reconstruction of the haemopoietic and immune systems after marrow transplantation. *B.M.T. 5:* 209–226.

Atkinson, K. et al. 1987. The development of the acquired immunodeficiency syndrome after bone-marrow transplantation. *The Medical Journal of Australia 147:* 510–512.

Balfour, H.H. et al. 1984. Cytomegalovirus vaccine in renal transplant candidates: Progress report of a randomized, placebo-controlled, double-blind trial. *Birth Defects 20:* 289–304.

Ball, E.D. et al. 1990. Autologous bone marrow transplantation for acute myeloid leukemia using monoclonal antibody-purged bone marrow. *Blood 75* (5): 1199–1206.

Band, J., and Maki, D. 1980. Steel needles used for intravenous therapy. *Archives of Internal Medicine 140:* 31–34.

Bar, B.M.A.M. et al. 1989. Host and donor erythrocyte repopulation patterns after allogeneic bone marrow transplantation analysed with antibody-coated fluorescent microspheres. *British Journal of Hematology 72:* 239–245.

Barge, A.J. et al. 1989. Antibody-mediated marrow failure after allogeneic bone marrow transplantation. *Blood 74* (5): 1477–1480.

Beelen, D.W. 1989. Acute toxicity and first clinical results of intensive postinduction therapy using a modified busulfan and cyclophosphamide regimen with autologous bone marrow rescue in first remission of acute myeloid leukemia. *Blood 74* (5): 1507–1516.

Bensinger, W. et al. 1989. Engraftment and transfusion requirements after allogeneic marrow transplantation for patients with acute non-lymphocytic leukemia in first complete remission. *B.M.T. 4:* 409–414.

Bowden, R.A., and Meyers, J.D. 1985. Infectious complications following marrow transplantation. *Plasma Therapy Transfusion Technology 6:* 285.

Brand, A. et al. 1984. Blood componenet therapy in bone marrow transplantation. *Seminars in Hematology 21* (2): 141–155.

Brandt, B. 1984. A nursing protocol for the client with neutropenia. *O.N.F. 11* (2): 24–28.

Brandt, S.J. et al. 1988. Effect of recombinant human granulocyte-macrophage factor on hematopoietic reconstitution after high-dose chemotherapy and autologous bone marrow transplantation. *N. Engl. J. Med. 318:* 869–873.

Brittingham, T.E., and Chaplin, H. 1957. Febrile transfusion reactions caused by sensitivity to donor leukocytes and platelets. *JAMA 165:* 819–825.

Buckner, C.D. et al. 1979. Protective environment for marrow transplant recipients. *Ann. Intern. Med. 89:* 893–901.

Buckner, C.D. et al. 1983. Early infectious complications in allogeneic marrow transplant recipients with acute leukemia: Effects of prophylactic measures. *Infection 11:* 243–250.

Burakoff, S.J. et al. 1983. Recapitulation of the immune response and haematopoietic system in bone marrow transplantation. *Clinics in Hematology 12* (3): 695–720.

Burdoch, S. et al. 1988. Differential T cell modulation of hematopoiesis is mediated at different levels of gene expression and is dependent upon alternatve IL-2 receptor (IL-2R) expression. *Blood 72:* 111a (suppl. 1).

Cahn, J.Y. et al. 1986. Autologous bone marrow transplantation (ABMT) for acute leukaemia in complete remission: A pilot study of 33 cases. *British Journal of Haematology 63:* 457–470.

Cahn, J.Y. et al. 1989. Autoimmune-like thrombocytopenia after bone marrow transplantation. *Blood 74* (8): 2771–2772.

Clark, R.A. et al. 1976. Defective neutrophil chemotaxis in bone marrow transplant patients. *J. Clin. Invest. 58:* 22.

Clift, F.A., Buckner, C.D., and Thomas, E.D. 1979. Gnotobiology in marrow transplantation. *Zentralbl. Bakteriol. 7* (suppl.): 255–264.

Conly, J.M. et al. 1989. A prospective, randomized study comparing transparent and dry gauze dressings for central renous catheters. *J. Inf. Dis. 159* (2): 310–319.

Davis, B.H. et al. 1989. Utility of flow cytometric reticulocyte quantification as a predictor of engraftment in autologous bone marrow transplantation. *American Journal of Hematology 32:* 81–87.

de Alarcon, P.A. et al. 1988. Pattern of response of magakaryocyte colony-stimulating activity in the serum of patients undergoing bone marrow transplantation. *Exp. Hematol. 16:* 316–319.

Deeg, H.J. et al. 1988. *A guide to bone marrow transplantation.* New York: Springer-Verlag.

Drutz, D.J. et al. 1985. Invasive fungal disease. *Conversation in Infection Control 6* (6): 1–12.

Engelhard, D., Marks, M.I., and Good, R.A. 1986. Infections in bone marrow transplant recipients. *J. Pediat. 108* (3): 335–343.

Epstein, J. 1990. Infection prevention in bone marrow transplantation and radiation patients. *NCI Monographs 9:* 73–85.

Erickson, J.M. 1990. Blood support for the myelosuppressed patient. *Seminars in Oncology Nursing 6* (1): 61–66.

Fauser, A.A. et al. 1988. Megakaryocytic colony-stimulating activity in patients receiving a marrow transplant during hematopoietic reconstitution. *Transplantation 46* (4): 543–548.

First, L.R. et al. 1985. Isolated thrombocytopenia after allogeneic bone marrow transplant and chronic thrombocytopenia syndromes. *Blood* 65 (2): 368–374.

Ford, R., and Eisenberg, S. 1990. Bone marrow transplant: Recent advances and nursing implication. *Nurs. Clin. North Am.* 25 (2): 405–422.

Ganong, W.F. 1985. Section VI. Circulation. Circulating Body Fluids. In Ganong, W.F. (ed.). *Review of Medical Physiology.* Twelfth Edition. Los Altos, CA: Lange Medical Publication, pp. 421–441.

Gee, A.P. 1990. Bone marrow purging and processing—A review of ancillary effects. In *Bone Marrow Purging and Processing.* Alan R. Liss, Inc.: 507–521.

Gianni, A.M. et al. 1989. Rapid and complete hemopoietic reconstitution following combined transplantation of autologous blood and bone marrow cells. A changing role for high dose chemo-radiotherapy? *Hematological Oncology* 7: 139–148.

Gmur, J.P. et al. 1990. Pure red cell aplasia of long duration complicating major ABO-incompatible bone marrow transplantation. *Blood* 75 (1): 290–295.

Golden, W. 1979. Routine protective isolation: Worth the trouble in neutropenic patients? *JAMA* 242 (19): 2045.

Goldstein, I.M. 1987. Phagocytic Cells: Chemotaxis and effector functions of macrophages and granulocytes. In Stites, D.P. et al. (eds.). *Basic and Clinical Immunology, Sixth Edition.* Norwalk, CT: Appleton & Lange, pp. 106–113.

Goodman, J.W. 1987. Immunoglobulins I: Structure & Function. In Stites, D.P., Stobo, J.D., and Wells, J.V. (eds.). *Basic and Clinical Immunology. Sixth Edition.* Norwalk, CT and Los Altos, CA: Appleton & Lange, pp. 27–36.

Griffin, J.P. 1986. Physiology of the hematopoietic system. In Griffin, J.P. (ed.). *Hematology and Immunology. Concepts for Nursing.* Norwalk, CT: Appleton-Century-Crofts, pp. 19–40.

Groopman, J.E. et al. 1987. Effect of recombinant human granulocyte-macrophage colony-stimulating factor on hematopoietic reconstitution after high-dose chemotherapy and autologous bone marrow transplantation. *N. Engl. J. Med. 319:* 593–598.

Guyton, A.C. 1986. *Textbook of Medical Physiology. 7th ed.* Phil.: Saunders.

Halliburton, P. 1986. Impaired immunocompetence. In Carrieri, V.K., Lindsey, A.M., and West, C.M. (eds.) *Pathophysiological Phenomena in Nursing. Human Responses to Illness.* Philadelphia, PA: W.B. Saunders Company, pp. 319–342.

Ho, W.G. et al. 1987. Bone marrow transplantation in patients with leukaemia previously transfused with blood products from family members. *British Journal of Hematology* 67: 67–70.

Juttner, C.A. et al. 1988. Early lympho-hemopoietic recovery after autografting using peripheral blood stem cells in acute non-lymphoblastic leukemia. *Transplantation Proc.* 20 (1): 40–43.

Kelleher, J., and Bochsel, P. 1989. Bone marrow transplantation. *Nurs. Clin. North Am.* 24 (4): 707–938.

Ketchel, S. and Rodriguez, B. 1978. Acute infections in cancer patients. *Seminars in Oncology* 5 (2): 167–179.

Korbling, M. et al. 1989. Disease-free survival after autologous bone marrow transplantation in patients with acute myclogenous leukemia. *Blood* 74 (6): 1898–1904.

Kurrle, E. et al. 1980. The efficiency of strict reverse isolation and antimicrobial decontamination in remission induction therapy of acute leukemia. *Blut* 40: 187–195.

Levine, A.S. et al. 1973. Protected environments and prophylactic antibiotics. *N. Engl. J. Med.* 288: 477–483.

Lindgren, P.S. 1983. The laminar air flow room: Nursing practices and procedures. *Nurs. Clin. North Am.* 18 (3): 553–561.

Livnat, S. et al. 1980. Analysis of cytotoxic effector cell function in patients with leukemia or aplastic anemia before and after marrow transplantation. *J. Immunol.* 124: 481.

Lubran, M.M. 1989. Hematologic side effects of drugs. *Annals of Clinical and Laboratory Science* 19 (2): 114–121.

Lum, L.G. 1987. The kinetics of immune reconstitution after human marrow transplantation. *Blood* 69 (2): 369.

Lum, L.G. 1990. Immune recovery after bone marrow transplantation. *Hematology/Oncology Clinics of North America* 4 (3): 659–675.

Lum, L. et al. 1986. The detection of specific antibody formation to recall antigens after human bone marrow transplantation. *Blood* 67: 582–587.

McCullough J. et al. 1984. Role of the blood bank in bone marrow transplantation. In *Advances in Immunobiology: Blood cell Antigens and Bone Marrow Transplantation.* NY: Alan R. Liss, pp. 379–412.

Mackinnon S. et al. 1988. Seronegative blood products prevent primary cytomegalovirus infection after bone marrow transplantation. *J. Clin. Pathol.* 41: 948–950.

Marsh, J.C. 1985. Chemical toxicity of the granulocyte. In Irons, R.D. (ed.) *Toxicology of the Blood and Bone Marrow.* New York, NY: Raven Press, pp. 51–63.

Messerschmidt, G.L. et al. 1981. Blood component irradiation prior to transfusion of allogeneic blood products in immunosuppressed patients. *Transfusion* 58 (5): 183a.

Messerschmidt G.L. et al. 1988. A prospective randomized trial of HLA-matched versus mismatched single donor platelet transfusions in cancer patients. *Cancer* 62: 795–801.

Meyers, J.D., and Atkinson, K. 1983. Infection in bone marrow transplantation. *Clinical Haematology* 12: 791.

Meyers, J.D., Flournoy, N., and Thomas, E.D. 1986. Risk factors for cytomegalovirus infection after human marrow transplantation. *J. Infect. Dis.* 153: 478–488.

Milliken, S.T., and Powles, R.L. 1990. Antifungal prophylaxis in bone marrow transplantation. *Reviews of Infectious Diseases* 12 (suppl. 3): 5374–5379.

Mulder, P.O.M. et al. 1989. Bleeding prophylaxis in autologous bone marrow transplantation for solid tumors. *Haemostasis* 19: 120–124.

Murohashi, I. et al. 1988. Effects of recombinant G-CSF and GM-CSF on the growth in methyl-cellulose and suspension of the blast cells in acute myeloblastic leukemia. *Leukemia Research* 12: 433–440.

Neuseef, W., and Maki, D. 1981. A study of the value of simple protective isolation in patients with granulocytopenia. *N. Engl. J. Med.* 304 (8): 448–453.

Nims, J.W., and Strom, S. 1988. Late complications of bone marrow transplant recipients: Nursing care issues. *Seminars in Oncology Nursing* 4 (1): 47–54.

Noel, D.R. et al. 1978. Does graft-versus-host disease influence the tempo of immunologic recovery after allogeneic human marrow transplantation? An observation on 56 long-term survivors. *Blood* 51: 1087.

Ogden, A.K. et al. 1990. Bone marrow transplantation in childhood leukemia using reverse isolation techniques. *Med. Ped. Onc.* 18 (1): 1–5.

Oncology Nursing Society. 1989. Module I Catheters. *Recommendations for Nursing Education and Practice*. Pittsburgh, PA: Oncology Nursing Society Press, Inc.

Oniboni A.C. 1990. Infection in the neutropenic patient. *Seminars in Oncology Nursing* 6 (1): 50–60.

Osterwalder, B. et al. 1988. Hematological support in patients undergoing allogeneic bone marrow transplantation. *Recent Results in Cancer Research* 108: 44–52.

Panzer S. et al. 1989. Immune thrombocytopenia more than a year after allogeneic marrow transplantation due to antibodies against donor platelets with anti-Pl[A1] specificity: Evidence for a host-derived immune reaction. *British Journal of Haematology* 71: 259–264.

Patterson J. et al. 1985. Analysis of rejection in HLA-matched T-depleted bone marrow transplants. *Experimental Hematology* 13 (suppl. 17): 117.

Peters, W. 1988. The effect of recombinant human neutropoietin (G-CSF) on hematopoietic reconstitution during autologous bone marrow transplantation. *ASH*, December 3.

Peters, N. 1990. Infectious complications of bone marrow transplant. The article reviewed. *Oncology*.

Petz, L.D. 1987. Immunologic problems associated with bone marrow transplantation. *Transfusion Medicine Reviews* 1 (2): 85–100.

Petz, L.D. 1989. Bone marrow transplantation. In Petz, L.D., and Svisher, S. (eds.). *Clinical Practice of Transfusion Medicine. Second edition*. N.Y.: Churchill Livingstone, pp. 485–508.

Phillips, G.L. 1988. The management of infections. In Deeg, H.J., Klingemann, H.G., and Phillips, G.L. (eds.) *A Guide to Bone Marrow Transplantation*. Berlin: Springer-Verlag, pp. 107–113.

Pizzo, P.A. 1989. Considerations for the prevention of infections complicatious in patients with cancer. *Reviews of Infectious Diseases* 11 (suppl. 7): s1551–s1563.

Plotkin, S.A. et al. 1984. Towne-vaccine-induced prevention of cytomegalovirus disease after renal transplants. *Lancet 1*: 528–530.

Pomeroy, C., and Englund, J.A. 1987. Cytomegalovirus: Epidemiology and infection control. *American Journal of Infection Control* 15: 107–119.

Postmus, P.E. et al. 1988. Graft-versus-host disease after transfusions of non-irradiated blood cells in patients having received autologous bone marrow. A report of 4 cases following ablative chemotherapy for solid tumors. *European Journal of Cancer and Clinical Oncology* 24 (5): 889–894.

Preisler, H.D., Goldstein, I.M., and Henderson, E.S. 1970. Gastrointestinal "sterilization" in the treatment of patients with acute leukemia. *Cancer* 26: 1076–1081.

Remington, J., and Schimpff, S. 1981. Please don't eat the salads. *N. Engl. J. Med.* 304 (7): 433–435.

Rowley, S.D. et al. 1987. CFU-GM content of bone marrow graft correlates with time to hematologic reconstitution following autologus bone marrow transplantation with 4-hydroperoxycyclophosphamide-purged bone marrow. *Blood* 80 (1): 271–275.

Rowley, S.D. et al. 1989. Correlation of hematologic recovery with CFU-GM content of autologous bone marrow grafts treated with 4-hydroperoxycyclophosphamide. Culture after cryopreservation. *B.M.T.* 4: 553–558.

Roy, D.C. 1990. Natural history of mixed chimerism after bone marrow transplantation with CD6-depleted allogeneic marrow: A stable equilibrium. *Blood* 75 (1): 296–304.

Rubin, M. et al. 1988. Gram-positive infections and the use of vancomycin in 550 episodes of fever and neutropenia. *Ann. Intern. Med.* 108: 30–35.

Saral, R. 1985. Viral infections in bone marrow transplantation recipients. *Plasma Therapy Transfusion Technology* 6: 275.

Schimpff, S.C. et al. 1975. Infection prevention in acute nonlymphocytic leukemia. *Ann. Intern. Med.* 82: 351–358.

Schuchter, L.M. et al. 1989. Herpes zoster infection after autologous bone marrow transplantation. *Blood* 74 (4): 1424–1427.

Siegel, S. et al. 1971. Protected environments in acute leukemia. *Blood* 38 (abstract): 803.

Slavin, S. et al. 1983. Total lymphoid irradiation (TLI) as part of the conditioning regimen for bone marrow transplantation in severe aplastic anaemia. In Gale, R.P. (ed.) *Recent Advances in Bone Marrow Transplantation*. New York NY: Alan R. Liss Inc.: 21.

Spitzer, G. et al. 1980. The myeloid progenitor cell—Its value in predicting hematopoietic recovery after autologous bone marrow transplantation. *Blood* 55 (2): 317–323.

Stedman, T.L. 1982. In J.V., Basmajian et al. (eds.) *Stedman's Medical Dictionary 24th edition*. Los Angeles: Williams & Wilkins, p. 708.

Steere, A., and Mallison, G. 1975. Handwashing practices for the prevention of nosocomial infections. *Ann. Intern. Med. 83* (5): 683–690.

Storb, R. 1989. Bone Marrow Transplantation. In DeVita, V.T. et al. (ed.) *Cancer: Principles and Practice of Oncology. 3rd Edition*. Philadelphia: J.B. Lippincott Company, pp. 2474–2489.

Storb, R., and Weiden, P.L. 1981. Transfusion problems associated with transplantation. *Seminars in Hematology 18* (2): 163–176.

Tafuri, A. et al. 1988. Stimulation of leukemic blast cells in vitro by colony-stimulating factors (G-CSF, GM-CSF) and interleukin-3 (IL-3): Evidence of recruitment and increased cell killing with cytosine arabinoside (ARA-C). *Blood 72*: 105a (suppl. 1).

Vadhan-Raj, S. et al. 1987. Effect of recombinant human granulocyte-macrophage colony-stimulating factor in patients with myelodysplastic syndromes. *N. Engl. J. Med. 317*: 1545–1552.

Visani, G. et al. 1990. Cryopreserved autologus bone marrow transplantation in patients with acute nonlymphoid leukemia: Chemotherapy before harvesting is the main factor in delaying hematological recovery. *Cryobiology 27*: 103–106.

Viz, L. et al. 1990. A prospective study of complications in Hickman right atrial catheters in marrow transplant patients. *J. of Parenteral and Enteral Nutrition 14* (1): 27–30.

Voogt, P.J. et al. 1990. Rejection of bone-marrow graft by recipient-derived cytotoxic T lymphocytes against minor histocompatibility antigens. *Lancet 335*: 131–134.

Wade, J.C., and Schimpff, S.C. 1988. Epidemiology and prevention of infection in the compromised host. In Rubin, R.H., and Young, L.S. (eds.) *Clincial Approach to Infection in the Compromised Host*. NY.: Plenum Medical Book Company, pp. 5–40.

Wessler, R. 1982. Care of the hospitalized adult patient with leukemia. *Nurs. Clin. North Am. 17* (4): 649–663.

Wingard, J. 1990. Management of infectious complications of bone marrow transplantation. *Oncology 4* (2): 69–75.

Winston, D.J. et al. 1982. Alveolar macrophage dysfunction in human bone marrow transplant recipients. *Am. J. Med. 73*: 859.

Witherspoon, R.P. et al. 1982. In vitro regulation of immunoglobulin synthesis after human marrow transplantation II. Deficient T and non-T lymphocyte function within 3-4 months of allogeneic, syngeneic, or autologous marrow grafting for hematologic malignancy. *Blood 59*: 844.

Wulff, J.C. et al. 1983. Transfusion requirements after HLA-identical marrow transplantation in 82 patients with aplastic anemia. *Vox Sang 44*: 366–374.

Yeager, A.M. et al. 1986. Autologous bone marrow transplantation in patients with acute nonlymphocytic leukemia, using ex vivo marrow treatment with 4-hydroperoxycyclophosphamide. *N. Engl. J. Med. 315* (3): 141–147.

Young, L.S. 1984. An overview of infection in bone marrow transplant recipients. *Clinical Haematology 13*: 661.

Chapter 7

Graft-Versus-Host Disease

Kathryn A. Caudell

Introduction

Graft-versus-host disease (GVHD) remains a major complication following allogeneic bone marrow transplantation and continues to reduce the survival rate in this patient population. GVHD is defined as "a consequence of the reaction initiated by a graft of immunologically competent lymphocytes introduced into a host that confronts the graft with a histocompatibility difference, yet unable to mount a similar immunological attack against the intrusive donor lymphoid system" (McDonald et al. 1986). More simply defined, GVHD results when the donor's T lymphocytes reject the tissue of the bone marrow recipient (Stream et al. 1980).

GVHD primarily affects the liver, skin, and gastrointestinal tract (Gale and Bortin 1987). Several interventions may minimize the risks of developing GVHD. These include (1) limiting marrow transplantation donors to those who have a human leukocyte antigen (HLA) genotypical identical sibling (Beatty et al. 1985), (2) infusing T cell-depleted bone marrow (Cooley et al. 1987;

Rohatiner et al. 1986; Mullbacher et al. 1988; Martin, Hansen, and Thomas 1984), and (3) administering immunosuppressive agents prophylactically (Storb et al. 1985; Thomas et al. 1975; Santos et al. 1983; Powles et al. 1980).

This chapter will discuss the incidence of GVHD, the pathophysiology, clinical manifestations, methods of diagnosis, medical and nursing management, and future directions. Several nursing care plans that are directed specifically at problems that may occur in a patient experiencing GVHD appear at the end of the text.

Incidence

The incidence of GVHD varies widely depending on the type of transplant. GVHD generally does not occur in syngeneic transplants, those in which the donor and recipient are identical twins, because the siblings are completely matched for all of the histocompatibility complex and for all genetic loci. Nor is it likely to occur in autologous transplants, those in which the patient serves as his own source of marrow. However, Hood and colleagues (1987) summarized a smattering of reports of GVHD-like phenomenon (primarily skin rashes, vesicles, and bullae) in both autologous and syngeneic transplants, and reported nine additional cases from their institution. Although the histologic and clinical evidence supporting the occurrence of GVHD in these groups is compelling, the authors also concluded that a drug-related etiology could not be entirely ruled out (Hood et al. 1987).

In allogeneic HLA genotypically identical sibling transplants, the occurrence of moderate to severe acute GVHD is reported to be about 45% (Bortin et al. 1989). Despite immunosuppressive therapy with cyclosporine either alone or in combination with methotrexate or steroids, several studies have shown that acute GVHD (including grades II to IV defined in Table 7.1) still develops in 20%–45% of HLA-matched bone marrow transplant patients (Weisdorf et al. 1990; Bortin et al. 1989; Storb et al. 1986a; Santos et al. 1987; Deeg et al. 1980a; Glucksberg et al. 1974; Thomas et al. 1976). However, clinical trials from several European institutions revealed that there was a decreased incidence and improved patient survival when cyclosporine was administered prophylactically (Powles et al. 1980; Hows et al. 1981; Barrett et al. 1982; Gratwohl et al. 1983).

Several risk factors have been identified that may predispose the patient to developing GVHD. These include a donor-recipient sex mismatch (an increased incidence is noted with female donors to male recipients), increased age of the patient, and the cumulative number of blood transfusions (Weisdorf et al. 1990; Bortin et al. 1989; Champlin 1984b). Although transfusion-related GVHD, a well-described phenomenon resulting from infusion of immunocompetent T cells, can occur; it is virtually nonexistent in BMT due to the use of irradiated blood products (Anderson and Weinstein 1990).

Incidence rates of GVHD in partially matched allogeneic transplants currently appears to be slightly greater than in HLA-matched transplants (Gingrich et al. 1988). However, few patients have undergone this therapy to date so that it is still early to predict if this trend will continue.

Incidence rates for chronic GVHD are reported to be between 30% and 45% (Wingard et al. 1989). Common risk factors for developing chronic GVHD include prior acute GVHD and increasing patient age (Wingard et al. 1989).

Currently, it is unclear why GVHD develops in some patients and not in others despite prophylactic therapy with immunosuppressive agents. Subtherapeutic serum concentrations of the immunosuppressive drugs may be one reason. Serum concentration variability among patients

Table 7.1. Clinical Stages of Acute GVHD

Stage	Skin	Liver	Gut
I	Maculopapular rash < 25% body surface	bilirubin 2–3mg/dl	Diarrhea 500–1000ml/day
II	Maculopapular rash 25–50% body surface	bilirubin 3–6mg/dl	Diarrhea 1000–1500ml/day
III	Generalized erythroderma	bilirubin 6–15mg/dl	Diarrhea > 1500ml/day
IV	Desquamation and Bullae	bilirubin > 15mg/dl	Pain or Pileus

Source: H.J. Deeg et al. 1984. Graft-versus-host disease: Pathophysiological and clinical aspects. *Annual Review of Medicine* 35: 11–24.

receiving the same drug dose is another possible explanation (Yee et al. 1988).

Pathophysiology

Acute GVHD

From the immunological standpoint, GVHD is initiated when (1) genetically determined histocompatibility differences exist between the bone marrow recipient and the bone marrow donor, (2) immunocompetent cells in the donor's bone marrow that can recognize the foreign histocompatibility antigens of the host and can therefore mount an immunological reaction against them are present, (3) the bone marrow recipient is unable to react against and reject the donor marrow (Billingham 1966). It is thought that the underlying mechanism of GVHD is alloaggression resulting from histocompatibility differences. It is unclear, however, what the exact immunological events are that cause the disease or bring about the other associated phenomena such as autoimmunity, immunodeficiency, and immune dysfunction.

GVHD is thought to be initiated by the donor's immunocompetent T lymphocytes reacting against the immunoincompetent recipient's tissues. Subsequently, lymphocyte-mediated damage occurs to the recipient's target cells or organs (Tsoi 1982). Histologically, the interaction of effector lymphocytes and target skin cells produces epidermal changes that occur during GVHD (Slavin and Santos 1972; Woodruff et al. 1976; Saxon et al. 1981).

The immunopathogenesis of acute GVHD can be divided into three phases: (1) an afferent or recognition phase, (2) a central or recruitment phase, and (3) an effector phase (Shulman et al. 1978; Sullivan 1986).

Recognition Mechanisms

In both animals and humans, the principal target organs of acute GVHD are the epithelium of the skin, the gastrointestinal tract, the small intra-

hepatic biliary ducts, and the lymphoid system. It is unknown, at this point, why these specific epithelial cells are recognized and targeted in the process of GVHD.

The range of alloaggression in acute GVHD appears to depend on the degree of antigenic disparity to non-HLA antigens between the donor and recipient, and/or the differences in the ability of donor lymphocytes to recognize and react immunologically to non-HLA antigens.

The targeted epithelial cells all have surfaces that have the ability to synthesize and express the major histocompatibility (MHC) class II (Ia) antigens in response to a stressor. The stimulus for this expression of Ia on keratinocytes, enterocytes, and bile ducts appears to be endogenous interferon that is released by T cells. Macrophages, which are stimulated by interferon, release the metabolite neopterin, an indicator of activated cell-mediated immunity (Wachter et al. 1989). Neopterin has been shown to predict the onset of GVHD. It is also important to note that rising neopterin levels are associated with marrow engraftment. Decreasing levels are noted during marrow aplasia and successful treatment of GVHD with steroids (Wachter et al. 1989). The clinical usefulness of measuring this substance is still under study.

Recruitment Mechanisms

During the recruitment phase, the injured keratinocytes produce a surface membrane–bound epidermal thymocyte activating factor (ETAF) which has characteristics similar to interleukin. ETAF is chemotactic for neutrophils, monocytes, and T cells and thus may amplify GVHD by recruiting alloreactive mononuclear cells and enhancing the secretion of interleukin-2 by T cells (Breathnach and Katz 1986).

Several nonspecific stimuli may also enhance GVHD by increasing immune recognition. For example, microorganisms may trigger GVHD (1) by sharing antigenic determinants with gut epithelial cells, (2) by reactivating latent viruses by chemotherapy or irradiation thereby inducing viral-associated antigens on cell surfaces to become targets for alloreactivity, and (3) because viral infections with Epstein Barr (EBV) or herpes simplex (HSV) may stimulate an anamnestic response in immune donor lymphocytes, which leads to the endogenous production of beta-interferon, Ia tissue expression, interleukin-2, and enhancement of GVHD (Unanue and Allen 1986; Gratoma et al. 1987). The use of a microbial-free environment through the use of laminar airflow (LAF) rooms, gut sterilization, antibiotics, and sterile food is the clinical attempt to eliminate the initiation or enhancement of GVHD through these mechanisms. Although problems with patient compliance with this strict regimen often interfere with its potential effectiveness, a beneficial effect (lower frequency of acute GVHD) in patients treated in this environment over those treated in conventional rooms has been described (Deeg 1988).

Effector Mechanisms

It has been suggested, based on data from experimental and morphologic studies, that acute GVHD is a cell-mediated phenomenon. Targeted epithelial cells undergo an individual cell necrosis frequently surrounded by satellite cell lymphocytosis (Weedon et al. 1979).

There is strong evidence that suggests that T cells mediate acute GVHD. Mice studies have demonstrated that GVHD does not occur when allogeneic fetal liver cells and spleen cells from neonatally thymectomized mice are infused in irradiated animals (Kernan et al. 1986).

Chronic GVHD

Chronic GVHD, on the other hand, has characteristics similar to the naturally occurring autoimmune collagen-vascular diseases such as scleroderma, systemic lupus erythematosus, and rheumatoid arthritis (see Table 7.2). Chronic GVHD exhibits more pronounced lasting inflammation and fibrotic changes in the affected organs. Chronic GVHD normally develops about three months following transplantation, but has

been reported to occur as many as two years later (Wingard et al. 1989). Chronic GVHD can occur following acute GVHD or may occur de novo. Affected target organs and clinical manifestations differ from those of acute GVHD and are described below (Klingemann 1988). Chronic GVHD is characterized by a complicated immunopathogenesis involving the interaction of alloimmunity and immune disregulation, which produces severe immunodeficiency and autoimmunity. Two dominant factors that have been associated with the development of chronic GVHD are prior acute GVHD and increasing patient age (Storb et al. 1983a; Sullivan 1986; Storb 1986).

Skin

The skin is the most frequently affected organ in chronic GVHD. Inflammatory changes occur early in the pathological course while fibrotic changes occur later. Lichenoid reactions with concurrent destruction of the epidermal basal layer and pilar units are frequent in chronic GVHD. The destructive fibrosing inflammatory reactions occur around the eccrine coils, deep dermal nerves, and in the subcutaneous fat. Skin biopsies demonstrate fibroplasia that may advance to epidermal atrophy, loss of cell dermal appendages, and fibrous remodeling of the reticular dermis with expansion into the subcutaneous fat (see Figure 7.1) (Sale and Shulman 1984; Shulman et al. 1978).

A localized, self-limiting variant form of chronic GVHD occurs in 20% of the patients. This form is manifested by clusters of small lesions or large areas with induration, hyper- or hypopigmentation, and peridermal atrophy. The inflammatory changes range from absent to mild while the deep reticular dermis demonstrates nodular fibrous remodeling. The lesions may expand and cause extensive depigmentation and scarring before they resolve (see Figure 7.2).

Gastrointestinal System

Gastrointestinal histopathology in chronic GVHD differs considerably from that of acute GVHD. Lichenoid inflammation with subsequent destruction of the mucosa and submucosal glands occurs

Table 7.2. Clinical Manifestations of Acute and Chronic Graft-Versus-Host Disease

Affected Organ	Acute	Chronic
Skin	Erythematous rash Exfoliation Bollous eruption Toxic epidermal necrolysis	Lichen planus–like eruption Scleroderma
Gastrointestinal tract	Diarrhea and abdominal cramps Vomiting	Malabsorption
Liver	Liver function abnormalities	Chronic active hepatitis
Other	Fever, malaise, weight loss, Eosinophilia, lymphophenia, positive direct Coombs' test	Weight loss Recurrent infection Prolonged impairment of immunity

Source: Lucas, C.F., and Barret, A.J. 1982. Bone Marrow Transplantation. *Update*: 2403.

in the esophageal area more so than in the stomach, intestine, and colon (McDonald et al. 1981).

Mouth

Eighty percent of the patients with chronic GVHD exhibit involvement of the mouth (Schubert and Sullivan 1990). The patients most frequently complain of pain, particularly if eating hot or warm foods, and dryness of the mucous membranes. Lichen planus-type lesions are commonly found on the buccal and labial mucosa, and frequently appear similar to oral candidiasis. Dental caries and periodontitis may occur due to xerostomia. Histopathological alterations observed include atrophy, necrosis of squamous cells, and mononuclear cell infiltration, all of which are characteristic of a lichenoid reaction (Klingemann 1988).

Eyes

Approximately 80% of patients with chronic GVHD will experience ocular involvement. Insufficient tear production occurs as a result of the "dry eye" or sicca syndrome which is present in chronic GVHD. The patients may complain of pain, burning, and photophobia. Keratitis and scarring may also result from the ocular sicca (Klingemann 1988; Calissendorff et al. 1989). Lymphoplasmacytic infiltrates have been found in glandular tissues such as the lacrimal glands, salivary glands, and submucosal glands. These in-

filtrates first accumulate around the ductal structures and eventually lead to fibrous destruction (Sale et al. 1981).

Lungs

In approximately 5%–10% of patients with chronic GVHD, lesions involving the bronchioles resulting in fibrous obliteration of the lumen occur and result in an obstructive small airway disease (see Figure 7.3) (Sullivan 1986; Ralph et al. 1984). The obstructive airway may be the result of depressed mucosal immunity and repeated infections compounded by aspiration from simultaneously occurring esophageal disease.

Vagina

Inflammation, sicca, adhesions, and stenosis of the vagina may occur in severe cases of chronic GVHD (Lorson et al. 1982). If any of these should occur, systemic immunosuppressive therapy is recommended, and surgery may be required in some instances. If these symptoms occur in the absence of chronic GVHD, lack of use or long-term complications of total body irradiation should be considered as causative factors (Klingemann 1988).

Neuromuscular System

Several patients with chronic GVHD have been observed to experience symptoms similar to those of myasthenia gravis, specifically muscular weak-

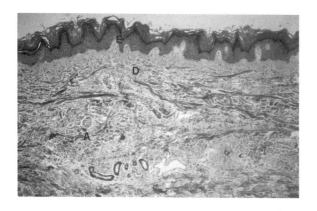

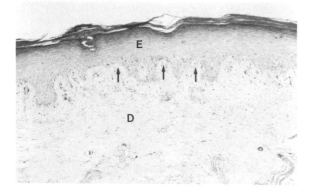

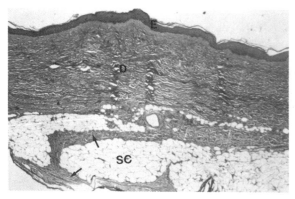

Figure 7.1. Top photo shows normal skin. E = epidermis, D = dermis, A = adnexal structures, SC = subcutaneous tissue. Center and bottom photos show progressive changes that occur with chronic GVHD. Lichenoid reactions with concurrent destruction of the epidermal basal layer (indicated by arrows on center photo) and pilar units are frequent in chronic GVHD. The destructive fibrosing inflammatory reactions occur around the eccrine coils, deep dermal nerves, and in the subcutaneous fat. Skin biopsies demonstrate fibroplasia that may advance to epidermal flattening and atrophy, loss of cell dermal appendages, and fibrous remodeling of the reticular dermis with expansion into the subcutaneous fat (bottom photo).

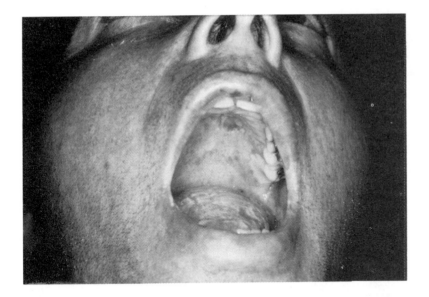

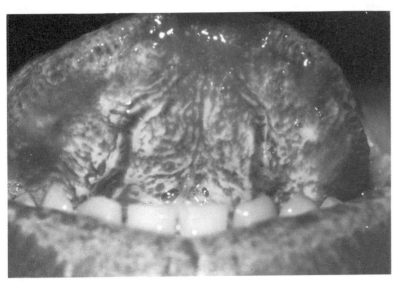

Figure 7.2. Lichen planus-type lesions are commonly found on the buccal (top) and labial mucosa (bottom), and frequently appear similar to oral candidiasis.

ness, repetitive nerve stimulation, response to edrophonium, and having antibodies against the acetylcholine receptor. These symptoms were noted to occur after tapering of corticosteroid therapy and were thought to be a result of immune dysregulation and donor-host alloreactivity. Polymyositis and peripheral neuropathy have also been observed in chronic GVHD (Klingemann 1988). (Neuromuscular effects are discussed further in Chapter 11.)

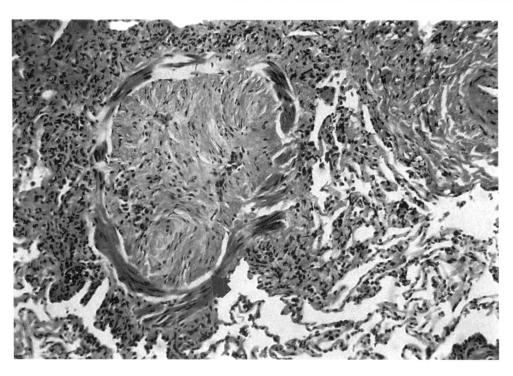

Figure 7.3. In approximately 5%–10% of patients with chronic GVHD, lesions involving the bronchioles resulting in fibrous obliteration of the lumen occur and result in an obstructive small airway disease (Sullivan 1986; Ralph 1984).

Graft-Versus-Leukemia Effect

During periods of acute GVHD, leukemia cells have been reported to disappear from recipients of allogeneic marrow transplants (Odom 1978). In allogeneic bone marrow recipients with GVHD grades II–IV the relapse rate is 2.5 times lower than in syngeneic recipients or in allogeneic recipients without GVHD (Weiden et al. 1979). Unfortunately patient survival was still similar in the two groups since the lower leukemia relapse rate was offset by higher mortality from complications of GVHD. Another analysis also showed similar results in that patients who developed acute and/ or chronic GVHD had a higher probability of remaining in remission (Weiden et al. 1981). Some studies have attempted to initiate GVHD by ad-

ministering additional donor T cells to reduce the incidence of relapse. This approach has had many limitations because control and prediction of the course of GVHD is currently extremely difficult (Thomas 1988).

Clinical Manifestations

Clinical manifestations differ between acute and chronic GVHD. These are described below and were summarized earlier in Table 7.2.

Acute GVHD

The median onset of GVHD is approximately 25 days after transplant. GVHD usually affects the skin, the liver, and the gastrointestinal tract

(Champlin and Gale 1984). The most common initial presenting manifestation is a maculopapular rash involving the palms, soles, trunk, and ears. Bullae, ulcerations, and epidermal necrosis may occur (see Figure 7.4), progressing to a generalized desquamation of the skin (Press 1987).

Liver function abnormalities that appear with GVHD include elevated alkaline phosphatase and bilirubin levels. The serum glutamic oxaloacetic transaminase (SGOT) may increase, but somewhat slower than the alkaline phosphatase and bilirubin levels (Sullivan 1983). Right upper quadrant pain, hepatomegaly, and jaundice also may be exhibited (Ford and Ballard 1988).

Patients who have gastrointestinal GVHD will usually experience skin and/or liver GVHD as well. Presenting symptoms of gut GVHD include nausea and vomiting, pain, anorexia, and a paralytic ileus (Sullivan 1983). Watery hemenegative

diarrhea usually develops, progressing to heme-positive diarrhea as more of the intestinal mucosal begins to slough (Ford and Ballard 1988). Several liters of diarrhea may be produced daily resulting in severe hypoalbuminemia and fluid and electrolyte imbalances. The severity of GVHD and the patient's response to treatment often are quantitated by measuring stool volumes (Sullivan 1983).

Chronic GVHD

Chronic GVHD is a complex syndrome whose clinical manifestations resemble naturally occurring collagen vascular disorders. Figure 7.5 lists the incidence of various clinical manifestations seen in the many forms of the disease. The skin is the most frequently affected system with greater

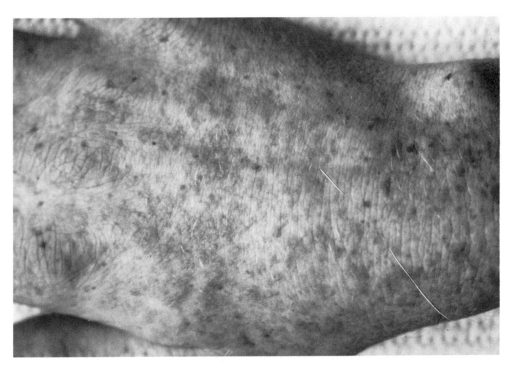

Figure 7.4. The most common initial presenting manifestation is a maculopapular rash.

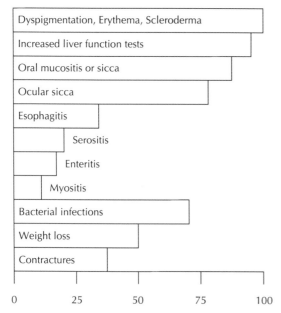

H.J. Deeg et al. 1984. Bone Marrow Transplantation: A Review of Delayed Complications, *British Journal of Haematology, 57*: 185. Reprinted with permission.

Figure 7.5.   Incidence of clinical manifestations in patients with extensive chronic GVHD.

than 95% of patients experiencing alterations in this organ (Deeg et al. 1984a). Patchy alopecia and mucous membrane and nail abnormalities may occur. Pruritis is an early symptom, while tightness and contractures characterize late symptoms. In addition, the patient may lose the ability to sweat, which returns after resolution of the GVHD (Sullivan 1983).

Chronic skin GVHD may begin with an erythema in the malar area, spreading to other areas. Integumentary lesions have been found to occur usually in sun exposed areas, although they have occurred occasionally in non-sun exposed areas. Insidious pigmentary changes may occur in some patients. In others, patchy hyper- or hypopigmentation, sometimes only in the periorbital area, sites of trauma, or undergarment area may develop. A mottled appearance of the skin

with faint, blotchy macular erythema has been observed. Hyperkeratotic, flat-topped perifollicular papules may also occur (see Figure 7.6).

Approximately 6 to 18 months after transplantation, the skin becomes progressively indurated and adheres to the underlying fascia. The dermis becomes thickened. Progressive skin involvement resembles scleroderma in which bronze-colored hyperpigmentation, hide bound skin, pressure point ulcerations and joint contractures occur (Shulman et al. 1980).

In 90% of individuals with chronic GVHD, liver disease occurs (Deeg et al. 1984a). The alkaline phosphatase may be five to ten times higher than normal, the SGOT three to six times higher, and either normal or moderately elevated bilirubin levels are evident. Chronic active hepatitis and severe cholestasis are also observed. Hepatic function improves within two to four weeks after therapy has begun, although high alkaline phosphatase and SGOT levels may persist for months (Sullivan 1983).

Those patients experiencing multiorgan chronic GVHD often have oral involvement. Pain and mucosal dryness are common manifestations. Lichenoid reactions, although similar in appearance to candidiasis, may appear as fine white reticular striae on the buccal mucosa, large plaques on the buccal surface and lateral aspect of the tongue (Schubert et al. 1983).

Ocular involvement is observed in 65–80% of the patients with extensive chronic GVHD (Buchsel 1986; Calissendorff et al. 1989). Patients may complain of dryness, burning, photophobia, and grittiness that results from lacrimal insufficiency.

Esophageal involvement has been observed in patients with extensive chronic GVHD (Sullivan 1981). Other areas of involvement that have been reported include the vagina (inflammation, adhesions, sicca, and stenosis) (Corson 1982), joints (arthralgias and synovial effusions), heart (pericardial effusions) (Sullivan et al. 1981a; Deeg et al. 1984a) and lungs (obstructive airway disease and pleural effusion) (Sullivan 1986; Ralph et al.

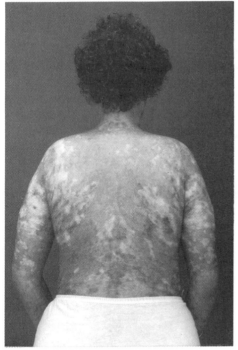

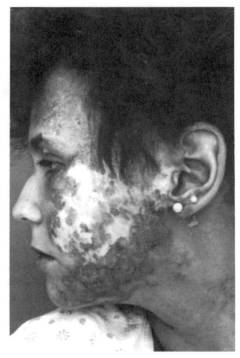

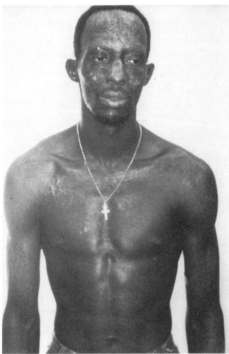

Figure 7.6. Chronic skin GVHD may begin with an erythema in the malar area spreading to other areas. Integumentary lesions have been found to occur usually in sun exposed areas, although they occasionally have occurred in non-sun exposed areas. Insidious pigmentary changes may occur in some patients. In others patchy hyperpigmentation, sometimes only in the periorbital area, sites of trauma, or undergarment area, may develop. A mottled appearance of the skin with faint, blotchy macular erythema has been observed. Hyperkeratotic, flat topped perifollicular papules may also occur.

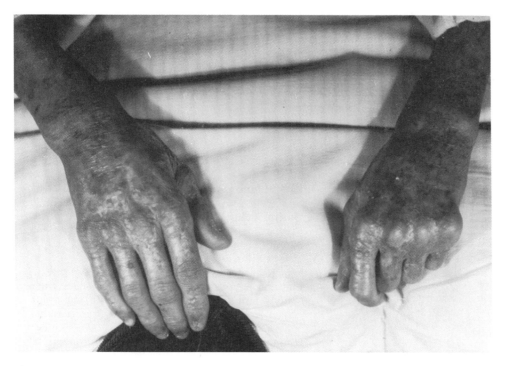

Figure 7.7. Approximately 6 to 18 months after transplantation, the skin becomes progressively indurated and adheres to the underlying fascia. The dermis becomes thickened. Progressive skin involvement resembles scleroderma in which bronze-colored hyperpigmentation, hide bound skin, pressure point ulcerations, and joint contractures occur.

1984; Deeg et al. 1984a). Table 7.3 summarizes the late effects seen in chronic GVHD.

Diagnosis, Grading, and Prognosis

The diagnosis of GVHD is made by the combination of clinical manifestations and histologic findings. The safest and simplest method is confirmation by skin biopsy. If the biopsy results are ambiguous, a repeat biopsy may be taken three to seven days later. If liver or gastrointestinal manifestations occur in the absence of skin rash, a "blind" biopsy can be taken from the forearm. These biopsies may help to establish the diagnosis

if biopsies of the other organs (i.e., gut or liver) are ambiguous or dangerous. Other sites that have been found helpful in establishing a diagnosis are the esophagus and muscle. If clinical manifestations exist in only one organ, multiple site biopsies can be obtained. It is unusual for GVHD to be isolated to only one site, except in chronic GVHD (Sullivan 1983).

The clinical stage (see Table 7.1) and grade of acute GVHD is based on the severity of organ dysfunction of the skin, liver, or gut. The incidence of moderate to severe (II–IV) acute GVHD in patients that have HLA-matched donors and have sustained engraftment is between 30%–50% (Weisdorf et al. 1990; Bortin et al. 1989). Of these patients, 30%–60% die either from GVHD or re-

Table 7.3. Late Effects of Bone Marrow Transplantation: Chronic Graft-Versus-Host Disease

Late Effect	Incidence Rate	Time Post-BMT (Days)	Signs and Symptoms	Nursing Management	Diagnostic Tools	Medical Treatment
Skin	95%	100–400	Rough, scaly skin Malar erythema Generalized rash Hypo/hyperpigmentation Dyspigmentation Premature graying Alopecia Joint contractures Scleroderma Loss of sweating	Use of nonabrasive soaps, lotions, sunscreen Cosmetic support, makeup, wigs Range-of-motion activities Patient/Family education Monitor compliance to treatment protocols	Skin biopsy positive for GVHD Karnofsky score	Lanolin-based creams Possible systemic immunosuppressive therapy with cyclosporin A, prednisone, Imuran
Liver	30%	100–400	Jaundice	Infection precautions until differential diagnosis is made Monitor LFTS Low-fat diet	Alkaline phosphates SGOT Bilirubin	Possible systemic immunosuppressive therapy with cyclosporin A, prednisone, Imuran
Oral	80%	100–400	Pain, burning, dryness, irritation, soreness, loss of taste Lichenoid changes, atrophy, erythema in oral cavity *Candida* infection Stomatitis Dental caries Xerostomia	Encourage soft, bland diet Dental hygiene education, soft toothbrush, flossing Saline rinses Dental medicine referral/recommendation Salivary gland stimulants, sugarless mints, artificial saliva	Labial mucosa biopsy positive for GVHD Secretory IgA levels Mouth culture positive for yeast organisms Mouth culture positive for bacterial and viral etiologies Radiographs	Possible systemic immunosuppressive therapy with cyclosporin A, prednisone, Imuran Artificial saliva Clotrimazole troches or nystatin Swish and Swallow Appropriate topical medication Topical fluoride treatment Appropriate dental therapy

Table 7.3. *Continued*

Ocular	80%	100–400	Grittiness, burning of eyes Dry eyes Sicca syndrome	Artificial tears Schirmer's tear test: if < 10 mm of wetting, refer to ophthalmologist	Keratoconjunctivitis Corneal ulceration Slit-lamp microscopy	Lacriset plugs Soft contact lens Punctal ligation for obliteration of tear duct outflow Keratoplasty Tarsorrhaphies
GI tract, esophagus	36%	100–400	Anorexia Difficulty eating Painful swallowing Retrosternal pain Weight loss Vomiting	Serial weights High-calorie food supplement Recommend nutritional counseling	Barium swallow of esophagus and small bowel follow-through	Esophageal dilatation Possible systemic immunosuppressive therapy with cyclosporin A, prednisone, Imuran Parenteral nutrition
Vagina	20%	100–400	Inflammation Stricture formation causing obstruction of menstrual flow Adhesions Dry vagina Painful intercourse Marital problems	Water-soluble lubricants Recommend sexual counseling and therapy	Papanicolaou smear	Vaginal stints Estrogen cream Surgical intervention

Source: Buchsel, P.C.: Long-term complications of allogeneic bone marrow transplantation: Nursing implications. *Oncol. Nurs. Forum* 13: 67, 1986.

lated infectious complications (Weisdorf et al. 1990).

The prognosis in GVHD depends on the overall severity of the disease. Additional factors that have been correlated with poor survival in patients developing acute GVHD include (1) older age of the patient, (2) refractory to random donor platelets, (3) lack of LAF isolation (Storb et al. 1983) and, (4) lack of complete response or resistance to GVHD treatment (Weisdorf et al. 1990).

In chronic GVHD, oral biopsies and lacrimal function studies facilitate staging the extent of the disease (Sullivan et al. 1981b). The Karnofsky performance scale has also been used to grade the severity of the disease (Sullivan 1985). Table 7.4 shows a classification system used for chronic GVHD.

Prior acute GVHD is a risk factor that has been identified for the development of chronic GVHD. The risk appears to increase with the increasing severity or grade of the prior acute GVHD. One factor that has been found to adversely influence survival in patients with chronic GVHD is the type of onset. The progressive onset from acute to chronic, without any resolution of

Table 7.4. Clinicopathological Classification of Chronic Graft-Versus-Host Disease

Limited chronic graft-versus-host disease:
Either or Both:
• Localized skin involvement
• Hepatic dysfunction (due to chronic GVHD)

Extensive chronic graft-versus-host disease:
Either:
• Generalized skin involvement;
or:
• Localized skin involvement or hepatic dysfunction due to chronic GVHD or both plus:
  —Liver histology showing chronic aggressive hepatitis, bridging necrosis, or cirrhosis; or
  —Involvement of eye (Schirmer's test with less than 5mm wetting); or
  —Involvement of minor salivary glands or oral mucosa demonstrated on labial biopsy; or
  —Involvement of any other target organ

Adapted from Shulman and colleagues.

acute GVHD correlates with the highest mortality (Wingard et al. 1989; Sullivan et al. 1981a). Other factors include persistent severe thrombocytopenia (Sullivan et al. 1982), lichenoid changes on skin histology, and elevation of serum bilirubin > 1.2mg/dL (Wingard et al. 1989). Factors that have not been found to be associated with development of chronic GVHD include patient and donor sex, donor-recipient sex mismatching, donor age, or transplantation either during leukemic remission or relapse (Sullivan 1983).

Medical Management

Prophylaxis

A variety of prophylactic therapy regimens are being utilized to prevent GVHD. These regimens can be single agents or a combination of agents. Single agents include methotrexate (Sullivan 1985), corticosteroids (Blume et al. 1980; Forman et al. 1982; Ringden et al. 1982), and cyclosporine (Powles et al. 1980; Tutschka et al. 1983). Combination agent protocols include methotrexate and cyclosporine (Storb 1986; Deeg et al. 1982; Deeg et al. 1984b), antithymocyte globulin (ATG), methotrexate and corticosteroids (Ramsay et al. 1982), and prednisone with three different cytotoxic agents: procarbazine, azathioprine or cyclophosphamide (Sullivan 1983).

Storb and colleagues (1985) studied the effectiveness of cyclosporine versus methotrexate in preventing acute and chronic GVHD, and examined each of their effects on long-term survival. Their data showed that the drugs were equivalent in almost all of the parameters examined. The projected survival of patients receiving cyclosporine was 62%, and 66% for those receiving methotrexate. Patients receiving cyclosporine did not exhibit impairment of hematopoietic engraftment or an increase in infection associated deaths. Analysis of studies by the International Bone Marrow Transplant Registry suggests that the occurrence of interstitial pneumonia in cyclosporine treated patients is reduced. The overall morbidity related to the incidence and severity of oral mucositis was also found to be reduced in these patients (Bortin 1983; Gale et al. 1982).

Cyclosporine has been found to cause a delayed red blood cell recovery. In vitro studies utilizing bone marrow derived from canine erythroid colonies show suppression of erythroid colony formation when cyclosporine was exogenously added. It was thought that this was due to either a direct suppression of erythroid precursors or by inhibition of an accessory cell (Deeg et al. 1980a and 1980b). Additional reported toxicities of cyclosporine are nephrotoxicity (Deeg et al. 1980a; Kennedy et al. 1983; Haus et al. 1983; Atkinson et al. 1983), hypertension (Loughran et al. 1985), hepatotoxicity (Keown et al. 1982), and neurological disturbances (Storb et al. 1988). No statistically significant differences have been observed between cyclosporine and methotrexate in regard to toxicities (Storb et al. 1988; Ringden et al. 1986; Biggs et al. 1986).

Several canine studies have shown a synergism between methotrexate and cyclosporine, where GVHD was reduced and long-term survival was impressively improved (Deeg et al. 1982; Deeg et al. 1984b). A study by Storb (1986b), based on the previous canine models showed that combination therapy with cyclosporine and methotrexate was superior to cyclosporine alone in three areas: (1) reducing GVHD, (2) reducing the incidence of fatal infections, and (3) increasing long-term survival. On the other hand, the incidence and severity of oral mucositis and transient elevations in serum bilirubin levels during the first 14 days after transplant were found to be higher. A follow-up analysis of patients at three to four and one-half years, however, demonstrated that the survival advantage was only maintained for patients with chronic myelogenous leukemia (Storb et al. 1989). Unfortunately, the early survival advantage seen in AML patients in longer follow-up was offset by an increase in leukemia relapses.

The combination of methotrexate, antithymocyte globulin, and prednisone has been found to be superior to methotrexate alone in preventing GVHD. However, no improvement in long-term survival was observed because the number of fatal infections was not reduced (Ramsay et al. 1982).

Several nonpharmacologic techniques have been evaluated in the attempt to reduce GVHD. Since the T cells have been identified as the principal cells responsible for the initiation of GVHD, several investigators have attempted to remove T cells from the donor marrow prior to transplantation. Several techniques capable of removing the T cells from the marrow include agglutination techniques, immunoabsorption columns, and treatment with anti-T cell monoclonal antibodies. These techniques have been found to reduce the incidence of GVHD; however, a significant incidence of engraftment failure resulting in the death of the patient has been observed with this therapy (Martin et al. 1985).

Studies examining germ-free mice have revealed a reduced incidence and mortality from GVHD (van Bekkum et al. 1974). Patients with aplastic anemia who were transplanted in LAF rooms had a lower incidence of grades II–IV acute GVHD than those transplanted outside of LAF rooms (23% and 39% respectively). Survival was also significantly improved for patients treated in LAF rooms (Storb et al. 1983a). There has been speculation that enterobacteria may have antigenic characteristics similar to those of gut mucosal epithelium and therefore may activate lymphocytes to react against the gut mucosa (Buckner et al. 1978). This has provided the rationale for the use of gut sterilization with nonabsorbable antibiotics.

Treatment

Established acute GVHD has been treated primarily with corticosteroids, although other immunosuppressive therapies have been used (i.e., cyclosporine, anti-T cell immunotoxins, antilymphocyte globulin, or antithymocyte globulin [ATG]) (Weisdorf et al. 1990). A prospective study examining the effectiveness of ATG and corticosteroids showed a decrease in GVHD although there was no improvement in survival (Doney et al. 1981). Patients have been found to improve with methylprednisolone (2mg/kg) or ATG (10–15mg/kg) (Sullivan 1985). Diminished clinical manifestations of GVHD have also been observed in patients receiving higher doses of corticosteroids. However, long-term survival has not improved in these patients as they continue to die from infections (Kendra et al. 1981).

Treatment of chronic GVHD often includes steroids, cyclosporine, and azathioprine alone or in combination (Wingard et al. 1989). Patients experiencing chronic GVHD also require skillful supportive care to manage infections, fluid and electrolyte imbalances, and nutritional deficits. Hyperalimentation, fluid replacement, transfusions, and antibiotic therapy are often necessary (Gauvreau et al. 1981; Parker and Cohen 1983). Ocular manifestations of chronic GVHD occur in approximately 80%–90% of patients, including keratoconjunctivitis, sicca, and corneal wasting. Patients are encouraged to use artificial tears as ocular damage may occur before the patient is symptomatic (Sullivan et al. 1984; Deeg et al. 1984a; Sullivan 1986).

Nursing Management

The nursing management of patients experiencing GVHD is complex and requires expert skills, knowledge, and creativity (Copel and Smith 1989; O'Quin and Moravec 1988; de la Montaigene et al. 1981). Careful assessment is required to identify its early clinical manifestations and to distinguish GVHD from other complications such as antibiotic or chemotherapy reactions, irritated bowel, infections, and radiation toxicity. An awareness of high-risk factors that may increase the likelihood of developing GVHD, and the identification of patients in this high-risk category is important so that scrupulous monitoring of these patients in particular can occur during the period when GVHD is most likely to occur.

Considering the three systems affected by GVHD, nurses should assess and monitor skin integrity, gastrointestinal function, and hepatic function. However, because the similar toxicities from chemotherapy, radiation, immunosuppressive agents, and antibiotics complicate this assessment, many factors need to be considered when assessing and planning care for bone marrow transplant patients.

Providing appropriate skin care is an important aspect of patient comfort and prevention of infection (McConn 1987). Placing oil in the bathwater or applying it after showering helps to decrease the skin dryness and to soothe the discomfort caused by pruritis. Antipruretic and steroid creams have been found to have marginal benefit for pruritis.

In some instances of acute GVHD, the rash may progress to bullae with subsequent desquamation of the outer epidermal layers. If this should occur, preventing infection and bleeding is important. To decrease discomfort caused by pressure points and to facilitate exudate absorption, silicon bead or low air-loss beds may be helpful. Covering the desquamated areas with Burrow's Solution (e.g., Domeboro) soaked gauze pads for approximately ten minutes serves as a means of debridement. Application of hydrogel dressings that have been painted with an antibiotic ointment has several advantages: It is nonadherent; absorbs wound exudate, bacteria, and odor; provides a physiologically moist environment; and is conducive to wound healing and tissue granulation (Caudell and Schauer 1989). Skin desquamation can be intensely painful requiring narcotic drips for pain control.

Acute GVHD can also effect the gastrointestinal system causing several liters of diarrhea per day. Strict monitoring of intake and output, daily weights, and serum electrolytes, such as sodium, chloride, and potassium, is essential. Loss of these electrolytes may cause metabolic alkalosis. Severe diarrhea combined with intestinal sloughing may also produce malabsorption and result in malnutrition. Therefore, hyperalimentation may be needed to provide the patient with adequate nutritional support. The patient may require placement on an NPO diet to further reduce gut activation. Visceral proteins such as prealbumin and albumin, the height and weight index, anthropometric measurements, and the creatinine height index are parameters that can be used to evaluate somatic and visceral protein measurements (Behnke 1986).

Should the patient experience moderate to severe diarrhea, he/she should be instructed to clean the perineal area thoroughly after each bowel movement. Sitz baths may be recommended to further cleanse the perineal area and to soothe irritated skin. The patient should be assessed regularly for rectal lesions.

Mucosal sloughing that occurs in severe gut GVHD can also produce gastrointestinal bleeding. All emesis and stool output should be regularly tested for occult blood. GVHD stools often appear mahogany colored and have a strong, foul odor. If gastrointestinal bleeding occurs, the hemaglobin and hematocrit should be monitored carefully and appropriate blood product therapy should be administered if needed.

In liver GVHD, the patient may experience right upper quadrant pain, hepatomegaly, jaundice, and elevated liver function studies (McDonald et al. 1981). The serum alkaline phosphatase and bilirubin levels should be monitored (Sullivan 1983). Although the serum SGOT may rise, it usually does so much slower. If a liver biopsy is performed to obtain an accurate diagnosis, careful assessment for bleeding is necessary. However, a liver biopsy may be contraindicated in the presence of thrombocytopenia.

Moderate to severe acute GVHD (grades II–IV) has been strongly correlated with the incidence of nonviral infection (Paulin 1987). Also, chronic GVHD has been found to be a major factor predisposing patients to infection (Englehard 1986). For these reasons, patients experiencing either acute or chronic GVHD should be thoroughly assessed for infection, and appropriate infection prevention measures should be included following discharge.

Patients who experience ocular sicca with resultant insufficient tear production should be advised to use artificial tears to prevent corneal erosion, perforation, and scarring. Sicca syndrome can also affect the mouth, genital tract, and the mucosa of the tracheobronchial tree. If the patient exhibits these symptoms, moisture enhancing measures to treat these various areas include frequent mouth care and adequate lubrication of the vagina prior to intercourse. The use of an air humidifier also may be recommended.

Nursing management of patients receiving medications to prevent or treat GVHD is also an important consideration. For instance, nurses are quite familiar with the complex management of patients receiving high-dose steroids but managing side effects of cyclosporine may be less familiar. These are discussed in other chapters in this section related to the affected system. The reader is also referred to two recent reviews of nursing management of the patient receiving cyclosporine in the pediatric and adult patient (Truog and Wozniak 1990; Klemm 1985).

Nursing management of the variety of complications common to patients with acute and/or chronic GVHD is challenging. Nursing management of the effects of acute and chronic GVHD often continues after the patient is discharged from the hospital and long-term effects of chronic GVHD are primarily within the realm of the ambulatory, community health, and long-term follow-up nursing staff (Buchsel and Kelleher 1989; Buchsel 1986). Principles of long-term management and nursing care of patients with chronic GVHD are discussed in greater detail in Part III of the text. Standardization of nursing care based on systematic study of effective nursing interventions for GVHD is in its infancy (Machak and Adams 1990). Nursing interventions and research focused on appropriate nursing interventions to treat the effects of GVHD is necessary and needs to correspond to the different and varied degrees of the disease until consistent GVHD prevention is a reality.

Future Directions

Despite HLA identical donor/recipient transplants and prophylactic immunosuppressive therapy, GVHD continues to be a significant problem in patients receiving allogeneic bone marrow transplants. The incidence of GVHD is still around 50% and is one of the major causes of transplant-related mortalities.

Research directed at investigating new drugs or drug combinations that can prevent or decrease the incidence of GVHD with minimal toxicities is ongoing. Cyclosporine combined with methotrexate has been found to reduce the incidence of GVHD to a greater extent than either drug alone (Storb 1986a). Similarly, another study compared methotrexate and prednisone to cyclosporine and prednisone and found the incidence of acute GVHD to be 28% in those patients who had received the cyclosporine combination (Deeg 1988). Because of this data, combinations of cyclosporine with prednisone or cyclosporine with methotrexate are suggested as the best prophylactic regimens currently available for GVHD (Deeg 1988). The immunosuppressive agent thalidomide has also been used to treat acute GVHD (Lims et al. 1988).

T cell-depleted donor marrow has been utilized to reduce the incidence of GVHD. T cells have been found to be the principal cells responsible for the initiation of GVHD. Depletion of T lymphocytes is normally performed prior to transplantation and has historically relied on monoclonal antibodies specific for T cell antigens (Rohatiner et al. 1986). Rosetting and lectin binding columns have also been employed (Reisner et al. 1983). Gliotoxin, a secondary fungal metabolite, irreversibly inhibits murine T cell proliferation (Mullbacher et al. 1988) and may also be used for T cell depletion.

Conclusion

Many research centers are currently investigating a variety of prophylactic and therapeutic regimens that will have the most efficacious effect on reducing the incidence, morbidity, and mortality from GVHD. Since the occurence of GVHD continues to afflict approximately half of allogeneic BMT patients, it is critical that nurses working in the area of transplantation understand the etiology and the physiological mechanisms of GVHD, and the temporal sequencing in which these pathophysiological events occur. Furthermore, it is essential that BMT nurses are sensitive to the negative effects that GVHD may have on their patient's body image, self-esteem, and sexuality.

References

Anderson, K.C., and Weinstein, H.J. 1990. Transfusion-associated graft-versus-host disease. *N. Engl. J. Med. 323* (5): 315–321.

Atkinson, K. et al. 1983. Cyclosporin A associated nephrotoxicity in the first 100 days after allogeneic bone marrow transplantation: Three distinct syndromes. *British Journal of Haematology 54:* 59.

Barrett, A.J. et al. 1982. Cyclosporin A as prophylaxis against graft-versus-host disease in 36 patients. *Br. Med. Jo. 285:* 162.

Beatty, P.G. et al. 1985. Marrow transplantation from related donors other than HLA-identical siblings. *N. Engl. J. Med. 313* (13): 765–771.

Behnke, M.C. 1986. Anorexia. In V.K. Carrieri, A.M. Lindsey, C.M. West (eds.). *Pathophysiological Phenomena in Nursing: Human Responses to Illness.* W.B. Saunders Company: Philadelphia: 110–111.

Biggs, J.C. et al. 1986. A randomized prospective trial comparing cyclosporine and methotrexate given for prophylaxis of graft-versus-host disease after bone marrow transplantation. *Transplant Proceedings 18:* 253.

Billingham, R.E. 1966. The biology of graft-versus-host reactions. *Harvey Lecture 62:* 21.

Blume, K.G. et al. 1980. Bone marrow ablation and allogeneic marrow transplantation in acute leukemia. *N. Eng. J. Med. 302:* 104.

Bortin, M.M. 1983. Pathogenesis of interstitial pneumonitis following allogeneic bone marrow transplantation for acute leukemia. In R.P. Gale (ed.). *Recent Advances in Bone Marrow Transplantation.* New York: Liss, pp. 445–460.

Bortin, M.M. et al. 1989. Factors influencing the risk of acute and chronic graft-versus-host disease in humans: A preliminary report from the IBMTR. *B.M.T. 4* (suppl. 1): 222–224.

Breathnach, S.M., and Katz S.I. 1986. Cell-mediated immunity in cutaneous disease. *Human Pathology 17:* 161–167.

Buchsel, P.C. 1986. Long-term complications of allogeneic bone marrow transplantation: Nursing Implications. *O.N.F. 13* (6): 61–70.

Buchsel, P.C., and Kelleher J. 1989. Bone marrow transplantation. *Nurs. Clin. North Am. 24* (4): 907–938.

Buckner, C.D. et al. 1978. Protective environment for marrow transplant recipients. A prospective study. *Ann. Intern. Med. 89:* 893.

Calissendorff, B. et al. 1989. Dry eye syndrome in long-term follow-up of bone marrow transplantation patients. *B.M.T. 4:* 675–678.

Caudell, K.A., and Schauer, V. 1989. A dressing used for GVHD skin desquamation. *O.N.F. 16* (5): 726.

Champlin, R.E., and Gale, R.P. 1984a. Role of bone marrow transplantation in the treatment of hematologic malignancies and solid tumors. Critical review of syngeneic, autologous, and allogeneic transplants. *Cancer Treatment Report 68:* 145–161.

Champlin, R.E., and Gale, R.P. 1984b. The early complications of bone marrow transplantation. *Seminars in Hematology 21* (2): 101–108.

Cooley, M.A. et al. 1987. T cell depletion of bone marrow cell grafting. Optimalization of conditions for depletion by anti-

CD2 and anti-CD8 monoclonal antibodies with rabbit complement, and for detection of residual T cell content. *Pathology* 19: 131.

Copel, L.C., and Smith, M.E. 1989. Oncology nurses' knowledge of graft-versus-host disease in bone marrow transplant patients. *Cancer Nursing 12* (4): 243–249.

Corson, S.L. et al. 1982. Gynecologic manifestations of chronic graft-versus-host disease. *Obstetrics & Gynecology 60:* 488.

de la Montaigne, M. et al. 1981. Standards of care for the patient with "graft-versus-host disease" post bone marrow transplant. *Cancer Nursing 4:* 191–198.

Deeg, H.J. 1988. Acute graft-versus-host disease. In H.J. Deeg et al. (eds). *A Guide to Bone Marrow Transplantation.* Berlin, Heidelberg: Springer-Verlag, pp. 86–98.

Deeg, H.J. et al. 1980a. Effect of Cyclosporin A (CyA) on marrow engraftment in vivo and on hematopoiesis in vitro. *Experimental Hematology 8:* 78 (abstr. 138).

Deeg, H.J. et al. 1980b. Cyclosporin A, a powerful immunosuppressant in vivo and in vitro in the dog, fails to induce tolerance. *Transplantation 29:* 230–235.

Deeg, H.J. et al. 1982. Cyclosporin A and methotrexate in canine marrow transplantation: Engraftment, graft-versus-host disease, and induction of tolerance. *Transplantation 34:* 30–35.

Deeg, H.J., Storb, R., and Thomas, E.D. 1984a. Bone marrow transplantation. A review of delayed complications. *British Journal of Haemotology 57:* 185–208.

Deeg, H.J., Storb, R., and Thomas, E.D. 1984b. Combined immunosuppression with cyclosporine and methotrexate in dogs given bone marrow grafts from DLA-haploidentical littermates. *Transplantation 37:* 62–65.

Doney, K.C. et al. 1981. Treatment of graft-versus-host disease in human allogeneic marrow graft reciepents: A randomized trial comparing antithymocyte globulin and corticosteroids. *American Journal of Hematology 11:* 1.

Englehard, D., Marks, M.I., and Good, R.A. 1986. Infections in bone marrow transplant recipients. *J. Pediatr.* March 108 (3): 335–346.

Ford, R., and Ballard, B. 1988. Acute complications after bone marrow transplantation. *Seminars in Oncology Nursing 4* (1): 15–24.

Forman, S.J. et al. 1982. Prevention and therapy of graft-versus-host disease (letter). *N. Engl. J. Med.* 307: 376.

Gale, R.P., and Bortin, M.M. 1987. Risk factors for acute graft-versus-host disease. *British Journal of Haematology 67:* 397–406.

Gale, R.P. et al. 1982. Bone marrow transplantation for acute leukemia in first remission. *Lancet 2:* 1006.

Gauvreau, J.M. et al. 1981. Nutritional management of patients with intestinal graft-versus-host disease. *Journal of the American Dietetic Association 79:* 673.

Gingrich, R.D. et al. 1988. Allogeneic marrow grafting with partially mismatched, unrelated marrow donors. *Blood 71* (5): 1375–1381.

Glucksberg, H. et al. 1974. Clinical manifestations of graft-versus-host disease in human recipients of marrow from HLA matched sibling donors. *Transplantation 18:* 295.

Gratoma, J.W. et al. 1987. Herpes virus immunity and acute graft-versus-host disease. *Lancet 1:* 471–473.

Gratwohl, A. et al. 1983. Cyclosporine in human bone marrow transplantation: Serum concentration, graft-versus-host disease, and nephrotoxicity. *Transplantation 36:* 40–44.

Griffin, J.P. (ed.). 1986. Alteration in protective mechanisms: Immune system disorders decreased. In *Hematology and Immunology. Concepts for Nursing.* Connecticut: Appleton-Century-Crofts, p. 120.

Haus, J.M. et al. 1983. Nephrotoxicity in bone marrow transplant recipients treated with Cyclosporin A. *British Journal of Haematology 54:* 69.

Hood, A.F. et al. 1987. Acute graft-vs.-host disease: Development following autologous and syngeneic bone marrow transplantation. *Arch. Dermatol.* 123: 745–750.

Hows, J. et al. 1981. Immunosuppression with Cyclosporin A in allogeneic bone marrow transplantation for severe aplastic anemia: Preliminary studies. *British Journal of Haematology 48:* 227.

Kendra, J. et al. 1981. Response of graft-versus-host disease to high doses of methylprednisolone. *Clinical Laboratory Haematology 3:* 19.

Kennedy, M.S. et al. 1983. Pharmacokinetics and toxicity of cyclosporine in marrow transplant patients. *Transplant Proceedings 15:* 2416 (suppl. 1).

Keown, P.A. et al. 1982. The effects and side effects of cyclosporine: Relationship to drug pharmacokinetics. *Transplant Proceedings XIV* (4): 659–661.

Kernan, N.A. et al. 1986. Clonable T lymphocytes in T cell-depleted bone marrow transplants correlate with development of graft-versus-host disease. *Blood 68:* 770–773.

Klemm, P. 1985. Cyclosporin A: Use in preventing graft-versus-host disease. *O.N.F. 12* (5): 25–32.

Klingemann, H.-G. 1988. Chronic graft-versus-host disease. In H.J. Deeg, H.-G. Klingemann and G.L. Phillips (eds.). *A Guide to Bone Marrow Transplants.* Berlin, Heidelberg: Springer-Verlag, pp. 156–169.

Lims, S.H. et al. 1988. Successful treatment with thalidomide of acute graft-versus-host disease after bone marrow transplantation. *Lancet* (January 16): 117.

Lorson, S.L. et al. 1982. Gynecologic manifestations of chronic graft-versus-host disease. *Obstetrics and Gynecology 60:* 488.

Loughran, T.P., Jr. et al. 1985. Incidence of hypertension after marrow transplantation among 112 patients randomized to either cyclosporine or methotrexate as graft-versus-host disease prophylaxis. *British Journal of Haematology 59:* 547.

Machak, M.E., and Adams, J. 1990. BMT standards update. *Oncology Nursing Society, Bone Marrow Transplantation Special Interest Group Newsletter 1* (1): 3.

Martin, P.J., Hansen, J.A., and Thomas, E.D. 1984. Preincubation of donor bone marrow cells with a combination of murine monoclonal anti-T cell antibodies without complement does not prevent GVHD after allogeneic marrow transplantation. *J. Clin. Immunol.* January 4 (1): 18–22.

Martin, P.J. et al. 1985. Effects of in vitro depletion of T cells in HLA identical allogeneic marrow grafts. *Blood* 66: 664–672.

McConn, R. 1987. Skin changes following bone marrow transplantation. *Cancer Nursing* 10 (2): 82–84.

McDonald, G.B. et al. 1981. Esophageal abnormalities in chronic graft-versus-host disease in humans. *Gastroenterology* 80: 914–921.

McDonald, G.B. et al. 1986. Intestinal and hepatic complications of human bone marrow transplantation. *Gastroenterology* 90: 460–477, 770–784.

Mullbacher, A. et al. 1988. Prevention of graft-versus-host disease by treatment of bone marrow with gliotoxin in fully allogeneic chimeras and cytotoxic T cell repertoire. *Transplantation* 46 (1): 120–125.

Odom, L.F. et al. 1978. Remission of relapsed leukemia during a graft-versus-host reaction: A "graft-versus-leukemia reaction" in man? *Lancet* 2: 537–540.

O'Quin, T., and Moravec, C. 1988. The critically ill bone marrow transplant patient. *Seminars in Oncology Nursing* 4 (1): 25–30.

Parker, N., and Cohen, T. 1983. Acute graft-versus-host disease in allogeneic marrow transplantation. A nursing perspective. *Nurs. Clin. North Am.* 18: 569.

Paulin, T. et al. 1987. Variables predicting bacterial and fungal infections after allogeneic marrow engraftment. *Transplantation* March 43 (3): 393–398.

Powles, R.L. et al. 1980. Cyclosporin A to prevent graft-versus-host disease in man after allogeneic bone marrow transplantation. *Lancet* 1: 327.

Press, O.W. 1987. Bone marrow transplant complications in Toledo. In L.H. Pereyra (ed.). *Complications of Organ Transplantation.* New York: Marcel Dekker: 399–424.

Ralph, D.D. et al. 1984. Rapidly progressive airflow obstruction in marrow transplant recipients. *American Review of Respiratory Disease* 129: 641–644.

Ramsay, N.K.C. et al. 1982. A randomized study of the prevention of acute graft-versus-host disease. *N. Engl. J. Med.* 306: 392.

Reisner, Y. et al. 1983. Transplantation for severe combined immunodeficiency with HLA-A, B, D, DR in compatible parental marrow cells fractionated by soy agglutinatin and sheep red blood cells. *Blood* 61: 341–348.

Ringden, O. et al. 1982. Experience with a cooperative bone marrow transplantation program in Stockholm. *Transplantation* 33: 500.

Ringden, O. et al. 1986. A randomized trial comparing use of cyclosporine and methotrexate for graft-versus-host disease prophylaxis in bone marrow transplant recipients with haematologic malignancies. *B.M.T.* 1:41.

Rohatiner, A. et al. 1986. Depletion of T cells from human bone marrow using monoclonal antibodies and rabbit complement. *Transplantation* 42: 73.

Sale, G.E. et al. 1981. Oral and ophthalmic pathology of graft-versus-host disease in man: Predictive value of lip biopsy. *Human Pathology* 12: 1022–1030.

Sale, G.E., and Shulman, H.M. (eds.). 1984. Pathology of bone marrow transplantation. *Masson Monograph in Diagnostic Pathology Series.* New York: Masson Publishing, Inc.

Santos, G.W. et al. 1983. Marrow transplantation for acute nonlymphocyte leukemia after treatment with busulfan and cyclophosphamide. *N. Engl. J. Med.* 309: 1347.

Santos, G.W. et al. 1987. Cyclosporine plus methylprednisolone versus cyclophosphamide plus methylprednisolone as prophylaxis for graft-versus-host disease: A randomized double-blind study in patients undergoing allogeneic marrow transplantation. *Clin. Transplantation* 1: 21–28.

Saxon, R. et al. 1981. Lymphocyte dysfunction in chronic graft-versus-host disease. *Blood* 58: 746.

Schubert, M.M. et al. 1983. Oral complications of bone marrow transplantation. In D.E. Peterson and S.T. Sonis (eds.). *Oral Complications of Cancer Chemotherapy.* Boston: Martinus Nijhoff, p. 93.

Schubert, M.M., and Sullivan, K.M. 1990. Recognition, incidence, and management of oral graft-versus-host disease. *NCI Monographs* 9: 135–143.

Shulman, H.M. et al. 1978. Chronic cutaneous graft-versus-host disease in man. *Am. J. Pathol.* 91: 545.

Shulman, H.M. et al. 1980. Chronic graft-versus-host syndrome in man. A long term clinicopathological study of 20 Seattle patients. *Am. J. Med.* 69: 204.

Slavin, R.E., and Santos, G.W. 1972. The graft-versus-host reaction in man after bone marrow transplantation: Pathology, pathogenesis, clinical features, and implications. *Clinical Immunological Immunopathology* 1: 472.

Storb, R. 1986. Graft-versus-host disease after marrow transplantation. In Meryman (ed.). *Transplantation: Approaches to Graft Rejection.* New York: Alan R. Liss, pp. 139–157.

Storb, R. et al. 1983a. Graft-versus-host disease and survival in patients with aplastic anemia treated by marrow grafts from HLA identical siblings. Beneficial effect of a protective environment. *N. Engl. J. Med.* 308: 302.

Storb, R. et al. 1983b. Predictive factors in chronic graft-versus-host disease in patients with aplastic anemia treated by marrow transplantation from HLA-identical siblings. *Ann. Intern. Med.* 98: 461.

Storb, R. et al. 1985. Marrow transplantation for chronic myelocytic leukemia. A controlled trial of cyclosporine versus methotrexate for prophylaxis of graft-versus-host disease. *Blood* 66: 698.

Storb, R. et al. 1986a. Marrow transplantation for severe aplastic anemia: Methotrexate alone compared with a combination of methotrexate and cyclosporine for prevention of acute graft-versus-host disease. *Blood* 68: 119–125.

Storb, R. et al. 1986b. Methotrexate and cyclosporine compared with cyclosporine alone for prophylaxis of acute graft versus host disease after marrow transplantation for leukemia. *N. Engl. J. Med.* 314 (12): 729–735.

Storb, R. et al. 1988. Cyclosporine vs. methotrexate for graft-versus-host disease prevention in patients given marrow grafts for leukemia: Long term follow-up of three controlled trials. *Blood* 71 (2): 293–298.

Storb, R. et al. 1989. Methotrexate and cyclosporine versus cyclosporine alone for prophylaxis of graft-versus-host disease in patients given HLA-identical marrow grafts for leukemia: Long-term follow-up of a controlled trial. *Blood* 73 (6): 1729–1734.

Stream P. et al. 1980. Bone marrow transplantation: An option for children with acute leukemia. *Cancer Nursing* 3 (3): 195–199.

Sullivan, K.M. 1983. Graft-versus-host disease. In K.G. Blume and L.D. Petz (eds.). *Clinical Bone Marrow Transplantation.* New York: Churchill Livingstone, pp. 98–101

Sullivan, K.M. 1985. Special care of the bone marrow transplant patient. In P.H. Wiernik et al. (eds.). *Neoplastic Diseases of the Blood.* New York: Livingstone, pp. 1124–1129.

Sullivan, K.M. 1986. Acute and chronic graft-versus-host disease in man. *International Journal of Cell Cloning* 4: 42–93.

Sullivan, K.M. et al. 1981a. Chronic graft-versus-host disease in 52 patients: Adverse natural course and successful treatment with combination immunosuppression. *Blood* 57: 267.

Sullivan, K.M. et al. 1981b. Day 100 screening studies predict development of chronic graft-versus-host disease. *Blood* 58: 176a (abstr.).

Sullivan, K.M. et al. 1982. Preliminary analysis of a randomized trial of immunosuppressive therapy of chronic graft-versus-host disease (abstr.). *Blood* 60: 173a.

Sullivan, K.M. et al. 1984. Late complications after marrow transplantation. *Seminars in Hematology* 21: 53–63.

Thomas, E.D. 1988. The future of marrow transplantations. *Seminars in Oncology Nursing* 4 (1): 74–78.

Thomas, E.D. et al. 1975. Bone marrow transplantation. *N. Engl. J. Med.* 292: 832–843; 895–902.

Thomas, E.D. et al. 1976. Total body irradiation in preparation for marrow engraftment. *Transplant Proceedings* 8: 591.

Truog, A.W., and Wozniak, S.P. 1990. Cyclosporin-A as prevention for graft-versus-host disease in pediatric patients undergoing bone marrow transplants. *O.N.F.* 17 (1): 39–44.

Tsoi, M.S. 1982. Immunological mechanisms of graft-versus-host disease in man. *Transplantation* 13: 459.

Tutschka, P.J. et al. 1983. Cyclosporin A to prevent graft-versus-host disease: A pilot study in 22 patients receiving allogeneic marrow transplants. *Blood* 61 (2): 318–324.

Unanue, E.R., and Allen, P.M. 1986. Editorial comment on the finding of Ia expression in nonlymphoid cells. *Laboratory Investigations* 55: 123–125.

van Bekkum, D.W. et al. 1974. Mitigation of secondary disease of allogeneic mouse radiation chimeras by modification of the intestinal microflora. *J.N.C.I.* 52: 401.

Wachter, H. et al. 1989. Neopterin as marker for activation of cellular immunity: Immunologic basis and clincial application. *Advances in Clinical Chemistry* 27 (1–2): 81–141.

Weedon, D. et al. 1979. Apoptosis: Its nature and implications for dermatopathology. *American Journal of Dermatopathology* 1: 133–144.

Weiden, P.L. et al. 1979. Antileukemic effect of graft-versus-host disease in human recipients of allogeneic marrow grafts. *N. Engl. J. Med.* 300: 1068–1073.

Weiden, P.L. et al. 1981. Antileukemic effect of chronic graft-versus-host disease. *Medical Intelligence* 304: 1529–1533.

Weisdorf, D. et al. 1990. Treatment of moderate/severe acute graft-versus-host disease after allogeneic bone marrow transplantation: An analysis of clinical risk features and outcome. *Blood* 75 (4): 1024–1030

Wingard, J.R. et al. 1989. Predictors of death from chronic graft-vs-host disease after bone marrow transplantation. *Blood* 74 (4): 1428–1435.

Woodruff, J.M. et al. 1976. The pathology of graft-versus-host reaction (GVHR) in adults receiving bone marrow transplants. *Transplant Proceedings* 8: 675.

Yee, G.C. et al. 1988. Serum cyclosporine concentration and risk of acute graft-versus-host disease after allogeneic marrow transplantation. *N. Engl. J. Med.* 319 (2): 65–70.

Chapter 8

Pulmonary and Cardiac Complications of Bone Marrow Transplantation

Terri J. Wikle

Introduction

Although the results of bone marrow transplantation (BMT) are improving in terms of both improved efficacy and fewer complications, pulmonary problems continue to be a major source of morbidity and mortality for about half of the patients who undergo allogeneic BMT. A lesser but significant number of autologous recipients are plagued by pulmonary problems as well (Fort and Graham-Pole 1989). Although the course is variable, about 50–75% of these patients will die of pulmonary complications (Hutchison and King 1983). Lung disease is the most common cause of death in patients receiving BMT, with interstitial pneumonitis accounting for about 40% of all transplant-related deaths (Weiner et al. 1986).

Patients who undergo BMT are normally screened pretransplant for underlying pulmonary disease by obtaining baseline pulmonary function tests. Poor pulmonary function often indicates underlying pulmonary disease. These patients are generally not eligible for BMT since pulmonary disease places the patient at too high a risk for the development of lethal pulmonary complications.

Baseline cardiac function should also be assessed in all patients who undergo BMT. Patients with a **cardiac ejection fraction** of $< 50\%$ are generally at too high a risk to undergo the process, and are therefore usually denied a BMT as a therapeutic option. Cardiac complications occur in about 25% of all patients who undergo allogeneic and autologous BMT, with a higher incidence in the autologous population. Cardiac complications, however, are rarely the cause of death in the BMT patient (Bearman et al. 1988).

Nurses play a vital role in the prevention, detection, and intervention of cardiopulmonary complications of bone marrow transplantation. Nurses caring for these patients must have a strong knowledge base of the medical, scientific, and nursing interventions necessary to deal with these often grave complications.

Pulmonary Complications of Bone Marrow Transplantation

Pathogenesis

In order to plan effective preventative measures, it is necessary to understand the many complex interacting factors that lead to the patient developing pulmonary **interstitial pneumonitis (IPn)**. IPn is a general term referring simply to an inflammatory process involving the intra-alveolar lining of the lung. A model is presented in Figure 8.1 to help sort out these factors (Bortin 1983). There are three major predisposing factors for the development of IPn in bone marrow transplant patients: (1) an immunosuppressed host, (2) lung damage; and (3) the presence of **opportunistic microorganisms** (Bortin 1983). Any of these three predisposing factors alone can lead to the development of IPn. In combination, the nurse can learn to appreciate the perilous position in which these patients are placed. Table 8.1 lists the common risk factors that predispose the BMT patient to the development of IPn.

Immunosuppression

A sequence of pre- and post-transplant events contributes to the patient's severe immunosuppressed state, leaving the patient vulnerable to pulmonary infection. These events occur as fol-

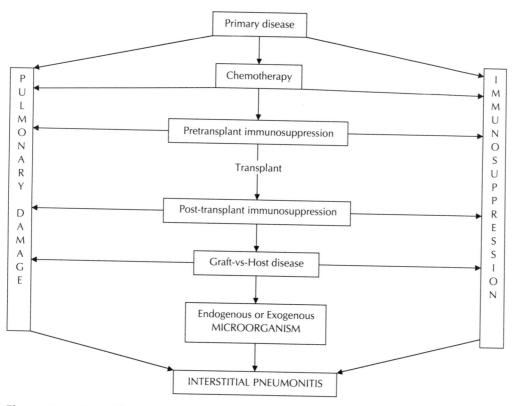

Figure 8.1. Possible Pathways for the Pathogenesis of Interstitial Pneumonitis

Table 8.1. Risk Factors for the Development of Interstitial Pneumonitis

1. Immunosuppressive agents (corticosteroids, MTX, cyclosporine)
2. High-dose cyclophosphamide prior to BMT
3. Graft-versus-host disease
4. Blood product transfusions (transmission of CMV infection)
5. High-dose rate of radiation therapy
6. High total lung dose of radiation therapy
7. Single-fraction radiation therapy
8. Total body irradiation
9. Increased age at time of transplant
10. Seropositivity to CMV pretransplant

lows. A significant number of patients with malignancies receive chemotherapy for remission induction and consolidation for weeks or months prior to transplant. This therapy has significant immunosuppressive activity. In addition, some cancers are, in and of themselves, immunosuppressive. The patient's pretransplant conditioning regimen also causes profound immunosuppressive effects. The immunosuppressive effects of the agents that are administered pretransplant are compounded by their ability to cause lung damage. Table 8.2 is a list of agents commonly administered pretransplant that cause both immunosuppression and pulmonary damage. Posttransplant immunosuppression with methotrexate, cyclosporine, antithymocyte globulin (ATG),

Table 8.2. Agents Associated with Interstitial Pneumonitis that are Immunosuppressive and/or Cause Lung Damage

Actinomycin	Irradiation[a]
BCNU	Melphalan
Bleomycin[a]	Methotrexate[a]
Busulfan	Mitomycin
Chlorambucil	Procarbazine
Cyclophosphamide[a]	Vincristine

[a]Frequent association.
Source: Bortin 1983; with permission.

and other immunosuppressive agents administered to prevent or treat graft-versus-host disease (GVHD) adds to and prolongs the patient's immunosuppressed state. In addition, GVHD has immunosuppressive effects.

BMT patients have multiple interacting factors that result in the virtual destruction of the patient's defenses against infection. Opportunistic pathogens are often found in the lungs of patients with IPn, suggesting that the severe and prolonged injury to the immune system may allow for the growth of these microorganisms. This may be especially true of lung tissue that is already damaged.

Lung Damage

The same sequence of events that leads to immunosuppression in the transplant patient also leads to lung damage. For example, patients with a history of leukemic infiltrates upon diagnosis have already suffered a pulmonary insult even if the infiltrates have resolved at the time of transplant. Patients may receive many of the chemotherapeutic agents listed in Table 8.2 at some time for either induction or consolidation therapy. Perhaps of greater importance is the fact that many of these drugs have been reported to interact with radiation by increasing the amount of damage to normal lung tissue (Bortin 1983). At the present time, many patients who undergo BMT are treated with cyclophosphamide and/or methotrexate along with total body irradiation (TBI); lung damage has been reported to be magnified when either of these drugs is administered in conjunction with irradiation to the lung (Bortin 1983).

Although it is well known and documented that irradiation injures the lungs, the precise role of TBI in the pathogenesis of IPn has yet to be clearly identified. Dose rates, the use of fractionated TBI, and the total dose received by the lung affects the patient's risk for the development of IPn. These factors will be discussed in further detail later in this chapter.

Finally, while the lung is not considered to be a primary target organ for GVHD, lung damage and decreased pulmonary function can occur with both acute and chronic GVHD.

Thus as shown in Figure 8.1 and Table 8.2, BMT patients have multiple and cumulative interacting factors that cause pulmonary injury. The fact that fungal and viral microorganisms are frequently found in the lungs of patients with IPn also suggests that damaged lungs provide an optimal environment for the growth of opportunistic pathogens.

Opportunistic Microorganisms

The finding of opportunistic microorganisms such as cytomegalovirus (CMV) and *Pneumocystis carinii* in the lungs of BMT patients with IPn does not prove that the organism is the cause of the patient's compromised pulmonary state. Damaged lungs in immunosuppressed patients with IPn simply provide a suitable environment for the overgrowth of opportunistic pathogens.

BMT patients are exposed to many endogenous or exogenous sources of CMV and other dangerous microorganisms. The presence of lung damage in an immunosuppressed host strengthens the hypothesis that these microorganisms are the causative agents. Therefore, infection is responsible for many cases of IPn. However, approximately 30–50% of IPn patients are categorized as "idiopathic," meaning no causative organism was isolated either through lung biopsy samples or, all too often, tissue obtained postmortem (Meyers et al. 1982).

Diagnosis of Pulmonary Interstitial Pneumonitis

IPn typically presents as a dry cough, dyspnea, fever with tachypnea, dry rales, restricted ventilatory capacity due to decreased pulmonary compliance, hypoxia, and bilateral diffuse interstitial or reticulonodual infiltrates on the chest x-ray. Prompt diagnosis and treatment is essential if the patient is to survive. Therefore, weekly chest x-rays are recommended for all BMT patients. The chest x-ray remains the major signpost of pneumonitis. Although no radiographic pattern of

pneumonitis is specific either for a particular disease process in the lungs or for a particular infectious agent, some x-ray findings are more characteristic of some diseases than of others. This helps simplify the process of differential diagnosis for the physician (Rubin 1988).

The basic principles by which infections should be diagnosed and treated are the same for BMT patients as for other high-risk patients. Intensive evaluation, including appropriate biopsies, should be performed in an attempt to identify specific pathogens responsible for the pulmonary process. If a specific pathogen is identified, then specific antibiotic therapy can be instituted. The rapidity with which a specific diagnosis is made and effective therapy is instituted is the most important, controllable variable in determining the patient's outcome. Specific diagnoses may be made by one of several approaches: sputum examination, invasive procedures designed to sample secretions from the lower respiratory tract and/or lung tissues, and open lung biopsy.

Conventional Sputum Examination

Examination of expectorated sputum for Gram stain and culture can sometimes be helpful in the diagnosis of pulmonary infections. It is important for the nurse to save sputum samples for diagnostic tests, especially if the patient has not expectorated secretions in the past. The Gram stain is helpful in the compromised host even if it only confirms that the sputum contains the patient's own normal flora. Unfortunately, in the immunocompromised BMT patient, particularly those who are also granulocytopenic, sputum samples are difficult to obtain due to a low white count, and may provide confusing information. Because of its limitations, other diagnostic techniques usually must be employed to determine the etiology of the IPn.

Transbronchial Biopsy (TBB)

Transbronchial biopsy is considered a "middle level" diagnostic technique that is employed in the less emergent situations where the diagnosis cannot be made by noninvasive approaches. TBB provides an actual biopsy of lung tissue during fiberoptic bronchoscopy. All transbronchial biopsies should be submitted for both culture and histologic exam. Bronchial alveolar lavage is also used in conjunction with TBB for an increase in diagnostic yield. This entails lavaging the diseased sections of the lung via the bronchoscope, and then submitting the lavage fluid for studies.

The patient must be closely monitored following TBB for signs of bleeding, infection of the pulmonary tree, and pneumothorax. TBB is often the procedure of choice over the more invasive and risky open lung biopsy, especially in patients who are severely thrombocytopenic, or in patients with a markedly compromised respiratory status. The nurse should always send the first sputum expectorated post-TBB since this may also increase the diagnostic yield of the procedure.

Open Lung Biopsy (OLB)

OLB is often instituted if the above mentioned procedures fail to establish a diagnosis, or if the patient continues to deteriorate despite other therapeutic measures. A BMT patient in this situation should be considered a diagnostic emergency, especially if the patient's hypoxemia is intensifying and the pulmonary infiltrates are spreading rapidly. BMT patients tolerate OLB poorly due to the need for general anesthesia, thoracotomy, and postoperative chest tube. Many BMT patients with IPn require mechanical ventilation following the procedure and therefore many thoracic surgery teams hesitate to operate on these patients. Because a specific pathogen is found in 50–70% of these patients, OLB continues to be an important diagnostic procedure in this patient population (Bortin 1983).

Whatever diagnostic procedure is employed, a detailed analysis of the lung material is carried out. The lung sample is Gram stained and cultured for aerobic and anaerobic bacterial pathogens, as well as mycobacteria, fungi, viruses, mycoplasmas, and the Legionella species. In addition, materials are processed with methenanine silver staining for Pneumocystis, and immunofluorescent staining for Legionella, CMV, and other organisms that are difficult to culture.

The noninfectious, "undiagnosed" cases are most likely due to drug or radiation toxicity, or some other pathologic process, which will be discussed in further detail later in this chapter. On the horizon are newer, less invasive techniques to aid in the rapid, sensitive, and specific identification of the CMV pathogen. These include viral culturing through centrifugation and identification with monoclonal antibodies, early antigen fluorescent foci, and in situ hybridization. The benefits of these newer tests are twofold: they decrease the need for an invasive procedure (OLB) as these can be obtained via bronchoalveolar lavage, and second, they increase the early and rapid diagnosis of CMV, which often responds better if specific therapy is implemented in an early stage of the infection (Chan et al. 1990).

In summary, the diagnosis of IPn is essential if appropriate therapeutic measures are to be successful in preventing progressive respiratory compromise in the BMT patient. Diagnosis is based on symptomatology, chest x-ray, tissue culture, and sometimes sputum examination. The BMT nurse plays an active role in early detection and treatment of IPn by frequently assessing the patient's pulmonary status during activity and at rest, and by reporting suspicious pulmonary findings as they occur.

Pulmonary Edema in the Bone Marrow Transplant Patient

Pulmonary toxicity developing early after BMT is probably due to the individual or collective effects of the pretransplant conditioning, chemotherapy, radiation therapy, and marrow infusion. These early effects are usually seen in the form of pulmonary edema seven to 28 days after BMT (Fort and Graham-Pole 1989). This syndrome is presumed to be due primarily to a leaky pulmonary vasculature. High-dose cytosine arabinoside (Ara-C), which is used in several pretransplant conditioning regimens, has been shown to cause capillary leakage of proteinlike serous fluid into the alveolar spaces (Cardozo et al. 1985). Total body irradiation (TBI), which is used pretransplant to condition many patients, causes similar capillary leakage. Radiation doses in excess of 1000cGy to the lung are associated with increased vascular permeability, alveolar wall edema, alveolar protein leakage, loss of pulmonary surfactant, and formation of an alveolar hyaline membrane.

Symptoms of pulmonary edema include tachypnea, rales, orthopnea, lethargy, restlessness, and if the patient experiences extreme hypoxemia, cyanosis. Nursing management of the BMT patient with pulmonary edema includes assisting the patient to maintain oxygenation, monitoring of weight and strict intake and output, and assisting the medical team with precise fluid management along with the judicious use of diuretics. With astute management, the patient can be assisted through this complication of the initial phase of BMT with complete resolution of the process.

Acute hemorrhagic pulmonary edema may also develop early. This is much less common than the edema caused by increased vascular permeability, and seems to be more frequently associated with patients receiving HLA-mismatched transplants (Hamilton et al. 1986). It is associated with hemorrhage into the alveolar sacs, low central venous pressure, fluid retention, hypotension, and renal failure. Once this complication develops, it is about 90% fatal.

Pulmonary edema may also arise secondary to myocardial damage due to prior chemotherapy, irradiation, or infection. Cardiac complications are discussed later in the chapter.

Pulmonary Infections Associated with BMT

Among the numerous causes of IPn, about two thirds of the patients with IPn have a documented infectious agent causing their pneumonitis (viral, bacterial, fungal, or protozoal), while other cases are attributable to the noxious effects of drugs

Table 8.3. Microorganisms Frequently Associated with Interstitial Pneumonitis

Aspergillus	Mycoplasma
Candida	Pneumococcus
Cryptococcus	Pneumocystis
Cytomegalovirus	Pseudomonas
Herpes simplex	Toxoplasma
Histoplasma	Varicella zoster
Klebsiella	

and/or radiation therapy. Infections are a major cause of pulmonary pathology following BMT. IPn from infectious causes usually occurs from day 30 to day 100 post-BMT, and approximately 50% of these cases are fatal.

The infections may take the form of intraalveolar lobar consolidation or involve the interalveolar linings, hence the name interstitial pneumonitis (IPn). The symptoms associated with infectious pulmonary infiltrates include dyspnea, tachypnea, cyanosis, dry rales, and a cough. These symptoms are a result of inadequate gas exchange, which results from the abnormal alveolar structure thus producing an alveolar/capillary block.

As mentioned previously, intensive evaluation, including appropriate biopsies, should be performed to identify the specific organism responsible for the pulmonary infection. Table 8.3 lists microorganisms that are commonly associated with interstitial pneumonitis. If a specific pathogen is identified, then the appropriate antibiotic/drug therapy should be instituted as soon as possible. If a specific pathogen cannot be found (idiopathic), or is not found because the patient cannot undergo the required diagnostic procedures, then broad spectrum antibiotics are usually administered to cover any or all potentially treatable microorganisms that could be causing the infection. The patient is usually treated with medications for all possible bacterial, fungal, protozoal, viral, and chlamydial infections. Caring for a patient who is being treated for all likely infectious sources can be one of the greatest challenges that a BMT nurse experiences. Venous access, renal compromise, and fluid overload may complicate the overall management of this type of patient due to the large number of medications that must be administered.

The objectives of therapy for the BMT patient with IPn are twofold: treat and/or reverse the causative factor(s), and maintain adequate ventilation/oxygenation. Unfortunately, the treatment of established IPn has been unsuccessful for the most part. This negative experience may partly reflect the irreparable pulmonary damage produced by the overwhelming number of pathologic organisms that are likely present in established pneumonia. For this reason, the effectiveness of any therapeutic modality is severely limited, and efforts at prevention of the pneumonia(s) appear to be more successful.

Bacterial Pneumonia

Bacterial pneumonia commonly occurs within the first six months post-BMT. Etiological factors include neutropenia, B cell immune deficiency, and chronic graft-versus-host disease. In normal individuals, the flora of the upper respiratory tract consists primarily of Gram-positive organisms that are relatively nonvirulent and are antibiotic sensitive. Because of the interaction between these bacteria and the specialized receptors on the surface of the upper respiratory tract, colonization with Gram-negative bacilli is prevented. In the immunocompromised BMT patient, this ecological system is disturbed, resulting in a high rate of colonization of the respiratory tract with Gram-negative organisms (Rubin 1988).

Bacterial infections usually take the form of consolidation of the alveolar sacs in the lungs. Both Gram-positive organisms such as *Staphylococcal aureus*, *Staphylococcal epidermidis*, and *Streptococcus pneumonia*, and Gram-negative organisms such as *Klebsiella*, and the *Pseudomonas* species are the common causative pathogens of pulmonary infections during immunosuppression. Patients with chronic GVHD have a higher incidence of pneumococcus pneumonia. *Legionella*, *Chlamydia*, *Mycobacteria*, and *Mycoplasma* are also more frequently isolated in these patients. Several resistant strains of Gram-positive organisms are more frequently seen late into the BMT patient's treatment. These Gram-positive organisms may be sensitive to vancomycin only.

The approach to therapy for pulmonary bacterial infections was mentioned earlier; if a specific pathogen is identified, then antibiotic therapy should be tailored according to the culture and sensitivity reports. Frequently, if the patient is neutropenic, he/she will require other antibiotic coverage as well to prevent superinfection. Double or triple antibiotic coverage is standard in these patients since there are a vast number of bacteria that may pose a threat. Prophylactic use of trimethoprim-sulfamethoxazole may lower the frequency of *Streptococcus pneumonia* and certain Gram-negative infections, but further study in this area is required. The present pneumococcal vaccine seems to offer no protection for the post-BMT patient with chronic GVHD due to the patient's inability to mount a normal immune response.

Although sometimes fatal, bacterial pneumonias are generally more sensitive to drug therapy than the viral, fungal, and protozoal infections. This is most likely due to the fact that the alveolar wall becomes increasingly thickened in the nonbacterial IPns, thus rendering the lung more resistant to treatment and repair.

Viral Pneumonia

Viral infections are the most commonly documented cause of IPn in the BMT patient population. Treatment of IPn from viral pathogens has been mostly ineffective. Most attempts to treat viral interstitial pneumonia have focused on cytomegalovirus (CMV) infections since the mortality rate of CMV pneumonia following BMT approaches 90% (Bortin 1983). CMV is the most common viral pathogen isolated in the allogeneic patient, and it is the etiologic agent responsible for about 50% of all cases of IPn post-BMT.

CMV infection usually presents six to eight weeks after BMT, either as multifocal disease suggestive of hematologic dissemination, or strictly localized in the lungs suggestive of airway dissemination. CMV pneumonitis may occur as: (1) a reactivation of latent CMV virus in the BMT recipient, (2) an acquired viral pathogen from an infected marrow donor, or (3) an acquired viral pathogen through a blood transfusion.

Prolonged immunosuppression seems to be the single most important factor in the development of CMV pneumonitis. This is supported by the increased incidence of CMV pneumonitis in patients who have received antithymocyte globulin for GVHD prophylaxis, and in patients being treated for acute GVHD with high-dose steroids. The patient's resistance to CMV infection is mediated by cellular immunity, and although the total number of WBCs and phagocytes may be normal in patients post-transplant, T and B cell mediated immune function may be reduced in BMT patients for up to two years. This is especially true of the allogeneic BMT population (Lum 1987).

The most promising current management for CMV infection post-BMT is by prophylaxis with immune globulin containing a high titer of CMV antibody. Intravenous immunoglobulin administered one week prior to, and for the first three to four months after BMT probably reduces the incidence of pneumonitis, although the data is conflicting. The use of CMV seronegative blood products in recipients who are seronegative, and who also have a seronegative donor has also assisted in decreasing the incidence of CMV infection. These prophylactic measures against CMV are generally isolated to allogeneic BMT patients since the incidence of CMV is relatively low in autologous transplant patients.

The use of various antiviral agents has shown little efficacy in preventing or treating CMV pneumonitis (Krowka 1985). Adenine arabinoside, an antiviral agent used in the treatment of herpes simplex viral encephalitis has been used with poor results in the treatment of proven CMV pneumonitis. Human leukocyte interferon is another antiviral agent that has been effective

against herpes-zoster infections and hepatitis B infections, but has been ineffective against CMV. The newest drug, gancyclovir (DHPG) is currently being used in clinical trials, and shows some promise in the treatment of biopsy-proven CMV pneumonitis. Some trials have shown an improved disease response when gancyclovir is used in conjunction with CMV immune globulin. Use of prophylactic gancyclovir and acyclovir may also prevent or decrease the severity of CMV infections; study in this area continues.

In summary, all regimens used to treat established CMV pneumonia after BMT have so far been unsuccessful. Due to the devastating effects of CMV pneumonitis, nurses can expect many new clinical trials in both the treatment and prevention of this grave complication of BMT.

Although CMV is the most common viral etiology of IPn, other viruses are occasionally implicated. These include adenovirus, Herpes simplex virus (HSV), and Varicella zoster (VZV). These viruses account for about 7-10% of the infectious cases of viral IPn (Fort and Graham-Pole 1989). Acyclovir prophylaxis has decreased the incidence of IPn caused by the herpes viruses, and has also reduced the severity of established infections. Epstein-Barr virus (EBV), respiratory syncitial virus (RSV), influenza, and parainfluenza infections are rare causes of IPn in BMT patients.

Fungal Pneumonia

The pulmonary fungal infections that occur in the BMT patient may be divided into three categories: (1) opportunistic infections caused by organisms that primarily invade the lung, e.g., Aspergillus species and Cryptococcus neoformas; (2) opportunistic infections that reach the lung either by way of the circulating blood from another site, or as organisms superinfecting a lung that was previously injured by a viral or bacterial process, e.g., the Candida species and the Aspergillus species; and; (3) systemic mycoses that resemble tuberculosis by lying dormant for many years after the initial infection but subsequently undergo reactivation during the patient's immunosuppressed state, e.g., blastomycosis, coccidioidomycosis, and histoplasmosis. This latter type of infection is rare in the transplant setting (Rubin 1988).

Of all the pulmonary fungal infections that occur in BMT patients, invasive aspergillosis is by far the most important in terms of both incidence and severity. *Aspergillus* accounts for about 10% of all the cases of IPn (Paulin et al. 1987). The *Aspergillus* species most commonly associated with invasive infections are *A. fumigatus* and *A. flavum*. A typical clinical setting for the development of invasive aspergillosis is the BMT patient with severe granulocytopenia or the patient with GVHD receiving high-dose corticosteroids who has received broad-spectrum antibiotics within the previous month.

The presenting clinical symptoms of invasive pulmonary aspergillosis are usually subtle, with persistent fever often being the sole manifestation. In time, a mild productive cough may develop, which may cause pleuritic-type chest pain. As the disease progresses, fever worsens, rales develop, and pulmonary infiltrates appear. Invasive pulmonary aspergillosis causes a necrotizing bronchopneumonia with or without a hemorrhagic infarction. It is not unusual to aspirate lung tissue while suctioning the intubated patient who has an invasive aspergillosis infection due to the necrotizing process. The most characteristic x-ray finding is that of a rapidly progressing nodular infiltrate, often cavitating, that frequently crosses lung fissures (Rubin 1988). Figure 8.2 shows close-ups of these cavitating lesions in a patient with invasive aspergillosis.

One of the most challenging aspects of an *Aspergillus* infection is its rapid spread to the central nervous system (CNS). CNS symptoms may be the nurse's first indication that *Aspergillus* is a threat, even while the primary pulmonary site of infection is relatively asymptomatic. Therefore, major emphasis is placed on early diagnosis via bronchial alveolar lavage or open lung biopsy in the patient with this type of infiltrate, even if the patient displays no signs of pulmonary compro-

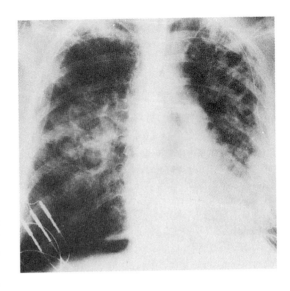

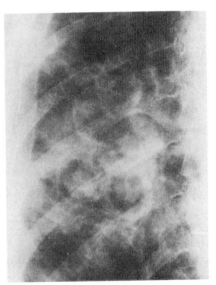

Source: Rubin 1988, with permission.

Figure 8.2.   X-ray of Cavitations Caused by *Aspergillus*

mise. Surgical wedge resection is sometimes performed in patients who have isolated, cavitating lesions in hope of removing the primary site of the infection.

Several transplant centers have suffered devastating epidemics of invasive pulmonary aspergillosis secondary to hospital air conditioning system contamination with *Aspergillus* spores. Protective environments, particularly laminar air flow, seem to decrease the incidence of *Aspergillus pneumonitis*, an important finding given the very high mortality rate of *Aspergillus* infections. At present, the most reasonable approach to early intervention is the empiric use of amphotericin B for the treatment of the neutropenic BMT patient who develops a fever that is unresponsive to broad-spectrum antibiotics after approximately seven days, although centers differ about when to start antifungal therapy. This alone may prevent pulmonary seeding of organisms such as the *Candida* and *Aspergillus* species via the circulating blood.

Presumptive therapy should be initiated in the BMT patient who has a clinical compatible syndrome and x-ray picture, and has either *A. fumigatus* or *A. flavus* isolated from their respiratory secretions (Rubin 1988). The treatment of choice for pulmonary fungal infections in the BMT patient is amphotericin B (Rubin 1988). However, successful treatment using amphotericin B is limited by the toxicity of the drug and the organism's intrinsic resistance to its antifungal activity. Maintenance doses of 0.6–0.7mg/kg/day are often used, but higher doses of up to 1.5mg/kg/day may be administered. Miconazole, 5-fluorocytosine (5-FC), or ketoconazole are unacceptable substitutes for amphotericin B. However, some experimental data do support the use of 5-FC, rifampin, or tetracycline in combination with amphotericin B. Because of the excessively high mortality rate associated with pulmonary aspergillosis, further study in the treatment and prevention of of this lethal fungus is warranted.

Parasitic Pneumonia

Two different opportunistic parasites are capable of producing IPn in the immunosuppressed BMT patient: *Pneumocystis carinii* and *Toxoplasma gon-*

dii. By far the most important is *P. carinii*. The typical x-ray appearance of pulmonary Pneumocystis infection is a diffuse interstitial alveolar pneumonia that often becomes confluent as the disease progresses. Usually the disease affects the lower lobes and is bilateral and symmetric. The patient usually presents with a nonproductive cough, tachypnea, hypoxemia, and a restrictive defect on pulmonary function testing. These symptoms may be present despite a normal chest x-ray. In such patients, a gallium scan can be useful in suggesting the presence of a *Pneumocystis* infection.

Prior to prophylaxis with trimethoprim-sulfamethazole (TMP-SMZ), *P. carinii* was a common cause of severe pneumonia in all immunocompromised patients. With the institution of TMP-SMZ prophylaxis, *Pneumocystis* accounts for less than 5% of IPn post-BMT. Inhaled pentamidine is now being used prophylactically in patients who have poor compliance in taking oral TMP-SMZ, or those patients with an allergy to TMP-SMZ. The advantage in using inhaled pentamidine is that it only requires monthly administration.

Although *P. carinii* rarely develops in patients who are receiving prophylaxis, infection carries a 30% mortality rate. This is presumably due to the emergence of resistant strains of the organism. In this unusual patient, intravenous TMP-SMZ is the drug of choice for initial treatment because it has less toxicity than pentamidine. The dosages are 20mg of trimethoprim/kg per day and 100mg of sulfamethazole/kg per day in four equally divided doses (Winston et al. 1983). Therapy is given for approximately 14 days. Using this approach, a therapeutic response is expected in about 70% of patients. Deaths are frequently associated with concomitant viral or fungal infections (Winston et al. 1983).

Toxoplasmosis is an uncommon cause of pneumonia in BMT patients. As a rule, if *Toxoplasmosis gondaii* does infect the lung, almost invariably other pathogens are also present, particularly one or more of the herpes group of viruses or *Pneumocystis*.

Drug-Induced Pulmonary Damage

Certain drugs used in the pre-BMT conditioning regimens are known to be pulmonary toxins, and may be implicated in some of the cases of idiopathic IPn. As previously mentioned, Table 8.2 lists chemotherapeutic agents most commonly associated with IPn. This toxicity may be an acute single-dose effect or a cumulative effect from the combination of different drugs the patient has received prior to transplant. Such toxicity becomes compounded when these drugs are used in conjunction with radiation therapy and other treatments such as oxygen therapy and positive pressure ventilation (Weiss et al. 1980; Bortin 1983). This additional lung damage may account for the difficulty in weaning the mechanically ventilated BMT patient.

Two clinical syndromes of drug-induced pneumonitis are recognized. The first is a subacute, progressive IPn characterized by fever, nonproductive cough, and dyspnea. This form begins weeks to months following BMT, and resembles a viral or *Pneumocystis* infection both clinically and on the chest x-ray. The second is a chronic interstitial fibrosis that occurs insidiously. Diagnosis is generally made by use of a gallium scan that is positive in the inflammatory form of the disease. Pulmonary function tests reveal progressive pulmonary restriction and a decreased diffusing capacity. Transbronchial or open lung biopsy is usually required for a diagnosis to be made (Rubin 1988).

Bleomycin is one of the most pulmonary-toxic chemotherapeutic agents currently in use. This is because of its tendency to bind to receptors found in large quantities distributed in the skin and in the lungs (Bortin 1983). Patients suffering from such toxicity present with a dry, hacky cough and exertional dyspnea that can progress to resting dyspnea, tachypnea, and cyanosis. The physical and x-ray findings may often be preceded by abnormal pulmonary functions tests (PFTs). Bleomycin causes pulmonary fibrosis, which appears to be dose related. This fibrosis can develop in up to 40% of patients at doses of greater than 150 units. This type of fibrosis is usually irreversible and often fatal (Weiss et al. 1980). The route of bleomycin administration may play a role in toxicity, with continuous infusion being less toxic than IV bolus or intramuscular therapy. The dose at which pulmonary toxicity occurs is much lower when combined with other pulmonary toxins, such as alkylating agents, radiation therapy, and high oxygen tensions to the lung (Ginsberg and Comis 1982).

One study of patients undergoing operative procedures necessitating elevated oxygen tensions during the procedure showed a 100% mortality in patients who had received cumulative doses of bleomycin between 200 and 400 units/m^2 (Weiss et al. 1980). The major cause of mortality in those patients was pulmonary fibrosis. Synergy also appears to exist between bleomycin and radiation therapy. The frequency of severe pulmonary toxicty when radiation is used with bleomycin is 35–50%, with 50% of those cases being fatal (Ginsberg et al. 1982). Currently there is no treatment for the pulmonary fibrosis caused by bleomycin. However, the occasional hypersensitivity reactions to bleomycin, seen as fever, eosinophilia, and diffuse pulmonary infiltrates, will often respond to corticosteroid therapy (Ginsberg et al. 1982).

The nitroureas (carmustine [BCNU], lomustine [CCNU], semustine [methyl CCNU], and chlorotocin) are pulmonary toxins with a reported incidence of pulmonary complications in about 20–30% of patients. The doses at which symptoms develop are unknown, but there is usually a six-month or greater delay from the time of drug exposure to the development of symptoms. Symptoms that are normally seen are progressive dyspnea, tachypnea, and a nonproductive cough. The patient's chest x-ray shows a reticulonodular pattern, pulmonary edema, and often pleural effusions. PFTs reveal a restrictive lung defect with hypoxemia and a decreased carbon monoxide diffusion capacity (DLCO). Tissue that is evaluated from open lung biopsy or upon autopsy shows interstitial fibrosis, alveolar septal thickening, and protein-filled alveoli. Although the outcome varies, and is probably dose-dependent, mortality secondary to nitrourea pulmonary toxicity ranges from 24–60%. Corticosteroids are of no benefit in the treatment of pulmonary toxicity from nitroureas.

Methotrexate produces a variable pulmonary toxicity that is independent of the dose the patient receives. Pulmonary damage can result from any route of administration. PFTs usually show hypoxemia, a decreased DLCO, and a restrictive defect. Methotrexate's toxic effects vary. A hypersensitivity drug reaction is the most common pulmonary toxic effect seen with methotrexate. Leucovorin does not seem to protect against the pulmonary toxicity. Fortunately, recovery usually occurs after the methotrexate is stopped. Corticosteroids appear to be of some benefit in the treatment of methotrexate-induced pulmonary toxicity, but do not induce a complete reversal of the pulmonary process.

The alkylating agents, cyclophosphamide, busulfan, chlorambucil, and melphalan, probably have additive toxicity when used in combination with bleomycin or carmustine (Weiss et al. 1980; Ginsberg et al. 1982). Cyclophosphamide can cause intra-alveolar inflammation and edema leading to fibrosis, with similar PFT changes to those seen with the nitroureas. Infiltration can lead to a complete "whiting out" of the entire lung. Fortunately, early drug cessation can lead to a complete clinical and radiological resolution (Weiss et al. 1980). As with methotrexate, the route of administration and total drug dose do not appear to determine how much toxicity the patient will suffer. Symptoms can begin while the patient is receiving cyclophosphamide, and may occur as late as eight years following therapy. Children who receive cyclophosphamide during their growth spurt can also experience a decrease

in their relative lung volume (Ginsberg et al. 1982).

Many transplant protocols use a combination of busulfan and cyclophosphamide, both of which can produce similar symptoms of hypoxemia and a restrictive ventilatory defect. These patients are especially at high risk for pulmonary toxicity, and should be monitored closely for pulmonary compromise. Onset of symptoms is insidious, and usually appears as cough, tachypnea, fever, and crepitant rales. Symptoms normally arise while the patient is on therapy, and often progress over weeks or months, unfortunately leading to a fatal outcome. Clinical improvement has been reported after discontinuing the busulfan, along with treating the patient with high-dose steroids. Busulfan is also associated with the loss of lung volume if given to children during their growth spurt (Ginsberg et al. 1982).

Melphalan rarely causes pulmonary toxicity, but may occasionally damage the alveolar epithelium by causing dysplasia that can progress to fibrosis. Proliferation of epithelial cells in the bronchi and alveoli, which then results in the infiltration of these areas with plasma is the presumed mechanism by which the damage occurs.

Cytosine arabinoside (ARA-C) can increase pulmonary vascular permeability leading to pulmonary edema as mentioned earlier in this chapter. This seems to correlate with the time course of drug administration, and not to the dose of the drug. In other words, the pulmonary toxic effects of ARA-C are increased if the drug is given in close proximity to other pulmonary toxins prior to the transplant conditioning regimen.

Although most drugs can cause toxicity through pulmonary parenchymal inflammation and fibrosis, procarbazine, like methotrexate causes pneumonitis through a hypersensitivity reaction. Permanent fibrosis can result if the hypersensitivty reaction is prolonged. Fortunately symptoms will usually resolve if the procarbazine is stopped.

The chemotherapy that BMT patients receive prior to transplant is administered in large doses over a short period of time. Despite the development of symptoms, the BMT patient is usually committed to receiving their full conditioning regimen since the transplant is the patient's most likely chance for cure. Therefore, with the exception of methotrexate for GVHD prophylaxis, chemotherapeutic agents are given in full doses, which may lead to the development of pulmonary or other serious symptomatology.

Radiation-Induced Pulmonary Damage

In addition to infections and chemotherapy-induced pulmonary toxicity, radiation therapy is a major cause of BMT-related pulmonary damage. The damage associated with total body irradiation usually develops two to three months after treatment (Bortin 1983; Gross 1977). Shielding the lungs, reducing the total dose exposure of TBI to 600cGy or less, fractionating the TBI over several days, and decreasing the dose delivery rate all seem to decrease the incidence of IPn. Unfortunately, many of these solutions are impractical. Lung shielding may also shield tumor cells and result in an increase risk of relapse. Many patients require greater than 600cGy in order to achieve the required immunosuppression and antineoplastic effects that TBI offers. Much research is presently focused on the elimination of TBI, and thus its toxicities, so that the patient would be conditioned pretransplant with chemotherapy only. However, this may significantly increase the patient's risk of cardiac and other serious complications.

Signs and symptoms of radiation-induced pneumonitis are progressive dyspnea, high spiking fevers, a nonproductive cough with occasional hemoptysis, and chest pain secondary to pleural inflammation. Radiation-induced pulmonary damage may resolve slowly, or progress to fibrosis. Late symptoms include cyanosis, clubbing of the nails, orthopnea, and chronic **cor pulmonale**. Scoliosis with a midline shift may result from loss of pulmonary volume in the irradiated field in patients who receive local irradiation as part of their pretransplant conditioning. Progressive fibrosis is seen as a "ground glass" appearance on chest x-ray, with hazy pulmonary markings. As fibrosis develops, linear streaked consolidation with an occasional midline shift occurs. Bronchiolectatic cysts may also develop in the fibrosed lung. Corticosteriods offer some benefit in chronic radiation fibrosis. Unfortunately, symptoms usually reappear with tapering of the steroids. The time course for resolution or progression of the radiation damage is related to the severity of the pulmonary insult (Gross 1977).

Graft-Versus-Host Disease (GVHD) and Pulmonary Damage

Thirty to seventy percent of allogeneic BMT patients develop GVHD as a complication. These patients are predisposed to lung infections because of the immunosuppression that accompanies GVHD and its treatment. Additionally, GVHD appears to have a direct effect on the pulmonary epithelium. The sicca syndrome of chronic GVHD, which is recognized to have other target organs, can also exert its effect on the lungs. This is demonstrated as a decrease in the production of IgA and reduced local humoral immunity. Because of the death of epithelial cells, ciliary function is decreased as are bronchial secretions. The bronchial mucosa is thus exposed. This results in a loss of its normal protective action, thus predisposing the patient to bronchopneumonia (Bortin et al. 1982).

A lymphocytic bronchitis can also occur concurrently with the development of acute GVHD. This type of syndrome can also be caused by ventilator trauma or viral infections. Signs and symptoms include dyspnea, tachypnea, and a nonproductive cough due to bronchospasm with occasional progressive airway obstruction. With this syndrome there is lymphocytic infiltration of the mucosa, submucosa, and mucularis, with necrosis of epithelial cells, loss of cilia, and decreased goblet cells. This decreased ciliary function will predispose the patient to the development of bronchopneumonia.

Bronchiolitis obliterans affects about 10% of chronic GVHD patients. It is characterized by loss of the elastic recoil in the lung tissue, with infiltration of the walls of the small bronchioles by acute and chronic inflammatory cells. The tissue in the upper airways remains normal. Granulomas can also plug the alveolar spaces secondary to the sicca syndrome seen in chronic GVHD (Ostrow et al. 1985). Clinically, the patient rapidly develops shortness of breath, inspiratory rales, a nonproductive cough, and airway obstruction. The patient's chest x-ray is usually normal except for mild hyperinflation. Unfortunately, the obstruction is irreversible, unresponsive to bronchodilators, mucolytic agents or steroids, and usually progresses to recurrent pneumothoraces and hypoxia leading to death.

Malignant Infiltration

With the increasing use of autologous BMT for solid tumors and hematologic malignancies involving the bone marrow, another theoretical source of pulmonary disease associated with transplantation is infiltration with malignant cells. Although bone marrow purging techniques are frequently used, the procedure may not be adequate to remove all malignant cells from the purged marrow. This occurs infrequently, but must be a part of the differential diagnosis in patients with diffuse pulmonary infiltrates after autologous BMT (Glorieux et al. 1986). Leukemic infiltration can also be associated with pulmonary compromise associated with fever.

Miscellaneous Pulmonary Complications

Another less common cause of lung disease associated with BMT is pulmonary embolism due to infusing fat particles and bone spicules from unfiltered bone marrow. This finding has been been detected at autopsy from patients dying from other causes, and the significance is uncertain.

Pulmonary veno-occlusive disease has also been documented (Hamilton et al. 1986). This is probably an unusual response to high-dose chemotherapy and TBI.

Acute pulmonary hemorrhage, a threat in these pancytopenic patients, may result from trauma (as from a diagnostic procedure or during intubation) or secondary to an underlying pulmonary condition such as aspergillosis. It is important to note that any of these causes may be complicated by an underlying infection in this group of patients, particularly if the patient has undergone endotracheal intubation as part of their overall pulmonary management (Rubin 1988).

An unusual cause of febrile pneumonitis syndrome is a leukoagglutination reaction. This syndrome is characterized by the abrupt onset of fever, rigors, tachypnea, nonproductive cough, and respiratory distress within the first 24 hours following the transfusion of a blood product. The clinical picture stems from the interaction in the blood between preformed antibodies and antigens. These antibodies may be directed against the patient's leukocytes. These reactions were most commonly seen following now rare granulocyte transfusions. Leukoagglutination reactions can best be avoided by using blood products that are washed, packed, filtered, or frozen/thawed if possible. All of these measures reduce or eliminate leukocytes in blood products.

Nursing Diagnosis, Planning, and Intervention for the BMT Patient with Interstitial Pneumonitis

It is obvious that all patients who undergo BMT are at risk for lethal pulmonary complications. The BMT nurse plays a key role in the prevention, detection, and treatment of patients who develop acute pulmonary complications. Pulmonary diseases are perhaps the most devastating of any that we deal with in this clinical setting.

Preventative Nursing Measures

An important preventative measure performed by the nurse is encouraging the patient to exercise despite an obvious decrease in energy level. This poses a great nursing challenge, especially when patients are isolated in a laminar air flow environment. Many transplant centers utilize a variety of exercise equipment, such as exercise bikes. Consultation with the physical therapy department to assist in the development of an appropriate exercise program may also be of some benefit. These types of activities aside from the pulmonary benefits may also improve the patient's state of mind, and may increase the motivation to participate in their own care.

Good pulmonary toilet should also be encouraged. This can be accomplished in the form of coughing and deep breathing every two to four hours, as well as the use of incentive spirometry. These two techniques can aid in the prevention of atelectasis, and thus facilitate gas exchange as each alveolus is filled (Ellis and Nowlis 1989). Caution should be taken with percussion and postural drainage in thrombocytopenic patients, since pulmonary trauma can occur.

Maintaining appropriate isolation techniques to avoid infections from exogenous sources is vital to the well being of the BMT patient. Isolation of the BMT patient from possible infection involves either minimal protection such as wearing masks, handwashing, and restricting visitor contact, to very strict isolation through the use of laminar air flow isolation rooms. Successful transplants are performed in both settings (Hutchison and King 1983). Since optimal isolation techniques are not known, practices vary from center to center. One fact seems certain; the use of laminar air flow does decrease incidence of aspergillosis while the patient is hospitalized. Isolation practices present an exciting challenge for further nursing research.

Finally, the BMT nurse will be involved in the prophylactic use of many of the agents already mentioned. The BMT nurse will continue to be involved in a variety of research protocols aimed at the prevention and treatment of IPn. This research is expected to continue for a long time, or until a treatment plan aimed at lowering the excessively high morbidity and mortality of these complications is found.

Nursing Assessment and Diagnosis of the BMT Patient with IPn

Continuous and astute nursing observation of the BMT patient for alterations in respiratory function is an essential component of the patient's nursing care plan. The BMT patient should have his or her lungs ascultated at least every eight hours since expeditious intervention is likely a key component in the patient's survival. Once impaired gas exchange develops, the patient's respiratory status should be assessed a minimum of every four hours. Symptoms of pulmonary dysfunction have already been mentioned in context with the specific disease entities. A sample nursing care plan is presented at the end of the text.

Care of the Intubated BMT Patient with Adult Respiratory Distress Syndrome (ARDS)

There are several causes of ARDS in the BMT patient population, including: (1) septic shock; (2) pulmonary infection, and/or IPn; (3) exposure to toxins, i.e., chemotherapy/radiation therapy; and (4) immunologic reactions. ARDS is usually a terminal event for the BMT patient with IPn, and is manifested by increased permeability of pulmonary capillaries to water and plasma proteins.

Management of the patient with ARDS involves: (1) finding and treating the "cause" of the process, (2) maintaining a pO_2 above 55mm Hg, and, (3) avoiding other potentially fatal complications.

These patients frequently will require endotracheal intubation and mechanical ventilation in order to maintain oxygenation. Maintenance of an adequate arterial pO_2 is accomplished by careful fluid and ventilator management. A variety of ventilators are used in BMT/intensive care units to aid in sustaining respirations for the BMT patient with IPn. Most of these ventilators work on the principle of positive pressure to inflate the lungs, but can be set to meet the individual needs of a particular patient with regard to the rate and depth of respirations, as well as the concentration of oxygen needed to maintain the pO_2. Close assessment of the arterial blood gases allows constant assessment and readjustment of the ventilator; frequently these patients require an invasive arterial pressure line, so that frequent blood gas measurements can be made.

Positive end-expiratory pressure (PEEP) has been demonstrated to improve the PaO_2 in the patient with ARDS (Spragg 1980). Applied during continuous mechanical ventilation, or during intermittent mandatory ventilation with continuous positive airway pressures (IMV/CPAP), PEEP may help decrease cardiac output by decreasing the venous return to the chest, thus leading to an increase in the pulmonary vascular resistance. BMT patients often require large amounts of PEEP and CPAP to maintain adequate oxygenation.

Since careful fluid management is so important to the treatment outcome, frequent measurement of the patient's cardiac output is required. This can be accomplished through the use of a Swan-Ganz thermodilutional catheter. Since a physiologic consequence of IPn is a shunting of venous blood through the nonventilated areas of the lungs, the Swan-Ganz catheter allows measurement of the extent of this shunting. Measurement of the pulmonary artery wedge pressures and cardiac output is mandatory in many of these patients. An adequate cardiac output, and a low pulmonary artery wedge pressure both help minimize the extravascular lung "water" that plagues these patients.

Unfortunately, despite all of the above described efforts, mortality approaches 70% in BMT patients with IPn who are intubated and receive > 50% oxygen for 24 hours or more (Rubin 1988). Very often the patient will quickly experience multisystem organ failure, further increasing the rate of mortality.

Despite heroic measures, ventilatory efforts are often futile. If a pneumonia develops, the patient and family will need emotional support. Most transplant patients and families fear pneumonia and may express worries of impending death. Additionally, the family, patient, and transplant team may have to face the possibility of life-support mechanisms if the pneumonia progresses (Hutchison and King 1983). The patients may be given the choice of less aggressive medical interventions if the causative agent(s) of the pneumonia is found to carry a poor prognosis. The BMT nurse is an important team member in clarifying information and supporting the patient and family in making difficult decisions. Living wills can be helpful in this situation in assisting the family and health care team to follow the patient's wishes about whether or not they wish to be placed or continued on mechanical life support.

This chapter would be remiss without mentioning the emotional impact that caring for the intubated BMT patient with ARDS has, not only on the nurse caring for the patient, but on the entire nursing staff. The human resources required to manage one of these patients are tremendous and rarely successful. Support groups for the transplant staff are often warranted following the death of one of these patients.

Cardiac Complications of Bone Marrow Transplantation

Cardiac complications of BMT are not uncommon, but rarely cause death in this patient population. In contrast to allogeneic BMT patients whose major complications are GVHD, interstitial pneumonitis, and hepatic veno-occlusive disease, cardiac complications have been reported to occur in about 40% of autologous patients, and ac-

Table 8.4. Risk Factors for the Development of Cardiac Complications Post BMT

1. History of anthracyclines
2. History of radiation therapy to the chest
3. Total dose of cyclophosphamide of > 150mg/kg
4. Cyclophosphamide as pretransplant conditioning, especially if patient has had ARA-C or 6-thioguanine
5. Cyclophosphamide and TBI as pretransplant conditioning
6. Sepsis
7. History of mitral valve disease
8. Cardiac ejection fraction of < 50%.

count for about 10% of the deaths associated with autologous BMT (von Herby et al. 1988). This incidence is attributable most likely to the regimen-related toxicity caused by high-dose antineoplastic drugs that these patients receive prior to transplantation. Although the occurrence is not that common, currently cardiac toxicity is one of the most limiting factors for BMT (Cazin et al. 1986). Therefore, all pre-BMT patients, especially those who have been heavily treated with anthracyclines or cyclophosphamide, and/or radiation to the chest, must be carefully screened prior to their acceptance for transplantation.

In high-risk cancers, bone marrow toxicity has been the most important factor limiting the use of adequate doses of chemo and/or radiation therapy for curative treatment. The use of BMT in cancer therapy permits intensified chemo- and/or radiation therapy with the promise of a cure in the treatment of leukemia, lymphomas, and a variety of solid tumors. However, toxic effects on other organs are now becoming manifest. This is certainly true for the heart, and may account for many of the cardiac complications that are seen in these patients (von Herby et al. 1988). Table 8.4 lists factors that place the BMT patient at risk for the development of cardiac complications.

Chemotherapy-Induced Cardiac Damage

The cardiotoxicity of doxorubicin (Adriamycin) is known to occur at doses greater than 450mg/m^2. Although it is infrequently used in pretransplant conditioning regimens, many leukemia and some solid tumor patients may have received a significant amount of doxorubicin for induction and/or consolidation therapy. Another anthracycline, daunorubicin, can also contribute to cardiac damage. Both of these agents have been shown to be correlated with cardiac failure in the BMT patient (von Herby et al. 1988). Even if these drugs are not used in the pretransplant conditioning regimens, history of their use may significantly increase the patient's risk of cardiac toxicity post-BMT.

The heart damage caused by anthracyclines is from a loss of myocardial fibrils, mitochondrial changes, and cellular degeneration. Necrosis of the cardiac fibers is often seen on autopsy in these patients, along with necrosis of the contraction bands in the heart. Chronic changes such as fibrosis are also common. The cardiac damage associated with anthracyclines is, for the most part, irreversible. Cells termed "adria" cells are often seen in patients who receive large doses of doxorubicin, and are characterized by a "clumping" of myocardial cell nuclei. These cells are often associated with severe cardiomyopathy.

Cardiac toxicity induced by anthracyclines may occur very early in the post-transplant period. This is most likely due to the pretransplant conditioning regimen adding to the cardiac insult. The period of marrow aplasia also places the patient under extreme physical stress, which may also contribute to the cardiac episode. Pulmonary edema may arise secondary to myocardial damage caused by anthracyclines. Symptoms the nurse should watch for are chronic weight gain, peripheral edema, tachycardia, dyspnea with exertion, orthopnea, rales, and rhonchi. At the first indication of cardiac difficulty the patient should have a cardiac ejection fraction measured to compare with the preadmission baseline study.

Unfortunately, if the chronic and cumulative damage associated with anthracyclines has occurred, supportive measures are rarely successful in reversing this progressive deterioration. Precise fluid management, and the judicious use of diuretics and digitalis, along with lowering the stress to the heart by resting the patient, presently seem to be the best approach.

Cardiac complications associated with cyclophosphamide (Cy) have been well documented at the doses used in the BMT setting (Kupari et al. 1990). Cy is an alkylating agent that has been shown to have both potent immunosuppressive properties and antineoplastic activity. It is a mainstay in most pretransplant conditioning regimens. Most BMT centers employ doses of 50–60mg/kg/day, with total pretransplant doses in the range of 120mg to 200mg. Cardiac complications rarely occur at doses below this. Cardiac damage may worsen if the patient has received other cardiotoxic drugs in the past such as high-dose cytasine arabinoside (ARA C) and 6-thioguanine, or total body irradiation.

Cy causes hemorrhagic myocardial necrosis, thickening of the left ventricular wall, serosanguinous pericardial effusions, and a fibrinous pericarditis. Autopsy results on these patients have shown many areas of myocardial necrosis along with fibrin microthrombi near the areas of capillary damage (Goldberg et al. 1986). These changes are usually seen at Cy doses that are greater than 150mg/kg, although damage has been reported at doses as low as 120mg/kg (Levine 1982; Kupari et al. 1990).

Clinical signs of Cy induced cardiac damage such as severe and often refractory congestive heart failure normally occur one to ten days following Cy administration (Goldberg et al. 1986). Symptoms are those associated with pulmonary edema, cardiomegaly, poor peripheral perfusion, and systemic edema. Decreased voltage is noted on the patient's electrocardiograph (ECG). The presence of sepsis appears to worsen the patient's cardiac dysfunction (Goldberg et al. 1986). These symptoms may progress to a hemorrhagic myocarditis, cardiac tamponade, and death. If symptoms occur prior to completion of the patient's course of Cy, the drug may be stopped and replaced with some other chemotherapeutic agent, usually nitrogen mustard.

Like the toxicity suffered with anthracyclines, little can be done to treat Cy-induced cardiac damage. Supportive care involves astute fluid management and the use of diuretics and digitalis. Pericardiocentesis, and the placement of a pericardial window are sometimes performed on patients who suffer from pericardial effusions since cardiac tamponade is a threat.

Of interest is that children seem to have a lower incidence of Cy-induced cardiac damage. Since children have a relatively smaller ratio of weight to body surface area than do adults, children may receive less Cy than adult patients. Also, obese patients are more likely to be overdosed when treated on a mg/kg basis; these patient's dosages may be calculated based on an ideal body weight rather than actual body weight.

Radiation-Induced Cardiac Damage

Heart muscle disease induced by radiation therapy is a well known entity. Lowered dose rates and fractionation of total body and/or total lymphoid irradiation (TLI) appears to lessen the cardiac toxicity seen in BMT patients. Most transplant centers now fractionate their TBI and TLI doses, and use dose rates that should not evoke cardiac damage if the radiation therapy were used by itself. Thus, pure radiation-induced cardiotoxicity is unlikely (von Herbay et al. 1988). However, there does seem to be a synergistic effect between chemotherapy and radiation.

BMT patients who are at highest risk for the development of radiation-induced cardiac damage are those patients who have received radiation to the chest prior to their transplant conditioning regimen, and who will then go on to receive TBI or TLI. Pretransplant patients who have borderline cardiac function prior to transplant may have their heart shielded for TBI in order to decrease their chances of suffering a fatal cardiac complication.

Cardiac irradiation has been associated with the development of pericardial effusions and constrictive pericarditis, thus predisposing the patient to the development of pulmonary edema. This toxicity may be triggered by the microvascular damage that is noted with Cy (von Herby et al. 1988). It is also possible that radiation therapy may have a synergistic effect with the hyperlipidemia that is caused by chronic corticosteriod therapy for GVHD (Chan et al. 1989). Supportive measures for radiation-induced cardiac damage are the same as those utilized with Cy toxicity.

In summary, the types of cardiac damage seen with regimen-related toxicity closely resemble one another regardless of the causative factor. Little can be done to reverse the clinical course that results from cardiac damage caused by high-dose chemotherapy and radiation therapy, although it is only fatal in about 10% of the cases. Many patients may suffer from mild, and often undetected cardiac toxicity. If the toxicity progresses, the patient will suffer from oliguria and fluid retention refractory to diuretics, cardiomegaly with persistent pericardial effusions, a fall in blood pressure, worsening pulmonary edema, cardiac collapse, and death. Research directed at improving and decreasing the toxicity of conditioning regimens is currently being conducted so that the risk of cardiac and other serious complications will lessen the threat of morbidity and mortality in patients who undergo BMT.

Cardiac Infections

Cardiac infections in BMT patients can affect the pericardium, endocardium, and the myocardium. *Candida albicans*, *Aspergillus*, *Pseudomonas*, *Clostridium*, *Streptococcus*, *Staphylococcus toxoplasma*, coxsackie virus, and adenovirus are the most common causative pathogens (Sale and Shulman 1984). Despite the patient's severe immunosuppressed state, cardiac infections are rather rare.

Noninfectious endocarditis also rarely occurs in these patients, and is usually secondary to subclavian central venous lines.

Bacterial Infections Affecting the Heart
Rarely, bacterial infections disseminating from the gut of the BMT patient seed the heart (Sale and Schulman 1984). These infections can cause microabscesses containing organisms such as *Pseudomonas* and *Clostridium*. *Streptococcus viridans*, an organism commonly found in the oral cavity, can also cause endocarditis if the patient has heart valves that are already damaged (Guzzetta 1987). This makes the pretransplant dental exam highly important. *Staphylococcus aureus* is a more virulent organism, and can attack normal heart valves.

The pathogenesis of acute infective endocarditis is related to the presence of a bacteremia caused by a highly virulent organism. Because 50–60% of the acute infections occur in patients without previous cardiac valvular deformities, several theories have been formulated to explain why some types of bacteria affect normal heart valves. One explanation is that *S. aureus* and other Gram-positive bacteria exhibit a unique property that permit them to adhere to the endothelial surface of the heart valve. More recently, infective endocarditis in some patients was believed to be related to the presence of a right atrial catheter (Martino et al. 1990). It appears that only a few highly virulent organisms are necessary to establish the infection (Guzetta 1984). Infections forming on the heart valves produce endothelial lesions called vegetations. The organisms lie deep in the layers of these vegetations. This explains why patients who receive adequate intravenous antimicrobial therapy may experience progressive valvular infection. Figure 8.3 shows infective endocarditis vegetations of the mitral valve (Guzzetta 1984).

Infective endocarditis often goes unnoticed in these patients. Clinical signs are fever, chills, cough, malaise, and headache. The patients temperature will normally range from 39.4–40 C. The

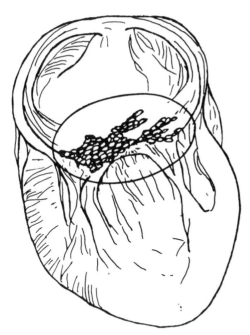

Reproduced by permission from Guzetta 1984.

Figure 8.3. Infective Endocarditis Vegetations (*circle*) of the Mitral Valve

BMT patient may already experience many of these symptoms early in the post-transplant period. More specific symptoms include a new murmur, a pericardial friction rub, and symptoms of congestive heart failure. Positive blood cultures may also be found. The ECG may show conduction or rhythm disturbances or even myocardial ischemic changes. An echocardiogram may reveal vegetations on the patient's heart valves. The patient should also be closely monitored for symptoms of an embolus since these vegetations can break away from the valves into the circulating blood.

Empiric, broad spectrum antibiotic therapy is especially important in the prevention and early treatment of this complication since sepsis is most commonly the cause. Removal of the central venous catheter may be necessary if it is considered a source of bacterial seeding . Intracardiac infections secondary to central venous catheters are

rare, but should not be ruled out if the patient is symptomatic. Precise fluid management is also essential in these patients. As a note, patients who survive this complication may require a heart valve replacement sometime in the future.

Fungal Infections Affecting the Heart

The deep-seated and disseminated fungal infections often caused by *C. Albicans* and *Aspergillus* produce multiple fungal emboli to many organs including the heart. Cardiac involvement by disseminated aspergillosis is rare and usually presents as a myocarditis, with subsequent involvement of the pericardium and the endocardium (Atkinson et al. 1984). Death from myocardial infarction secondary to *Aspergillus* embolization to the coronary arteries has also been reported in patients following BMT (Laszewski et al. 1988).

The predominant form of cardiac involvement with *Aspergillus* is pericarditis. Pathogenesis of the infection appears to include initial myocardial involvement with eventual spread to the pericardium. Spread to the heart appears to be by direct invasion from infected lung tissue lying adjacent to the heart, or by fungus in the circulating blood from involved pulmonary veins (Laszewski et al. 1988). Involvement of the endocardium is common in patients who have widespread aspergillosis since thromboemboli disseminate from the primary source. It is these fungal microemboli that can cause a myocardial infarction if they become lodged in the coronary arteries.

Symptoms of fungal endocarditis closely resemble those seen with bacterial endocarditis. There is also great difficulty in diagnosing aspergillosis of the heart. In most cases of aspergillosis some radiographic or clinical sign or symptom of a respiratory infection or pleuritis is usually evident even when the patient's blood cultures are negative. Spread to the heart by embolization may occur even if the patient has no signs of a primary pulmonary infection. The patient may simply complain of substernal chest pain that is refractory to pain medications. Further cardiac work-up may reveal an ECG with ischemic changes, an abnormal echocardiogram, and elevated cardiac isoenzymes. If the ischemia continues, the patient will most likely develop congestive heart failure and/or cardiac arrest and die.

Fortunately, aspergillosis of the heart remains a rare complication of BMT. The difficulty in diagnosing aspergillosis prior to the patient's death has been well recognized, as well as the importance of early detection so that appropriate treatment and possible cure can occur. For these reasons, the empiric use of antifungal therapy, i.e., amphotericin B, has been widely advocated in the immunosuppressed BMT patient who remains febrile and symptomatic despite the use of antibacterial therapy. Supportive measures also include precise fluid management, the use of digitalis if needed, judicious use of diuretics, and the use of nitroglycerin for chest pain relief.

There are increasing numbers of case reports of fungal infections affecting the endocardium, myocardium, and pericardium of post-BMT patients. This suggests that disseminated aspergillosis or candidiasis needs to be included in the differential diagnosis of chest pain and ECG changes in the immunocompromised BMT patient for early detection and successful treatment to be possible.

Viral Infections Affecting the Heart

Viral infections of the heart are rare and not well documented in the literature. The viruses most frequently documented are the coxsackie virus and adenovirus. Although CMV infections frequently occur in BMT patients, rarely does this virus affect the heart. Viruses, when they do occur, generally attack the myocardium, sometimes causing irreversible myocardial damage. Since viral infections are difficult to detect, they are often mistaken for drug and/or radiation toxicity (Sale and Schulman 1984). Symptoms resemble those seen in all infective endo/myocarditis patients, such as those symptoms associated with decreased myocardial contractility, diminished cardiac output, and secondary pulmonary edema. Supportive measures are the same as well. Little

can be offered in the way of antiviral therapy, especially since most viral infections of the heart go undetected.

Nonbacterial Thrombotic Endocarditis (NBTE)

Although not commonly recognized as a complication of BMT, nonbacterial thrombotic endocarditis (NBTE) has been described by a large autopsy study to occur more frequently in BMT patients (7.7%) than either the general population (1.9%) or in patients who had diseases that would have made them eligible for but who did not receive BMT (1.8%) (Patchell et al. 1985b).

The pathogenesis of NBTE is not completely understood, although it is thought to be a manifestation of disseminated intravascular coagulopathy (DIC) (Davis and Patchell 1988; Olney et al. 1979). Clinical evidence diagnostic of NBTE is uncommon and may be difficult to differentiate from findings of other sequelae of BMT. For example, DIC manifests as thrombocytopenia and an elevated prothrombin time. In the BMT patient these same findings can result from the myelosuppressive preparatory regimen and liver GVHD (Jerman and Fick 1986; Patchell et al. 1985b). It is often difficult to detect with an echocardiogram, and murmurs are rare. In many cases, the vegetations are small and may be impossible to auscultate (Jerman and Fick 1986; Patchell et al. 1985b).

Several as yet unproven etiologies for NBTE have been proposed. First, the conditioning regimen with chemoradiotherapy may damage the cardiac endothelium, causing increased susceptibility for thrombus formation (Patchell et al. 1985b; Wiznitzer et al. 1984). For example, high-dose cyclophosphamide has been documented to cause changes and necrosis in endocardial connective tissue (Slavin and Woodruff 1974). Second, during the infusion of marrow, thrombus formation may occur as a large bolus of donor cells, platelets, and fibrin enter the recipient's circulation (Patchell et al. 1985b). Lastly, GVHD has been associated with cardiac necrosis and other effects (i.e., hypercoagulability) (Slavin and Woodruff 1974) that in combination may predispose BMT patients to develop NBTE .

Cerebrovascular accidents due to NBTE are an important cause of morbidity in BMT recipients. Emboli to the CNS and heart may manifest as seizures and focal neurologic or myocardial dysfunction (Rosen and Armstrong 1973). Anticoagulation might be able to prevent the associated morbidity (Jerman and Fick 1986), however this is currently an unlikely therapy for a BMT patient. Since prevention seems unlikely and antemortem diagnosis is rare, nursing care would not differ from what has already been described.

Graft-Versus-Host Disease and Cardiac Damage

Evidence for GVHD affecting the heart is conflicting. An acute inflammatory reaction involving the endocardium has sometimes been associated with the onset of severe, acute GVHD. Animal studies have shown chronic inflammation involving the valves, and in rare instances, the myocardium and the coronary arteries. Most recent autopsy studies of GVHD have shown that myocardial abnormalities were present in about half of the animals, but consisted only of interstitial edema and sparse lymphocyte infiltration (Sale and Schulman 1984). The relationship between GVHD and cardiac problems in man remains controversial. Concentric intimal sclerosis of the major coronary arteries has been seen in some BMT patients with chronic GVHD. These changes are most likely due to the same processes that cause scleroderma in patients with chronic GVHD. It is unclear whether the cause of these changes is a viral infection or the late, toxic effects of the pretransplant conditioning regimen. However, there is anecdotal evidence that chronic GVHD may be associated with coronary atherosclerosis. Whether this is due to the GVHD itself, or to the hyperlipidemia caused by high-dose corticosteroid therapy is unclear (Chan et al. 1989). More

recently cyclosporine has also been found to be associated with elevated cholesterol levels in allogeneic transplant patients (Luke 1990).

Nursing Diagnosis, Planning, and Intervention for the BMT Patient with Cardiac Complications

Keen assessment and identification of BMT candidates who may be at risk for the development of cardiac complications should be included in the patient's nursing history prior to initiating the patient's pretransplant conditioning regimen. Table 8.4 listed factors that may put the patient at risk for the development of cardiac complications. It is essential for the transplant team to know what chemotherapy and radiation therapy the patient has received in the past. Pretransplant baseline studies should include a cardiac ejection fraction and a 12-lead ECG. Auscultation of heart and lung sounds should be performed upon patient admission, and at least every eight hours throughout the patient's transplant hospitalization.

Twelve-lead electrocardiograms are suggested prior to each dose of Cy and anthracyclines if these drugs are a part of the patient's pretransplant conditioning regimen. Some centers monitor the patient via bedside cardiac monitors throughout the patient's course of Cy and for 24 hours following its completion. A follow-up 12-lead ECG should also be done seven days after Cy administration (Hutchison and King 1983). If ECG changes occur, the physician should be notified at once. Twice daily weights on the days the patient who receives Cy is also a frequent practice.

Nursing assessment for murmurs, friction rubs, and breath sounds is key in the early detection of infective endocarditis. Comfort measures for fever management, appropriate antibiotic administration, and balancing rest with activity are also important. Frequent assessment for signs of cardiac tamponade (including tachycardia, distended neck veins, and a positive pulsus paradoxus) should also be included in the BMT nurses' initial and ongoing assessments. Detection of these symptoms should result in prompt medical intervention. The nurse should prepare for the patient to undergo pericardiocentesis if cardiac tamponade occurs.

For the patient with cardiac-induced pulmonary edema and/or congestive heart failure, the primary nursing focus should be on maintaining oxygenation and resolution or reduction of edema. These patients may require endotracheal intubation and the use of CPAP/PEEP, or may simply need a small amount of oxygen delivered by nasal cannula. It is important to reduce stressors to the patient's heart; rest periods between procedures can be helpful. Strict intake and output, close monitoring of the patient's electrolytes, administering diuretics as ordered, and weighing the patient at least daily are essential in managing the patient's fluid balance. Transplant patients have a tendency to become fluid overloaded despite cardiac problems, due to the excessive amounts of blood products and medications they receive. It is important to administer the patient's medications in as small a fluid volume as possible.

For the patients in congestive heart failure, frequent skin care and evaluation is needed, especially if the patient has excessive peripheral edema. If the patient is on digitalis therapy, the nurse should monitor the patient's drug levels, and watch for signs of digitalis toxicity. These symptoms include, nausea, anorexia, headache, bigeminy and ectopic beats, confusion, and a pulse deficit. These symptoms should be reported as soon as possible to the physician. A sample nursing care plan for the BMT patient with fluid volume excess appears later in the text.

It is important to note that since cardiac complications are infrequently seen in the BMT patient population, cardiology consultants can be extremely helpful in the overall management of these patients. Currently, cardiac toxicity remains a limiting factor in escalating therapies for BMT. It has therefore been suggested that transplantation should be done as early as possible so that pretransplant patients will not have received excessive doses of cardiotoxic drugs that will further increase their risk of developing serious cardiac complications.

References

Atkinson, J.B. et al. 1984. Cardiac fungal infections: Review of autopsy findings in 60 patients. *Human Pathology* 15: 935–942.

Bearman, S.I. et al. 1988. Regimen-related toxicity in patients undergoing bone marrow transplantation. *J. Clin. Oncol.* 6 (10): 1562-1568.

Bortin, M.M. et al. 1982. Factors associated with interstitial pneumonitis after bone marrow transplantation. *Lancet 1*: 437.

Bortin, M.M. 1983. Pathogenesis of interstitial pneumonitis following allogeneic bone marrow transplantation for acute leukemia. In Gale, R.P. (ed.). *Recent Advances in Bone Marrow Transplantation*. New York: Alan R. Liss, pp. 445–460.

Buja, L.M. et al. 1976. Cardiac pathologic findings in patients treated with bone marrow transplantation. *Human Pathology* 7: 15–45.

Chan, K.W. et al. 1989. Coronary artery disease following bone marrow transplantation. *B.M.T.* 4: 327–330.

Chan, K.W. et al. 1990. Pulmonary complications following bone marrow transplantation. *Clincis in Chest Medicine* 11 (2): 323–332.

Cardozo, B.L. 1985. Interstitial pneumonitis following bone marrow transplantation: Pathogenesis and therapeutic considerations. *European Journal of Cancer and Clinical Oncology* 21: 43.

Cazin, B. et al. 1986. Cardiac complications after bone marrow transplantation. *Cancer* 57: 2061–2069.

Davis, D.G., and Patchell, R.A. 1988. Neurologic complications of bone marrow transplantation. *Neurologic Clinics* 6 (2): 377–383.

Ellis, J.R., and Nowlis, E.A. 1989. *Supporting Oxygenation. Nursing: A Human Needs Approach*. Houghton Mifflin Company: 788–797.

Fort, J.A., and Graham-Pole, J. 1989. Pulmonary complication of bone marrow transplantation. In Johnson, F.L., and Pochedlym, C. (eds.). *Bone Marrow Transplantation in Children*. New York: Raven Press, Ltd., p. 397.

Ginsberg, S.J., and Comis R.L. 1982. The pulmonary toxicity of antineoplastic agents. *Seminars in Oncology 9*: 35–51.

Glorieux, P. et al. 1986. Metastatic interstitial pneumonitis after autologous bone marrow transplantation: A consequence of reinjection of malignant cells. *Cancer 58* (9): 2136–2139.

Goldberg, M.A. et al. 1986. Cyclophosphamide cardiotoxicity: An analysis of dosing as a risk factor. *Blood 68* (5): 1114–1118.

Gross, S.J. et al. 1982. The pulmonary toxicity of antineoplastic agents. *Seminars in Oncology 9* (1): 34–51.

Gross, N.J. 1977. Pulmonary effects of radiation therapy. *Ann. Intern. Med. 86*: 81–92.

Guzetta, C.E. 1984. The person with infective endocarditis. In Guzetta, C., and Dorsey, B.M. (eds.). *Cardiovascular Nursing: Body Mind Tapestry*. St. Louis: Mosby, pp. 661–691.

Hamilton, P.J. et al. 1986. Bone marrow transplantation and the lung. *Thorax 41* (7): 497–502.

Hutchison, M., and King, A. 1983. A nursing perspective on bone marrow transplantation. *Nurs. Clin. North Am. 18* (3): 511–520.

Jerman, M.R., and Fick, R.B. (1986). Nonbacterial thrombotic endocarditis associated with bone marrow transplantation. *Chest 90*: 919–922.

Krowka, M.J. 1985. Pulmonary complications of bone marrow transplantation. *Chest 87* (2): 237–46.

Kupari, M. et al. 1990. Cardiac involvement in bone marrow transplantation: electrocardiographic changes arrythmias, heart failure and autopsy findings. *B.M.T. 5*: 91–98.

Laszewski, M. et al. 1988. Aspergillus coronary embolization causing acute myocardial infarction. *B.M.T. 3*: 229–233.

Levine, A.S. 1982. *Cancer in the Young*. New York: Masson Publishing USA, Inc.: 735–737.

Link, H. et al. 1986. Lung function changes after allogeneic bone marrow transplantation. *Thorax 41* (7): 508–512.

Luke, D.R. 1990. Longitudinal study of cyclosporine and lipids in patients undergoing bone marrow transplantation. *J. Clin. Pharmacol. 30*: 163–169.

Lum, L.G. 1987. The kinetics of immune reconstitution after human marrow transplantation. *Blood 69* (2): 369.

Martino, P. et al. 1990. Catheter-related right-sided endocarditis in bone marrow transplant recipients. *Reviews of Infectious Diseases 12* (2): 250–257.

Meyers, J.D. et al. 1983. Biology of interstitial pneumonia after marrow transplantation. In Gale, R.P. (ed.). *Recent Advances in Bone Marrow Transplantation*. New York: Alan R. Liss, Inc., pp. 406–421.

Meyers, J.D. et al. 1982. Nonbacterial pneumonia after allogeneic marrow transplantation: A review of ten years' experience. *Review of Infectious Diseases 4*: 119.

Minow, R.A. et al. 1977. Adriamycin cardiomyopathy: Risk factors. *Cancer 39*: 1397–1402.

Olney, B.A. et al. 1979. The consequences of the inconsequential: Marantic (nonbacterial thrombotic) endocarditis. *Am. Heart J. 98*: 513–522.

Ostrow, D. et al. 1985. Bronchiolitis obliterans complication after bone marrow transplantation. *Chest 87* (6): 828–830.

Patchell, R.A. et al. 1985a. Neurologic complications of bone marrow transplantation. *Neurology 35*: 300–306.

Patchell, R.A. et al. 1985b. Nonbacterial thrombotic endocarditis in bone marrow transplant patients. *Cancer 55*: 631–635.

Paulin, T. et al. 1987. Variables predicting bacterial and fungal infections after allogeneic marrow engraftment. *Transplantation 48* (8): 393–398.

Pecego, R. et al. 1986. Interstitial pneumontis following autologous bone marrow transplantation. *Transplantation 42* (5): 515–517.

Rosen, P., and Armstrong, D. 1973. Nonbacterial thrombotic endocarditis in patients with malignant neoplastic diseases. *Am. J. Med. 54*: 23–29.

Rubin, R. 1988. Pneumonia in the immunocompromised host. In Fishman, A.P. (ed.). *Pulmonary Diseases and Disorders*. New York: MacGraw Hill Co., pp. 1745–1760.

Sale, G.E., and Shulman, H.M. 1984. In Sale G.E and Shulman, H.M. (eds.). *The Pathology of Bone Marrow Transplantation*. Chicago: Masson Publishing USA, Inc., pp. 193–194.

Slavin, R.E., and Woodruff, J.M. 1974. The pathology of bone marrow transplantation. *Pathol. Annu. 9*: 291–344.

Spragg, R.G. 1980. Adult Respiratory Distress Syndrome. In Bordow, R.A., Stool, E.W., and Moser, K.M. (eds.). *Manual of Clinical Problems in Pulmonary Medicine*, Boston: Little, Brown and Company, pp. 252–253.

Weiner, R.S. et al. 1986. Interstitial pneumonitis after bone marrow transplantation: assessment of risk factors. *Ann. Intern. Med. 104*: 168–175.

Weiss, B.R. et al. 1980. Cytotoxic drug-induced pulmonary disease: update 1980. *Am. J. Med. 68*: 259–266.

Winston, D.J. et al. 1983. Treatment and prevention of interstitial pneumonia associated with bone marrow transplantation. In Gale, R.P. (ed.). *Recent Advances in Bone Marrow Transplantation*. New York: Alan R. Liss, Inc., pp. 425–444.

Wiznitzer, M. et al. 1984. Neurologic complications of bone marrow transplantation in childhood. *Ann. Neurol. 16*: 569–76.

von Herbay, A. et al. 1988. Cardiac damage in autologous bone marrow transplant patients: An autopsy study. *Klinische Wochenschrift 66*: 1175–1181.

Chapter 9

Gastrointestinal Complications of Bone Marrow Transplantation

Karen S. Vanacek

Introduction

A wide spectrum of gastrointestinal (GI) complications are frequently seen in all types of bone marrow transplant (BMT) patients. Although these complications tend to present some of the earliest challenges for transplant nurses, certain GI disorders may continue to plague patients as late problems, requiring specialized nursing management as well.

GI complications occur on a continuum from mild, temporary disturbances to protracted, life-threatening situations. In general, all upper and lower GI problems are attributable to one, several, or all of the following causes (Wolford and McDonald 1988), including:

- effects of the high-dose chemotherapy and/or radiotherapy (conditioning regimen) delivered pretransplantation
- infection involving any part of the GI tract or liver
- acute or chronic graft-versus-host disease (GVHD) (seen in allogeneic transplant patients)

- side effects of other medications or treatments used during the transplant treatment process.

The impact of these contributing factors, either alone or in combination, varies greatly among BMT patients. For many, however, the GI sequelae of bone marrow transplantation are among the most uncomfortable and distressing aspects of the entire treatment. Risk of sepsis from widespread mucosal disruption, risk of end organ damage from conditioning therapies or GVHD, and the resultant profound nutritional deficits all have an impact on the patient's well-being and overall treatment results. Transplant nurses play a vital role in the early detection, monitoring, and delivery of available treatments and comfort measures aimed at managing these problems during the entire treatment course.

Impact of Conditioning Regimens

High-dose conditioning regimens generally cause GI problems that are more severe in nature and tend to persist longer than those arising from standard dose regimens. The combined effects of intensive chemotherapy and TBI cause more GI mucosal damage than either one of these components alone (McDonald et al. 1986; Ford and Ballard 1988). The most common toxic effects from conditioning regimens include mucositis, nausea and vomiting, diarrhea, dysphagia, xerostomia, taste changes, abdominal pain, GI bleeding, and anorexia. However, only preliminary information is available to clearly qualify and quantify the nature of several of these uncomfortable problems (Chapko et al. 1989). The intensity of GI side effects is contingent on the toxic properties of the treatment regimen used and the patient's individual response. Prior treatment with cytotoxic agents may also have an impact on the outcome of GI effects seen.

The nursing complexities in caring for BMT patients experiencing GI problems evolving from multiple etiologies are discussed below. A "top to bottom" approach to the alimentary canal is used for presentation of information. Specific nutritional implications are integrated into each problem discussion. Global nutritional issues in bone marrow transplantation are discussed in a separate section at the end of the chapter.

Upper Gastrointestinal Complications

Severe oral complications occur in approximately 75% of allogeneic transplant patients and in a smaller percentage of autologous and syngeneic patients (Carl and Higby 1985). Esophageal complications can also be problematic. The etiology of these complications is multifactoral, involving not only the direct stomatoxic effects of the conditioning regimen used, but also the indirect effects of myelosuppression and GVHD.

Direct Stomatotoxicity: Conditioning Regimens

Oropharyngeal mucositis is seen with many conditioning regimens, particulary those including TBI (Dreizen et al. 1979; Seto et al. 1985; Barrett

1986; Kolbinson et al. 1988). Mucositis generally manifests itself when 1000–2000cGy are delivered to the head and neck area (Carl 1983).

Oral mucositis generally begins as swelling, soreness, and whitening of the mucosa (pseudomembrane formation). In approximately three days, cheilitis, glossitis, and stomatitis may ensue, with continued reddening of the mucosa, pain, and sloughing of the pseudomembranes (Dreizen et al. 1979). Ulcerations occur most frequently on the buccal/labial mucosa and tongue (Kolbinson et al. 1988), but may appear anywhere from the lips to the esophagus. Mucositis tends to worsen within the first two weeks after therapy, but generally resolves within three weeks (Champlin and Gale 1984). Clinically, patients may encounter difficulty eating and swallowing, and oral pain can be severe.

One group of researchers recently studied the time course and variation in transplant related mucositis and pain in more detail (Chapko et al. 1989). Descriptive findings demonstrated that pain and mucositis commenced just prior to transplant but did not peak until the second week post-transplant. Post-transplant pain was also found to be significantly related to the use of a higher dose fraction of TBI (1575cGy versus 1200cGy). Finally, although gender and age were not related to the magnitude of mucositis in this study, its severity was higher in patients with hematologic malignancy as compared to aplastic anemia, thus reflecting the use of TBI in the first study group. A similar time course for mucositis was also reported by others (Eilers et al. 1988).

Several high-dose chemotherapeutic agents, in particular, are also thought to be associated with more severe mucositis. Cyclophosphamide and cytosine arabinoside are known to precipitate mucositis in approximately 50% of patients (Carl and Higby 1985). Other drugs that are known mucositis culprits are etoposide, melphalan, and thiotepa (Kaye 1982; Mascret et al. 1985; Herzig et al. 1987; Williams et al. 1987; Deeg et al. 1988). Methotrexate, used as GVHD prophylaxis post-transplant, can produce or accentuate already existing mucosal breakdown (Barrett 1986; Dahllof et al. 1988).

Infections of the Oral Cavity/ Esophagus

BMT recipients are susceptible to a wide variety of upper gastrointestinal infections, which can affect the oral cavity and esophagus. Bacterial, viral, or fungal pathogenic organisms may cause or further aggravate mucositis. Such infections may appear early in the transplant process or after discharge during the long period of immune reconstitution.

Bacterial Infections

Bacterial pathogens in the oral cavity can cause not only localized infections, but can also enter the systemic circulation, resulting in septicemia. As most BMT recipients will experience major disruptions in mucosal lines of defense due to TBI and/or chemotherapy, the normal host flora and pathogens of the oral cavity or of the esophagus are often suspected when systemic infection occurs. Patients with preexisting peridontal disease or poor dentition can become seriously infected after receiving profoundly myelosuppressive therapy (Dahllof et al. 1988).

Although many infections in cancer patients are caused by their own endogenous flora, 47% of the infections are nosocomial (Robichaud and Hubbard 1987). It is known that hospitalized patients frequently experience a shift in their oropharyngeal organisms to predominantly Gram-negative organisms. A variety of bacterial infections can occur in BMT recipients during the myelosuppressive period from organisms such as Gram-negative bacilli, Gram-positive staphylococci and streptococci. While Gram-negative organisms are still seen in transplant patients (Champlin and Gale 1984) increasing attention is being given to the problems of staphylococcal (Pizzo et al. 1984), and streptococcal organisms (Cohen et al. 1983; Bostrom and Weisdorf 1984; Ferretti et al. 1988) in BMT and other myelosuppressed patients. Staphylococcal infections (primarily coagulase-negative staphylococci), in particular are more prominent pathogens now in BMT patients due to increased use of indwelling right atrial catheters, gut colonization with these organisms, and antibiotic use (Peterson et al. 1987).

Gram-negative bacterial infections in the mouth usually present as creamy, raised, shiny, nonpurulent erosions on an erythematous foundation; Gram-positive staphylococcal and streptococcal infections appear as dry, raised, wartlike, yellowish-brown round plaques (Brager and Yasko 1984).

Bacterial esophagitis can occur in the early post-transplant period as a mixed infection, along with viral and fungal pathogens (Walsh, et al. 1986; McDonald et. al. 1985). As oropharyngeal microbes normally reside on the mucosal surface of the esophagus, definitive diagnosis is obtained by a biopsy specimen that has large numbers of bacteria mixed with necrotic epithelial cells (McDonald et al. 1985).

Viral Infections

Oral herpes simplex virus (HSV) infections frequently occur in allogeneic BMT patients. The average time to initial onset and diagnosis is 8–12 days (Kolbinson et al. 1988; Strohl 1989). Oral HSV also occurs often in autologous BMT patients, although a comparative incidence of the infection rate in both groups of patients has not been reported (Montgomery et al. 1986).

HSV infections can occur because of primary exposure to the virus or more often from reactivation of the latent virus. Common sites of reactivation in BMT patients include oral and esophageal mucosa. Estimated reactivation rates are reported to be 80% or higher (Meyers et al. 1980; Saral et al. 1983; Montgomery et al. 1986). A BMT patient with a high HSV titer (1:8 or greater) is an example of a patient at "high risk" for reactivation (Poland 1989).

Oral HSV lesions can occur anywhere in the mouth or on the lips. They can be classically discrete and vesicular in appearance, present with pain, or assume a stomatitis or "ulcerlike" appearance. In one study of early oral changes following BMT (Kolbinson et al. 1988), it was noted that patients with positive HSV oral cultures had a predisposition for more severe ulcerative changes, a longer duration of these changes, and more severe oral pain.

Because oral HSV lesions can take on an appearance similar to other oral infections and/or direct conditioning regimen toxicity, definitive diagnosis is obtained by viral culture. Use of prophylactic antiviral therapy during BMT has lessened the incidence and severity of lesions. However, without appropriate therapy, oral HSV lesions can progress rapidly, becoming a major source of morbidity (Saral 1989). HSV can disseminate to the lungs, liver, or central nervous system in an immunocompromised patient. Other viral infections that have been reported to affect the oropharyngeal mucosa less frequently include cytomegalovirus (CMV) and varicella zoster virus (VZV) (Kolbinson et al. 1988).

Viral esophagitis is another serious complication that can occur in BMT patients. In allogeneic patients, it can be seen between days 30 and 75 (Wolford and McDonald 1988). HSV and CMV are the major pathogens implicated in viral esophagitis (McDonald et al. 1985). Nausea and vomiting are prominent symptoms (Spencer et al. 1986; Apperly and Goldman 1988), and fever and dysphagia can also occur. Diagnosis is made by esophageal biopsy and culture. Definitive diagnosis for CMV esophagitis is particularly important because dissemination may occur if the patient is receiving immunosuppressants for GVHD (McDonald et al. 1986). Unlike CMV infections in allogeneic transplant patients, life-threatening CMV disease is uncommon in autologous transplant patients (Wingard et al. 1988). Stricture formation may be a late complication of severe HSV esophagitis (Wolford and McDonald 1988).

Fungal Infections

Oral fungal infections are extremely common in both autologous and allogeneic transplant patients. *Candida albicans* is most frequently impli-

cated, however, other species such as *Candida tropicalis* can also be seen (Dreizen et al. 1979). *Candida* is a ubiquitous organism and can live harmlessly in the normal host (Robichaud and Hubbard 1987). However, positive cultures in myelosuppressed BMT patients are meaningful and require treatment. Other types of GI fungal infections seen in severely immunocompromised BMT patients include *Aspergillus* and *Mucopmycosis*.

An additional risk for fungal infection in the BMT patient is the prolonged use of broad-spectrum antibiotic therapy and widespread mucosal disruption from conditioning regimen toxicities or GVHD. The clinical manifestation of oral candidiasis includes yellowish or whitish curdlike patches on the tongue and buccal mucosa, which, when scraped, show erythematous ulcerated mucosa underneath (Brager and Yasko 1984). Other typical complaints of patients with oral candidiasis include burning, pain, or dysguesia.

Fungal esophagitis can occur in any BMT patient although some researchers report a decreasing incidence due to prophylactic and empiric antifungal therapies (McDonald et al. 1986; Wolford and McDonald 1988). In allogeneic patients, fungal esophagitis can occur either early, during granulocytopenia, or late (after discharge), during the time of immune recovery (Meyers 1986). A variety of *Candida* and *Aspergillus* species have been isolated (Wolford and McDonald 1988).

Clinical manifestations of fungal esophagitis include dysphagia, presence or absence of oral candidiasis, heartburn, epigastric pain, GI bleeding, or fever (McDonald et al. 1985; McDonald et al. 1986). Diagnosis is made by endoscopic brushings, biopsies, and cultures.

Treatment of Direct Stomatotoxicity and Oral/Esophageal Infection

As mucositis is frequently compounded by the presence of oral and/or esophageal infections in BMT patients, major goals of treatment include appropriate antimicrobial therapy, meticulous oral hygiene, and pain control.

Bacterial infections in granulocytopenic BMT patients are treated with broad-spectrum intravenous antibiotics, typically a penicillin, aminoglycoside, and vancomycin. Even in the absence of a positive culture, antibiotic coverage is always rapidly initiated in a neutropenic BMT patient with the first fever spike. Patients remain on antibiotic therapy throughout the entire neutropenic period. Antibiotics may be changed or adjusted pending antibiotic levels or organism sensitivity/resistance or toxicity of the particular regimen in use.

The treatment of oral and esophogeal HSV in BMT patients may be either prophylactic in nature or for documented HSV infections. Because the HSV reactivation rate is high in BMT patients, some researchers advocate treating all seropositive BMT patients with prophylactic intravenous acyclovir, starting three days prior to transplant and continuing until the patient is discharged (Saral 1989). When acyclovir prophylaxis is not used, the drug is either initiated empirically for highly suspicious lesions or upon determination of a positive culture. The dose of intravenous acyclovir is typically 5mg/kg every eight hours. Uncommonly, HSV resistance to acyclovir has been reported in immunocompromised patients (Wong and Hirsch 1984).

Ganciclovir and foscarnet are currently under investigation for the treatment of CMV infections (Erice et al. 1987; Ringden et al. 1987; Laskin et al. 1987; Reed et al. 1988). Other studies have been aimed at prevention of CMV infections in the BMT patient through therapeutic strategies such as the use of blood products from seronegative donors for seronegative recipients (Bowden et al. 1986), prophylaxis with intravenous CMV hyperimmune globulin (Condie and O'Reilly 1984), and CMV hyperimmune globulin plus oral acyclovir (Einsele et al. 1988).

Oral antifungal prophylaxis is frequently employed in BMT patients. Antifungal troches (i.e., clotrimazole 10mg p.o. 5x/day) slowly dissolved in the mouth or antifungal suspensions (i.e., nystatin 30ml, 100,000u/ml, swish and swallow 3x/day) are used. More recent research has focused on oral fluconazole, a promising new agent used for antifungal prophylaxis in autologous and allogeneic transplant patients (Millikin et al. 1989). For patients unable to comply with routine use of these agents, creative antifungal popsicle formulations have been devised (Brager and Yasko 1984). Intravenous amphotericin B (0.6–1.0mg/kg/day for three to six weeks) (McDonald et al. 1986) is the standard treatment of invasive fungal esophagitis.

Oral and dental care is an extremely important component of supportive care in BMT patients due to their high susceptibility to infection from these sources during the period of profound myelosuppression (Carl and Higby 1985). Ideally, the patient should undergo a thorough dental evaluation and cleaning pretreatment. Dental problems that should be addressed and corrected (Dahllof et al. 1988; NIH Consensus Development Conference Statement 1989) include:

- poor oral hygiene
- peridontal abscesses (soft-tissue abscesses)
- periapical pathology (infrabony cysts or abscesses)
- dental caries
- third molar pathology (impacted wisdom teeth)
- oral infections
- poorly fitting dental prostheses
- orthodontic appliances (removal necessary)

Ideally, any required dental extractions should be performed in ample time prior to therapy.

Many suggestions for oral hygiene and oral pain palliation for cancer patients exist in the dental and nursing literature (Dreizen et al. 1979; Beck 1979; Daeffler 1980; Owen et al. 1981; Carl 1983). Yet there are few randomized, controlled studies that indicate the superiority of one oral care strategy over another. Currently, no drug or oral care strategy exists that completely prevents mucositis in BMT patients. Of recent note are two blind, randomized studies in BMT patients that investigated the impact on oral infection and mucositis of a broad-spectrum antimicrobial mouth rinse, chlorhexidine gluconate. One study of chlorhexidine use resulted in significant reductions in the incidence and severity of oral mucositis and significant reduction in total oral *Streptococci* and oral *Candida* (Ferretti et al. 1988). The other study, however, showed no significant advantage from chlorhexidine in the reduction of mucositis or oral infection, although there was a trend noted towards lessened oral candidiasis in the chlorhexidine users (Weisdorf et al. 1989). In the latter study's discussion of the data (Weisdorf et al. 1989), it was suggested that chlorhexidine may be more beneficial for oral mucosa less injured from chemotherapy. Although dosing and rinsing schedules were the same for both studies, the overall intensity of mucositis seen in the Weisdorf (1989) study was greater. Additional research is needed to clarify further the role of chlorhexidine in BMT patients.

Oral care regimens for BMT patients include vigorous, frequent oral rinsing to decrease the pathogen load in the oral cavity. Saline rinses every two to three hours can be instituted. Routine soft toothbrushing with toothpaste and flossing are recommended, although their practice during profound granulocytopenia and thrombocytopenia are discouraged. Toothettes® or gauze-covered tongue blades can be used at such times. Dilute peroxide and saline rinses (i.e., 1:4 concentration) or weak bicarbonate solution (1 tsp. in 8oz. H₂O) followed by saline can be done if oral crusting/debris is present (Goodman and Stoner 1985). Dentures should be removed before oral hygiene. Thorough oral evaluation, using a bright light, should be performed on each shift and suspicious lesions should be cultured. Lip lubricant should be applied frequently. Oral antifungal agents should be used after oral cleaning procedures to maximize their effectiveness. Patients should also be reminded to rinse after emetic episodes as mucositis can be aggravated by acidic gastric secretions.

When moderate to severe mucositis is present, oral suction should be readily available as patients may not be able to swallow secretions or to expectorate after oral rinsing. Dentures or other oral prostheses should be left out entirely. Systemic and topical analgesics most likely will be required to promote patient comfort and compliance with oral hygiene. Topical anesthetics available to palliate minor discomfort from mild mucositis (i.e., Dyclone® 0.5% swish and expectorate; Xylocaine® 2% viscous swish and expectorate; Cetacaine® spray—one second spray) are often ineffective when mucositis is severe (Carl and Higby 1985). Oral analgesics may not be tolerated during periods of GI distress. Continuous infusions, intermittent boluses, and patient-controlled devices to deliver intravenous morphine are often necessary and can be carefully titrated to match the patient's need for pain control.

Dietary modifications for mild mucositis include providing the patient with a soft, bland diet that contains high protein/calorie nutrients and that avoids overly dry, hot, or acidic foods (i.e., toast, crackers, citrus juices). For severe mucositis, parenteral nutrition is usually required as the patient may not even be able to tolerate clear liquids.

Salivary Gland Changes

In addition to mucositis, bilateral parotitis (inflammation of the parotid glands) and partial xerostomia (dry mouth) are frequently reported in patients after TBI (Thomas et al. 1975; Dreizen et al. 1979; Carl and Higby 1985). The parotitis from TBI is characterized by tender transient "mumpslike" swelling that resolves spontaneously in 24–48 hours. One study on early oral changes following BMT reported that salivary viscosity, xerostomia, and patients' subjective complaints of dryness changed most significantly in the first two weeks after transplant (Kolbinson et al. 1988). TBI was cited as the probable major etiologic factor, and interestingly, xerostomia persisted for the entire 5-week study period.

Salivary glands are highly sensitive to radiation exposure and the acinar cells of the parotid gland are affected more than the mucinous acinar cells in other areas of the mouth (Carl 1983). Saliva, in turn, becomes scant, tenacious, and ropy. Its normal functions of cleansing the oral cavity and assisting food in its passage down the alimentary canal are greatly compromised. In addition, the pH of remaining saliva becomes more acidic, thus altering normal patterns of microbial flora and further aggravating mucositis (Carl 1983). The incidence of oral and gingival infections in patients experiencing xerostomia increases significantly.

Salivary gland dysfunction is also attributable to causes other than TBI in transplant patients. Autologous transplant recipients undergoing combined alkylating agent therapy can experience transient xerostomia, which gradually improves over time. Methotrexate, used to combat GVHD, was reported in one study as a possible contributor to salivary gland damage in allogeneic recipients (Barrett 1986). Other variables causing xerostomia include chronic GVHD (Barrett and Bilous 1984), chemotherapy (Kolbinson et al. 1988), medications (such as certain antiemetics and diuretics), and mouth breathing.

Treatment of Salivary Gland Problems and Nursing Implications

The goals of xerostomia treatment in transplant recipients include: (1) stimulation of any existing salivary flow, (2) lubrication and hydration of oral tissues, (3) prevention of oral infections and tooth decay, (4) comfort, and (5) management or prevention of nutritional deficits related to this problem.

Rigorous oral hygiene, both during and after the transplant hospitalization, is necessary to decrease the incidence of oral pathogens. Regular dental care post-transplant including oral evaluation and fluoride treatments are important in the prevention and treatment of xerostomia-related problems such as dental caries and peridontal disease (Schubert et al. 1983). Routine soft brushing with toothpaste and flossing by the patient are recommended, although their practice during profound granulocytopenia and thrombocyto-

penia is discouraged. Sterile water or saline rinsing should be performed at frequent intervals. Dentures or other prostheses should be removed often to assure thorough oral cleaning. Lips can be kept lubricated with any of a variety of emollients such as lip balm, cocoa butter, lanolin, petrolatum, Blistex®, or K-Y® jelly. Patients with xerostomia should have a daily oral inspection for signs of oral infection. Education for home care should also include continuance of oral inspections using a bright light. A variety of artificial saliva products are currently available for patient use if tolerated (Salivart®, Xero-lube®, Ora-lube®, Moistir®). Frequent sips of water or non-acidic juices (i.e., apricot, grape, or apple) are also helpful.

Unnecessary trauma to the oral mucosa can be avoided with several simple dietary modifications. These include avoidance of hot, spicy foods, alcohol, and rough, or excessively dry foods. Patients should also avoid mucosal irritants such as commercial mouthwashes that contain alcohol, toothpicks, and cigarette smoking. Foods that are replete with sauces or gravies or are otherwise high in water content promote the easiest swallowing. Consultation with a dietician for the family member in charge of home food preparation may be helpful before discharge.

Occasionally, sialorrhea (excess salivation) or drooling is seen in transplant patients due to their inability to handle oral secretions, as a result of painful mucositis, or dysphagia (Champlin and Gale 1984). Hand-held oral suction should be made available to the patient along with head-of-bed elevation to prevent aspiration.

Taste Changes

Dysguesia (abnormal taste) and hypoguesia (diminished taste) are frequently reported in cancer patients (DeWys and Walters 1975; Carson and Gormican 1977; Huldij et al. 1986). Factors thought to predispose cancer patients, in general, to taste problems include tumor extent, trace metal abnormalities such as zinc deficiency, mucosal and salivary gland damage from chemotherapy and radiation, and oral infection (Strohl 1983).

Taste alterations are also commonly experienced by BMT patients (Cunningham et al. 1983). Etiologies of taste changes in BMT patients include TBI, chemotherapeutic agents, oral candidiasis, and antibiotics. Although temporary in nature, these changes can significantly contribute to anorexia. Taste changes have been observed to persist in BMT patients for several weeks after transplant (Barale et al. 1982).

Treatment of Taste Changes and Nursing Implications

Management of taste alterations includes identifying the nature of the taste problem and providing dietary modifications to improve the flavor and palatability of the BMT patient's diet. Patients generally report a varied spectrum of taste disturbances, including meat aversion, intolerance of sweets, loss of food flavor, or bitter/metallic taste. Offering samples of different foods is helpful in identifying the most accepted foods. Enhancing flavor through seasonings, sauces, and gravies is also useful, provided that the patient's oral mucosa is not overly irritated. As patients can experience much frustration in finding desirable foods, patience and frequent supportive encouragement are required from caregivers.

Impact of GVHD on the Oral Cavity and Esophagus

The oral manifestations of acute GVHD have not been well documented (Kolbinson et al. 1988). Painful desquamation, mucosal ulceration, erythema, plaques, and lichenoid keratoses have been noted (Barrett and Bilous 1984; Kolbinson et al. 1988). More clinical descriptions of oral changes from chronic GVHD are available (Rodu and Gockerman 1983; Sullivan et al. 1984; Atkinson et al. 1989); it affects the oral mucosa in about 80% of patients with the extensive form of the disease (Corcoran-Buchsel 1986). These authors have described clinical manifestations of oral GVHD including mucosal atrophy, ulceration, salivary gland fibrosis, erythema, and lichen planus-like lesions. The most common sites of involvement include the buccal mucosa and lateral tongue; lichenoid lesions may also appear elsewhere in the oral cavity or on the lips (Corcoran-Buchsel 1986). Lip biopsy is used to diagnose this syndrome (Sale et al. 1981). Analysis of labial saliva IgA concentrations has been used to differentiate between the xerostomia and salivary changes due to GVHD and TBI; saliva IgA concentrations have been found to be depressed in patients with chronic GVHD (Izutsu et al. 1985).

Approximately 10% of patients with extensive chronic GVHD have esophageal involvement characterized by dysphagia, pain, weight loss, and aspiration (McDonald et al. 1981; Wolford and McDonald 1988). Radiographically, webbing, ring formation, and strictures are seen (Deeg and Storb 1986).

Treatment of Oral/Esophageal GVHD and Nursing Implications

Medical treatment for oral chronic GVHD may include the use of such agents as prednisone, azothiaprine, cyclosporine, and Decadron 0.25% mouth rinses (Corcoran-Buchsel 1986; Deeg and Storb 1986; Deeg et al. 1988). The use of thalidomide and ultraviolet radiation (PUVA) for more resistant disease has also been reported (Deeg et al. 1988).

The nursing care of patients experiencing oral chronic GVHD involves monitoring for oral changes and oral infections, and management of oral pain and xerostomia. Many patients are at risk for opportunistic oral infections due to the use of immunosuppressive therapies. Early subtle clues of oral chronic GVHD include patient complaints of dysguesia and oral pain/burning when eating warm foods or toothbrushing (Corcoran-Buchsel 1986). Frequent oral assessment, culturing of suspicious lesions, education of the patient in meticulous oral hygiene, and management of oral pain/xerostomia are necessary. These patients also require routine dental care and flouride rinsing as they are at increased risk for caries and peridontal disease from chronic xerostomia.

The medical management of esophageal chronic GVHD manifestations involves treatment with immunosuppressants, possible esophageal dilations, and antireflux measures (Wolford and McDonald 1988). Nursing care involves education of patients in antireflux positioning (i.e., Fowler's position) and dietary modifications for dysphagia. Small, frequent feedings are suggested, as well as avoiding of foods that are too dry, spicy, hot, or rough in texture. Aspiration precautions should be instituted and suction should also be available when severe dysphagia is present. Alternating intake of liquids and solids may be helpful. Patients should remain upright after meals. In the setting of severe esophageal stricture, invasive nutritional support may be necessary.

Nausea and Vomiting

Management of nausea and vomiting in the BMT patient is not well described. Much work still needs to be done to understand nausea and vomiting patterns of various conditioning regimens, to develop antiemetic protocols used to combat vomiting from highly emetic combination chemotherapy regimens, and to evaluate the use/impact of non-pharmacologic interventions. Aspects of nausea and vomiting and care strategies are outlined below.

Overview of Emetic Physiology

Nausea is an uncomfortable feeling in the stomach that frequently precedes vomiting. It may be continuous or "wave-like" in nature and is typically accompanied by diaphoresis, pallor, and tachycardia. Vomiting, on the other, hand, is a mechanical act of emptying the stomach contents, orchestrated by variations in intra-abdominal pressure and conducted by respiratory and abdominal musculature. Retching refers to forceful, continuous, synchronized muscular efforts occuring before or after vomiting; emesis production may or may not occur. The different components

of the emetic response frequently occur together in varying degrees of intensity. However, they can also occur independently of each other.

Vomiting is modulated by the vomiting center (VC) located in the medulla oblongata of the brain. The VC receives afferent inputs from other areas of the brain and body, including the chemoreceptor trigger zone (CTZ), cerebral cortex and limbic region, vagal and visceral nerves, and the vestibulocellular apparatus (Wickham 1989). The CTZ is located in the floor of the fourth ventricle of the brain. Chemoreceptors in the CTZ sense noxious chemicals or other substances in the blood or CSF which, in turn, send impulses to the VC. A variety of purported neurotransmitters or neuromodulators have been implicated in the emetic response (i.e., dopamine, serotonin, acetylcholine, histamine, enkephalins); these substances and their precise roles in the emetic response are still under investigation (Borison and McCarthy 1983; Craig and Powell 1987).

Chemotherapy is one example of a noxious substance sensed by the CTZ that, in turn, stimulates the VC. Emotions, patient perceptions, and sensations are examples of stimuli arising from the cerebral cortex/limbic system. Motion sickness arises from the vestibulocellular connection to the VC. Irritation or damage to the abdominal viscera and abdominal distention can stimulate vomiting through visceral or vagal nerve pathways. Certain medications such as antibiotics, steroids, and high doses of abdominal irradiation are examples of such gastrointestinal irritants.

In general, nausea and vomiting can occur surrounding the immediate treatment period or can be protracted in nature. Nausea and vomiting can also be anticipatory or conditioned, occuring for some patients in response to certain perceived noxious stimuli in their environment (Duigon 1986).

Etiologies of Nausea and Vomiting in the BMT Patient

Nausea and vomiting in the transplant patient can occur for a variety of reasons, including effects of conditioning regimens, organ damage, acute

GVHD, and adverse side effects of other supportive medications. Overall, nausea and vomiting in the transplant patient can be much worse and more protracted in nature than in patients receiving standard-dose chemotherapy (Schryber et al. 1987; Ford and Ballard 1988). Outcomes of unremitting nausea and vomiting include severe electrolyte disturbances, Mallory-Weiss tears, major nutritional deficits, aspiration (with a resulting pneumonia), psychological problems, and prolonged hospitalization (Lazlo 1983).

In the early allogeneic transplant period (days 0–15), chemoradiation or other supportive medications are the likely source of nausea and vomiting (Wolford and McDonald 1988). Such medications include cyclosporine, methotrexate, trimethoprim-sulfamethoxazole, narcotics, antibiotics (both oral nonabsorbable and parenteral), and hyperalimentation (Cunningham et al. 1983; Klemm 1985; Wolford and McDonald 1988). Chemoradiation may cause varying degrees of nausea and vomiting, but these effects of conditioning generally do not last beyond two weeks (Spencer et al. 1986). High-dose cyclophosphamide had been reported to cause moderate to severe nausea and vomiting (Fetting et al. 1983). High-dose combined alkylating agent regimens used for autologous solid tumor recipients are moderately to severely emetogenic, especially the administration of high-dose carmustine (Owen et al. 1981), and busulfan. In general, the nausea and vomiting from high-dose chemotherapy is worse than that from TBI.

One study investigated the variations in degree and time of nausea in two groups of allogeneic transplant recipients (Chapko et al. 1989). Considerable unrelieved nausea was reported. Variability in nausea was largely attributed to differences in conditioning regimens. Aplastic anemia patients who received higher doses of cyclophosphamide (200mg/kg) experienced more nausea pretreatment than did patients with hematologic malignancies treated with a lower cyclophosphamide dose (120mg/kg) and TBI. Higher dose fractions of TBI (1575cGy versus 1200cGy) were associated with more nausea. Conversely, higher post-transplant nausea was seen in the hematologic malignancy group, partially resulting from frequent opioid administration for severe mucositis. Neither gender nor age was significantly related to magnitude of nausea in this study. Clearly, more research is necessary to determine specific antiemetic programs for specific conditioning regimens.

Etiologies of nausea and vomiting seen later in the allogeneic transplant course include acute GVHD and viral GI infections, with average onsets of day 34 and 54 respectively (Wolford and McDonald 1988). Uncontrollable retching may be seen early in the course of intestinal GVHD, but it generally subsides despite continuation of other severe GI symptomatology (McDonald et al. 1986). Other reported reasons for vomiting in BMT patients include encephalitis, subdural hematomas, septicemia, adrenal insufficiency, cholecystitis, pancreatitis, or liver disease (McDonald et al. 1986; Wolford and McDonald 1988). Etiologies of protracted vomiting in autologous transplant patients are not well described.

Unknown physiologic reasons for vomiting have been reported in BMT patients (Spencer et al. 1986). In many instances, psychological causes are implicated. Just the fact that many transplant candidates have already undergone highly emetogenic chemotherapy programs pretransplant raises the suspicion that a very high incidence of conditioned vomiting exists in this group. Other psychological manifestations such as anxiety, depression, and pain may have significant implications for protracted nausea and vomiting in the BMT population, yet remain largely unexplored.

Treatment of Nausea and Vomiting and Nursing Implications

Appropriate treatment of nausea and vomiting in the BMT patient involves assessment of etiologic factors and the timing of their occurrences. Transplant nurses play a key role in characterizing the nature, duration, and intensity of this problem so that appropriate interventions can be made.

A multiplicity of antiemetics are available for the management of therapy-induced emesis (see Table 9.1). Unfortunately, no one antiemetic exists that is able to completely prevent or ablate nausea and vomiting. As many conditioning regimens have moderate-to-high emetogenic potential, antiemetic therapy should be liberally used in these patients. Combination antiemetic regimens are recommended for the best control of emesis; agents should be combined that have different mechanisms of action, nonoverlapping toxicities, demonstrated efficacy as single agents, and demonstrated ideal administration routes/schedules (Gralla et al. 1987).

Studies are underway to further define superior antiemetic regimens that can be used with

Table 9.1. Antiemetics Used In the Transplant Setting

Drug/Class	Mechanism of Action	Standard Dosage* Range	Duration of Action	Side Effects/ Comments
Antihistamines Diphenhydramine (Benadryl®)	H1 histamine blocker, CNS depression, anticholinergic action	25–50mg IV or PO q 4–6h	3–6 hours	Blurred vision, urinary retention, drowsiness, dry mouth; frequently used to counteract extrapyramidal reactions from other antiemetics
Butyrophenones Droperidol (Inapsine®)	Dopamine antagonist (CTZ)	a. 5–15mg IV × 1 then 2–7.5mg q 2h × 6–8h post-chemotherapy b. 1mg IV q 1h × 6 doses	2–4 hours	Extrapyramidal reactions, sedation, hypotension, tachycardia
Benzodiazepines Lorazepam (Ativan®)	CNS depression, anxiolytic	1–2.5mg/m² IV q 4h 1–4mg PO q 4h	4 hours	Sedation, hypotension, bad dreams, hallucinations, amnesia, perceptual disturbances, urinary incontinence; sedative effects may be longer than antiemetic duration of action
Cannabinoids Dronabinol (Marinol®)	Unknown	5–19mg/m² PO q 4–6h	4–6 hours	Sedation, hallucinations, dysphoria, depression, headache, poor concentration, anxiety, tachycardia, orthostatic hypotension, dry mouth, altered perception of reality
Substituted Benzamides Metoclopramide (Reglan®)	Dopamine antagonist (CTZ), both central and peripheral effects; enhanced gastric emptying	a. 2–3mg/kg IV q 2–3h × 2–5 doses b. 3mg/kg IV × 1 then 1–2mg/kg q 2–3h × 2–4 doses	2–3 hours	Extrapyramidal reactions, sedation, headache, fatigue, restlessness, diarrhea, tachycardia

Table 9.1. *Continued*

Phenothiazines Perphenazine (Trilafon®)	Dopamine antagonist (CTZ), may suppress VC	5mg IV q 4–6 hrs 4mg PO q 4–6 hrs	4–6 hours	Extrapyramidal reactions, dry mouth, dizziness, headache, drowsiness, anxiety, constipation, urinary retention, hypotension, tachycardia, nasal congestion, hepatotoxicity
Prochlorperazine (Compazine®)		5–20mg PO or IV q 4–6 hrs	4 hours	
Promethazine (Phenergan®)		12.5–25mg IV q 4–6 hrs	4 hours	
Thiethylperazine (Torecan®, Norzine®)		10mg PO q 6–8 hrs	4–6 hours	
Chlorpromazine (Thorazine®) Miscellaneous		10–25mg PO q 4–6 hrs	4–6 hours	
Scopolamine	Anticholinergic effect	1 transdermal patch (placed behind ear) q 72h	3 days	Dry mouth, tachycardia, fatigue, dilated pupils

Adapted from Brager and Yasko, 1984; Craig and Powell, 1987; Wickham, 1989; and personal communication with C. Gilbert, RPh, B.S., 1989.

*The doses have been reported in the literature. However, the author does not assume responsibility for dosing schedules. Various combinations, alternate schedules, and doses may be used at different transplant centers.

specific conditioning regimens in BMT patients (Vanacek and Gilbert 1989). Current studies done in the cancer chemotherapy population at large reflect newer antiemetic strategies such as the use of higher doses of prochlorperazine, metoclopramide drips, and serotonin antagonists (Merrifield and Chaffee 1989).

It is important to assess the patient's previous experience with nausea and vomiting associated with cytotoxic treatment, medications used that were helpful, patient history of dystonic reactions or other unpleasant side effects, and any interventions that were found to be useful. It is also important to plan the antiemetic program in conjunction with the anticipated emetogenic potential for treatment.

A quiet, restful environment should be maintained while the patient is undergoing treatment. Achieving of sedation with an antiemetic program

is beneficial, as it helps the patient sleep through periods of nausea (Wickham 1989). Patients should be monitored closely for dystonic reactions if higher doses of medications such as phenothiazines or metoclopramide are used. Other nursing measures that may be helpful include encouraging the patient to refrain from heavy oral intake during therapy and providing simple distraction techniques such as music.

The treatment of nausea and vomiting caused by acute GVHD or viral infections involves treating the underlying disorder. More specific information on therapeutic strategies for these disorders is covered elsewhere in the text.

Nausea and vomiting caused by the various supportive medications used in transplant patients can be partially ameliorated by the use of antiemetics (Cunningham et al. 1983). As many of them are essential to the patient's care and may not be able to be discontinued, the intravenous form of a particular drug may be warranted.

Anticipatory nausea and vomiting (ANV) and protracted vomiting are more difficult to treat in BMT patients. The best treatment of ANV is prevention of its development by appropriate drug management of vomiting from the beginning of chemotherapy (Craig and Powell 1987). There are reports that ANV that has already occurred is more responsive to behavioral interventions such as hypnosis, systematic desensitization, guided imagery, and progressive muscle relaxation than to standard antiemetics (Nesse et al. 1980; Morrow and Morrell 1982; Redd and Andrykowski 1982; Cotanch 1983). The treatment of protracted vomiting remains difficult. Anecdotal antiemetic approaches that have been tried with varying degrees of success include the use of scopolamine patches, or the use of dronabinol or lorazepam on an around-the-clock schedule (personal communication, Gilbert 1989). The results of a recent study showing that aerobic exercise on a regular basis helps decrease nausea (Winningham and MacVicar 1988) may also be an interesting area for further research and clinical application in BMT recipients. Overall, more nursing research needs to be directed at this very difficult problem in the transplant population.

Lower Gastrointestinal Complications

Diarrhea/Enteritis

Diarrhea in the BMT patient can be a result of direct conditioning regimen-induced mucosal damage, acute or chronic GVHD, intestinal infection, side effects of certain transplant-related supportive medications, or an underlying GI problem (i.e., polyps or irritable colon). More than one source of intestinal dysfunction can contribute to any diarrhea seen. Each source of diarrhea is discussed in more detail below.

Direct Intestinal Toxicity From Conditioning Regimens

It has been noted that within ten days of combined cyclophosphamide/TBI delivery, diffuse mucosal changes can occur all along the intestinal tract; degeneration, flattening or necrosis of intestinal crypt cells, and abnormalities of intestinal villous architecture appear (McDonald et al. 1986). Clinical manifestations of this damage are abdominal cramps, pain, anorexia, and watery diarrhea; these symptoms may persist for two to three weeks (Champlin and Gale 1984). Intestinal bleeding also may be seen if the damage is extensive. Concomitant thrombocytopenia further exacerbates this problem. As intestinal mucosal surfaces and villi are denuded, the patient incurs difficulty with malabsorption of drugs and nutrients (Guyotat et al. 1984).

Other high-dose chemotherapeutic drugs used in the transplant setting are also more likely to be associated with intestinal toxicity. These drugs include thiotepa, etoposide, cytosine arabinoside, melphalan, and methotrexate (Mascret et al. 1985; Williams et al. 1987; Herzig et al. 1987; Deeg et al. 1988). High-dose chemotherapy with autologous bone marrow transplantation also has been reported to result in malabsorption and damage to mucosal integrity, sometimes not fully recovering by the time of hospital discharge (Matthey et al. 1989). Non-chemotherapy medications that may further contribute to diarrhea include metoclopramide, oral/parenteral antibiotics, oral magnesium, and antacids (Gauvreau 1985).

Impact of GVHD on the Intestines

For allogeneic transplant patients, acute GVHD is a major source of morbidity and mortality. Although acute GVHD involves organs other than the GI tract (i.e., skin and liver), diarrhea can be one of the first manifestations of the disease. Typically, the diarrhea is profuse, green, watery, and contains mucus strands, protein, and cellular debris (McDonald et al. 1986). Cramping before bowel movements, nausea and vomiting, and anorexia are also symptoms. Diarrhea is usually negative for occult blood in the early stages but soon becomes positive for blood as intestinal mucosal sloughing occurs (Ford and Ballard 1988). Severe GI bleeding may ensue if the patient does not respond to immunosuppressive therapy. Acute GVHD onset is between days 20 and 60, but mismatched marrow recipients may have an even earlier onset after the completion of therapy (Wolford and McDonald 1988).

Diagnosis of intestinal GVHD is made by clinical findings, radiologic studies, abdominal ultrasound, and intestinal biopsy. A clinical staging system for acute GVHD is available that quantifies the severity of the disease by volumes of diarrhea seen (see Tables 9.2 and 9.3). High-volume diarrhea may persist for weeks with this disorder; irreversible damage to the intestines may result.

Chronic GVHD may also have intestinal manifestations, although intestinal involvement with chronic GVHD is much less common than in acute GVHD (Deeg et al. 1984; Atkinson et al. 1989). Intestinal fibrosis has been reported in some patients (Shulman et al. 1980). Signs and symptoms may include malabsorption, persistent steatorrhea, weight loss despite good oral intake, or nausea and vomiting (Nims and Strom 1988).

Intestinal Infections

Diarrhea may be caused by bacterial, fungal, viral, or parasitic infections in BMT patients. In allogeneic transplant patients in particular, these infections may occur concomitantly with GVHD and conditioning regimen damage. Thus, there may be further aggravation of intestinal disruption with significant morbidity and mortality resulting.

The prolonged use of antibiotics predisposes the transplant patient to an overgrowth of Gram-negative bacteria and fungal organisms. These infections are more likely to occur early in the transplant process (Champlin and Gale 1984). Breaks in the intestinal mucosal lines of defense subject the patient to a risk of sepsis. The use of immunosuppressants and the presence of granulocytopenia further complicate the infection risk.

Pseudomembranous enterocolitis from *Clostridium difficile* is an example of a pathogenic gut infection that arises in BMT patients after broad-spectrum antibiotics alter the normal balance of gut flora (Jones et al. 1988). Fever, diarrhea, and pain are presenting symptoms.

Opportunistic viral pathogens, including CMV, HSV, adenovirus, rotavirus, and coxsackievirus have been implicated in infectious gastroenteritis occuring later in the transplant process (Yolken et al. 1982). CMV infections occur most commonly and may resemble GVHD in presenting signs and symptoms (Jones et al. 1988; Wolford and McDonald 1988). Adenovirus is thought to have an endogenous source, with reactivation occuring during immunosuppression (Shields et al. 1985).

Examples of opportunistic intestinal parasitic infections that may affect BMT patients include

Table 9.2. Clinical Stages of Acute Graft-Versus-Host Disease

Stage	Skin	Liver	Gut
+	Maculopapular rash < 25% body surface	Bilirubin 2–3mg/dl	Diarrhea 500–100ml/day
++	Maculopapular rash 25%–50% body surface	Bilirubin 3–6 mg/dl	Diarrhea 1000–1500ml/day
+++	Generalized erythroderma	Bilirubin 6–15mg/dl	Diarrhea > 100ml/day
++++	Desquamation and bullae	Bilirubin >15 mg/dl	Pain or ileus

Source: McDonald, G.B. et al. 1986. Intestinal and hepatic complications of human bone marrow transplantation, Part I. Elsevier Science Publishing Co., Inc., with permission.

Table 9.3. Clinical Grades of Acute Graft-Versus-Host Disease Severity

Grade	Degree of Organ Involvement
1	+ to ++skin rash; no gut involvement; no liver involvement; no decrease in clinical performance
2	+ to +++ skin rash; + gut involvment or + liver involvement (or both); mild decrease in clinical performance
3	++ to +++ skin rash; ++ to +++ gut involvement or ++ to +++ liver involvement (or both); marked decrease in clinical performance
4	Similar to grade 3 but with ++ to ++++ organ involvement and extreme decrease in clinical performance

Source: McDonald, G.B. et al. 1986. Intestinal and hepatic complications of human bone marrow transplantation, Part I. Elsevier Science Publishing Co., Inc., with permission.

Giardia lamblia, Cryptosporidia, or *Strongyloides* (McDonald et al. 1986; Nims and Strom 1988). These infections may be quiescently present in the patient pretransplant and activate to become more problematic and symptom-producing with the transplant and immunosuppression (McDonald et al. 1986).

Diagnosis of intestinal infections in BMT patients is generally made by stool culture, stool examination (i.e., for ova and parasites), or endoscopic exam and biopsy.

Treatment of Diarrhea/Enteritis and Nursing Implications

Treatment of diarrhea in the BMT patient is directed at (1) identifying and treating the underlying cause, (2) controlling any fluid/electrolyte and acid/base imbalances that may result, (3) providing symptomatic relief for the patient, and (4) protecting the skin in the rectal area from severe excoriation and breakdown.

The patient experiencing diarrhea due to conditioning regimen toxicity may obtain partial relief from symptoms with antidiarrheal agents such as diphenoxylate hydrochloride with atropine sulfate (Lomotil®) or other opioid drugs. However, these medications should be used with caution and only after appropriate stool cultures have been analyzed to rule out intestinal infections. In the setting of severe intestinal dysfunc-

tion/bleeding, they may be contraindicated altogether. Auscultation of bowel sounds and constant observation for signs of ileus should be performed.

Fluid and electrolyte status should be monitored closely and replaced as necessary. Strict intake and output, daily weights, and cardiovascular parameters generally provide nurses with data for assessing volume status. The rectal area should be cleaned and dried thoroughly after each diarrheal episode; hair dryers on a low cool setting are useful for rapid drying. The entire perineal and perirectal area should be inspected carefully during each shift. Bed-bound, incontinent patients need to be checked at frequent intervals. Moisture barrier creams or ointments should be used preventatively (i.e., Desitin®, Carrington® Moisture Barrier Cream, equal parts admixture of petrolatum:zinc oxide:cornstarch) and should be applied after rectal cleansings. Frequent warm water sitz baths or tub soaks are soothing and help assure that the rectal area is kept as clean as possible. Washcloths should be used cautiously to clean the rectal area as they may cause increased irritation with frequent use; soft gauze, mild aloe cleansing sprays, or a soapy gloved hand can be used instead. Powders applied to the rectal area may "cake" and further macerate the already compromised skin. Dietary modifications for diarrhea in this situation include a bland, low residue diet with avoidance of lactose-containing products, spices, caffeinated beverages, and fruit juices. Sodas, Gatorade®, bouillon, pudding, creamed soups, pasta, cooked white potatoes, and white breads are better tolerated.

Medical treatment of acute GVHD is covered in more detail in Chapter 7. Preventative therapy generally involves short-course methotrexate combined with cyclosporine, although other current research strategies include the use of antithymocyte globulin, monoclonal antibodies, methylprednisolone, and thalidomide (Deeg and Storb 1986; Thomas 1988).

Patients experiencing acute GVHD must be closely monitored by transplant nurses. Since nausea and vomiting may accompany voluminous diarrhea, severe volume deficits and electrolyte disturbances can be seen. Antidiarrheal agents are generally not helpful in this setting (Parker and Cohen 1983). Superinfection with enteric pathogens may occur. Thus, stool cultures are obtained and sent to the laboratory. In the setting of GI bleeding, platelet counts, hematocrits, and coagulation studies should be monitored closely. Dietary modifications include keeping the patient NPO except for required oral medications to allow the GI tract to rest and heal. Parenteral nutrition is alternatively used. When the disease begins to improve, a special GVHD diet (Gauvreau et al. 1981) can be instituted to facilitate a slow, gradual adaptation to oral intake (see Table 9.4).

Medical treatment for enteric infections involves administration of organism-specific antimicrobial therapy. Oral vancomycin or metronidazole is used to treat *Clostridium difficile* infections. Acyclovir is used to treat HSV. Ganciclovir and foscarnet are under study for CMV infections, as previously mentioned. Treatment for other opportunistic viral infections is extremely limited (Deeg et al. 1988); a risk factor identified for adenovirus infection is the presence of GVHD (Shields et al. 1985). Other antibiotics may be used in treating intestinal parasites. Family members and sexual partners also need to be examined and treated.

Perirectal Lesions

Any lesion in the perirectal or perineal area of a BMT patient warrants culturing and extremely close observation and follow-up. The effects of the conditioning regimens and frequent diarrhea can also result in perirectal breakdown. Organisms causing these infections include aerobic and anaerobic Gram-negative bacilli, *Streptococci, staphylococci, Candida,* and HSV. The dangers of such lesions in the myelosuppressed BMT patient are that they may progress rapidly, invade tissues, and result in sepsis and death. Risk factors for the development of rectal lesions in BMT patients include severe prolonged granulocytopenia, rectal mucosal damage from conditioning therapy, diarrhea or constipation, presence of rectal fissures or hemorrhoids, or unnecessary rectal trauma.

Rectal infections may take on various clinical presentations (Yeomans 1986). Bacterial infections may rapidly appear as a raging, painful cellulitis. HSV infections may appear as discrete vesicles or small ulcers that progress to confluent ulceration. *Candida* infection may present as itchy, shiny, red areas. As the inflammatory response of these patients is greatly suppressed, pus formation is absent. Fever, rectal pain, or pain upon defecation are early warning signals that need careful evaluation and monitoring. In particular, it has been noted that point tenderness and poorly demarcated induration are the early consistent findings of bacterial abscess (Barnes et al. 1984).

Treatment of Perirectal Lesions and Nursing Implications

Medical management of acute perirectal inflammatory lesions includes broad-spectrum antibiotic therapy, and possibly even surgical incision or drainage (Barnes et al. 1984; Shaked et al. 1986). Perirectal HSV is treated with intravenous acyclovir. Topical fungal infections may be treated with antifungal creams; severe invasive infections are treated with intravenous amphotericin B.

Nursing care involves preventative measures and meticulous local skin care. The perirectal area should be examined carefully during each shift for signs of infection. Cultures should be sent on suspicious lesions. Even in the absence of lesions, the BMT patient should perform routine rectal care, particularly after bowel movements. Rectal care procedures vary widely among institutions and different soaps or antiseptic cleansing solutions may be used (i.e., chlorhexidine gluconate, povidone iodine solution, etc.). When skin decontamination strategies are used, antimicrobial

Table 9.4. Intestinal GVHD Diet Progression

Phase	Average Number of Patient Days on Phase*	Clinical Symptoms	Diet	Clinical Symptoms of Diet Intolerance
1 NPO†	16	GI cramping, large volumes watery diarrhea, GI protein losses, depressed serum albumin, severely reduced transit time, small bowel obstruction or diminished bowel sounds, nausea and vomiting	Oral: NPO IV: 1.8 × BEE;‡ kcal/day Adults: 2gm protein/kg IBW# 500cc fat emulsion Children: 2.5–3.0gm protein/kg IBW# 250cc fat emulsion/day (maximum 4gm fat/kg IBW)	
2 Introduction of oral diet	9	Minimal GI cramping, diarrhea less than 1 L./day, improved transit time (minimum 1 1/2 hr), infrequent nausea and vomiting	Oral: isosmotic, low-residue beverages initially allow 60cc every 2–3 hr IV: as for Phase 1	†Stool volume or diarrhea †Emesis †Abdominal cramping
3 Introduction of solids	9	Minimal or no GI cramping formed stool	Oral: allow introduction of solid foods, 1 every 3–4 hrs Foods are: a. minimal lactose b. low fiber c. low fat (20–40gm/day) d. low total acidity e. without gastric irritants IV: as for Phase 1	As in Phase 2
4 Expansion of diet	45	Minimal or no GI cramping formed stool	Oral: a. minimal lactose b. low fiber c. low total acidity d. no gastric irritant If stools indicate fat malabsorption: e. low fat (40gm/day for adults) IV: as needed to meet nutritional requirements	As in Phase 2

Table 9.4. *Continued*

| 5 Resumption of regular diet | — | No GI cramping, normal stool, normal transit time, normal albumin | Oral: progress to regular diet by introducing restricted foods 1/ day to assess tolerance: a. acid foods with meals b. fiber-containing foods c. lactose-containing foods; order of addition will vary, depending on individual tolerances and preferences patients no longer exhibiting steatorrhea should have the fat restriction liberalized slowly IV: Discontinue when oral nutritional intake meets estimated requirements | as in Phase 2 |

*Based on 16 patients who progressed beyond intestinal GVHD diet —Phase 1.
†NPO = *nil per os;* nothing by mouth.
‡BEE = basal energy expenditure.
#IBW = ideal body weight.
Reprinted by permission from *Journal of the American Dietetic Association,* Vol. 79: 673, 1981.
Gauvreau et al. Nutritional management of patients with intestinal graft-versus-host disease. © American Dietetic Association.

ointments may also be applied to the rectal area (Lindgren 1983). When strict decontamination procedures are not in effect, simple soap and water cleansing followed by thorough drying can be practiced. The underlying principle in performing consistent rectal care is to remove potentially pathogenic organisms from the rectal area. Patients can be educated by nurses in rectal self-care. However, they need to be monitored for compliance and effectiveness of their cleansing techniques. Back-up nursing assistance is required if the rectal area appears inadequately cleansed or if the patient is weak and debilitated.

As constipation and diarrhea are risk factors for the development of rectal lesions, attempts should be made to eliminate or minimize these problems. Warm water sitz baths are an ideal strategy for patients with hemorrhoids, fissures, frequent diarrhea, and/or perirectal breakdown to help keep the rectal area scrupulously clean.

When deep rectal wounds or cellulitis develop, wound care becomes more complicated.

Once lesions appear in the perirectal area, healing is impaired due to the effects of chemoradiation and resulting granulocytopenia. Other factors that adversely affect wound healing include pressure, obesity, steroids, bacterial contamination of the site, malnutrition, vitamin and mineral deficiencies (Vitamin C, thiamine, zinc, magnesium), anemia, and hypoxia (Sieggren 1987). The goal of nursing care in this situation is to keep existing wounds as clean as possible (to prevent further breakdown) and to modify as many of the above variables as is realistically possible.

Established rectal lesions need frequent cleansing in BMT patients to prevent colonization with other microbes and resulting superinfection. A variety of soaps, antiseptics, and surfactant cleansers are available (see Table 9.5), however, they have not been adequately studied in the BMT population to ascertain superiority in wound care. Based on a review of studies involving use of these agents in non-BMT patients, one author (Fowler 1987) raises the issue of many antiseptic solutions

Table 9.5.   Cleansing Agents

Antiseptic: inhibits bacterial growth when applied to living tissue
    Antimicrobial: agent that destroys microorgansims or suppresses their multiplication or growth.
    Bactericidal: a substance that destroys bacteria
      1. Povidone-iodine: an antibacterial substance reported to be active against bacteria, spores, fungi, and viruses: liberates 10% free iodine
      2. Chlorhexidine gluconate: a topical bactericidal agent effective against Gram-negative and Gram-positive organisms and some fungi
      3. Sodium hypochlorite: solution with antimicrobial action for cleansing and disinfecting wounds; liberates elemental chlorine, which is irritating to tissue
      4. Acetic acid: solution used as bactericidal shown to be specifically effective against *Pseudomonas aeruginosa*
      5. Hydrogen peroxide: an oxidizing agent; on contact with tissue, releases molecular oxygen and a brief antimicrobial action; the mechanical (fizzing) release of oxygen has a cleansing effect; organic matter can reduce its effectiveness

Mild skin-wound cleanser: a nonirritating liquid preparation (or product to be used with water) that assists in the removal of foreign material, does not delay wound healing, and may contain an antimicrobial ingredient
    Surfactant: wetting agent beads that break down the surface action between water and oil
      1. Shur Clens: a nonionic surfactant wound cleanser
      2. Cara-Klenz: a blend of selected moisturizers and sodium lauryl sulfate, which provides cleansing, emulsifying, and detergent actions
      3. PharmaClens: nonionic surfactant, sterile nonpyrogenic wound cleanser containing no sodium lauryl sulfate
      4. Puri-Clens: a wound deodorizer/cleanser containing methylbenzethonium chloride in a soothing base

Source: Fowler, E.M. Equipment and products used in management and treatment of pressure ulcers. *Nursing Clinics of North America* 22: 450, 1987, with permission.

possibly impairing wound healing due to damage of tissue not protected by the epidermis, and recommends that cleaning with a gentle surfactant cleanser or soap and water may be more beneficial. Frequent sitz baths followed by thorough drying and air exposure are also helpful in keeping superficial wounds or excoriations as clean as possible in order to promote healing. When evidence of severe breakdown is noted in the perirectal area, heavy ointments and creams should be avoided, unless a lesion needs treatment for a specific infection (i.e., topical antifungal cream). Ointments do not allow drainage or evaporation from the skin and obscure thorough rectal assessment. Ointments are better used as a preventative approach in the patient at risk for perirectal excoriation from diarrhea.

Deeper wounds or ulcers are the most complex to treat and are a source of continual concern in the neutropenic transplant patient. If necrotic tissue is present in the wound, debridement strategies are generally necessary (i.e., wet-to-dry dressings with a prescribed solution or frequent irrigations) to loosen necrotic tissue. Debridement procedures continue until a pink granulation base is seen; wounds should be checked every eight hours (Fowler 1987). Consultation with a wound care clinical nurse specialist or enterostomal therapist is recommended to devise a wound care protocol that can be consistently followed by the staff. As a variety of wound care products are now available on the market, the nurse specialist can aid in the selection and proper use of these products.

Measures to prevent undue rectal pressure and rectal trauma should also be instituted. Patients should be encouraged to lie on their sides for air exposure and turn frequently in bed. It is advisable that female BMT patients refrain from wearing nylon underpants; cotton underpants are recommended instead. Rectal temperatures, suppositories, and enemas are contraindicated. If dressings need to be applied to lesions on the buttocks, special care is to be given to the skin to avoid tape excoriation. For bed-bound, critically ill transplant patients, a variety of different air therapy beds are available to relieve skin pressure. Nutritional strategies aimed at providing adequate calories/protein/vitamins, minerals and trace elements for healing should be continued.

Pain control in the BMT patient experiencing painful rectal lesions is of paramount importance to provide adequate around-the-clock comfort and to facilitate the patient's tolerance of frequent rectal cleaning procedures. For severe pain, morphine continuous infusions are recommended. A patient-controlled analgesia pump may have the additional benefit of providing individualized relief for breakthrough pain, by providing boluses of analgesics before rectal care is performed. The transplant nurse should be constantly wary of constipation, however, if the patient is receiving opioids. Bowel sounds should be auscultated at regular intervals.

Gastrointestinal Bleeding

Transplant patients are at significant risk for gastrointestinal bleeding, particularly during times of severe thrombocytopenia. Mucosal damage from radiation and/or chemotherapy, alimentary tract infection, and GVHD are all risk factors for this problem. Frequent uncontrollable retching episodes place the patient at risk for esophageal tears with subsequent bleeding. The presence of refractory thrombocytopenia (severely low platelet counts despite platelet transfusion therapy), in particular, places the patient at extreme risk for spontaneous GI bleeding.

Treatment of GI Bleeding and Nursing Implications

Patients at risk for GI bleeding are observed closely for signs of overt or occult bleeding. Stools and emesis should be frequently tested for occult blood. Patients with "heartburn-type" symptoms or esophagitis are frequently placed on antacids and/or sucralfate on a regular schedule to protect mucosa from continued irritation from gastric secretions/reflux. Histamine receptor antagonists (i.e., cimetidine, ranitidine) are used infrequently due to their myelosuppressive effects (Gauvreau 1985).

Oral GI bleeding can generally be managed with such interventions as Amicar® mouth rinses or presoaked gauze, Surgicel®, Gelfoam®, topical Thrombostat® soaked gauze, or silver nitrate sticks. Oral suction should be readily available. The patient should be closely monitored for difficulty with breathing.

When frank GI bleeding is noted, medical interventions are aimed at maintaining hemodynamic stability and finding and treating the bleeding source. Platelet counts, hematocrits, and coagulation studies are monitored closely. Sudden hematocrit drops may reflect significant internal bleeding. Parameters for more frequent platelet transfusions (i.e., maintaining the platelet count at 50,000) or platelet drips may be instituted. Amicar® drips may also be initiated in the setting of refractory thrombocytopenia.

Endoscopic procedures, surgery, or angiography used for the management of bleeding sites/vessels may or may not be performed depending on the medical team's appraisal of risks versus benefits for the patient (Wolford and McDonald, 1988).

Gastrointestinal Decontamination

One special and controversial issue in the care of BMT patients is the use of gastrointestinal decontamination. Decontamination involves using prophylactic, nonabsorbable antibiotics to achieve either total GI decontamination or partial decontamination. Total decontamination aims to completely suppress microbes in the GI tract whereas selective decontamination suppresses known infection-inducing aerobic bacteria and yeast but leaves anaerobic bacteria intact (Heimdahl et al. 1984). Anaerobic microbes are responsible for colonization resistance of the digestive tract, a phenomenon that prevents antibiotic-resistant nosocomial pathogens from gaining entry into the GI tract and remaining there (Schmeiser et al. 1988). Total GI decontamination has most often been used in a strict protective environment to prevent environmental pathogens from rapidly reconstituting the alimentary tract (Schimpff 1980; Heidt and Vossen 1985). Examples of nonabsorbable antibiotics that have been used in varying combinations include: neomycin, tobramycin, gentamicin, polymyxin B, bacitracin, vancomycin, amphotericin B, nystatin, nalidixic acid, cefamandole, cotrimoxazole, and norfloxacillin (Lindgren 1983; Heimdahl et al. 1984; Heidt and Vossen 1985; Skinhoj et al. 1987; Schmeiser et al. 1988).

There is only limited information demonstrating the superiority of one of these approaches over another (Schmeiser et al. 1988). Some authors (Heidt and Vossen 1985) conclude from their review of previous studies that selective GI decontamination is as effective as total GI decontamination in infection prevention, but that total GI decontamination in a strict protective environment may be more effective in preventing GVHD. Bacterial contamination in BMT patients is thought to influence the development of GVHD because immunocompetent cells from the donor crossreact with antigens on bacteria, which are shared with the patient's tissues (Deeg et al. 1988). Thus, if bacterial sources could be removed, then theoretically, GVHD could be ameliorated. Some studies reflected this idea, noting lower incidence, delayed onset of GVHD, and improved survival in certain BMT patients who received prophylactic nonabsorbable antibiotics in a strict protective environment (Moller et al. 1982; Storb et al. 1983).

There are inherent roadblocks in gastrointestinal decontamination procedures. Patients experiencing severe chemoradiation mucosal toxicity may not be able to comply with the antibiotic regimen due to nausea or difficulty swallowing. The antibiotics have an unpleasant taste. Antibiotic schedules can be rearranged and antiemetics and pain relief measures can be provided in an effort to facilitate compliance (Lindgren 1983). Nonabsorbable antibiotics may also cause or aggravate diarrhea. Total decontamination with protective isolation, although beneficial in reducing infection rates, is costly and labor-intensive. Also, when patients are not able to comply with an entire course of therapy, rapid recolonization with more harmful or resistant GI pathogens may place the patient at high risk for a more serious infection. A recent nonrandomized study in allogeneic and syngeneic BMT patients showed that total decontamination in a strict protective environment was superior to selective decontamination with just "barrier nursing" (Schmeiser et al. 1988). These authors were also in agreement with others (Skinhoj et al. 1987) that the initial higher cost was justified by a lower usage of systemic antibiotics in the total decontamination group. Other researchers, however, question the usefulness of gastrointestinal oral nonabsorbable antibiotics particularly in autologous transplant patients (Chastagner et al. 1989). They suggested that a lower negligible incidence of Gram-negative infection in their transplant population and less toxic mucosal therapy may have contributed to their success with fecal flora suppression using parenteral antibiotics. Research will continue to define the best antimicrobial prophylaxis methods for all types of BMT patients.

Liver Complications in BMT Patients

Etiologies of liver dysfunction are varied in BMT patients. Veno-occlusive disease (VOD), GVHD, drug-induced liver injury, infection, and recurrent tumor involvement of the liver are all probable etiologic factors (Deeg et al. 1988). The pathogenesis, treatment, and management of liver GVHD and VOD are discussed in detail in chapters 7 and 10 respectively. Only the nutritional implications of VOD are addressed here. Other remaining etiologies of liver complications are briefly outlined below.

Liver Infection

Bacterial and fungal liver infections are generally seen early in the post-transplant granulocytopenic period, whereas viral liver infections are seen later due to time needed for viral replication to occur after a latent state (Wolford and McDonald 1988). In the allogeneic population in particular, viral infections reported most commonly with non-A, non-B hepatitis being the most frequent infection (Deeg et al. 1988). All transplant patients are at risk for the development of non-A, non-B hepatitis due to the high frequency of blood transfusions used. Screening for hepatitis B from blood transfusions is routinely practiced. Screening procedures for hepatitis C (a type of non-A, non-B hepatitis) have more recently become available. Chronic hepatitis B infection pretransplant has been reported to result in active viral replication during immunosuppression posttransplant, with resulting fulminant hepatitis when the immune system recovers (Wolford and McDonald 1988). As viral hepatitis pretransplant is a risk factor for VOD development post-transplant, a routine part of transplant eligibility workup includes evaluation and recognition of these problems before delivery of the conditioning regimen.

Other viral etiologies that can cause liver dysfunction in the allogeneic transplant patient include HSV, VZV, adenovirus, and Epstein-Barr virus (McDonald et al. 1986). Diagnoses of viral infections of the liver are obtained from liver biopsy. Liver function tests may reflect variably elevated serum transaminase levels.

Bacterial and fungal infections can result in liver abscesses, causing pain and fever. Bacterial infections are generally not common due to antibiotic prophylaxis and empiric antibiotic therapy; fungal infections of the liver are part of widespread fungal disease and are associated with fever, hepatomegaly, and an elevated alkaline phosphatase (McDonald et al. 1986). Diagnostic techniques include ultrasound, CT scans, magnetic resonance imaging (MRI), fine needle aspiration of suspected lesions, and liver biopsy.

Drug-Induced Liver Injury

In addition to the hepatotoxic effects of the conditioning regimens, certain medications delivered to BMT patients have potential for liver dysfunction. Some of these medications include cyclosporine, azothiaprine, ketoconazole, amphotericin B, antithymocyte globulin (ATG), methotrexate, and other antibiotics (i.e., piperacillin, ticarcillin, gentamicin, tobramycin, trimethoprim-sulfamethoxazole, cefazolin, cephalexin, cefotaxime, cephalothin) (Klemm 1985; Gauvreau 1985; Deeg et al. 1988; Wolford and McDonald 1988). The aforementioned list is not all-inclusive, however, because of the dynamic evolution of new drugs and therapeutic strategies used in BMT patients. Total parenteral nutrition may also affect the liver by causing increases in liver function tests, hepatomegaly due to fatty changes, cholestasis, and rare liver failure; careful monitoring helps to detect and minimize these complications (Sax and Bower 1988).

Treatment of Liver Dysfunction and Nursing Implications

Therapies for treating bacterial, fungal, HSV, VZV, and CMV infections have been addressed earlier. Drugs which are suspected hepatotoxins may be withheld or the dosages may be modified, depending on the severity of the liver dysfunction.

Nursing management of BMT patients experiencing liver dysfunction involves close monitoring of trends in liver function tests (i.e., serum bilirubin, SGOT, SGPT, alkaline phosphatase), serum ammonia, and coagulation studies. Deviations from normal values or progressively worsening trends should be reported immediately. As encephalopathy occurs with progressive liver dysfunction, the patient's level of consciousness and potential for aspiration should be monitored and appropriate safety precautions should be instituted. As abnormal fluid shifts and renal dysfunction from poor renal perfusion may occur concomitantly with a failing liver, the patient's BUN, creatinine, volume status, abdominal girth, and electrolytes also need to be monitored. More detailed nursing management strategies for the patient experiencing fluid and electrolyte problems from VOD are outlined in a separate chapter.

Management of abdominal pain from liver injury is difficult in the transplant patient as great care and caution needs to be exercised in any medications selected for use. The metabolism of many narcotics, anxiolytics, and sedatives is prolonged in the setting of liver dysfunction. The optimum narcotics to use for pain management in this setting should be short-acting and given in small doses (i.e., morphine and hydromorphone); sedatives or anxiolytics that are renally cleared should be used preferentially over those that are metabolized by the liver (Ford et al. 1983).

Nutritional Management of Veno-Occlusive Disease

Veno-occlusive disease (VOD) is a transplant-related liver toxicity clinically characterized by right upper quadrant pain, rising serum bilirubin/jaundice, sudden weight gain, ascites, hepatomegaly, and hepatic encephalopathy. This disorder can occur one to three weeks post-transplant and may be associated with significant morbidity and mortality for the transplant patient.

The nutritional implications of VOD involve ample support to prevent catabolism yet maintenance of fluid and sodium restrictions to prevent further ascites formation. A balance must be achieved, however, to promote adequate intravascular volume and renal perfusion; prerenal azotemia may develop from intravascular volume de-

pletion (O'Quinn and Moravec 1988). Methods to accomplish this goal include concentrating TPN solutions, restricting oral and sodium intake, and changing or concentrating intravenous medications mixed in saline to dextrose solutions.

The use of lipid emulsions in patients with liver disease is debated; parenteral combinations of dextrose, amino acids, and lipids can be delivered as long as the patient is monitored carefully (Ford et al. 1983; Darbinian and Schubert 1985). In the setting of a rising serum ammonia and VOD-induced hepatic encephalopathy, parenteral solutions of high-branched chain amino acids may be used (Darbinian and Schubert 1985). Oral protein intake may also need to be restricted.

Diuretics such as spironolactone or small doses of furosemide may be used as well to decrease the volume of ascites and maintain adequate renal perfusion; furosemide must be used cautiously, however, due to its unpredictable effect on sodium balance and its rapid depletion effects on intravascular volume (Ford et al. 1983; Deeg et al. 1988).

Global Nutritional Issues in BMT Patients

Problem-specific nutritional strategies that transplant nurses can employ have been addressed earlier in this chapter. The remaining nutritional issues for transplant patients include the use of low-microbial diets and the role of parenteral and enteral nutrition.

The Use of Low-Microbial Diets

A common protective isolation strategy used by many transplant centers is the institution of some type of low-microbial or sterile diet. These diets are utilized for the purpose of protecting the patient from exposure to virulent pathogens from foodstuffs at a time when normal host defenses are greatly compromised (Pizzo 1982). For instance, it is well known that certain foods, particularly fresh fruits and vegetables, harbor pathogens such as *Pseudomonas aeruginosa* (Bodey 1984).

There is wide variation, however, in how transplant diets are developed and administered. In general, transplant diets that have been used include the sterile diet, the low-microbial diet, and the modified house diet. Sterile diets include germ-free foodstuffs that are microbiologically tested. Sterility is achieved by autoclaving, canning, prolonged oven-baking, or irradiation (Dezenhall et al. 1987). Low-microbial diets include well-cooked foods or foods containing a minimum number of pathogens (bacteria and fungi). Modified house diets are the most liberal and are essentially regular diets without fresh fruits or vegetables.

In a recent survey of 30 transplant centers (Denzenhall et al. 1987), several researchers noted some interesting findings and trends in BMT dietary practices. Data indicated a trend away from strict sterile diets to the use of more lenient diets such as low-microbial or modified house diets. The researchers also noted that the most frequently reported food service problems were those relative to the development of a sterile food service system. These problems include: high cost, lack of standardized guidelines, inadequate or inappropriate facilities, difficulty educating kitchen personnel, and low patient acceptance of sterile food items. Another finding included variation in the practice of biologic monitoring of foods (even when LAF rooms were used); of the nine centers reponding, five centers did not practice bacteriologic monitoring. Of these five centers, three centers had LAF rooms, one center had a clean air environment, and one center had standard isolation rooms. Clearly, wide variation exists in current transplant dietary practices.

Other authors have reviewed the use of sterile and low-microbial diets used in isolation environments and summarized knowledge gained from previous studies (Aker and Cheney 1983). These authors reported a lack of randomized studies done to determine superiority of either low-microbial or sterile diets used for BMT patients in LAF and protective isolation environments. They suggest that there may be a protective benefit of limiting potentially pathogenic foods in immunocompromised patients, irrespective of the isolation strategy used. Furthermore, it was noted from their review that sterile food is not required when oral nonabsorbable antibiotics are used; however, patient compliance with these antibiotic routines is frequently problematic. The authors warn that even if low-risk foods are used, the patient may still become colonized with an antibiotic-resistant organism if it is present in the food.

More research is necessary to better define the optimum low-microbial dietary practices for BMT patients. Cost factors in relationship to the therapeutic outcome should also be examined. The collaborative relationship between the transplant nurse and the transplant dietician is critical in effectively implementing any strategies used. Patients and family members require education in the rationale and importance of the selected dietary practice used during hospitalization.

Parenteral and Enteral Nutrition: Nursing Issues

Nutritional Assessment

Poor oral intake with a subsequent debilitated nutritional state is the central nutritional concern in BMT patients. All of the gastrointestinal complications, such as mucositis, GVHD, fever, infection, enteritis, diarrhea, xerostomia, dysguesia, nausea and vomiting, and organ damage predispose the BMT patient to severe metabolic disorders, catabolism, and an almost certain inability to meet nutritional requirements both during and even frequently after the hospital stay. Energy needs in the initial 30–50 day post-transplant period have been estimated to be 170% of the basal energy expenditure and approximately 130–140% at the time of discharge; protein requirements are twice the Recommended Daily Allowance (Aker et al. 1983). Nutritional consequences are further compounded by the fact that many transplant candidates are already nutritionally compromised pretransplant from malignancy, previous cancer treatments, emotional stress, and a whole host of preexisting gastrointestinal complaints.

Baseline nutritional assessment of the BMT patient is critically important to define the nature and extent of nutritional deficiencies in order to rapidly prepare for and intervene with nutritional strategies aimed at preventing further deterioration during a very stressful treatment. If the patient is well nourished pretransplant, the goal of nutritional care is to maintain that status.

The transplant nurse and dietician should work collaboratively with other transplant team members in an ongoing fashion to promote optimum nutrition. Baseline nutritional parameters that the nurse can use to evaluate the BMT patient are outlined in Table 9.6.

Parenteral Nutrition

Total parenteral nutrition (TPN) is a frequently utilized supportive care strategy for BMT patients. It is often practiced from the onset of the transplant hospitalization (Petz and Scott 1983) and is often required by even initially well-nourished patients (ASPEN 1986; Weisdorf et al. 1987). Some authors note that if parenteral nutrition is delayed in BMT patients, it is difficult to "catch-up," particularly as resultant organ dysfunction after the treatment impedes tolerance of fluids and high concentrations of proteins, carbohydrates, and fat (Cunningham et al. 1983). In addition, nutritional deprivation in the immediate post-transplant period may have a detrimental effect on the marrow graft (Stuart and Sensenbrenner 1979).

TPN and energy requirements for the BMT patient have been the focus of numerous studies (Schmidt et al. 1980; Hutchinson et al. 1984; Weisdorf et al. 1984; Szeluga et al. 1985; Cheney et al. 1987; Weisdorf et al. 1987; Michallet et al. 1989). One early study showed advantages of using prophylactic TPN in well-nourished BMT patients, including rapid hematologic recovery (Weisdorf et al. 1984). However, the authors noted that overall improvement in survival, relapse, GVHD, sepsis and length of hospital stay were not found to be statistically significant.

A more recent, larger randomized trial in well-nourished BMT patients (n = 137; 104 allogeneic, 1 syngeneic, 32 autologous) evaluating the effects of prophylactic TPN (starting one week prior to transplant) has shown significant improvements in overall survival, time to relapse, and disease-free survival in the experimental TPN group (Weisdorf et al. 1987). The control group in this study received 5% dextrose maintenance fluid, electrolytes, minerals, trace elements, and vitamins; 61% of these patients required intravenous nutritional support prior to discharge. Further multivariate analysis of the data by the researchers in this study showed that TPN has a significant influence on survival and relapse, independent of the type of transplant, risk category for relapse, and the incidence of GVHD (in allogeneic patients). Variables not found to be significant between the two groups included engraftment, duration of hospitalization, incidence of GVHD, and bacteremia.

Another smaller prospective randomized study (n = 57 evaluable patients) compared the efficacy of nutritional support in BMT patients receiving TPN versus an enteral feeding program (Szeluga et al. 1987). The two areas of the study had comparable numbers of allogeneic patients, and fewer autologous patients. Both groups began treatment on day −1 and continued the study through day +28 unless discharge, death, or treatment failure ensued. TPN patients were permitted to eat as desired. The enteral feeding program was individualized to the patient, involving such strategies as counseling, positive reinforcement, meal-to-meal menu selection, between meal snacks, commercial supplements, or tube feedings. Enteral patients also received a daily vitamin-mineral supplement. Enteral patients who had inadequate oral protein intake were sup-

Table 9.6. Nursing Nutritional Assessment for the BMT Patient

History and Physical Assessment

Diagnosis
Age, sex, educational level
Other outstanding medical problems (i.e., diabetes mellitus, hyperthyroidism, etc.)
Conditioning regimen used for BMT
Previous cytotoxic treatments or surgeries
Height, weight, percentage deviation from ideal body weight
Hydration status
Condition of oral cavity/teeth
Activity level/exercise tolerance
Presence of GI problems; anorexia, nausea and vomiting, stomatitis, dysphagia, xerostomia, diarrhea,
  constipation
Psychological factors: anxiety, pain, depression, etc.
Current medications

Dietary History

Dietary practices at home; meal patterns
Household members (including person responsible for food preparation)
Ethnic background
Food allergies
Food preferences/aversions
Practice of any nonconventional dietary strategy (i.e., macrobiotic diet, high-dose vitamin therapy, etc.)
Ability to feed self
Income

Laboratory Data

Albumin, serum transferrin
WBC, hematocrit, hemoglobin, platelets
Sodium, potassium, carbon dioxide, chloride, glucose
BUN, creatinine
Magnesium, calcium, phosphorus
Total Bilirubin, SGOT, SGPT, alkaline phosphatase, LDH
PT, PTT

plemented with IV amino acids until their oral protein intake met study standards or until treatment failed. If oral intake was inadequate after ten days, nasoenteric feedings were instituted. If the minimum protein intake could not be met in these patients despite the aforementioned strategies or if the enteric route was contraindicated, patients were given TPN. Findings shared by the authors included that TPN was associated with more days of diuretic use, more frequent hyperglycemia, and more frequent venous access cath-

eter removal due to catheter-related complications; less frequent hypomagnesemia was seen in the TPN group. No significant difference in the rate of hematologic recovery, length of hospitalization, or survival were seen. However, nutrition-related costs were 2.3 times greater in the TPN group. In patients being fed by nasogastric tubes, the only complication seen was occasional occlusion requiring tube replacement. The authors conclude that TPN was not clearly superior to an individualized enteric feeding program; they recommend that TPN be reserved for those patients failing enteral feeding.

A very recent prospective, randomized hyperalimentation study (n = 22) involved solid tumor autologous bone marrow transplant recipients who received an intensive chemotherapy regimen (Mulder et al. 1989). This study suggested that hyperalimentation with total parenteral nutrition (TPN) and partial parenteral plus enteral nutrition by tube feeding (PPN/EN), if providing 25 grams of nitrogen and twice the basal caloric requirement, were comparable and effective in maintaining body weight and balance of nitrogen in these patients. Although no statistically significant differences were found between the two groups regarding hyperglycemia, infection, and fever, the number of patients with positive blood cultures was twice as high in the PPN/EN group. The authors suggested that further research be done to investigate the possibility that nasogastric tubes might enhance bacteremia in these patients. Additionally, the PPN/EN group had significantly fewer days of diarrhea, suggesting that enteral tube feedings in this study may have had a beneficial gastrointestinal effect after intensive chemotherapy.

Studies will continue to clarify the best, yet most cost-effective nutritional support strategies possible. This is particularly important as the overall therapeutic outcome of bone marrow transplantation continues to improve for patients. Nasoenteric tube feedings may be possible in select groups of BMT patients. However, this method of feeding is frequently controversial. It is also contraindicated because of severe mucositis, esophagitis, GI tract irritation, severely low platelet counts, risk of aspiration, severe diarrhea, and paralytic ileus, or intestinal hypomotility (Moe et al. 1985; ASPEN 1987). Protracted nausea and vomiting can also make tube placement and retention extremely difficult. Nonetheless, issues of nutritional support continue to warrant careful scrutiny.

Issues in Parenteral Nutrition Administration in BMT Patients

Clinical goals of TPN administration include the prevention of a negative nitrogen balance and loss of lean body mass, without overloading patients with excessive fluids or nutrients (Cunningham et al. 1983). The availability of different concentrations of amino acid, dextrose, and lipid solutions allows the dietician, TPN pharmacist, and physician to tailor a TPN regimen specific to the dynamic nutritional needs of the transplant patient. Volumes of TPN meet but do not go beyond maintenance fluid requirements ($1500ml/m^2$ of body surface area) (Aker et al. 1983).

The role of the nurse in caring for the transplant patient on TPN includes delivery of the solutions, and monitoring of the patient for tolerance of the TPN solution and any resultant adverse complications. The availability of silastic right atrial catheters has facilitated easy administration of TPN in the transplant patient. Dual lumen right atrial catheters have been noted to be superior to single lumen right atrial catheters in the delivery of TPN (Sanders 1982; Aker et al. 1982). Other researchers have recently noted that patients who arrive at their transplant center with a previously inserted right atrial catheter do not routinely need to have the catheter replaced; routine insertion of double lumen catheters in patients where bone marrow transplantation is anticipated was recommended (Peterson et al. 1987). Of possible interest to the transplant nurse is another recent study that examined the rate of catheter sepsis in surgical patients when triple-lumen percutaneous central venous catheters were inserted (McCarthy et al. 1987). These researchers found significant incidence of systemic sepsis and local entry site infections; it was recommended that these catheters not be used in patients receiving long-term TPN.

The transplant nurse should exercise meticulous care in the maintenance of aseptic technique when handling right atrial catheters and the delivery of hyperalimentation. Institutional policies and procedures should reflect current research on infection control in parenteral nutrition. General guidelines in hyperalimentation administration include changing TPN tubing every 24–48 hours, maintaining a closed system, and avoiding blood draws through TPN tubing (except in emergency situations or when changing or discontinuation of tubing is planned (Williams 1985). Microorganisms that have been associated with septicemias occuring during TPN include *Staphylococci, Enterococci*, fungi (especially *Candida* species), Gram-negative bacilli, and *Corynebacterium* species (Williams 1985).

Data is not currently available from controlled studies in which infection rates and the risk of using TPN cannulas for multiple purposes in highly susceptible populations are compared with those using central parenteral nutritional cannulas for parenteral nutrition therapy alone (Williams 1985). When parenteral nutrition cannulas are used for multiple purposes in the BMT patient, careful maintenance and care should be used to minimize infection risk.

Other complications seen during TPN administration in the BMT patient are varied because of the possible impact of concomitant metabolic disturbances seen from organ system dysfunction and other medications administered. Hyperglycemia, for example, may result because of TPN and concurrent steroid therapy and/or sepsis. Hypoglycemia may result from abruptly stopping the solution or excess insulin administration. Hypokalemia and hypomagnesemia may result despite supplementation of these electrolytes because of the effects of parenteral antibiotics, amphotericin B, and diarrhea. Hypermagnesemia, hyperkalemia, and hyperphosphatemia may result because of renal failure. Suddden weight gain may reflect impending veno-occlusive disease or volume overload, whereas significant volume depletion may occur because of protracted vomiting or voluminous diarrhea.

The transplant nurse should be aware of all possible etiologies for these metabolic disturbances seen in the BMT patient on TPN. Routine serum chemistries, careful assessment of volume status, and electrolyte supplementation as ordered are performed. Hyperglycemia may require management by frequent serum glucose checks and urine glucose checks with the addition of insulin to the TPN bag and/or a sliding scale insulin schedule. Hypoglycemia can be avoided by properly tapering off solutions as ordered. Management of fluid excess may require diuresis and concentration of medications (antibiotics) to the minimum volume in which the drug can be given. Some researchers (Cheney et al. 1987) indicate that a shift of fluid from the intracellular to the extracellular compartment occurs during the first four weeks after marrow grafting; administration of TPN can result in such fluid shifts. Strict intake and output and daily weights need to be monitored. Constant weight fluctuations are often reflective of difficulty managing fluids rather than actual gains and losses in body mass.

Cycling of TPN (i.e., administration over 10–18 hours) can be successfully accomplished in BMT patients in order to create a daily infusion-free period (Reed et al. 1983). In this way the catheter can be used for the administration of other important medications and blood products, which the nurse may encounter difficulty scheduling when the TPN is infusing continuously. Also it may allow the patient to be temporarily disconnected to be "free" from intravenous lines.

Parenteral Nutrition After Discharge

Inability to sustain a caloric and protein intake necessary to meet required energy needs is not unusual in many BMT patients at the time of discharge. Anorexia is often seen because of continued gastrointestinal complications and/or medications used to manage these complications.

Outpatient home parenteral nutrition is a therapeutic option that has been used in various non-BMT settings successfully (Dudrick et al. 1984; Gouttebel et al. 1987) and has also been studied in allogeneic BMT patients (Lenssen et al. 1983).

In a retrospective analysis of 246 BMT patients, researchers noted that parenteral nutrition (PN) after discharge was used in 65% of all patients (Lenssen et al. 1983). Indications for PN included GVHD, stomatitis, esophagitis, nausea and vomiting not associated with fever or GI lesions, anorexia and malaise associated with fever or viral syndrome, or failure to thrive not associated with any gastrointestinal or clinical symptoms. Stomatitis was the central reason for PN among adults and failure to thrive among adolescents and children in this study. GVHD was another reason frequently cited; PN provided most of the nutrition during the weeks of acute GVHD and rehabilitation of gut GVHD. Transplanted leukemia patients required outpatient PN more frequently than aplastic anemia patients; the authors attributed this finding to transplant-related complications such as GVHD and infection, and not necessarily the conditioning regimen. Children under 12 years required outpatient PN for a significantly longer duration than adolescents or adults. Patients in this study required outpatient PN for a median time ranging from 10–15 days, however some patients were on PN much longer. There are no reported studies on the use of home PN in autologous BMT patients, although these patients also frequently have eating problems at the time of discharge.

Cost/benefit analysis of outpatient PN has also been addressed in several studies. Although the costs of outpatient PN are considerable, some authors (Gouttebel et al. 1987) report that this strategy still reduces annual costs by 50–70%; other benefits cited include its medical efficiency, avoidance of prolonged hospitalization, and social benefits for patients who regain a more normal life at home. Others (Lenssen et al. 1983) noted that the cost of outpatient PN is only a fraction of the cost of an intensive care bed for a BMT patient; the daily cost of maintaining an outpatient on PN at their center is approximately one-sixth the cost of maintaining a patient in the hospital on PN.

Oral Intake

Oral intake is frequently encouraged as tolerated during a transplant patient's hospitalization, even with the concurrent use of TPN. During times of acute GI stress, however, oral intake should not be forced or overly emphasized (Moe et al. 1985) as this can severely discourage the patient and become a psychological deterent when eating is difficult or impossible.

In a study on food intake patterns in one BMT center (Gauvreau-Stern et al. 1989), researchers noted that beverages were the most frequently requested item, followed by bread items and cooked fruits and vegetables; patients ingested 60% of their total calories from oral intake on the day prior to discharge. Oral intake becomes a major focus of nursing efforts, particularly when the patient is approaching discharge. TPN is usually stopped when the patient demonstrates ability to eat without significant GI distress. Also of critical importance is the patient's ability to maintain a prescribed oral fluid intake to prevent dehydration. In this way, subsequent hospital readmissions for intravenous hospitalization can be prevented.

The role of nursing in enhancing oral intake is critical throughout the treatment process. Nurses can identify barriers to eating such as protracted nausea, food aversions, depression, medications causing GI disturbances, and other GI complications that may plague the patient. They can coordinate a plan of care that includes monitoring of daily oral food and fluid intake, nutritional strategies aimed at GI symptom management, and patient/family education and support. As families frequently find support from hearing that other patients in addition to their loved one is having difficulty eating, simple nutrition classes and support groups may be helpful. It has been noted that oral intake frequently improves more rapidly when patients are able to eat "home-cooked" foods rather than only institutionalized foods (Petz and Scott 1983). Nurses, physicians, and dieticians should collaborate closely in mobilizing any and all resources available to enhance oral intake in the BMT patient.

Summary

Numerous gastrointestinal complications can plague the BMT patient during and after the transplantation process. Etiologies of these complications are numerous, and involve the combined impact of treatment, myelosuppression/immunosuppression, GVHD, and other supportive therapies. Transplant nurses are confronted by immense challenges in this setting as management of these complications is labor-intensive, difficult, and often costly.

All of these complications profoundly affect the patient's nutritional status. A summary care plan at the end of the text briefly outlines key outcomes and interventions. More nursing research is necessary to provide information on the best ways to provide gastrointestinal symptom management and to enhance nutritional intake in this population.

References

Aker, S.N. et al. 1982. Nutritional support in marrow graft recipients with single versus double lumen right atrial catheters. *Experimental Hematology* 10: 732–737.

Aker, S.N. et al. 1983. Nutritional assessment in the marrow transplant patient. *Nutritional Support Services* 3: 22–37.

Aker, S.N., and Cheney, C.L. 1983. The use of sterile and low microbial diets in ultraisolation environments. *Journal of Parenteral and Enteral Nutrition* 7: 390–397.

Apperly, J.F., and Goldman, J.M. 1988. Cytomegalovirus: Biology, clinical features, and methods for diagnosis. *B.M.T.* 3: 253–264.

A.S.P.E.N. Board of Directors. 1986. Guidelines for use of total parenteral nutrition in the hospitalized patient. *Journal of Parenteral and Enteral Nutrition* 10: 441–445.

A.S.P.E.N. Board of Directors. 1987. Guidelines for the use of enteral nutrition in the adult patient. *Journal of Parenteral and Enteral Nutrition* 11: 435–439.

Atkinson, K. et al. 1989. Consensus among bone marrow transplanters for diagnosis, grading, and treatment of chronic graft-versus-host disease. *B.M.T.* 4: 247–254.

Barale, K.V. et al. 1982. Primary taste thresholds in children with leukemia undergoing marrow transplantation. *Journal of Parenteral and Enteral Nutrition* 6: 287–290.

Barnes, S.G. et al. 1984. Perirectal infections in acute leukemia. Improved survival after incision and debridement. *Ann. Intern. Med. 100:* 515–518.

Barrett, A.P. 1986. Oral complications of bone marrow transplantation. *Aust. N.Z.J. Med.* 16: 239–240.

Barrett, A.P., and Bilous, A.M. 1984. Oral patterns of acute and chronic graft-versus-host disease. *Arch. Dermatol.* 120: 1461–1465.

Beck, S. 1979. Impact of a systematic oral care protocol on stomatitis after chemotherapy. *Cancer Nursing* 2: 185–199.

Bodey, G. 1984. Current status of prophylaxis of infection with protected environments. *Am. J. Med.* 76: 678–684.

Borison, H.L., and McCarthy, L.E. 1983. Neuropharmacology of chemotherapy-induced emesis. In Lazlo, J. (ed.). *Drugs, chemotherapy-induced emesis: Focus on metoclopramide*, Vol. 25 (suppl. 1). Balgowah, NSW, Australia: ADIS Press Australasia Pty Limited (Inc. NSW), pp. 8–34.

Bostrum, B., and Weisdorf, D. 1984. Mucositis and streptococcal sepsis in bone marrow transplant recipients. *Lancet 1:* 1120–1121.

Bowden, R.A. et al. 1986. Cytomegalovirus immune globulin and sero-negative blood products to prevent primary cytomegalovirus infection after marrow transplant. *N. Engl. J. Med.* 314: 1006–1010.

Brager, B.L., and Yasko, J. 1984. *Care of the client receiving chemotherapy.* Reston, Virginia: Reston Publishing Co.

Carl, W. 1983. Oral complications in cancer patients. *Am. Fam. Physician* 27: 161–170.

Carl, W., and Higby, D. 1985. Oral manifestations of bone marrow transplantation. *Am. J. Clin. Oncol.* 8: 81–87.

Carson, J.A., and Gormican, A. 1977. Taste acuity and food attitudes of selected patients with cancer. *J. Am. Dietetic Association* 70: 361–365.

Champlin, R.E., and Gale, R.P. 1984. The early complications of bone marrow transplantation. *Seminars in Hematology* 21 (2): 101–108.

Chapko, M.K. et al. 1989. Chemoradiotherapy toxicity during bone marrow transplantation: Time course and variation in pain and nausea. *B.M.T.* 4: 181–186.

Chastanger, P. et al. 1989. Role of parenteral antibiotic therapy in gastrointestinal tract flora suppression. A study in children with high-dose chemotherapy an autologous bone marrow transplantation. *B.M.T.* 4: 393–398.

Cheney, C.L. et al. 1987. Body composition changes in marrow transplant recipients receiving total parenteral nutrition. *Cancer* 59: 1515–1519.

Cohen, J. et al. 1983. Septicemia caused by viridans streptococci in neutropenic patients with leukaemia. *Lancet 1:* 1452–1454.

Condie, R.M., and O'Reilly, R. 1984. Prevention of cytomegalovirus infection by prophylaxis with an intravenous, hyperimmune, native, unmodified cytomegalovirus globulin. *Am. J. Med.* 76: 134–141.

Corcoran-Buchsel, P. 1986. Long-term complications of allogeneic bone marrow transplantation: Nursing implications. *O.N.F.* 13: 61–69.

Cornbleet, M.A., Leonard, R.C., and Smyth, J.F. 1984. High-dose alkylating agent therapy: A review of clinical experiences. *Cancer Drug Delivery 1* (3): 227–235.

Cotanch, P.H. 1983. Relaxation training for control of nausea and vomiting in cancer patients. *Cancer Nursing 6*: 277–283.

Craig, J.B., and Powell, B.P. 1987. Review: The management of nausea and vomiting in clinical oncology. *Am. J. Med. Sc.* 293 (1): 34–44.

Cunningham, B.A. et al. 1983. Nutritional considerations during marrow transplantation. *Nurs. Clin. North Am.* 18: 585–595.

Daeffler, R. 1980. Oral hygeine measures for patients with Cancer, II. *Cancer Nursing 3*: 427–432.

Dahllof, G. et al. 1988. Oral condition in children treated with bone marrow transplantation. *B.M.T.* 3: 43–51.

Darbinian, J., and Schubert, M.M. 1985. Special management problems. In Lenssen, P. and Aker, S.N. (eds.). *Nutritional assessment and management during marrow transplantation: A resource manual.* Seattle: Fred Hutchinson Cancer Center, pp. 63–79.

Deeg, H.J. et al. 1988. *A guide to bone marrow transplantation.* Berlin, Heidelberg: Springer-Verlag.

Deeg, H.J., and Storb, R. 1986. Acute and chronic graft-versus-host disease: Clinical manifestations, prophylaxis and treatment. *J.N.C.I.* 76: 1325–1328.

Deeg, H.J. et al. 1984. Bone marrow transplantation: A review of delayed complications. *British Journal of Haematology* 57:185–208.

DeWys, W.D., and Walters, K. 1975. Abnormalities of taste sensation in cancer patients. *Cancer 36*: 1888–1896.

Dezenhall, A. et al. 1987. Food and nutrition services in bone marrow transplant centers. *J. Am. Diet. Assoc.* 87: 1351–1353.

Dreizen, S. et al. 1979. Oral complications of bone marrow transplantation. *Postgrad. Med.* 66: 187–193, 196.

Dudrick, S.J. et al. 1984. 100 patient-years of ambulatory home total parenteral nutrition. *Ann. Surg.* 199: 770–781.

Duigon, A. 1986. Anticipatory nausea and vomiting associated with cancer chemotherapy. *O.N.F.* 13 (1): 35–40.

Eilers, J. et al. 1988. Development, testing, and application of the oral assessment guide. *O.N.F.* 15 (3): 325–330.

Einsele, H. et al. 1988. Significant reduction of cytomegalovirus (CMV) disease by prophylaxis with CMV hyperimmune globulin plus oral acyclovir. *B.M.T.* 3: 607–617.

Erice, A. et al. 1987. Ganciclovir treatment of cytomegalovirus disease in transplant recipients and other immuno-compromised hosts. *JAMA* 257: 3082–3087.

Ferretti, G.A. et al. 1988. Control of oral mucositis and candidiasis in marrow transplantation: A prospective, double-blind trial of chlorhexidine digluconate oral rinse. *B.M.T.* 3: 483–493.

Fetting, J.H. et al. 1983. The course of nausea and vomiting after high-dose cyclophosphamide. *Cancer Treat. Rep.* 66: 1487–1493.

Ford, R., and Ballard, B. 1988. Acute complications after bone marrow transplantation. *Seminars in Oncology Nursing 4* (1): 15–24.

Ford, R. et al. 1983. Veno-occlusive disease following marrow transplantation. *Nurs. Clin. North Am.* 18: 563–567.

Fowler, E.M. 1987. Equipment and products used in the management and treatment of pressure ulcers. *Nurs. Clin. North Am.* 22: 449–461.

Gauvreau, J.M. 1985. Drug-induced interactions. In Lensenn, P. and Aker, S.N., (eds.). *Nutritional assessment and management during marrow transplantation: A resource manual.* Seattle: Fred Hutchinson Cancer Center, pp. 15–29.

Gauvreau, J.M. et al. 1981. Nutritional management of patients with intestinal graft-versus-host disease. *J. Am. Diet. Assoc.* 79: 673–677.

Gauvreau-Stern, J.M. et al. 1989. Food intake patterns and foodservice requirements on a marrow transplant unit. *J. Am. Diet. Assoc.* 89: 367–372.

Gilbert, C. 1989. personal communication. Clinical Pharmacist, Bone Marrow Transplant Program/Duke University Medical Center.

Goodman, M.S., and Stoner, C. 1985. Mucous membrane integrity, impairment of: Stomatitis. In McNally, J.C., Stair, J.C., and Somerville, E.T., (eds.). *Guidelines for cancer nursing practice.* Oncology Nursing Society, Orlando, Florida: Grune and Stratton, Inc., pp. 178–182.

Gouttebel, M.C. et al. 1987. Ambulatory home total parenteral nutrition. *Journal of Parenteral and Enteral Nutrition* 11: 475–479.

Gralla, R. et al. 1987. The management of chemotherapy-induced nausea and vomiting. *Med. Clin. North Am.* 71 (2): 289–301.

Guyotat, D. et al. 1984. Intestinal absorption tests after bone marrow transplantation. *Exp. Hematol.* 12 (suppl. 15): 118–119.

Heidt, P.J., and Vossen, J.M. 1985. Prevention of infection. In van Bekkum, D.W., and Lowenberg, B. (eds.). *Bone marrow transplantation, biological mechanisms and clinical practice.* New York: Marcel Dekker, Inc. pp. 475–511.

Heimdahl, A. et al. 1984. Selective decontamination of alimentary tract microbial flora in patients treated with bone marrow transplantation. A microbiological study. *Scan. J. Infect. Dis.* 16: 51–60.

Herzig, R.H. et al. 1987. Phase I-II studies with high-dose N, N', N'' -triethylene thiosphosphoramide and autologous marrow transplantation in patients with refractory malignancies. In Gale, R.P., and Champlin, R. (eds.). *Progress in bone marrow transplantation.* New York: Alan R. Liss, Inc., pp. 889–901.

Huldij, A. et al. 1986. Alterations in taste appreciation in cancer patients during treatment. *Cancer Nursing 9:* 38–42.

Hutchinson, M.L. et al. 1984. Energy expenditure estimation in recipients of marrow transplants. *Cancer 54:* 1734–1738.

Izutsu, K.T. et al. 1985. Graft-versus-host disease-related secretory immunoglobulin A deficiency in bone marrow transplant recipients: Findings in labial saliva. *Lab. Innvest. 52:* 292–297.

Jones, B. et al. 1988. Gastrointestinal inflammation after bone marrow transplantation: Graft-versus-host disease or opportunistic infection? *A.J.R. 150:* 277–281.

Kaye, S. 1982. Intensive chemotherapy for solid tumours—current clinical applications. *Cancer Chemother. Pharmacol. 9:* 127–132.

Klemm, P. 1985. Cyclosporin A: Use in preventing graft-versus-host disease. *O.N.F. 12:* 25–32.

Kolbinson, D.A. et al. 1988. Early oral changes following bone marrow transplantation. *Oral Surg. Med. Oral Pathol. 66:* 130–138.

Laskin, R.L. et al. 1987. Ganciyclovir for the treatment and suppression of various infections caused by cytomegalovirus. *Am. J. Med. 83:* 201–208.

Lazlo, J. 1983. Nausea and vomiting as major complications of cancer chemotherapy. In Lazlo, J. (ed.). *Drugs, chemotherapy-induced emesis: Focus on metaclopromide* Vol. 25 (Suppl. 1). Balgowah, NSW, Australia: ADIS Press Australasia Pty Limited (Inc. NSW), pp. 1–7.

Lenssen, P. et al. 1983. Parenteral nutrition in marrow transplant recipients after discharge from the hospital. *Exp. Hematol. 11:* 974–981.

Lindgren, P.S. 1983. The laminar air flow room. *Nurs. Clin. North Am. 18:* 553–561.

Mascret, B. et al. 1985. Phase I-II study of high-dose melphalan and autologous marrow transplantationn in adult patients with poor-risk non-Hodgkin's lymphomas. *Cancer Chemother. Pharmacol 14:* 216–221.

Matthey, F. et al. 1989. Effect of high-dose conditioning therapy prior to autologous bone marrow transplantation (ABMT) on intestinal permeability, (abstract). *B.M.T. 4* (suppl. 2): 29.

McCarthy, M.C. et al. 1987. Prospective evaluation of single and triple lumen catheters in total parenteral nutrition. *Journal of Parenteral and Enteral Nutrition 11:* 259–262.

McDonald, G.B. et al. 1981. Esophageal abnormalities in chronic graft-versus-host disease in humans. *Gastroenterology 80:* 914–921.

McDonald, G.B. et al. 1985. Esophageal infections in immunocompromised patients after marrow transplantation. *Gastroenterology 88:* 1111–1117.

McDonald, G.B. et al. 1986. Intestinal and hepatic complications of human bone marrow transplantation, parts I-II. *Gastroenterology 90:* 460–477, 770–784.

Merrifield, K.R., and Chaffee, B.J. 1989. Recent advances in the management of nausea and vomiting caused by antineoplastic agents. *Clinical Pharmacy 8:* 187–199.

Meyers, J.D. 1986. Infections in bone marrow transplant recipients. *Am. J. Med.* (suppl.) 81: 27–38.

Meyers, J.D., Flournoy, N., and Thomas, E.D. 1980 Infection with herpes simplex virus after marrow transplantation. *J. Infect. Dis. 142:* 338–346.

Michallet, M. et al. 1989. Nutritional assessment of allogeneic BMT patients: Role of parenteral nutrition and protein intake, (abstract). *B.M.T. 3* (suppl. 1): 309.

Milliken, S. et al. 1989. Fluconazole versus polyenes as oral anti-fungal prophylaxis in autologous and allogeneic bone marrow recipients, (abstract). *B.M.T. 4* (suppl. 2): 27.

Moe, G. et al. 1985. Enteral management. In Lensenn, P. and Aker, S.N., (eds.). *Nutritional assessment and management during marrow transplantation: A resource manual.* Seattle: Fred Hutchinson Cancer Center, pp. 31–44.

Moller, J. et al. 1982. Protection against graft-versus-host disease by gut sterilization? Clinical experience with bone marrow transplantation in protective isolation. *Exp. Hematol. 10:* 101–102.

Montgomery, M.T. et al. 1986. The incidence of oral herpes simplex virus infection in patients undergoing cancer chemotherapy. *Oral Surg. Oral Med. Oral Pathol. 61:* 238–242.

Morrow, G.R., and Morrell, C. 1982. Behavioral treatment for the anticipatory nausea and vomiting induced by cancer chemotherapy. *N. Engl. J. Med. 307* (24): 1476–1480.

Mulder, P.O. et al. 1989. Hyperalimentation in autologous bone marrow transplantation for solid tumors: Comparison of total parenteral versus partial parenteral plus enteral nutrition. *Cancer 64:* 2045–2052.

National Institutes of Health Consensus Development Conference Statement. 1989. *Oral complications of cancer therapies: diagnosis, prevention, and treatment.* 7: 1–32.

Nesse, R.M. et al. 1980. Pre-treatment nausea and cancer chemotherapy: A conditioned response? *Psychosom. Med. 42:* 33–36.

Nims, J., and Strom, S. 1988. Late complications of bone marrow transplant recipients: Nursing care issues. *Seminars in Oncology Nursing 4* (1): 47–54.

O'Quinn, T., and Moravec, C. 1988. The critically ill bone marrow transplant patient. *Seminars in Oncology Nursing 4* (1): 25–30.

Owen, H., Klove, C., and Cotanch, P.H. 1981. Bone marrow harvesting and high-dose BCNU therapy: Nursing implications. *Cancer Nursing June:* 199–205.

Parker, N., and Cohen, T. 1983. Acute graft-versus-host disease in allogeneic marrow transplantation. *Nurs. Clin. North Am. 18:* 569–577.

Peters, W.P. et al. 1986. High-dose combination alkylating agents with autologous bone marrow support: A phase I trial. *J. Clin. Oncol.* 4: 646–654.

Peterson, F.B. et al. 1987. Fate of right atrial catheters inserted prior to arrival at a transplant center. *Journal of Parenteral and Enteral Nutrition* 11: 263–266.

Petz, L.D. 1983. Development. In Blume, K.G. and Petz, L.D. (eds.). *Clinical Bone Marrow Transplantation*. New York: Churchill Livingstone, Inc., pp. 15–32.

Petz, L.D., and Scott, E.P. 1983. Supportive Care. In Blume, K.G. and Petz, L.D. (eds.). *Clinical Bone Marrow Transplantation*. New York: Churchill Livingstone Inc., pp. 177–213.

Pizzo, P.A. et al. 1982. Microbiological evaluation of food items. *J. Am. Diet. Assoc.* 81: 272–279.

Pizzo, P.A. et al. 1984. Approaching the controversies in antibacterial management of cancer patients. *Am. J. Med.* 76: 436–448.

Poland, J. 1989. Differential diagnosis of oral HSV infection. *Nursing Acumen* 1: 3.

Redd, W.H., and Andrykowski, M.A. 1982. Behavioral interventions in cancer treatment: Controlling aversion reactions to chemotherapy. *J. Consult. Clin. Psychol.* 50: 1018–1029.

Reed, E.C. et al. 1988. Ganciclovir treatment of cytomegalovirus infection of the gastrointestinal tract after marrow transplantation. *B.M.T.* 3: 199–206.

Reed, M. et al. 1983. Cyclic parenteral nutrition during bone marrow transplantation in children. *Cancer* 51: 1563–1570.

Ringden, O. et al. 1987. A pilot trial using foscarnet for cytomegalo-virus infections in marrow transplant recipients. In Gale, R.P. and Champlin, R. (eds.). *Progress in bone marrow transplantation*. New York: Alan R. Liss, Inc., pp. 589–593.

Robichaud, K.J., and Hubbard, S.M. 1987. Infection. In Groenwald, S.L. (ed.). *Cancer Nursing Principles and Practice*. Boston: Jones and Bartlett Publishers, pp. 221–243.

Rodu, B., and Gockerman, J.P. 1983. Oral manifestations of the chronic graft-v.-host reaction. *JAMA* 249: 504–507.

Sale, G.E. et al. 1981. Oral and ophthalmic pathology of graft-versus-host disease in man: Predictive values of lip biopsy. *Hum. Pathol.* 12: 1022–1030.

Sanders, J.E. 1982. Experience with double lumen right atrial catheters. *Journal of Parenteral and Enteral Nutrition* 6: 95–99.

Santos, G., and Kaizer, H. 1982. Bone marrow transplantation in acute leukemia. *Seminars in Hematology* 19 (3): 227–239.

Saral, R. 1989. Morbidity from HSV infection: Yesterday, today and tomorrow. *Nursing Acumen* 1: 2.

Saral, R. et al. 1983. Acyclovir prophylaxis against herpes simplex infection in patients with leukemia. *Ann. Intern. Med.* 99: 773–776.

Sax, H.C., and Bower, R.H. 1988. Hepatic complications of total parenteral nutrition. *Journal of Parenteral and Enteral Nutrition* 12: 615–618.

Schimpff, S. 1980. Infection prevention during profound granulocytopenia. *Ann. Intern. Med.* 93: 358–361.

Schmeiser, T. et al. 1988. Antimicrobial prophylaxis in neutropenic patients after bone marrow transplantation. *Infection* 16: 19–24.

Schmidt, G.M. et al. 1980. Parenteral nutrition in bone marrow transplant recipients. *Exp. Hemat.* 8: 506–511.

Schryber, S., LaCasse, C.R., and Barton-Burke, M. 1987. Autologous bone marrow transplantation. *O.N.F.* 14: 74–80.

Schubert, M.M. et al. 1983. Oral complications of bone marrow transplantation. In Peterson, D.E., and Sonis, S.T. (eds.). *Oral Complications of Cancer Chemotherapy*. Boston: Martinus Nijhoff Publishing, pp. 93–112.

Seto, B.G. et al. 1985. Oral mucositis in patients undergoing bone marrow transplantation. *Oral Surg. Oral Med. Oral Path.* 60: 493–497.

Shaked, A.A., Shinar, E., and Freund, H. 1986. Managing the granulocytopenic patient with acute perianal inflammatory disease. *Am. J. Surg.* 152: 510–512.

Shields, A.F. et al. 1985. Adenovirus infections in patients undergoing bone-marrow transplantation. *N. Engl. J. Med.* 312: 529–533.

Shulman, H.M. et al. 1980. Chronic graft-versus-host syndrome in man. A long-term clinicopathological study of 20 Seattle patients. *Am. J. Med.* 69: 204–217.

Sieggren, M.Y. 1987. Healing physical wounds. *Nurs. Clin. North Am.* 22: 439–447.

Skinhoj, P. et al. 1987. Strict protective isolation in allogeneic bone marrow transplantation: Effect on infectious complications, fever, and graft-versus-host disease. *Scand. J. Infect. Dis.* 19: 91–96.

Spencer, G.D. et al. 1986. A prospective study of unexplained nausea and vomiting after marrow transplantation. *Transplantation* 42: 602–607.

Storb, R. et al. 1983. Graft-versus-host disease and survival in patients with aplastic anemia treated by marrow grafts from HLA-identical siblings. Beneficial effects of a protective environment. *N. Engl. J. Med.* 308: 302.

Strohl, R.A. 1983. Nursing management of the patient experiencing taste changes. *Cancer Nursing* 6: 353–359.

Strohl, R. 1989. Herpes simplex virus infection in the bone marrow transplant patient: Nursing considerations. *Nursing Acumen* 1: 1,5.

Stuart, R.K., and Sensenbrenner, L.L. 1979. Adverse effects of nutritional deprivation on transplanted hematopoietic cells. *Exp. Hematol.* 7: 435–442.

Sullivan, K.M. et al. 1984. Late complications after marrow transplantation. *Seminars in Hematology* 21: 53–63.

Szeluga, D.J. et al. 1985. Energy requirements of parenterally fed bone marrow transplant recipients. *Journal of Parenteral and Enteral Nutrition* 9: 139–143.

Szeluga, D. et al. 1987. Nutritional support of bone marrow transplant recipients: A prospective, randomized clinical trial comparing total parenteral nutrition to an enteral feeding program. *Cancer Research* 47: 3309–3316.

Thomas, E.D. et al. 1975. Bone marrow transplantation. *N. Engl. J. Med.* 292: 832–843, 895–902.

Thomas, E.D. 1988. The future of marrow transplantation. *Seminars in Oncology Nursing* 4 (1): 74–78.

Vanacek, K., and Gilbert, C.1989. A randomized, double blind antiemetic study in autologous bone marrow transplant patients. Oncology Nursing Society (in progress).

van Bekkum, D.W. 1984. Conditioning regimens for marrow grafting. *Seminars in Hematology* 21 (2): 81–90.

Walsh, T.J., Belitsos, N.J., and Hamilton, S.R. 1986. Bacterial esophagitis in immunocompromised patients. *Arch. Intern. Med.* 146: 1345–1349.

Weisdorf, D.J. et al. 1989. Oropharyngeal mucositis complicating bone marrow transplantation: Prognostic factors and the effect of chlorhexidine mouth rinse. *B.M.T.* 4: 89–95.

Weisdorf, S.A. et al.1984. Total parenteral nutrition in bone marrow transplantation: A clinical evaluation. *J. Pediatr. Gastro. Nutr.* 3: 95–100.

Weisdorf, S.A. et al. 1987. Positive effct of prophylactic total parenteral nutrition on long-term outcome of of bone marrow transplantation. *Transplantation* 43: 833–838.

Wickham, R. 1989. Managing chemotherapy-related nausea and vomiting: The state of the art. *O.N.F.* 16: 563–574.

Williams, W. 1985. Infection control during parenteral nutrition therapy. *Journal of Parenteral and Enteral Nutrition* 9: 735–745.

Williams, S. et al. 1987. A phase I-II study of bialkylator chemotherapy, high-dose thiotepa, and cyclophosphamide with autologous bone marrow reinfusion in patients with advanced cancer. *J. Clin. Oncol.* 5: 260–265.

Wingard, J.R. et al. 1988. Cytomegalovirus infection after autologous bone marrow transplantation with comparison to infection after allogeneic bone marrow transplantation. *Blood* 71: 1432–1437.

Winningham, M.L., and MacVicar, M.G. 1988. The effect of aerobic exercise on patient reports of nausea. *O.N.F.* 15: 447–450.

Wolford, J.L., and McDonald, G.B. 1988. A problem-oriented approach to intestinal and liver disease after marrow transplantation. *J. Clin. Gastroenterol.* 10 (4): 419–433.

Wong, K.K., and Hirsch, M.S. 1984. Virus infections in patients with neoplastic disease. *Am. J. Med.* 76: 464–478.

Yeomans, A.C. 1986. Rectal infections in acute leukemia. *Cancer Nursing* 9 (6): 295–300.

Yolken, R.H. et al. 1982. Infectious gastroenteritis in bone marrow transplant recipients. *N. Engl. J. Med.* 306: 1009–1012.

Chapter 10

Renal and Hepatic Complications

Bruce Ballard

Introduction

The kidneys and liver are both organs involved with the processing of blood. Complications of the renal and hepatic systems from bone marrow transplantation cause interrelated disruptions in homeostasis and present unique challenges to the nurse managing a bone marrow transplant patient. In this chapter normal renal and hepatic function will be briefly reviewed followed by a description of renal failure, acute tubular necrosis (ATN), radiation nephritis, hemorrhagic cystitis, and veno-occlusive disease of the liver. Principles of assessment and management of each of these complications will also be described. Manifestations of liver GVHD are described in Chapter 7.

Impact and Incidence of Renal Failure in Bone Marrow Transplant

Renal insufficiency in any patient is significant, and is uniquely so in the bone marrow transplant population. Renal insufficiency (defined as a dou-

bling of baseline creatinine) is a common complication of transplantation, occurring in as many as 50–64% of all hospitalized transplant patients (Ballard 1989; Kone et al. 1988), primarily due to circulatory problems, drug-induced toxicities, and infections (Deeg et al. 1988). Renal insufficiency is a dynamic pathological process and exists on a continuum ranging from mild to severe. While most cases of this insufficiency are mild, the problem is still significant, since it may compromise administration of optimal therapies required for the transplant patient. Also, even a subtle decrease in renal function may herald a more complicated clinical course involving renal failure, fluid and electrolyte imbalance, and multiorgan failure.

In the allogeneic transplant patient, there is a threat of graft-versus-host disease (GVHD). Although the kidneys are rarely the target of this pathologic process, drugs used to prevent or treat this complication can cause significant renal impairment (Deeg et al. 1988). For instance, cyclosporine, a drug commonly used for GVHD prophylaxis, is renally excreted, disruptive to renal blood flow even at low blood levels, and nephrotoxic at high levels. The resulting renal impairment may very well limit the use of the drug and cyclosporine doses are often reduced, if not withheld altogether (Kennedy et al. 1985; Yee et al. 1985; Kennedy et al. 1983). In addition to cyclosporine, there are many other drugs, such as methotrexate, antibiotics, and more recently, biological response modifiers that depend, in part, on adequate renal function for the best therapeutic response.

Clinicians often wrestle with the paradox of striving to optimize their patient's renal function, while continuing therapies that impair renal function. There is an art to this management, and astute, proactive nursing practice is a vital component in that art.

Normal Renal Anatomy, Physiology, and Function

Basic renal functions may be summarized as an attempt to maintain homeostasis in body water and electrolytes, and to distribute them within the body's various fluid compartments. The renal regulation of acid-base balance and hormonal functions are but some of these homeostatic actions. The clearance of the metabolic waste products of cellular metabolism and the removal of therapeutic drugs is the body's attempt to maintain a balanced state. Each of these is accomplished by altering the composition of the blood (Goodinson 1984).

The kidneys, viewed as a factory, use arterial blood as raw material. After altering, adjusting, and improving the quality of the blood, the kidneys send this improved product out to the rest of the body tissues. At the same time, they direct unwanted materials out of the blood in the form of urine. The primary function of the kidneys is not to make urine, but to make clean, appropriately constituted blood. Improved blood is the product and urine is just the by-product. This distinction may seem trivial, but when discussing renal impairment, the focus by clinicians on urine output often clouds this distinction.

Urine Formation

Urine formation is accomplished by the four processes of **filtration, absorption, secretion,** and **excretion.** These occur in the nephron, the basic functional unit of the kidneys (see Figure 10.1).

The first step is filtration. Renal arterial blood branches down into the capillary tuft of the glomerulus. Filtering here occurs by size—substances small enough move through the porous capillary walls. Blood cells, plasma proteins, and any substances bound to protein are not normally cleared by this filtration. Water, electrolytes, blood urea nitrogen (BUN), and creatinine filter very well, and become part of the filtrate that moves out of the glomerulus and into the space surrounded by Bowman's capsule. The rate at which this filtrate is produced is the **glomerular filtration rate** (GFR), normally about 100ml per minute in the adult. All fluid and materials not filtered at the glomerulus are passed downstream into the network of capillaries that surrounds the renal tubules (Stark 1988a).

Bowman's capsule is an extension of the renal tubules, and the filtrate begins its passage through them at this point. The purpose of the tubules is to modify the filtrate by absorption and secretion. The inner lumen of each tubule is lined with epithelial cells that do this work. As the filtrate passes through the renal tubules, material and water is absorbed back into the blood stream via the capillaries surrounding the tubules. At the same time, the process of secretion is occurring, with the passage of substances from these capillaries into the lumen of the tubule (Stark 1988a).

The collecting ducts continue the processes of absorption and secretion and pass the resultant urine to the ureters, bladder, and the urethra for excretion.

Absorption and secretion are active processes that substantially alter the character and com-

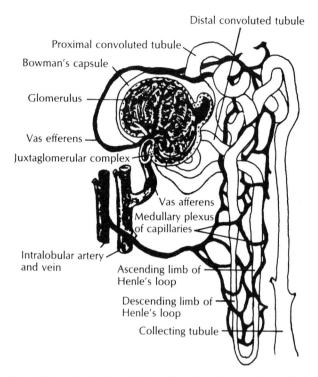

Distal convoluted tubule

Proximal convoluted tubule

Bowman's capsule

Glomerulus

Vas efferens

Juxtaglomerular complex

Vas afferens
Medullary plexus
of capillaries

Intralobular artery
and vein

Ascending limb of
Henle's loop

Descending limb of
Henle's loop

Collecting tubule

From Schottelius, B.A. and Schottelius, D.D. 1973. *Textbook of Physiology, ed. 17.* C.V. Mosby Co., with permission.

Figure 10.1.   Illustration of the Nephron and its Associated Blood Supply

position of the urine. These activities provide the body with the proper balance of water, electrolytes, and acid-base balance. Average GFR is 100ml per minute, and the urine output is 2 to 3ml per minute (Stark 1988a).

Determinants of Renal Function

For the kidneys to fulfill their functions, they must be able to perform each of the processes outlined above. If any determinant of renal function is impaired (see Table 10.1), renal insufficiency results (Epstein 1981). Good renal perfusion is necessary for adequate filtration. Adequate intravascular volume, cardiac output, and a patent renal vasculature are necessary to allow enough blood to reach the glomerulus with enough force to allow filtration to occur.

Table 10.1.   Determinants of Renal Function

Renal perfusion—filtration
    Intravascular volume
    Cardiac output
    Renal vasculature
Tubular function—secretion, absorption
    Tubular epithelial cells
    Tubular lumen
Postrenal structure—excretion
    Ureters
    Bladder
    Urethra

For secretion and absorption to occur, tubular function must be unimpaired. Normal tubular function is a product of healthy tubular epithelial cells and a tubular lumen free from obstructive debris. For excretion to occur, the postrenal structures of the ureters and bladder must be patent and unobstructed.

Acute Renal Failure

Classification

Acute renal failure is generally classified into three types, based on the etiology of the failure (Stark 1988c). The first is termed prerenal. It is a common misconception that prerenal failure is not in fact renal failure, but is simply a state that occurs just before a true renal failure. This misconception may hinder the appropriate nursing assessment and management of the patient with prerenal failure. Prerenal failure has, as its etiology, inadequate glomerular filtration due to inadequate delivery of blood to the nephron or lack of the proper pressure differential across the capillary wall. The causes generally are not in the nephron itself but previous to it. These include such clinical states common in transplantation such as hypovolemia, congestive heart failure, or septic shock. Prerenal failure is true renal failure because the kidneys fail to perform the necessary functions to maintain homeostasis.

Intrarenal failure originates at the level of the nephron. Clogged or damaged tubules or a toxic injury to the tubular epithelial cells can prevent the appropriate functions of absorption, secretion, and, at times, filtration. Nephrotoxicity secondary to aminoglycosides is a prime example.

Postrenal failure originates below the level of the kidney. If postrenal structures are obstructed, several processes ensue that hinder tubular filtrate processing, and renal failure is the end result. Tumor masses may at times be a factor in this type of renal failure.

Table 10.2. Etiology of Renal Failure in BMT

Prerenal conditions
  Hypovolemia
    Dehydration
    Third-spaced fluid
    VOD
    Hemorrhage
  Impaired circulation of blood volume
    Septic shock
    Congestive heart failure
    Cardiotoxic effects
  Renal vascular constriction
    Pressor drugs
Intrarenal conditions
  Acute tubular necrosis
    Nephrotoxic drugs
    Prolonged ischemia
  Tumor lysis syndrome
    Massive tumor lysis
  Postrenal obstruction
    Hemorrhagic cystitis

Adapted from: Ford and Ballard, 1988, with permission.

Etiologies in the Bone Marrow Transplant Patient

Renal insufficiency in the bone marrow transplant patient can arise from any of the types of renal failure discussed above (see also Table 10.2). Considering the clinical problems that predominate in this population, it is not surprising that the majority of renal problems have prerenal and intrarenal etiologies (Zager et al. 1989). Disruption of a normal fluid distribution in the body's compartments is a common problem, as are exaggerated sensible and insensible losses from the body. Also, nephrotoxic drugs (antibiotics and cyclosporine) are a common therapy for these patients, predisposing them to acute tubular necrosis, an intrarenal class of renal failure.

Other intrarenal problems possible for this group are syndromes secondary to massive cell lysis such as **tumor lysis syndrome**, rhabdomyolisis, and hemolysis from blood component administration, or more recently reported reinfusion of autologous marrow (Smith et al. 1987). Each of these problems involves the obstruction of renal tubules by the products of the cell lysis particular to them (Hou and Cohen 1985).

Prerenal Failure

The most common type of renal insufficiency seen in the bone marrow transplant patient is prerenal failure (Zager et al. 1989). The etiology of the prerenal state is usually multifactorial and complex to assess and diagnose. As a rule, it arises from one of the following: hypovolemia, impaired circulation of blood volume, or vascular constriction that alters renal blood flow. It is not uncommon for several processes to coexist.

Hypovolemia

Hypovolemia results from dehydration, when body losses are greater than intake. Common etiologies of hypovolemia in the bone marrow transplant patient are fever, diuresis, gastrointestinal losses from severe mucositis, diarrhea, or hemorrhage. Another cause of hypovolemia is "third spacing" of fluid. This is the shift of fluid from the vascular system to other body compartments that occurs commonly with the problems of septic shock, capillary leak syndrome, and veno-occlusive disease.

Impaired Circulation of Blood Volume

A prerenal failure may also arise from impaired circulation of blood, even if an adequate volume exists. This is a common problem in septic shock resulting from profound neutropenia, where the mean arterial pressure is too low for adequate perfusion of the nephron. Congestive heart failure, which often occurs in transplant from cardiotoxic drugs that have damaged the myocardium, is another situation where the blood volume is more than adequate, the ability of the heart to pump enough of it to perfuse the kidneys is impaired.

Renal Vascular Constriction

Lastly, during acute crises, transplant patients may be on pressor doses of drugs such as dopamine, where the vasoconstriction of the renal arteries restricts the flow of blood to the nephron. Renal artery vasoconstriction is also seen to a lesser, but significant, degree with other drugs, such as cyclosporine and amphotericin, both commonly administered to the bone marrow transplant patient.

The commonality among these problems is an insufficient blood volume delivered to the nephron or filtered at the glomerulus. Without adequate GFR, the blood altering work of the kidney cannot be accomplished.

Determining the etiology of prerenal problems is the key to appropriate intervention. Prerenal problems are generally reversible by correcting the underlying cause of the prerenal failure. In contrast, intrarenal problems exacerbated by the existence of a profound or prolonged prerenal state result in a more severe course, both in recovery time and in the restriction of therapies necessary for these patients.

Acute Tubular Necrosis

Acute tubular necrosis (ATN) is the most common type of intrarenal failure seen in the bone marrow transplant patient. ATN is renal failure caused by damage in or destruction of the renal tubules. If the insult is limited to the tubular epithelial cell layer, without damage to the underlying tissues, recovery is possible in time. Generally, the epithelial cell layer regenerates and begins functioning sufficiently to carry on the demands placed on it in one to five weeks.

Etiology of ATN in the Bone Marrow Transplant Patient

In the bone marrow transplant population, the most common cause of ATN is the use of nephrotoxic drugs. These include amphotericin B, cyclosporine, aminoglycosides, and acyclovir (Deeg et al. 1988; Yee et al. 1985). Each of these drugs damages the tubular cells and/or tends to crystallize in a concentrated filtrate and deposit in the tissues. The tubular lumens become clogged due to the debris of tubular cell destruction and the swelling of the tubular wall caused by the insulting agent. Filtrate cannot pass through the tubule. With no movement of filtrate, GFR is reduced or stopped. Even if debris is cleared by the healing process, it takes time for new tubular cells to become established and functional. Until this occurs, the renal functions of absorption and secretion cannot take place, necessitating therapies such as hemodialysis.

A second cause of ATN is an ischemic insult to the tubule. Since the oxygen supply to the renal tissue is the same that supplies the glomerulus, if impairment of the blood supply is profound and prolonged, renal tissues become anoxic. Severe anoxia may cause a necrosis of nephrons and their associated vasculature. In the bone marrow transplant patient, this may be more common than is usually appreciated. The bone marrow transplant patient commonly experiences fever and is often on steroidal drugs, both of which increase metabolism and, therefore, oxygen demand. Increased oxygen demand at a time of decreased supply predisposes tissue to anoxic insult. If the anoxic insult is severe enough, chances of recovering renal function are severely reduced.

Phases of ATN

ATN has three phases: oliguric, diuretic, and recovery (Stark 1988c). During the oliguric phase, little if any urine is produced because the tubules are generally clogged by the edematous epithelial cell lining and debris from cell destruction. During the diuretic phase, dilute urine is increasingly produced as a result of the clearance of the tubular lumen. This clearance allows GFR to occur at a time of impaired tubular function. Concentration of the filtrate is a function of the tubules and collecting ducts. Until they are functioning properly, GFR proceeds without the required reabsorption of water. This also explains why the quantity of urine may seem sufficient while the quality is poor. Epithelial cells are also required for the task of secretion, which is vital for the clearance of metabolic waste products and the removal of metabolized drugs. The last phase of ATN, recovery, is characterized by the ability of the nephron to concentrate the filtrate via absorption and to clear waste products and drugs out of the blood via secretion.

Within this classification of the phases of ATN there is variability in both timing and severity of each phase. It is not unusual for the oliguric phase to be absent. This is common for cases of ATN caused by nephrotoxic drugs. Nonoliguric ATN is often called "high output" renal failure due to the typical clinical picture of profuse urine volume at a time of poor waste product clearance (Dixon and Anderson 1985).

Radiation Nephritis

More recently, a clinical and pathological process affecting the kidneys has been described (Guinan et al. 1988) that may result from radiation damage. Nearly half of the young patients studied in the series described by Guinan and colleagues (1988) (median age of six) developed hemolytic anemia and renal insufficiency at five months post-transplant. The patients were treated with allogeneic or autologous transplant for acute lymphoblastic leukemia or neuroblastoma. The multiagent conditioning regimens combined with TBI in these patients were suspected as possible synergizers of the radiation effects to the kidneys resulting in this clinical syndrome.

Acute Hemolytic Reaction

Rapid onset acute renal failure has occurred following infusion of autologous marrow. Investigation of this problem has centered on both the condition of the patient at the time of reinfusion and on the marrow processing and storage materials (like DMSO) (Smith et al. 1987). Much is still unclear about this situation but management is similar to other forms of renal failure.

The nurse should be alert for signs of hemolytic reactions by testing the urine for blood either fresh or hemolyzed by inspection and dipstick. If there is a sudden onset of hematuria and significant change in urine volume in the hours after marrow reinfusion, prompt action must be taken. If hemolysis is determined, rapid hydration and the use of mannitol is necessary to allow the movement of hemoglobin through the renal tubules and out of the body.

In summary, the following characteristics of renal failure are common after bone marrow transplant. Renal failure is generally acute in nature. On resolution of the problems that produced the renal insufficiency, kidney function should recover. Mild impairment is common, especially that of prerenal failure etiology. ATN is the most common type of intrarenal failure and is often of the nonoliguric type. It is most common for insufficiency to occur in the first three weeks after transplant, yet it may occur at any time.

Nursing Assessment of Renal Function

When discussing the renal status of the bone marrow transplant patient, it is important to keep in mind concurrent medical issues. Renal insufficiency rarely exists in isolation from other clinical problems. It tends to arise at a time of multiorgan failure. If renal insufficiency is the only major clinical problem, it is generally easy to support the patient through its course. Unfortunately, this is seldom the case.

Renal insufficiency is not usually a primary conditioning toxicity. Figure 10.2, describing the interrelationships between some of the postconditioning toxicities, shows that the major problem in keeping the kidneys functioning properly is keeping the other organs at optimum perform-

ance. Lines from each of the conditioning-related toxicities may be drawn to factors that affect some element of renal function discussed here. It is the task of the nurse to understand the implications of each and to use the appropriate assessment tools to assist in the management of the patient whose renal system is impaired.

The nursing assessment (see Table 10.3) of the renal status of the bone marrow transplant patient includes five areas:

1. blood chemistries, which help determine the fluid and electrolyte balance, the level of vital organ functions, and the acid-base balance;

2. urine assessment, which helps determine the level of renal tubular function and/or damage;

3. fluid balance assessment, which determines the compartmental distribution of fluid in the body;

4. pharmacologic agents, to examine the contributors to renal dysfunction, mental status changes, and renal system demands; and

5. mental status assessment, which elucidates neurological effects of renal impairment.

Blood Chemistries

Serum sodium assessment helps determine the patient's free water balance. Appropriate fluid quantity and quality therapy is based on this calculation.

Serum CO_2 assessment helps in estimating the acid-base balance and determining the existence of the anion gap. If the CO_2 is low, it indicates a metabolic acidosis. If the calculated anion gap is high, it can indicate sepsis, ketoacidosis, or uremia. An acidosis without a significant anion gap is indicative of a renal tubular acidosis (RTA). This is common in patients receiving cyclosporine or amphotericin B, and is easily treatable.

Potassium assessment is important. In renal insufficiency, hyperkalemia would be expected, but in the bone marrow transplant patient receiving cyclosporine or amphotericin B, potassium wasting in the urine is common. Potassium

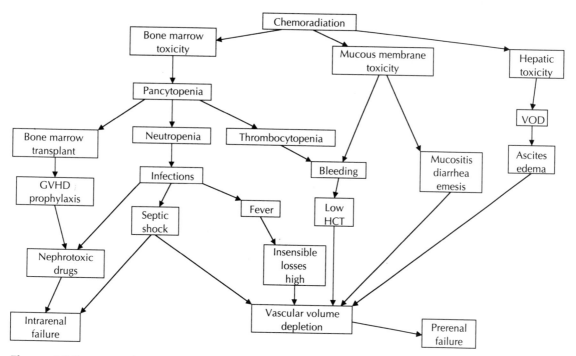

Figure 10.2. Interrelationship of Post-Transplant Patient Problems as Potential Contributors to Renal Failure

wasting results in hypokalemia, which often requires aggressive intravenous potassium replacement.

Serum blood urea nitrogen (BUN) is a complex value to interpret for bone marrow transplant patients. Since the rate of BUN production is a function of several factors, not the least of which is the patient's metabolic rate, the levels may be elevated with even a slight decrease in GFR. The addition of steroids to the patient's drug profile or the presence of blood in the GI tract can significantly increase the production of BUN without any significant alteration in kidney function.

Serum creatinine is a better gauge of kidney function than is BUN. It can indicate a change in GFR, yet, it is not diagnostic of the etiology of the renal insufficiency by itself.

The most important aspect of serum creatinine and BUN is the baseline measurement for that patient compared with the degree and rate of change from the baseline. A doubling of any given creatinine level means a 50% decline in renal functioning. This is an important concept. Consider the patient whose creatinine on the previous day was 1.2mg/dl. If the morning creatinine rises to 1.5mg/dl the response is different than if that same patient had a creatinine the day before of 0.7mg/dl. In the first case, we note a moderate increase in creatinine and continue to monitor the patient accordingly. In the second case, we realize that in the past 24 hours there has been a loss of more than half of the patient's renal function and a quick complete assessment and change in therapy may be needed.

This follow-up should be directed at collecting information necessary to determine whether the etiology of the renal insufficiency is prerenal or intrarenal. Urine studies help in this regard.

Table 10.3. Differential Findings in Acute Renal Failure

Test	Prenatal Findings	Intrarenal Findings Typical to ATN
Urine		
Specific gravity	> 1.015	≤ 1.010
Sodium	< 10 to 20mEq/L	> 20 to 40mEq/L
Sediment	MOD hyaline and finely granular casts	Dirty brown granular casts and epithelial cells
Volume output	Oliguria or anuria	Nonoliguric most common, but oliguria or anuria possible, especially if also prerenal
Blood		
Bun	Increased	Increased
Creatinine	Increased	Increased
Potassium	Increased or normal	Oliguric phase: increased Diuretic phase: decreased
Bun/Creatinine	> 10/1	< 10/1
Physical exam		
Blood pressure	Low BP, often with orthostatic drop in SBP and > in HR	Varies with volume status
Neck veins	Flat	Varies with volume status

Urine Assessment

Volume

Examination of the urine quantity and quality indicates the adequacy of renal tubular function and the type of renal insufficiency. Assessment should include the measurement of urine volume for a single shift plus the previous 24-hour period. A decrease in this volume coupled with an increase in serum creatinine suggests that renal insufficiency is present. However, other assessments are needed to further determine a prerenal or intrarenal etiology of the failure.

Specific Gravity

Since the tubular functions of secretion and absorption alter the filtrate character, abnormal values can be expected for urine electrolytes and specific gravity (Stark 1988b). Values typical of particular types of renal failure may be found.

Also, urine sediment, determined by urinalysis, can be diagnostic of tubular damage.

A healthy tubule has the ability to concentrate urine if it senses inadequate intravascular volume. It does this by reabsorbing filtered water back into the capillaries surrounding the tubules, creating a concentrated urine, typically greater than 1.020. If the tubules have been sufficiently damaged, as in ATN, this ability is lost and the urine specific gravity tends to be similar to that of the blood it filters. The specific gravity of blood is about 1.010.

As an example, consider how one might distinguish between a prerenal condition or intrarenal damage in the patient whose urine volume is down and morning serum creatinine is elevated. A routine specific gravity measurement in the high range indicates that the tubules are working well and a prerenal condition would be suspected. We know this because it takes the tubular function of absorption to accomplish this state. A damaged tubule cannot concentrate urine.

Urine Sodium

In a prerenal state, the kidneys attempt to increase blood volume by resorbing sodium as well as water. This tends to deplete the tubular filtrate of sodium, yielding a low urine sodium, typically less than 20mEq/liter. If the tubules are damaged, as in ATN, resorption of sodium is less efficient and urine sodium levels will be high, typically greater than 50mEq/liter (Espinel and Gregory 1980; Lam and Kaufman 1985).

The kidneys may inaccurately sense an intravascular depletion. Sensors in the kidneys measure pressure and flow but the kidneys are unable to tell whether the low renal blood flow is a result of true volume depletion from decreased cardiac output, as in CHF, or from vasoconstrictive drugs which are restricting renal arterial blood flow. The urine sodium and specific gravity may indicate what the kidney senses is happening as well as the status of the renal tubules, but more information is necessary to complete the picture. The determination of fluid distribution is helpful in this regard.

Urine Sediment

Urine casts are also diagnostic of tubular damage. If large amounts of renal tubular cell casts are passed out of the tubules, they may be seen in the urine under microscopic examination.

Fluid Balance

Fluid balance should be considered from two perspectives; the total body fluid and the distribution of that fluid within the body. Change in total body fluid is easily determined from changes in weight of the patient. For example an overnight change in body weight is not a change in the amount of muscle or fat; it is a change in the amount of fluid in the body. Explanations for changes in weight may be found in the intake and output records and by taking into consideration insensible losses, which may be profuse in a febrile patient. Other less obvious factors causing a disturbance in fluid balance may be depletion due to the decreased intake when mucositis is present or loss due to a high volume of emesis. These are significant factors in the early post-transplant patient.

Each of these assessments helps explain the amount of, or changes in, body fluid. They do not describe how that fluid is distributed in the body. From the kidney's standpoint, it is vital to determine whether the intravascular volume is sufficient. This determination guides therapy to prevent or reverse prerenal failure and reestablish homeostasis. It may be that the replacement of an adequate blood volume is the quickest and easiest intervention for the patient. Physical assessment is key in this evaluation.

Significant depletion of the patient's intravascular volume produces significant orthostatic changes in blood pressure and heart rate. Even a patient who spends a major portion of the day in bed should be able to compensate for postural changes in vital signs within 60 to 90 seconds. Measurement of orthostatic vital signs are significant in confirming a prerenal state due to hypovolemia. A finding of significant postural changes in blood pressure and heart rate, coupled with the findings discussed in this chapter is generally definitive of hypovolemia, without the need for invasive monitoring.

The level of intravascular fluid can be determined by assessing for distended neck veins in Trendelenburg's position, and by a cardiac exam listening for signs of fluid overload. Pulmonary edema as a result of fluid overload may be manifest by rales in the lungs, or if severe, by frothy sputum, respiratory distress, signs of fluid on the chest x-ray, or abnormal arterial blood gases. Each of these will support the case that fluid has left the vascular space and gone to the interstitial spaces in the lungs.

The bone marrow transplant patient, especially one who has veno-occlusive disease (discussed later), can sequester enormous amounts of fluid in the abdominal cavity, which will result in engorged organs and, at times, ascites (McDonald et al. 1986). Changes in abdominal girth and sudden weight gain indicates fluid that is not available for renal perfusion. An increase in abdominal girth without a concomitant rise in weight usually indicates a decrease in intravascular volume.

Pharmacological Considerations

Impaired renal function may be a result of the drugs. In turn, the drugs we give can be affected by impaired renal function. If a change in renal function is noted, it is important to look at the patient's drug profile and make appropriate adjustments. The adjustments are aimed at preventing toxic side effects of drugs that will be poorly excreted (Bennett 1988).

Assessment of the drug profile may also disclose a potential etiology of the renal insufficiency. If diuretics were aggressively used around the time of onset of renal insufficiency, assessment for signs of hypovolemia should occur. An elevation in BUN may reflect the increased metabolic rate seen with steroids. High-dose pressors such as dopamine constrict the renal arteries, causing a prerenal condition. Not all offending medications can be stopped. Some may be necessary to sustain life, but accounting for renal insufficiency may require adjustments in drugs or dosages to avoid compounding the problem.

Mental Status

The patient suffering severe renal impairment often exhibits mental status changes that must be monitored. Blood urea nitrogen (BUN) and other waste products can build up in the blood and cause uremic encephalopathy. Nonrenal etiologies for mental status changes are common, so other causes must also be evaluated (see Chapter 11).

For instance, since the kidneys metabolize many drugs, a review of the drug profile may reveal the source of mental status changes. This may be true for some drugs even if the kidney is not the major site of that drug's metabolism. Many narcotics are metabolized by the liver, yet the metabolites are cleared by the kidney. It is often the case, especially if both renal and hepatic function are impaired, that the metabolites cause the changes in mental status.

Management of Renal Insufficiency

The management of renal insufficiency in the bone marrow transplant patient requires a multidisciplinary approach involving at least the nurse, doctor, pharmacist, and nutritionist. The goal of management is to improve or maintain renal function while allowing the other organs to function properly.

Assessment

The first step in this management is assessment. Proper diagnosis directs proper treatment. For the nurse, the concepts and actions discussed above give the physician the information necessary to establish the proper treatment. The nurse is often first to have the information because the nursing assessment involves the collection of weight, intake and output, abdominal girth, postural blood pressure and heart rate, lung exam, urine specific gravity, and the other indices vital to therapeutic decisions.

Correcting Vascular Volume Disequilibrium

The next management step involves the correction of any vascular volume disequilibrium. This may require the use of diuretics or volume replacement. Whether replacement takes the form of crystalloid or colloid is determined by concurrent problems and the unique needs of the patient.

Correcting Electrolyte Imbalance

Along with this intravascular volume correction comes the correction of any electrolyte imbalances. This involves the correction of free water excess or deficit and adjustment of electrolytes in the intravenous fluids to match calculated losses and correction of any deficit or excess.

Minimizing Nephrotoxins

Adjustment of, or the removal of, nephrotoxic drugs must be attempted. This is often easier said than done in this population, given the requirements for such essential drugs as amphotericin B and cyclosporine. The decision to reduce or to maintain such therapy is based on the unique needs of the patient.

Treating Infections

To manage the renal problems that often arise in the bone marrow transplant patient, infections must be adequately treated. This may seem to contradict the previous paragraph. Yet the most severely malfunctioning kidneys are those of the patient suffering septic shock receiving pressor doses of dopamine.

Hemorrhagic Cystitis

Incidence

Bladder toxicity occurs in up to 24% of BMT patients (Miyamura et al. 1989). It is most often a primary toxicity from the conditioning regimen due primarily to the use of cyclophosphamide (Cy). Fortunately, it is usually preventable and/or responsive to conservative treatment.

Etiology

The etiology of the problem from Cy is acrolein, a metabolite of Cy that is toxic to the transitional epithelium of the bladder and ureters. This metabolite produces partial or complete ulceration of the bladder mucosal tissue. Small vessels in the underlying tissue hemorrhage into the bladder (Champlin and Gale 1984; Sale and Shulman 1984).

Another etiology is from adenovirus infection of the bladder mucosa causing hematuria. Some investigators have found an association between the two, which tend to coexist in the same patient (Miyamura et al. 1989).

Presentation and Clinical Course

Hemorrhagic cystitis may present immediately with the administration of Cy or be delayed, sometimes for months after the Cy course. It is most commonly seen at the time of Cy administration and presents as hematuria either by dipstick examination or as an obvious red-tinged urine with blood clots. It may also present as dysuria or frequency. It is generally responsive to the treatment measures instituted and resolves within a day or two of the end of the Cy (Champlin and Gale 1984).

In its severe form, larger and more deeply invasive ulcerations extend into the vascular tissue underlying the bladder mucosa (Sale and Shulman 1984). Bleeding may develop into a severe life-threatening problem. Also, since the blood often clots in the bladder, painful obstruction of bladder outflow may result.

Prevention

The prevention of hemorrhagic cystitis involves measures to decrease the toxicity of the metabolite. Three-way irrigation catheters are placed and 100-500ml/hour of fluid continuously irrigates the bladder from the start of Cy until at least 24 hours after the last dose or until the urine shows no evidence of blood. The goal of this maneuver is to dilute and remove the toxic substance from contact with the sensitive bladder tissue as fast as possible (Hutchinson and Itoh 1983).

Another preventive measure is the use of aggressive intravenous hydration with fluids at twice the usual maintenance rate. This aggressive hydration causes a rapid and dilute filtrate to pass through the ureters, thus preventing prolonged contact of the metabolite with epithelium. Vigorous hydration requires close monitoring of the patient. It is very common for the patient to develop either an overhydrated state or, if diuretics are used to force diuresis, a prerenal vascular state may result. Measures discussed in the previous section of this chapter are useful in determining the appropriate therapies for the patient situation.

The use of drugs to prevent cystitis is becoming more common. Mesna is an example of a drug that binds acrolein and prevents the damage it produces (Deeg et al. 1988). Since it acts at the time of the Cy administration, there is no benefit to its use once hemorrhagic cystitis has occurred.

Treatment

Treatment of cystitis involves many of the same therapies used for prevention. Continuous bladder irrigation at 500ml to 2 liters/hour will generally be sufficient to clear developing clots and prevent obstruction. Infusing platelets to maintain high platelet levels is also very important. At times cystoscopy is required, and cautery of bleeding ulcerative areas may be attempted. Unfortunately this is usually not a long-term solution due to the diffuse, wide-spread pathology associated with the problem. The instillation of chemicals into the bladder, such as mucomyst, is also used and may benefit the patient. Some of these chemicals can harden in the bladder if irrigation is insufficient. For this reason, the nurse must pay close attention to this aspect during their use.

Veno-Occlusive Disease of the Liver

Introduction

The major task of the liver is to alter the quality of blood. It attempts to maintain homeostasis by clearing waste products and drugs from the body. **Veno-occlusive disease** of the liver (VOD) is the most common liver problem that arises after bone marrow transplant, and has serious potential effects on the bone marrow transplant patient (Deeg

et al. 1988). It is discussed here since it is so intimately involved with the disruption of normal renal function and the fluid and electrolyte balance of the patient.

VOD is a distinct disease involving the blood vessels of the liver. This disease has a specific syndrome that manifests clinically with great variation in severity, affects several other organ systems, requires close attention, and alters the clinical management of the patient. In addition, it is associated with significant mortality.

VOD is a complex topic and is confusing to many. Part of the reason for this is that VOD means different things to different people. To the pathologist looking at liver tissue through the microscope, VOD is distinct and specific damage to liver tissue. To the clinician, it is a patient who is jaundiced, encephalopathic, with a distended abdomen, experiencing complex fluid and electrolyte problems. Both views are correct. Both are VOD. The pathologist looks at the cause of the clinical syndrome that nurses observe clinically.

Incidence and Risk Factors

The incidence of VOD in the bone marrow transplant population is about 21% (Grandt 1989; Deeg et al. 1988; McDonald et al. 1985; Ford et al. 1983). Most incidence studies predate the current use of higher toxicity conditioning regimens. Because of this the incidence may increase as conditioning becomes more intense in attempts to prevent the present high rate of relapse.

Table 10.4 summarizes the known risk factors predisposing a patient to develop VOD. The single most significant risk factor is the presence of liver abnormalities at the time of conditioning therapy. Whether the cause of abnormalities is viral hepatitis, tumor infiltrates, or infections, the finding of an elevated bilirubin and/or liver enzymes, predicts an increased risk for VOD. This is such a significant finding that, if at all possible, bone marrow transplant is postponed until liver function tests return to normal. This is often the case, for instance, with the patient with liver function

Table 10.4. Risk Factors Predisposing VOD

Liver abnormalities
Intense conditioning regimen
High-dose rate radiation
Leukemia versus aplasia
Malignancy other than ALL
Allogeneic versus autologous and syngeneic
  second transplant
Age > 15

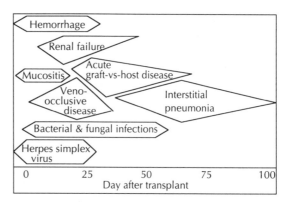

From Ford and Ballard, 1988, with permission.

Figure 10.3. Time of Occurrence of Acute Complications After Bone Marrow Transplantation

abnormalities from non-A, non-B hepatitis. Of the other potential risk factors for developing VOD, age and a higher dose-rate of radiation are the most significant (McDonald et al. 1984; Jones et al. 1987).

The desire to minimize risk factors, if possible, before proceeding with bone marrow transplant results from the significant morbidity and mortality associated with the disease. Table 10.5 summarizes two studies of the outcome of VOD in bone marrow transplant patients. According to these studies, about half of the patients with VOD recover. The other half die with VOD present. In those who have VOD at death, VOD is the direct cause of death in the majority (McDonald et al. 1985; Jones et al. 1987).

While the clinical symptoms of VOD arise in the time period shown in Figure 10.3, the liver insult actually occurs well before the clinical symptoms manifest.

Etiology of VOD

The etiology of VOD is usually the chemotherapy and radiation conditioning therapy for the bone marrow transplant. Interestingly, using a single conditioning agent generally does not bring on the disease. Yet, given in combination, there

Table 10.5. Outcome of Patients with VOD

	McDonald	Jones
Resolved	55%	48%
Died with VOD	45%	47%

seems to be a synergistic effect producing hepatic damage well beyond that produced by any single agent (McDonald et al. 1986).

Onset and Resolution

In contrast to other acute complications, VOD appears at any time after the start of conditioning, with its peak onset in the second week after bone marrow transplant. Recovery of hepatic function occurs about three weeks after the onset of jaundice (McDonald et al. 1985).

Pathophysiology

VOD is a disease of the small blood vessels in the liver. It is characterized by an occlusion in the venous outflow tract of the liver, hence its name, veno-occlusive disease. The clinical syndrome is a logical extension of the pathophysiological changes that occur.

Normal Hepatic Physiology

Normal hepatic blood flow comes from two major sources: the majority from the portal vein, which emerges from the spleen and intestines, and most of the rest from the hepatic artery, which supplies oxygenated blood to the hepatic tissues. The blood flows down into smaller and smaller vessels and eventually into the hepatic sinuses (see Figure 10.4). The sinuses are thin-walled vessels of endothelial tissue that empty into a central collecting vein. These sinuses are lined by hepatocytes, the cells most involved in processing products in the blood as they pass through the sinuses on a path toward the venules. Blood flow out of the liver then moves from these sinusoids into central veins, which lead to larger hepatic venules and eventually into the vena cava (Kaldor 1988).

Hepatic Venule Occlusion

The two areas of hepatic injury from VOD are the hepatic venules and the hepatocytes that line the sinusoids. As the hepatocytes metabolize and process the chemotherapeutic agents passing through the liver, the by-products, which tend to be toxic, are dumped into these small vessels. The endothelial linings of the sinuses and hepatic veins are damaged by the toxicity of these metabolites. The eventual result is impaired blood flow through the sinuses secondary to an obstruction of the hepatic veins. This obstruction results from several processes (McDonald et al. 1986).

First, the tissue is swollen from the chemo/radiation insult. Second, fibrin is deposited in the injured area in an attempt to stabilize and heal the area. This fibrin presents an impediment to the passage of cellular debris and exfoliated hepatocytes that have died from the conditioning toxicities. The process becomes self-perpetuating as the blood flow becomes impaired and the tissue is deprived of the oxygen necessary to support the tissue. Pressure and fluid backs up into, and previous to, the sinusoids. The entire liver becomes engorged as venous outflow becomes more and more occluded. Anoxia leads to further injury and necrosis of hepatic tissue with the result that hepatic blood flow and function is even more impaired. It is from this occluded flow that all the resultant clinical problems stem (McDonald et al. 1986).

These points suggest the first of three concepts basic to understanding the clinical pattern of VOD. VOD causes a disruption in the body's normal fluid distribution and flow patterns leaving the wrong fluid in the wrong place. The body's compensatory actions often become overwhelmed or counterproductive. Simplified to its basic elements, VOD repeats, in multiple areas, the problems of impaired flow, improper distribution, and inadequate and inappropriate compensation.

Consequences of Impaired Hepatic Blood Flow

Impaired hepatic blood flow has several consequences. The liver becomes swollen. As the pressure in the hepatic vasculature exceeds its ability

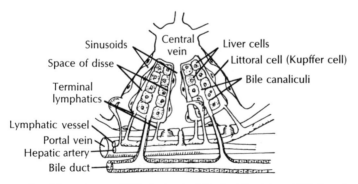

Sinusoids
Space of disse
Terminal lymphatics
Lymphatic vessel
Portal vein
Hepatic artery
Bile duct
Central vein
Liver cells
Littoral cell (Kupffer cell)
Bile canaliculi

Reprinted from Guyton 1986, *Textbook of Medical Physiology*, W.B. Saunders, with permission.

Figure 10.4. Basic Structure of a Liver Lobule

to keep the fluid inside the capillary bed, sodium and protein-rich fluid drip off the surface of the liver into the peritoneal cavity. For many patients this fluid is absorbed by the lymphatic system at the rate it is produced. If it becomes too profuse, this compensatory maneuver is inadequate, and ascites may accumulate.

Restricted blood flow through the liver also causes pressure in the portal system, engorging the mucosal vessels of the small intestine. A further consequence of poor flow is the renal tubules' strong reabsorption of sodium and water (Cade et al. 1987; McDonald et al. 1985).

Each of these conditions presents its own set of problems, yet the primary effect is to shunt vital blood away from the liver tissue. This consequence has the most serious implications because the shunting of blood, if severe and prolonged, can prevent the delivery of oxygen to the hepatic tissue. Without oxygen and the ability to carry off the hepatically metabolized substances, liver cells start to die, tissue necroses, and this destruction adds to the problems already existent. Liver enzymes start to reflect hepatic dysfunction, and the overall metabolic capability of the liver can become severely impaired (Shulman et al. 1980).

Consequences of Impaired Hepatic Function

As hepatic function falls, the ability to remove drugs and the body's metabolic wastes becomes impaired. The patient becomes jaundiced, as bilirubin is not processed out of the body. Impaired production of coagulation factors also can develop with a resultant coagulopathy.

Clinical Complications of VOD

Since VOD is set in motion at the conditioning stage of transplant treatment, the early processes occur well before the clinician can see overt signs and symptoms. Also, VOD exists on a continuum. Some cases are very mild and some severe, depending on the degree of hepatic damage. These points, plus the multitude of other clinical problems potentially occurring simultaneously, makes diagnosis of VOD somewhat problematic. A definitive diagnosis is possible by needle biopsy, but the risk to the thrombocytopenic patient from hemorrhage generally precludes this procedure. It is often necessary to make the diagnosis based on clinical signs and symptoms.

Clinical Diagnosis of VOD

Studies have demonstrated that a clinical diagnosis of VOD can be made based on as few as three or four criteria. McDonald and colleagues (1984) showed that the presence of hyperbilirubinemia, hepatomegaly or right upper quadrant pain, and significant weight gain were highly correlated with the presence of VOD as confirmed by biopsy. In fact, he showed that if the patient was in the first three weeks after bone marrow transplant, and if these signs could not be explained by other mechanisms, the finding of any two of these three was sufficient to confirm the diagnosis 89% of the time. Conversely, McDonald and colleagues (1984) also showed that in the absence of two of the three, there was a 92% chance that VOD did not exist. Other studies have used much the same criteria and had similar results.

This seems valid when one constructs a frequency chart (see Figure 10.5) of the VOD patient's signs and symptoms. The most frequent four symptoms are the ones used in the clinical diagnosis and occur in the majority of patients with the disease.

Common Additional Clinical Findings

Abdominal Distention

In addition to those findings used in the clinical diagnosis, a vast array of other common findings are associated with VOD (see Figure 10.6). The congested GI mucosa, liver, spleen, and ascites all lead to abdominal distention. Severe enlarge-

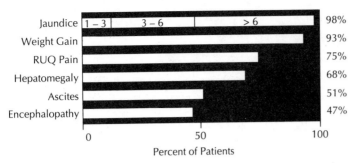

From G. McDonald, et al. The clinical course of 53 patients with veno-occlusive disease of the liver. *Transplantation* 39 (6): 604. © Williams and Wilkins, 1985.

Figure 10.5. Clinical Features of Patients with Veno-occlusive Disease of the Liver

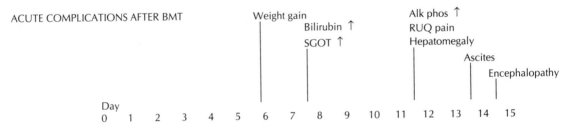

From Ford and Ballard, 1988, with permission.

Figure 10.6. Occurrence of VOD Symptoms

ment of the abdomen can impair respiratory efforts such that full ventilatory movement is impaired and painful. Circulation of blood to the vital organs of the abdominal cavity may be impaired if the intraperitoneal pressure becomes too great. This is believed by some to account for at least some of the impaired renal function common with VOD (McDonald et al. 1985).

Edema, Hyponatremia, Hypoalbuminemia

Water reabsorption by the renal tubules tends to produce a free water excess, which is manifest by hyponatremia. In addition, the leak of serum proteins into the peritoneal space produces hypoalbuminemia, reducing the oncotic pressure within the vascular space. This is compounded further by the renal reabsorption of sodium, increasing

total body sodium. The result of too much total body sodium, too much free water (which dilutes the serum sodium concentration to hyponatremic levels), and a serum oncotic pressure, invariably is the movement of water out of the capillaries into the interstitial space, or edema.

Encephalopathy

The shunting of blood away from the liver coupled with a loss of hepatic cells often causes the liver to inadequately metabolize metabolic waste products and the metabolites of drugs. These materials can build up in the blood and cause hepatic encephalopathy, which is clinically manifest as lethargy, confusion, and disorientation. These are also common findings in other hepatically-impaired patients.

Renal Insufficiency

Several forces operate against proper renal function in the patient suffering from VOD. While many VOD patients never show impaired renal function, some will have concomitant findings of renal insufficiency. One study of 77 bone marrow transplant patients who required hemodialysis found that all but four had a bilirubin greater than 2mg/dl at their first dialysis. Half had a bilirubin greater than 2mg/dl more than ten days before first dialysis (Ballard et al. 1990). This finding is suggestive of concomitant VOD and renal failure.

Prerenal factors, as discussed earlier in this chapter, and the impairment of the liver's metabolism of nephrotoxic drugs seem to be the etiology of the concurrent renal failure. For instance, several prerenal factors are common to the VOD patient (see Figure 10.7). Most important is the loss of fluid from effective circulation due to an engorged liver, GI mucosa, and spleen. Ascites and edema rob the kidneys of needed intravascular volume. The use of diuretics and the restriction of IV or oral fluids, while often necessary actions, may overshoot the intended target and deplete the already tenuous intravascular status. If the intraperitoneal pressure becomes too great, venous return may become impaired, and further restrict the already poor hepatic and renal blood flow.

The kidneys' response to these conditions is, in effect, to add fuel to the fire. Filtered sodium and water are reabsorbed at the renal tubules, urine output drops, clearance of metabolic waste products decreases still further, and weight gain continues.

In addition to the prerenal conditions is the potential that the kidneys may fall victim to nephrotoxic levels of hepatically metabolized drugs. Chief among these is cyclosporine, which is so common to this population (Yee et al. 1984). This close relationship between the kidneys and liver is a major concern and the focus of most of the clinical intervention directed at VOD.

Treatment of VOD

There is at present no definitive treatment to prevent or reverse VOD. Research attempts are directed at protecting the hepatic tissue from the initial conditioning insult or to prevent the deposition of fibrin on the insulted venules. Some of these approaches may hold promise for future prophylaxis or treatment measures, but at present, the clinical effort is directed toward supportive and symptomatic management of the patient until VOD has run its course and the regenerative capabilities of the liver have had a chance to repair the damage from the disease.

Supportive and Symptomatic Management of VOD Complications

The management of VOD entails preventing the development of the extremes of the complications and the maintenance of optimal vital organ function. The key is a thorough assessment that includes the knowledge of the patient's baseline information and the degree of change from this baseline. From this knowledge base comes the plan to manage the clinical problems.

The symptomatic management of VOD entails efforts to:

1. Maintain fluid and electrolyte balance,
2. Minimize the adverse effects of ascites,
3. Adjust drugs to reflect impaired hepatic and renal function,
4. Avoid compounding encephalopathy with drugs that alter mental status,
5. Attend to coagulopathy.

The overall goals of these tasks are to:

1. Improve the impaired flow of blood through the liver and kidneys,
2. Redistribute body fluids appropriately,
3. Assist the body's compensatory efforts, and
4. Counter inappropriate compensatory actions that the body institutes.

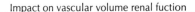

Impact on vascular volume renal fuction

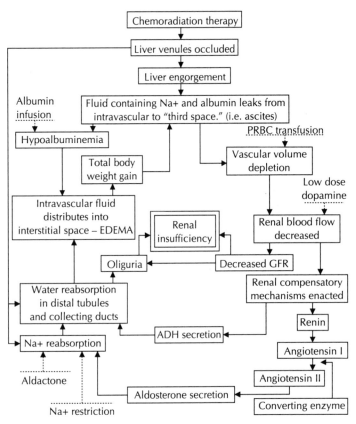

Dotted lines indicate the major clinical interventions used to manage this condition.

Figure 10.7. Impact of Veno-occlusive Disease on Renal Function

Maintaining Fluid and Electrolyte Balance

The maintenance of fluid and electrolyte balance requires a good assessment of total body fluid status through evaluation of weight, intake and output, and estimated insensible losses. The next task is to assess the distribution of that fluid in the body. Nursing assessment is an essential role in this task. The performance of postural blood pressure and heart rate, abdominal girth, lung exam, estimation of changes in peripheral edema, and the collection of urine for analysis, are vital in determining the distribution of fluid in the body. With this information one can determine the effect of the fluid distribution on the renal, pulmonary, or cardiac status of the patient.

Hypertransfusion of RBCs

Though not a universal finding, it is common for the VOD patient to be intravascularly depleted. Much of the crystalloid intravenous fluid given to the VOD patient has an end point outside the vascular space. For this reason, packed red blood cells are often recommended to maintain the intravascular fluid volume. This may generally require the elevation of the patient's hematocrit to levels well above normal values.

It is common to find the goal of this hypertransfusion of red blood cells to be a hematocrit of 40 or higher. This helps maintain a high osmotic pressure within the vascular space, which in turn draws extravascular interstitial fluid back into the vessels. If there is a finding of postural hypotension, another approach that may be more individualized for the patient is to transfuse to a level that relieves postural hypotension.

If intravascular volume is excessive, and it also is desired to hypertransfuse the patient, it is common to give a combination of packed red blood cells followed by a diuretic. This maneuver is especially effective in the patient with pulmonary edema that coexists with renal insufficiency of a prerenal etiology. The increased osmotic forces within the blood will draw pulmonary fluid into the vascular space to be removed by the diuretic.

Intravenous Albumin

Salt-poor albumin is also used to increase the oncotic pressure in the vascular space and to replace serum proteins that are lost into the peritoneal cavity with ascites (McDonald et al. 1985). The use of this controversial therapy varies among different institutions. Some believe that the half-life of salt-poor albumin in the vascular space for the VOD patient is so short that the benefits do not justify the impact that the leak out of the vessels into third space areas effects. Also, the cost of the product for such a brief potential benefit may seem unjustified. There are no definitive studies on this topic with the VOD patient. Generally, the infusion of this colloid is used to moderate levels, unless problems clearly develop (Epstein 1981).

Treating Sodium Imbalance

The treatment of elevated total body sodium levels requires a restriction of sodium intake plus the initiation of sodium diuresis. Spironolactone is effective in this regard, though it has its limitations and risks. It is only available as an oral drug, and effective sodium diuresis generally starts 36 to 72 hours after starting the drug and may persist for 24 to 36 hours after stopping doses. It also puts the patient at risk for hyperkalemia. Care must be used if renal insufficiency develops (Conn 1972).

Minimizing Movement of Fluid into Interstitial Compartments

The limitation of sodium intake, achieving sodium diuresis, hypertransfusion, and the salt-poor albumin all help to minimize fluid in the interstitial spaces. This has its most important impact on the prevention or treatment of pulmonary fluid excess.

Altering Renal Hemodynamics

The reversal of impaired renal hemodynamics must first be addressed by a correction in the intravascular volume disequilibrium. Renal hemodynamics may then be improved with the use of "renal dose" dopamine (defined as 1–2 micrograms/kg/minute), which will act to dilate the renal arteries, improve renal blood flow, and, therefore increase GFR. As GFR is improved, the kidneys are better able to regulate fluid and electrolytes, acid-base balance, and the metabolism and excretion of waste products and drugs.

Minimizing Effects of Ascites

In those cases of VOD in which ascites is a significant problem, it is often the intent of clinicians to reduce ascitic fluid that has accumulated. There are several ways to reduce ascitic fluid or to reduce the amount of fluid that has become sequestered in the abdominal organs. The removal of fluid by the aggressive use of diuretics, dialysis, or directly tapping the fluid via serial paracentesis, are all effective. Yet whatever method is used, the underlying process that allowed the ascites to form in the first place persists, and the ascites inevitably reaccumulates. This reaccumulation is always at the expense of the intravascular volume and invariably leads to renal impairment (Cade et al. 1987). Whether or not to remove fluid, and how much fluid to remove, must be based on a careful assessment of the benefit-risk ratio for the individual situation.

Adjusting Drugs In Altered Hepatic and Renal Function

The hepatic impairment found in VOD requires an adjustment in drugs that are hepatically metabolized. Narcotics are a common example. Resulting mental status changes from use of narcotics in the VOD patient may necessitate stopping or reducing the drugs in an attempt to prevent compounding hepatic encephalopathy. Narcotics and sedatives with shorter half-lives and fewer metabolites should be considered if these drugs are needed for patient comfort. For example, lorazepam is preferable to valium for sedation. Also hydromorphone has a shorter half-life and requires conversion to significantly fewer metabolites than morphine.

Treatment of Coagulopathy

The coagulopathy associated with VOD is managed by several measures. Vitamin K replacement and regular infusions of platelets when required, will generally be sufficient to prevent severe bleeding problems. If severe coagulopathy exists, strict attention to the prevention of bleeding is required. This includes prophylaxis against stress ulcers and the avoidance of invasive procedures.

Summary

The clinical issues discussed in this chapter are complex and present a challenge to the nurse caring for the transplant patient. Much of the nursing assessment and action required goes beyond that typical to the normal oncology patient. There is often some element of critical care nursing required for these patients, especially those who are experiencing severe renal or hepatic dysfunction. It has been the focus of this chapter to impress upon caregivers the significance of the nursing process in the overall management of these critical issues in order to improve the quality of complex care required by the transplant patient. A sample care plan summarizing salient features of nursing care appears at the end of the text.

References

Badr, K., and Ichikawa I. 1988. Prerenal failure: A deleterious shift from renal compensation to decompensation. *N. Engl. J. Med. 319* (10): 623–629.

Ballard, B.D. 1989. Incidence and outcomes of renal insufficiency and renal failure after bone marrow transplant. Unpublished data.

Ballard, B.D. et al. 1990. Characteristics of bone marrow transplant patients with renal failure requiring hemodialysis. Unpublished data.

Bennett, W.M. 1988. Guide to drug dosing in renal failure. *Clinical Pharmacokinetics 15:* 326–354.

Cade, R. et al. 1987. Hepatorenal syndrome. *Am. J. Med. 82:* 427–438.

Champlin, R.E., and Gale, R.P. 1984. The early complications of bone marrow transplantation. *Seminars in Hematology 21* (2):101–108.

Conn, H.O. 1972. The rational management of ascites. *Progress in Liver Disease 4:* 269–288.

Deeg, H.J. et al. 1988. *A guide to bone marrow transplantation.* NY: Springer-Verlag, p. 123–139.

Dixon, B.S., and Anderson, R.J. 1985. Nonoliguric acute renal failure. *American Journal of Kidney Diseases 6* (2): 71–80.

Epstein, M. 1981. The rational approach to the management of ascites. *Drug Therapy October:* 17–27.

Espinel, C.H., and Gregory, A.W. 1980. Differential diagnosis of acute renal failure. *Clinical Nephrology 13* (2): 73–77.

Ford R. et al. 1983. Veno-occlusive disease following marrow transplantation. *Nurs. Clin. North Am. 18* (3): 563–568.

Goodinson, S.M. 1984. Renal function: An overview. *Nursing 2* (29): 843–852.

Grandt, N.C. 1989. Hepatic veno-occlusive disease following bone marrow transplantation. *O.N.F. 16* (6): 813–817.

Guinan, E.C. et al. 1988. Intravascular hemolysis and renal insufficiency after bone marrow transplantation. *Blood 72* (2): 451–455.

Hou, S.H., and Cohen, J.J. 1985. Diagnosis and management of acute renal failure. *Acute Care 11*: 59–84.

Hutchinson, M.M., and Itoh, K. 1983. Nursing care for the patient undergoing bone marrow transplantation for acute leukemia. *Nurs. Clin. North Am. 17* (4): 697–711.

Jones, R.J. et al. 1987. Veno-occlusive disease of the liver following bone marrow transplantation. *Transplantation 44* (6): 778–783.

Kaldor, P.K. 1988. Anatomy and Physiology of the gastrointestinal system. In Kinney, M.R. et al. (eds.). *AACN'S Clinical Reference for Critical Care Nursing*. New York: McGraw-Hill.

Kennedy, M.S. et al. 1983. Acute renal toxicity with combined use of amphotericin B and cyclosporine after marrow transplantation. *Transplantation 35* (3): 211–215.

Kennedy, M.S. et al. 1985. Correlation of serum cyclosporine concentration with renal dysfunction in marrow transplant recipients. *Transplantation 40* (3): 249–253.

Kone, B.C. et al. 1988. Hypertension and renal dysfunction in bone marrow transplant recipients. *Quarterly Journal of Medicine, New Series 69* (260): 985–995.

Lam, M., and Kaufman, C.E. 1985. Fractional excretion of sodium as a guide to volume depletion during recovery from acute renal failure. *American Journal of Kidney Diseases VI* (1): 18–21.

Mars, D.R., and Treloar, D. 1984 Acute tubular necrosis—pathophysiology and treatment. *Heart & Lung 13* (2): 194–201.

McDonald, G.B. et al. 1984. Veno-occlusive disease of the liver after bone marrow transplantation: Diagnosis, incidence, and predisposing factors. *Hepatology 4* (1): 116–122.

McDonald, G.B. et al. 1985. The Clinical course of 53 patients with veno-occlusive disease of the liver after marrow transplantation. *Transplantation 39* (6): 603–608.

McDonald, G.B. et al. 1986. Intestinal and hepatic complications of human bone marrow transplantation. Part I. *Gastroenterology 90*: 460–477.

Miyamura, K. et al. 1989. Hemorrhagic cystitis associated with urinary excretion of adenovirus type II following allogeneic bone marrow transpalntation. *B.M.T. 4*: 533–535.

Sale, G.E., and Shulman, H.M. 1984. Pathology of other organs. In Sale, G.E., and Shulman, H.M. (eds.). *The Pathology of Bone Marrow Transplantation*. New York: Masson, p. 192–198.

Shulman, H.M. et al. 1980. An analysis of hepatic veno-occlusive disease and centrilobular hepatic degeneration following bone marrow transplantation. *Gastroenterology 79*: 1178–1191.

Shulman, H.M., and McDonald, G.B. 1984. Liver disease after marrow transplantation. In Sale, G.E., and Shulman, H.M. (eds.). *The Pathology of Bone Marrow Transplantation*. New York: Masson p. 104–135.

Smith, D.M. et al. 1987. Acute renal failure associated with autologous bone marrow transplantation. *B.M.T. 2*: 195–201.

Stark, J.L. 1988a. Renal anatomy and physiology. In Kinney, M.R. et al. (eds.). *AACN'S Clinical Reference for Critical Care Nursing*. New York: McGraw-Hill p. 843–859.

Stark, J.L. 1988b. Renal System Assessment. In Kinney, M.R. et al. (eds.). *AACN'S Clinical Reference for Critical Care Nursing*. New York: McGraw-Hill p. 860–872.

Stark, J.L. 1988c. Acute Renal Failure. In Kinney, M.R. et al. (eds.). *AACN'S Clinical Reference for Critical Care Nursing*. New York: McGraw-Hill p. 873–885.

Yee, G.C. et al. 1984. Effect of hepatic dysfunction on oral cyclosporine pharmacokinetics in marrow transplant patients. *Blood 64* (6): 1277–1279.

Yee, G.C. et al. 1985. Cyclosporine-associated renal dysfunction in marrow transplant recipients. *Transplant. Proc. 17* (4): 196–201.

Zager, R.A. et al. 1989. Acute renal failure following bone marrow transplantation: A retrospective study of 272 patients. *American Journal of Kidney Disease 13*: 210–216.

Chapter 11

Neurologic and Neuromuscular Complications of Bone Marrow Transplantation

Deborah Kryspin Meriney

Introduction

Neurologic and neuromuscular complications occur in 59–70% of patients undergoing a bone marrow transplant and result in a 6% fatality rate (Davis and Patchell 1988; Patchell et al. 1985; Wiznitzer et al. 1984). In many cases, neurologic complications occur insidiously, manifesting symptoms so general that they may be easily mistaken for the sequelae of prolonged isolation, bedrest, or the sedative side effects of certain medications.

Because neurologic deficits may render individuals incapable of self-care to varying degrees, either temporarily or permanently (Mitchell et al. 1984), the impact of neurologic and neuromuscular deficits on the patient, family, health care team and resources, is significant. Therefore, early assessment for complications may help prevent or ameliorate potentially severe neurological impairment.

The neurologic system is at risk for injury throughout the transplant process. Pretransplant conditioning with chemo- and radiotherapy may result in neurotoxicity. Post-transplant, neurologic and neuromuscular complications may result from infections occurring during the immunodeficient period, toxicities of antibiotics and immunosuppressive agents, or from therapies administered to control graft-versus-host disease (GVHD). Additionally, system failure in other organs may lead to metabolic encephalopathy and impair neurologic function.

Each potential source of neurological and neuromuscular injury will be discussed roughly in the order in which it might appear during the transplant process and will include risk factors, assessment, and treatment.

Chemoradiotherapy Pre-transplant Conditioning

Neurospecific diagnostic testing prior to bone marrow transplantation is limited to a lumbar puncture primarily in patients with acute lymphocytic leukemia or in those who are suspected to have central nervous system disease. Patients undergoing BMT for a malignant brain tumor may also have a computerized tomography (CT) scan, but this test is not part of the routine pre-BMT screening. Due to the lack of specific, quantitative neurological tests, it is essential that a history and physical assessment be obtained in order to establish a baseline for future comparison.

Chemotherapy used in the conditioning process places the patient at risk for neurological injury. Common drugs and their toxicities include: etoposide (VP-16) and associated peripheral neuropathy in 1–2% of cases (Barnhart 1988), carmustine (BCNU) and rare instances of neuroretinitis, and busulfan and the possible development of myasthenia gravis (Barnhart 1988).

Intrathecal and standard doses of cytosine arabinoside (ARA-C), a cell-cycle specific antimetabolite capable of intensive myelosuppression, are associated with myelopathy and peripheral neuropathy (Dunton et al. 1986). High-dose cytosine arabinoside (HDARAC), used as part of the pre-BMT conditioning regimen for leukemia (Champlin et al. 1989), is potentially toxic to the central nervous system as it readily crosses the blood brain barrier, and has a long half-life in the cerebrospinal fluid (CSF) (Walker and Brochstein 1988). Neurotoxicity is the most severe adverse effect of this drug and may necessitate cessation of therapy (Bolwell et al. 1988). Specific neurotoxicities include: headache, somnolence, personality changes, memory loss, intellectual impairment, confusion, slurred speech, stupor, coma, or seizures. Other unique ARA-C-related neurotoxicities include cerebellar dysfunction, hearing loss, encephalopathy, peripheral neuropathy, severe expressive aphasia, Guillain-Barre syndrome and a Parkinsonian-like movement disorder (Johnson et al. 1987; Luque et al. 1987; Borgeat et al. 1986; Cersosimo et al. 1987). In most cases, the syndromes were reversed after cessation of the drug.

The most common type of neurotoxicity, cerebellar dysfunction (Walker and Brochstein 1988), is seen only with high-dose regimens of

3g/m^2 every 12 hours, for a cumulative dose of 24–36 grams (Bolwell et al. 1988; Iacobini et al. 1986; Nand et al. 1986). Cerebellar manifestations include ataxia, dysarthria, dysdiadochokinesia, nystagmus, intention tremors, muscle weakness, truncal dysmetria, and incoordination (Champlin et al. 1989; Bolwell et al. 1988; Peters et al. 1988; Spriggs et al. 1988).

The major factor in predisposition to ARA-C related neurotoxicity is age (Champlin et al. 1989; Bolwell et al. 1988; Peters et al. 1988). Central nervous system (CNS) toxicity occurs in approximately 3–7% of treated patients overall, yet the incidence increases three to sixfold for patients over 50 years (Peters et al. 1988). Abnormal liver function, a shortened interval between courses (Pies 1981), and preexisting progressive neurological dysfunction also place in the patient at risk (Nand et al. 1986). Dose adjustments of HDARAC in the elderly and other patients at risk may be recommended (Champlin et al. 1989; Walker and Brochstein 1988). In addition, assessment of neurologic status must be performed on all patients prior to receiving HDARAC (Gottleib et al. 1987; Conrad 1986). Cerebellar manifestations accompanied by nystagmus result in termination of treatment (Gottleib et al. 1987; Sylvester et al. 1987; Conrad 1986), while withholding chemotherapy for 24 hours is required if nystagmus alone is present (Barnett et al. 1987).

Total body irradiation (TBI) may cause fatigue and weakness, occasional confusion, and has a high incidence of late onset of cataracts, which are usually correctable by surgery. Other effects of TBI (i.e., leukoencephalopathy (LEC) and vascular complications), which occur as a result of its use in combination with other treatments or as late effects are discussed later in this chapter.

Central Nervous System Infections

Central nervous system infection is a common neurologic complication of bone marrow transplant, occurring in 7–14% of patients (Davis and

Table 11.1. Windows of Infection

First:	Related to granulocytopenia 0–1 month after BMT Organisms: bacteria, viruses, fungi
Second:	Related to immunosuppression 1–12 months after BMT Organisms: viruses, parasites

Patchell 1988; Patchell et al. 1985; Wiznitzer et al. 1984). Heightened susceptibility is evident during two windows of infection following BMT. The characteristics of these two windows are listed in Table 11.1.

The first window occurs one month post-transplant, and corresponds to the period of granulocytopenia. During this time, bacterial, fungal, and viral infections predominate. The second window lasts from one month until one year post-transplant, correlating with prolonged immunosuppression, and more commonly gives rise to viral and parasitic infections (Davis and Patchell 1988; Applebaum and Thomas 1985; Patchell et al. 1985; Rogers 1985).

Bacterial Infections

Meningitis is the most common neurologic manifestation of bacterial infection, caused primarily by conventional bacteria or *Listeria monocytogenes*, *Streptococcus pneumoniae*, *Klebsiella pneumoniae*, *Escherichia coli* and alpha-Streptococci (Davis and Patchell 1988; Peeters et al. 1989; Wiznitzer et al. 1984). Contiguous spread from paranasal and paratympanic areas has been documented (Davis and Patchell 1988; Francke 1987).

Due to myelosuppression, the body is infrequently able to mount an inflammatory response, and therefore, meningeal inflammation is not commonly seen (Callaham 1989). Most patients present with fever (78%) and headache (58%), yet both Callaham (1989) and Francke (1987) observed that a substantial number of patients were without symptoms of CNS infection. When present, signs of bacterial meningitis include: changes in mental status, **meningismus**, lethargy, increasing confusion, or seizures (Francke 1987).

Preventative measures are those generally recommended during immunosuppression, including a private hospital room, protective isolation, and a low bacterial diet devoid of fresh fruits, vegetables, and salads (Remington and Schimpff 1981). Nonabsorbable antibiotics to sterilize the gut may be effective if they are tolerated by patients who may already have gastrointestinal irritability from transplant conditioning or other therapies (Ford and Eisenberg 1990; van den Broek 1988).

Fungal Infections

Fungal infections account for 50–57% of all CNS infection in BMT recipients, and are by far most frequently caused by *Aspergillus fumigatus* (Milliken and Powles 1990; Hara et al. 1989; Davis and Patchell 1988). The organism gains access to the CNS through hematogenous spread from the lungs, skin, or gastrointestinal tract, or by direct extension from the cranial sinuses (Hara et al. 1989; Davis and Patchell 1988; Wingard et al. 1987). *Aspergillus* may cause brain abscesses, and in 86% of cases, altered consciousness in the form of progressive obtundation is the presenting sign (Davis and Patchell 1988). Focal neurologic findings like sudden **hemiparesis** and seizures have also been documented.

The *Candida* species are another common cause of fungal infection in the bone marrow transplant patient (Meyers 1990; Milliken and Powles 1990), causing **meningoencephalitis** and brain abscesses (Lew 1989).

Cryptococcus, an organism ubiquitous in animals and the soil, is acquired by patients prior to hospitalization (Deeg 1984). These infections are normally asymptomatic and heal in the lungs of persons with properly functioning immune systems. Although about 50% of patients with cryptococcal meningitis are not immunosuppressed, these infections may be life-threatening to neutropenic patients following BMT. In addition to the associated pneumonia, the organism may become disseminated and infect the central nervous system, causing meningoencephalitis and its usual manifestations.

The only established treatment for otherwise fatal fungal infections in patients who remain febrile despite broad spectrum intravenous antibiotic therapy is the intravenous administration of amphotericin B (Milliken and Powles 1990). Presently, clinical trials are underway to establish the efficacy of new antifungal medications, such as fluconazole (Pfizer, Groton, CT), which may be more effective and less toxic than the present regimen (Brammer 1990).

Viral Infections

Viral complications are most commonly due to the herpes group, notably cytomegalovirus (CMV) and varicella-zoster virus (VZV) (Zaia 1990; Davis and Patchell 1988). Herpes zoster infections are potentially severe, with great risk of dissemination, and develop in 30-50% of patients undergoing allogeneic bone marrow transplantation (Perren et al. 1988). Herpes zoster is caused by reactivation of VZV first acquired in childhood as chicken pox. After resolution of the chicken pox, VZV may lie dormant in the posterior root ganglion of the spinal nerve or in a cranial nerve ganglion (Perren et al. 1988). The outbreak characteristically occurs along the dermatomes and may cause potentially severe neuralgias (Wacker et al. 1989; Perren et al. 1988).

Herpes simplex reactivates in up to 80% of bone marrow transplant recipients (Ford and Eisenberg 1990). Fortunately, however, infection is usually localized and rarely fatal (Winston et al. 1988). Prophylaxis with acyclovir, an antiviral agent, is often initiated prior to BMT; this has significantly reduced the incidence of serious viral infections.

Viral encephalitis is associated with systemic viral dissemination (Patchell et al. 1985; Wiznitzer et al. 1984). Infection with herpes zoster or simplex encephalitis often results in a fatal outcome (Atkinson et al. 1980; Locksley et al. 1985; Patchell et al. 1985; Wiznitzer et al. 1984). Common clinical manifestations of encephalitis include headache and altered sensorium. However, progressive **obtundation, ataxia** (Wiznitzer et al. 1984), and other focal neurologic abnormalities have also been reported.

Other causative organisms of viral encephalitis include cytomegalovirus (CMV), and, rarely, adenovirus (Ford and Eisenberg 1990; Davis et al. 1988). Because these viruses may be latent in the bone marrow transplant recipient prior to transplantation, encephalitis is often the result of reactivation of the virus under the conditions of immunosuppression (Meyers 1988). Other routes of spread include the nasopharyngeal or oro-fecal route (Davis et al. 1988; Davis and Patchell 1988). Blood products have also been implicated as sources of infection of the adeno- and cytomegaloviruses (Davis et al. 1988; Meyers 1988).

CMV encephalitis clinically resembles the signs of general viral encephalitis. Similarly, neurologic signs of a fatal case of meningoencephalitis manifested by the adenovirus have been described as headache, lethargy, and seizures (Davis et al. 1988).

Serologic screening of blood products and organ donors can eliminate transmission of CMV in those who have never been infected (Bowden et al. 1986; Winston et al. 1988). The use of intravenous ganciclovir has some efficacy against CMV if administered prophylactically or before the onset of pneumonia (Winston et al. 1988).

Parasitic Infections

The only identified parasitic pathogen of the CNS during BMT thus far is *Toxoplasma gondii* (Davis and Patchell 1988). Despite the fact that greater than 50% of the United States population may be carriers, significant infection with this organism in bone marrow transplant recipients is rare (Davis and Patchell 1988; Derouin et al. 1985). It is hypothesized that *P. carinii* prophylaxis pretransplant may also protect patients from reactivation of latent *Toxoplasma* infection (Derouin et al. 1985).

Although carriers of the parasite may be totally asymptomatic (Meredith 1987), an immunosuppressed individual who is infected, whether through acquisition by ingestion (Holland 1989) or reactivation of the virus, generally has a poor prognosis. The organism has a propensity for the central nervous system, with a usually fatal course in the patient who is immunosuppressed from disease or therapies used to prevent or treat GVHD (Davis and Patchell 1988; Meredith 1987).

Clinically, toxoplasmosis may manifest itself as a diffuse encephalopathy or meningoencephalitis, or as single or multiple enlarging mass lesions (Holland 1989; Davis and Patchell 1988). The signs are characteristic of a progressive neurologic disorder. Development of diffuse muscle pain, disorientation, and myoclonic twitching, have been reported (Meredith 1987). Ackerman et al. (1986) have observed the following symptoms: bifrontal headache, nuchal rigidity, Parkinsonian tremor, clouded sensorium, agitation, severe tremors, hemiparesis, and seizures. In the case study described by Ackerman et al. (1986), symptoms were reversed with treatment. Of special interest is that one of the drugs used to treat toxoplasmosis, Pyrimethamine, is known to decrease leukocyte and platelet counts (McCabe and Oster 1989).

Since the acquisition of toxoplasmosis is a late infection, most likely to occur long after the patient is discharged from the hospital, teaching by the inpatient nurse in anticipation of discharge, or by the clinic or the community nurse should focus on avoiding possible sources of the pathogen. Instructions to patients should include the following: careful hand washing after touching uncooked meat; washing fruits and vegetables, which may be contaminated with *Toxoplasma gondii*; and avoiding contact with cat feces or litter-boxes because parasite eggs can develop in the intestines of cats.

A patient hospitalized with toxoplasmosis should be placed on seizure precautions with frequent neurologic assessments. Any changes in neurologic status should be reported. Toxoplasmosis is contagious and appropriate isolation procedures should be instituted.

Neurologic Complications of Antibiotic Therapy

Many antibiotics used to treat infection are neurotoxic. Aminoglycosides are known to adversely affect the eighth cranial nerve, which is responsible for hearing and balance. Other antibiotics, either alone or in combination with aminoglycosides can potentiate neurologic deficits (Barnhart 1988). Toxicities include **ototoxicity** (tinnitus, hearing loss, loss of balance), acute muscular weakness, headache, dizziness, paresthesias and fatigue (Barnhart 1988). Table 11.2 lists some commonly used antibiotics and their neurologic side effects.

Nurses administering these therapies should be cognizant of individual and potentiated effects, appropriate neurologic assessments, and appropriate interventions to prevent or minimize toxicity. In addition, nurses should be aware of where the drug is metabolized, and concomitant conditions, such as decreased renal function, which will interfere with drug metabolism thereby exacerbating toxicity. Accordingly, serum and urine creatinine, intake and output, and daily weights need to be monitored in those patients receiving antibiotics metabolized by the kidneys. Drugs metabolized in the liver require close attention to liver function tests.

Metabolic Encephalopathy

Metabolic encephalopathy is the single most common neurological complication, occurring in approximately 37% of patients undergoing bone marrow transplantation (Davis and Patchell 1988; Patchell et al. 1985). It is caused by multiple organ failure (Davis and Patchell 1988; Patchell et al. 1985) and is usually associated with terminal

Table 11.2. Antibiotics and Their Neurotoxic Effects

Antibiotic	Neurotoxic Effects
Amikacin	Ototoxicity-eighth cranial nerve: hearing loss, loss of balance, or both. May cause acute muscular paralysis and apnea after treatment with aminoglycosides.
Cefoperazone	none reported
Ceftazidine	headache, dizziness, rarely-paresthesias
Gentamicin	Eighth cranial nerve—hearing and balance. Dizziness, vertigo, tinnitus, hearing loss—especially with renal impairment, dehydration, and other ototoxic drugs.
Piperacillin	Headache, dizziness, fatigue
Vancomycin	Rare vertigo, tinnitus, dizziness, hearing loss, with concomitant ototoxic drug administration or decreased renal function

events. Most frequently it is caused by hypoxia or ischemia, followed by hepatic failure, and renal failure with associated uremia and electrolyte imbalances (Davis and Patchell 1988; Patchell et al. 1985).

Another encephalopathic syndrome, idiopathic hyperammonemia, is seen after high-dose chemotherapy, and its abrupt development is associated with a grave prognosis (Mitchell et al. 1988). Clinically, the condition is characterized by a severe, sudden alteration in mental status and respiratory alkalosis in association with markedly elevated serum ammonia. It is usually apparent in the absence of liver dysfunction or any other identifiable cause, and progresses to coma and subsequent death (Mitchell et al. 1988).

In every case of encephalopathy, astute neurological assessment, monitoring of laboratory values, providing hydration, safety precautions, dialysis, oxygen therapy, and support for the family and patient are important interventions, usually with the goal of palliation.

Neurologic Complications of Immunosuppressive Agents

Immunosuppressive therapies are an integral part of bone marrow transplantation. Their role is in prevention of graft rejection and in the prophy-laxis and treatment of graft-versus-host disease (Walker and Brochstein 1988). Neurotoxic effects may be the sequelae of CNS infection resulting from prolonged immunosuppression, or may be a direct effect of the immunosuppressant agents. Table 11.3 summarizes the drugs, their action, and their use in BMT.

Cyclosporine

Cyclosporine (CyA) is a potent immunosuppressant with little myelocytic toxicity, used in BMT to reduce the incidence and severity of GVHD (McGuire et al. 1988). CyA makes the host tolerant of the allograft by selective inhibition of the T helper cells, while sparing T suppressor cells. The drug is administered intravenously usually the day before marrow infusion and continued for several weeks until recovery from chemo-radiotherapy-induced gastrointestinal toxicity (McGuire et al. 1988). At that time, an oral form is administered.

Neurologic complications occur in 10–25% of treated patients (Adams et al. 1987; DeGroen et al. 1987). Major side effects of the drug have been reported as tremors in 16–50% of patients, grand mal seizures in 5.5% (Deierhoi et al. 1988), and depression (Morris 1981). In addition, paresthesias have been noted in 29% of patients receiving CyA (McGuire et al. 1988), as well as quadriparesis, cerebellar ataxia and coma (Deierhoi et al. 1988). Burning dysesthesias of palms

Table 11.3. Immunosuppressive Therapies and Their Roles in BMT

Immunosuppressant	Action	Use in BMT	Neurologic Complications
Cyclosporine	Inhibits T helper cells	Reduces incidence and severity of GVHD	Confusion, tremors, seizures, paresthesias, muscle weakness, cerebellar ataxia, coma, LEC
Methotrexate	Antifolate metabolite; immunosuppressant	BMT prophylaxis and GVHD treatment	Aseptic meningitis, somnolence, transverse myelopathy, seizures, strokelike syndrome, confusion
High-dose cytosine arabinoside	Cell-cycle specific antimetabolite; causes intense myelosuppression	Pre-BMT conditioning	Cerebellar dysfunction, periph. neuropathy, Guillain-Barre syndrome, Parkinsonism, encephalopathy
Corticosteroids	Suppresses immune response at all levels	GVHD prophylaxis	Agitation, psychosis, seizures, steroid myopathy, increased intracranial pressure
Antithymocyte globulin	Lymphocyte-specific immunosuppressant	Prevents allogeneic bone marrow graft rejection	Headache, seizures
OKT-3 monoclonal antibody	Binds all immunocomponents of post-thymic T lymphocytes	Acute rejection treatment and GVHD prophylaxis	Headache, tremors, aseptic meningitis
Azathioprine	Immunosuppressive antimetabolite	Prevents graft rejection	No direct neurotoxic effects

and soles of feet have also been documented (Berden et al. 1985).

Conditions related to the transplant process may increase patient response to the side effects of CyA. For example, BMT patients are predisposed to the development of seizures related to previous chemotherapy and irradiation, which may lower their seizure threshold (Thomas et al. 1975; Walker and Brochstein 1988). Therefore, the potential for seizures due to CyA is increased in BMT recipients. Depression as a side effect of CyA may exacerbate depression related to the transplant process that the patient may already be experiencing.

The probability and severity of side effects is related to CyA levels in the blood. A bolus dose of CyA, which causes a rapid increase in the serum level, will result in greater toxicity (Deierhoi et al. 1988; McGuire et al. 1988) than a continuous infusion. Another factor precipitating seizures includes the simultaneous use of CyA and high-dose prednisone (Polson et al. 1985).

Hypomagnesemia has been reported to be strongly associated with CyA-neurotoxicity. CyA disrupts renal tubular function, which results in renal magnesium wasting (June et al. 1985). The occurrence of grand mal seizures in patients on CyA is strongly associated with magnesium levels two standard deviations below normal values (Adams et al. 1987). Normalization of the magnesium levels usually results in cessation of the seizures. In addition, extremely high serum CyA levels were recorded at the onset of seizure activity (Deierhoi et al. 1988; Adams et al. 1987; Rubin and Kang 1987).

Another effect of the drug, which may have neurologic implications, is its ability to engender hypertension (McGuire et al. 1988). Fortunately, it may be well controlled with medication. Although the role of magnesium is not implicitly stated, hypomagnesemia is proven to be linked to hypertension (June et al. 1986). Therefore, hypertension may result from CyA-induced hypomagnesemia.

Infrequently, a form of leukoencephalopathy (LEC) (described later) may be caused by CyA. Clinical presentation shows confusion and cortical blindness, which may progress to coma (DeGroen et al. 1987). Pathologic white matter degeneration and EEG slowing are present.

Another syndrome found in BMT patients consisted of ataxia and tremor, and occasional paresis and mental status changes, in the absence of CT or EEG abnormalities (Atkinson et al. 1984). The etiology is postulated to be a reaction to CyA, either caused or enhanced by hypomagnesemia (Thompson et al. 1984). Uncommonly, CyA may cause visual hallucinations (Katirji 1987) or neuropathy (DeGroen et al. 1987).

Neurological sequelae of CyA therapy are usually not permanent. Complete symptom resolution for all neurologic complications, including severe encephalopathy has been achieved with a decrease in the dosage or withdrawal of the drug (Walker and Brochstein 1988).

Care of the patient receiving CyA includes preferably continuous administration of the drug and daily monitoring of magnesium levels, with magnesium replacement as necessary (Thompson et al. 1984). Cyclosporine levels should also be monitored at least weekly. Administration of CyA in a bolus dose, or to patients with poor renal function requires close neurological supervision,

seizure precautions as necessary, and the monitoring of intake and output, weight, blood urea nitrogen, and creatinine levels. Frequent monitoring of vital signs and administration of antihypertensive medication as needed is extremely important, as post-BMT thrombocytopenia places the patient with high blood pressure at risk for a cranial bleed.

Predischarge teaching should include avoiding refrigeration of oral cyclosporine; using opened containers of CyA within two months, and preparing CyA in a glass container, as the drug potentially may stick to plastic (Barnhart 1988). Additionally, foods high in magnesium (nuts, soybeans, cocoa, seafood, whole grains, dried beans, and peas) are recommended (Lums 1973).

Methotrexate

Methotrexate (MTX), an antifolate metabolite, is an effective immunosuppressant used primarily in BMT for prophylaxis and treatment of GVHD (Walker and Brochstein 1988; Thomas et al. 1975). Neurotoxicity is a well documented complication, and may be acute or chronic, depending on the dose and route of administration (Balis and Poplack 1989).

For GVHD prophylaxis, intravenous MTX is usually given thrice weekly during the first week post-transplant, and once weekly thereafter in a dose of $10mg/m^2$. Neurologic symptoms associated with intravenous high-dose methotrexate (HDMTX) include acute somnolence, fatigue, confusion, disorientation, seizures, or increased intracranial pressure during or after administration (Bleyer 1988). Adults seem to have a higher incidence of HDMTX-induced sedation than children. Seizures rarely have been documented during the infusion (Bleyer 1977). The toxicity is thought to be mediated by lysis of tumor cells in the CNS, and may cause cerebral edema. It is rapidly reversed by the administration of systemic corticoids (Bleyer 1988).

HDMTX may also produce a strokelike syndrome in adults and children (Allen and Rosen

1978; Bleyer 1981; Walker et al. 1986), which typically occurs five to six days after completing a course of the drug (Walker and Brochstein 1988). Patients present with an altered mental status, usually accompanied by hemiparesis and other focal findings, such as aphasia, dysarthria, and cranial nerve and gaze palsies (Bleyer 1981; Walker and Brochstein 1988). The signs may vacillate between alternate sides of the body. Without treatment, the syndrome resolves within 48–72 hours, and usually without residual effects or fear of recurrence during subsequent MTX treatments (Walker and Brochstein 1988). The etiology and pathogenesis of this syndrome is unknown. CT scan and lumbar puncture results are normal; EEG shows solely some slowing (Walker and Brochstein 1988).

Recipients of BMT for a hematologic malignancy are given a single dose of MTX intrathecally (IT-MTX), just prior to BMT (Walker and Brochstein 1988). Acute effects of IT-MTX are manifested as aseptic meningitis and transverse myelopathy. Aseptic meningitis occurs in approximately 10% of patients receiving IT-MTX (Walker and Brochstein 1988). Aseptic meningitis mimics bacterial meningitis but occurs soon after the injection, with symptoms of headache, photophobia, fever, meningismus, nausea and vomiting, and lethargy (Bleyer 1977; Bleyer 1981). The syndrome is self-limiting, and symptoms resolve within a few days. Analgesia may be administered for headaches. Patients who develop meningitis may not necessarily experience the syndrome with subsequent injections (Walker and Brochstein 1988). No risk factors for this syndrome have been identified.

Transverse myelopathy occurs rarely, and is the result of multiple intrathecal MTX injections (Bleyer 1981; Gagliano and Costanzi 1976). It presents within 48 hours of administration, but may be delayed for up to two weeks (Walker and Brochstein 1988). The presence of CNS leukemia or prior irradiation may predispose patients to the myelopathy; other risk factors remain unclear (Luddy and Gilman 1973). By an unknown mech-

anism, the patients experience back pain, which may or may not radiate to the legs. These symptoms are followed by a loss of sensation, bowel and bladder dysfunction, and paraplegia (Bleyer 1981; Walker and Brochstein 1988). Spinal cord necrosis without striking vascular or inflammatory change is seen (Skullerud and Halvorsen 1978). There is no treatment for this myelopathy. Symptoms may be permanent, but are generally reversible after the drug is discontinued or the dosage is reduced (Bleyer 1981). This form of neurotoxicity appears related to the concentration and duration of MTX in the CNS (Pizzo et al. 1979).

Leukoencephalopathy, discussed later, is a delayed effect of MTX administration, and one with the most severe consequences. MTX-induced neurotoxicity seems limited to those patients undergoing BMT for a hematologic malignancy (Walker and Brochstein 1988). A possible explanation may be that these syndromes, with the exception of the stroke syndrome, are related to prolonged exposure to high CNS drug concentrations and previous irradiation (Balis and Poplack 1989).

Nurses must be cognizant of the potential for neurotoxicity related to MTX administration. Frequent neurologic assessments should be part of the daily care. When neurotoxicity from MTX is diagnosed or suspected, the drug should be discontinued, in favor of alternative therapies.

Corticosteroids

Glucocorticoids suppress the immune response at all levels, and are used for GVHD prophylaxis (Baxter and Forsham 1972). However, they disadvantageously may permit uncontrolled spread of infection or superinfection, as well as adversely affect metabolism (Walker and Brochstein 1988).

Neurologically, mental status changes may develop. These range from euphoria or agitation (in 40% of patients) to psychosis. Risk factors are not related to age, previous psychiatric illness, or previous steroid use (Hall et al. 1979; Walker and

Brochstein 1988). Steroid psychosis, when present, correlates with the total dose, usually greater than 40mg prednisone daily (Greeves 1984). Females are slightly more susceptible.

Mental symptoms may occur at any time during steroid treatment (Greeves 1984). Withdrawal of the drug is the most effective way to treat mental status changes, although the disease for which the steroids are being administered, and the necessity for a gradual tapering of the dose may make this difficult (Walker and Brochstein 1988). Alternatively, phenothiazines or butyrophenones may be used to treat unwanted symptoms.

Steroid myopathy is characterized by symmetrical involvement of proximal muscles (Walker and Brochstein 1988). Although a mild degree of weakness is seen in all patients receiving steroidal therapy for two to three weeks, prolonged administration is directly related to the severity of myopathy (Janssens and Decramer 1989). Patients may be unable to rise from a chair, brush hair, or climb stairs, and the myopathy may potentially progress to involve respiratory muscles (Walker and Brochstein 1988).

The treatment for these complications is withdrawal of the drug or the use of nonfluorinated steroids, which have a lower tendency towards causing myopathy (Walker and Brochstein 1988). Complete symptom resolution can be expected weeks to months after the drug is discontinued (Janssens and Decramer 1989).

Antithymocyte Globulin

Antithymocyte globulin (ATG) is a lymphocyte-specific immunosuppressant, which may be used to prevent allogeneic bone marrow graft rejection (Malilay et al. 1989). No specific neurologic complications have been documented. Headaches and seizures, potential effects listed on the package insert, occur less than 5% of the time (Walker and Brochstein 1988).

OKT-3 Monoclonal Antibody

OKT-3, a monoclonal antibody, which binds to post-thymic T lymphocytes, is efficacious in GVHD prophylaxis and in treating acute rejection after allogeneic BMT (Filipovich et al. 1987). General neurologic side effects include headaches and tremors in 25% and 10% of recipients, respectively (Thistlethwaite et al. 1987; Walker and Brochstein 1988). The patient usually does not experience the side effects after the first or second dose of the drug. OKT-3 represents one of many pharmacologic attempts to control graft-versus-host disease. Because no modality has been proven most effective, multicenter research trials continue different treatment modalities that work in theory or in vitro, in the hopes of finding the best drug. As a result, OKT-3 is not universally administered.

A CNS syndrome specifically associated with OKT-3 has been identified (Walker and Brochstein 1988). A form of aseptic meningitis may develop two to seven days after the initiation of therapy (Roden et al. 1987; Thistlethwaite et al. 1987). Symptoms include fever, headache, photophobia, and meningismus. This clinical syndrome resolves without residua or treatment in two to three days, and does not require the cessation of OKT-3 therapy. The pathogenesis of this treatment-related inflammation is unknown (Walker and Brochstein 1988). It is extremely important that it be distinguished from a serious CNS infection.

Azathioprine

Another drug used to prevent graft rejection is azathioprine, an immunosuppressive antimetabolite that is metabolized to mercaptopurine (Walker and Brochstein 1988). Direct neurotoxic effects have not been seen with this drug.

Summary

With the number of successful bone marrow transplants increasing, we can expect to see more patients suffering from neurotoxicity related to modalities necessary for their survival.

Leukoencephalopathy

Leukoencephalopathy (LEC) is a degenerative lesion occurring in the white matter of the CNS in approximately 7% of patients receiving cranial irradiation and intrathecal chemotherapy (Frytak et al. 1989; Thompson et al. 1986). The onset is approximately three to five months after bone marrow transplantation (Thompson et al. 1986).

LEC is characterized by severe neurologic degeneration resulting in permanent neurologic disability or death (Johnson et al. 1987). Clinically, LEC presents as lethargy, slurred speech, ataxia, seizures, abnormal EEG, confusion, dysphagia, akinetic mutism, spasticity, aphasia, decerebrate posturing, and coma (Balis and Poplack 1989; Devinsky et al. 1987).

The development of LEC is most closely associated with pretransplant treatment with cranial irradiation in combination with intrathecal methotrexate (IT-MTX) and/or high-dose intravenous methotrexate (HDMTX), and usually IT-MTX post-transplant (Mohrmann et al. 1990; Thompson et al. 1986).

Administration of MTX after total body irradiation contributes directly to the development of LEC (Johnson et al. 1987). The risk of developing LEC also seems heightened if the patient has received a high dose of cranial irradiation (> 2000cGy) (Thompson et al. 1986); if the MTX is given either during or after radiation (Frytak et al. 1989); and if the cumulative dose of MTX is high (Thompson et al. 1986).

Speculation as to the causality of these mechanisms centers around these hypotheses: (1) CNS irradiation alters the kinetics of the CNS, causing accumulation of large amounts of antifolate in certain areas of the brain (Bleyer, 1981); and (2) radiation may disrupt the blood-brain barrier, allowing systemically administered MTX to enter the brain (Frytak et al. 1989; Devinsky et al. 1987); or (3) radiation increases the vulnerability of the white matter to the effects of IT-MTX and/or HDMTX (Rubenstein et al. 1975). Also, a positive risk was found with the development of LEC

in BMT patients with ALL; LEC in the patient with acute nonlymphocytic leukemia is rare (Davis and Patchell, 1988).

LEC is not found to be associated with age, sex, acute or chronic GVHD, or bone marrow status at the time of transplant (Thompson et al. 1986). Nor has a causal link been established between LEC and bacterial infections, nutrition, CNS leukemia, or systemically circulating drugs other than MTX (Price and Jamieson 1975).

Despite a study by Price and Jamieson (1975), which concluded that benzyl alcohol is not a causative factor in the development of LEC, benzyl alcohol has been found to have neurotoxic effects (Conrad 1986). Therefore, its use in reconstituting MTX should be avoided. Alternatively, Elliott's B solution may be used (Humphrey et al. 1979). Combining MTX with hydrocortisone, and using a standard dose of MTX in patients three years and older, may help decrease the neurotoxicity (Humphrey et al. 1979; Bleyer 1977). An MTX dose based on body surface area is discouraged in persons older than three years because the cerebrospinal fluid volume is constant after that age. Additionally, judicious use of radiation therapy is essential to preventing relapse and minimizing the potential development of devastating LEC (Thompson et al. 1986).

Vascular Complications

Mineralizing microangiopathy, a complication of radiation therapy, causes dystrophic calcification of CNS grey matter (Davis et al. 1986). This degeneration usually is apparent approximately ten months after radiation therapy, and occurs much more frequently than LEC. Identified risk factors for the development of this dystrophy include a young age (less that ten years at the time of radiation), duration of survival after radiotherapy, and the number of CNS leukemic relapses after radiation therapy (Price 1979). The clinical manifestations are less evident than those of LEC, and include focal seizures, poor muscle coordination, abnormal EEG, perceptual motor disability and behavioral disorders (Packer et al. 1987).

While radiation to the cranium is directly related to the development of the dystrophic calcification, it has not yet been established whether chemotherapy influences the process. One study implies that certain doses of MTX and cytosine arabinoside influence the progression of the lesion, but that their role is contributory rather than engendering (McIntosh et al. 1977).

Because mineralizing microangiopathy is not easily controlled, neurologic examinations are important for all patients receiving radiation therapy and chemotherapy, especially those in high-risk groups. If clinical symptoms appear, a head CT may be valuable in early diagnosis of the lesion (Davis et al. 1986). Although mineralizing microangiopathy causes permanent destructive changes in the brain, its effect on neuropsychological functioning has not yet been established (Packer et al. 1987). One study showed that four out of five children who had received a BMT and underwent neuropsychological testing had abnormal results. Although IQ scores were within the normal range, deficiencies were found in auditory skills, visual-motor skills, and motor function (Wiznitzer et al. 1984). It was not revealed whether these children had mineralizing microangiopathy. Since it most commonly affects children, research needs to be done to determine the long-term sequelae.

Cerebrovascular complications, the third most common neurologic complication, have been found in 6–28% of patients undergoing BMT (Mohrmann et al. 1990 and 1987; Patchell et al. 1985; Wiznitzer et al. 1984). Subarachnoid hemorrhages and infarcts occur with equal frequency. Interestingly, parenchymal hemorrhages are rare, despite extremely low platelet counts in all bone marrow transplant patients (Davis and Patchell 1988).

Cerebral infarcts are most commonly associated with endocarditis (Patchell 1985). BMT recipients have a higher incidence of developing endocarditis than those with similar diseases who do not undergo BMT, most likely resulting from the additive effects of prior chemoradiotherapy (Wiznitzer et al. 1984). For a review of nonbacterial thrombotic endocarditis (NBTE) and its etiology in bone marrow transplant, the reader is referred to Chapter 8, on pulmonary and cardiac complications.

Cerebrovascular accidents due to NBTE are an important cause of morbidity in BMT recipients. Emboli to the CNS and heart may also manifest as seizures and focal neurologic or myocardial dysfunction (Rosen and Armstrong 1973). Therefore, nurses must institute seizure precautions and assess the patient's neurologic status frequently. Monitoring of the DIC screen, especially fibrinogen and fibrin degradation product may aid in the diagnosis, and treatment with anticoagulation may prevent the associated morbidity (Jerman and Fick 1986).

Neurologic Complications of Graft-Versus-Host Disease

For a complete discussion of GVHD, the reader is referred to Chapter 7. In relation to neurologic complications, it is important to know that primary CNS involvement of GVHD has not been recognized (Nelson and McQuillen 1988). Peripheral nerve inflammatory disease is a rare, if ever, clinically recognized complication of GVHD. Acute GVHD is not associated with neurologic dysfunction, therefore, this section of the chapter will be devoted to the neurologic manifestations of chronic GVHD.

Chronic GVHD is the result of a cell-mediated response of donor lymphocytes against host antigens (Nelson and McQuillen 1988). The cell-mediated and humoral limbs of the immune system are both impaired, and this may give rise to myositis and myasthenia gravis. The target antigens in chronic GVHD have not been identified, with the exception of the acetylcholine receptor in the myasthenia gravis (Nelson and McQuillen 1988).

Myositis

Myositis, like chronic GVHD, is more common in older patients (Slatkin et al. 1987). It has not been seen in autologous or syngeneic BMT recipients (Nelson and McQuillen 1988); these populations are also not at risk for developing GVHD. Those at greatest risk have undergone BMT for aplastic anemia (Slatkin et al. 1987).

The muscle is a target organ in GVHD (Anderson et al. 1982). Moderate to severe muscle weakness is the remarkable clinical presentation, which is indistinguishable from idiopathic polymyositis in symptomatology, pathology, and serology (Nelson and McQuillen 1988; Urbano-Marquez et al. 1986). In most cases, prednisone administration may improve strength (Reyes et al. 1983; Sullivan and Parkman 1983). Azathioprine has also been used with some efficacy (Reyes et al. 1983; Sullivan and Parkman 1983).

The progression or resolution of the chronic GVHD is the most important factor in determining the severity of the myositis (Nelson and McQuillen 1988). If the GVHD improves, the muscle weakness will resolve proportionately; and the converse is true.

Care of the patient with myositis focuses on safety. Teaching patients and family the etiology of the weakness and requiring the patient to ambulate or get out of bed with assistance only, is very important. Encouraging range of motion exercises and fostering as much independence in self care as possible, are essential for physical and psychological coping.

Myasthenia Gravis

A rare complication of chronic GVHD, myasthenia gravis, is the result of an antibody-mediated response specifically against the acetylcholine receptor (Grau et al. 1990). Its presentation is very similar to the autoimmune variety of myasthenia gravis. Symptoms include dysarthria, ptosis, diplopia, dysphagia, and weakness of facial and limb muscles (Bolger et al. 1986). It may progress to involve the muscles of respiration, ultimately leading to failure.

Treatment with steroids, azathioprine, and pyridostigmine is appropriate (Grau et al. 1990). Respiratory failure may necessitate intubation. Plasmapheresis and continued drug therapy have been successful in reversing the condition, allowing extubation (Bolger et al. 1986). The cessation of immunosuppressive therapy may precipitate a return of myasthenic symptoms (Bolger et al. 1986; Nelson and McQuillen 1988). In some cases, patients may be maintained on low doses of immunosuppressive therapy.

Although most patients with GVHD and myasthenia gravis have aplastic anemia as their primary disease (Nelson and McQuillen 1988), it is unclear which patients with GVHD are at risk for developing myasthenia gravis (Bolger et al. 1986).

Nursing care for patients with myasthenia gravis includes teaching the importance of compliance with medication regimes, and encouragement to seek immediate medical attention in the event of any abnormal neurological symptoms. Safety precautions and frequent neurologic examinations are important. Psychological support for the patient and family may be necessary to facilitate coping with this setback. Creative methods of communication with the intubated patient are also a necessity.

Central Nervous System Relapse of Disease

One of the major causes of treatment failure in allogeneic BMT for acute leukemia is a recurrence of the leukemia, which occurs in 5-75% of patients (Kelch et al. 1990; Mohrmann et al. 1990; Champlin and Gale 1987). Acute lymphoblastic leukemia is associated with a higher rate of CNS relapse (approximately 13%) than acute nonlymphoblastic leukemia (approximately 2%)

(Thompson et al. 1986). Relapse of leukemia after BMT generally represents a failure of the preparative chemotherapy or TBI to eradicate the patient's leukemic clone or may be due to a continued leukemogenic stimuli of the patient's cells on donor cells (Kelch et al. 1990; Ganem et al. 1989). Generally, the risk of relapse is greatest in those patients with advanced disease who undergo transplantation.

The CNS may be the site of relapse, regardless of whether the patient had previous CNS involvement. CNS leukemia can cause systemic relapse (Bleyer 1989). A recent study indicates an increased risk for post-BMT CNS complications in patients with pre-BMT CNS disease (Ganem et al. 1989).

Secondary Malignancy in the Central Nervous System

While chemotherapy and radiotherapy are important in bone marrow ablation prior to transplantation, they impose a risk, though small, that patients will develop a secondary malignancy (Applebaum and Thomas 1985). The etiology seems to be multifactorial and includes chemoradiotherapy treatments before the transplant, the preparative regimen, Epstein-Barr Virus (EBV) infection, immunosuppression, and chronic GVHD (Lishner et al. 1990; Ochs 1989). Characteristic of these secondary malignancies is a long latency period after initial exposure to chemoradiotherapy, a mean of 5–9 years (Ochs 1989; Champlin and Gale 1987).

Following BMT for the treatment of a hematologic malignancy, patients have developed leukemia of donor cell origin (Ochs 1989), lymphoproliferative disorders, including Hodgkin's Disease (Serota et al. 1983), and solid tumors, such as glioblastoma multiforme, adenocarcinoma, and squamous cell carcinoma (Deeg 1984; Lishner et al. 1990). Total body irradiation may

play a role in the development of solid tumors following BMT (Ochs 1989). Gliomas are the most common form of secondary malignancy following radiation therapy in children; meningiomas are the most common in adults (Ochs 1989).

Secondary gliomas are multifocal in origin and their abrupt clinical manifestation is characterized by seizures, increased intracranial pressure, or significant motor disability (Ochs 1989). Carcinomas may develop in radiation ports (such as the thyroid, basal cell, and parotid gland) of children who have undergone previous radiation therapy (Ochs 1989).

Patients and families must be made aware of the potential for secondary malignancy following BMT, and the importance of frequent medical check-ups. Support must be offered to the patient and family if relapse or secondary malignancy occur. If the prognosis is poor, hospice care may be appropriate.

Nursing Care of the Bone Marrow Transplant Patient with Neurologic Complications

A nursing care plan that addresses actual or potential sequelae of BMT-related neurologic complications can be found later in this text. These problems may be manifested by LEC, mineralizing microangiopathy, infections, immunosuppressive therapies, metabolic encephalopathy, myositis, myasthenia gravis, or CVA. The focus of care relates to the early detection of neurologic dysfunction and post-discharge teaching in an effort to ameliorate or prevent further impairment. If neurologic complications occur, nursing efforts must be directed at safety and teaching patients and families measures to preserve and support independence in self care. An interdisciplinary approach that involves physical and occupational therapy may be necessary to optimize patient functioning. This plan of care can serve as a framework to develop an individualized approach to the patient with actual or potential neurologic disturbance.

Summary

As the number of bone marrow transplant recipients increases, the likelihood that they will experience complications from the treatment also increases. Literature review reveals a paucity of medical and nursing research specifically dealing with the neurologic sequelae of bone marrow transplant. When one considers that neurotoxicity may have a significant impact on an individual's ability to engage in self-care (Cammermeyer 1983), thus threatening an individual's independence, neurologic impairment has far-reaching implications for medical, nursing, and self-care. Nurses must be alert to these potential complications, and, through assessment and teaching, prevent or ameliorate their effects.

Acknowledgement: I would like to thank Stephen Meriney for the patience, support, and encouragement, without which this would not have been possible.

References

Ackerman, Z. et al. 1986. Cerebral Toxoplasmosis complicating bone marrow transplantation. *Isr. J. Med. Sci.*, 22: 582–586.

Adams, D.H. et al. 1987. Neurological complications following liver transplantation. *Lancet 1*: 949–951.

Allen, J.C., and Rosen, G. 1978. Transient cerebral dysfunction following chemotherapy for osteogenic sarcoma. *Ann. Neurol. 3*: 441–444.

Applebaum, F.R., and Thomas, E.D. 1985. Treatment of acute leukemia in adults with chemoradiotherapy and bone marrow transplantation. *Cancer 55*: 2202–2209.

Atkinson, K. et al. 1980. Varicella-zoster virus infection after marrow transplantation for aplastic anemia or leukemia. *Transplantation 29*(1): 47–50.

Atkinson, K. et al. 1984. Cyclosporine-associated central nervous system toxicity after allogeneic bone marrow transplantation. *Transplantation 38*: 34–37.

Balis, F.M., and Poplack, D.G. 1989. Central nervous system pharmacology of antileukemic drugs. *Am. J. Pediatric Hematol./Oncol. 11* (1): 74–86.

Barnett, M.J. et al. 1987. A phase II study of high-dose cytosine arabinoside in the treatment of acute leukaemia in adults. *Cancer Chemother. Pharmacol. 19*: 169–171.

Barnhart, E.R. 1988. *Physician's Desk Reference*. New Jersey: Medical Economics Co.: 744, 779-780, 1007, 1166, 1217, 1768, 1879–1881, 1914.

Baxter, J.D., and Forsham, P.H. 1972. Tissue effects of glucocorticoids. *Am. J. Med. 53*: 573–589.

Berden, J.H.M. et al. 1985. Severe central nervous system toxicity associated with cyclosporin. Letter. *Lancet 1*: 219–220.

Bleyer, W.A. 1977. Clinical pharmacology of intrathecal methotrexate. II. An improved dosage regimen derived from age-related pharmacokinetics. *Cancer Treat. Rep. 61*: 1419–1425.

Bleyer, W.A. 1981. Neurologic sequelae of methotrexate and ionizing radiation: A new classification. *Cancer Treat. Rep. 65*: 89–98 (suppl. 1).

Bleyer, W.A. 1988. Central nervous system leukemia. *Pediatric Clin. North Am. 35* (4): 789–814.

Bleyer, W.A. 1989. Biology and pathogenesis of CNS leukemia. *Am. J. Pediatr. Hematol./Oncol. 11* (1): 57–63.

Bolger, G.B. et al. 1986. Myasthenia gravis after allogeneic bone marrow transplantation: Relationship to chronic graft vs. host disease. *Neurology 36*: 1087–1091.

Bolwell, B.J. et al. 1988. High dose cytarabine: A review. *Leukemia, 2*: 253–260.

Borgeat, A. et al. 1986. Peripheral neuropathy associated with high dose Ara-C therapy. *Cancer 58* (4): 852–854.

Bowden, R.A. et al. 1986. Cytomegalovirus immune globulin and seronegative blood products to prevent primary cytomegalovirus infections after bone marrow transplantation. *New Engl. J. Med. 314*: 1006–1010.

Brammer, K.W. 1990. Management of fungal infection in neutropenic patients with fluconazole. *Haematologie und Bluttransfusion 33*: 546–550.

Callaham, M. 1989. Fulminant bacterial meningitis without meningeal sign. *Ann. Emerg. Med. 8* (1): 90–93.

Cammermeyer, M. 1983. A growth model of self care for neurologically impaired people. *J. Neurosurg. Nurs. 15*: 299–305.

Cersosimo, R.J. et al. 1987. Acute cerebellar syndrome, conjunctivitis, and hearing loss associated with low-dose cytarabine administration. *DICP 21* (10): 798–803.

Champlin, R.E. et al. 1989. Treatment of acute myelogenous leukemia in the elderly. *Sem. Oncol. 16*: 51–56.

Champlin, R.C., and Gale, R.P. 1987. Bone marrow transplantation for acute leukemia: Recent advances and comparison with alternative therapies. *Sem. Hematol. 24*: 55–67.

Conrad, K.J. 1986. Cerebellar toxicities associated with cytosine arabinoside: A nursing perspective. *O.N.F. 13*: 57–59.

Davis, D. et al. 1988. Fatal Adenovirus meningoencephalitis in a bone marrow transplant patient. *Ann. Neurol. 23*: 385–389.

Davis, D., and Patchell, R.A. 1988. Neurologic complications of bone marrow transplantation. *Neurol. Clin. 6:* 377–387.

Davis, P.C. et al. 1986. CT evaluation of effects of cranial radiation therapy in children. *Am. J. Roentgenol. 147*(3): 587–592.

Deeg, H.J. 1984. Bone marrow transplantation: A review of delayed complications. *Br. J. Haematol. 57:* 185–208.

DeGroen, P.C. et al. 1987. Central nervous system toxicity after liver transplantation. *N. Engl. J. Med. 317:* 861–866.

Deierhoi, M.H. et al. 1988. Cyclosporine neurotoxicity in liver transplant recipients: Report of three cases. *Transplant. Proc. 20* (1): 116–118.

Derouin, F. et al. 1985. Early diagnosis of Toxoplasmosis after bone marrow transplantation. *Exp. Hematol. 13:* 73 (suppl. 17).

Devinsky, O. et al. 1987. Akinetic mutism in a bone marrow transplant recipient following total-body irradiation and amphotericin B chemoprophylaxis. *Arch. Neurol. 44:* 414–417.

Dunton, S.F. et al. 1986. Progressive ascending paralysis following administration of intrathecal and intravenous cytosine arabinoside. *Cancer 57:* 1083–1086.

Filipovich, A.H. et al. 1987. Graft-versus-host disease prevention in allogeneic bone marrow transplantation from histocompatible siblings. A pilot study using immunotoxins for T cell depletion of donor bone marrow. *Transplantation 44* (1): 62–69.

Ford, R., and Eisenberg, S. 1990. Bone marrow tranplant. Recent advances and nursing implications. *Nurs. Clin. N. Am. 25* (2): 405–422.

Francke, E. 1987. The many causes of meningitis. *Postgrad. Med. 82* (2): 175–178, 181–183, 187–188.

Frytak, S. et al. 1989. Leukoencephalopathy in small cell lung cancer patients receiving prophylactic cranial irradiation. *Am. J. Clin. Oncol. 12* (1): 27–33.

Gagliano, R.G., and Costanzi, J.J. 1976. Paraplegia following intrathecal methotrexate. *Cancer 37:* 1663–1668.

Ganem, G. et al. 1989. Central nervous system relapses after bone marrow transplantation for acute lymphoblastic leukemia in remission. *Cancer 64* (9): 1796–1804.

Gottlieb, D. et al. 1987. The neurotoxicity of high dose cytarabine arabinoside is age related. *Cancer 60:* 1439–1441.

Grau, J.M. et al. 1990. Myasthenia gravis after allogeneic bone marrow transplantation: Report of a new case and pathogenic considerations. *B.M.T. 5*(6): 435–437.

Greeves, J.A. 1984. Rapid-onset steroid psychosis with very low dosage of prednisolone. Letter. *Lancet 1:* 1119–1120.

Hall, R.C.W. et al. 1979. Presentation of the steroid psychoses. *J. Nerv. Ment. Dis. 167:* 229–236.

Hara, K.S. et al. 1989. Disseminated Aspergillus terreus infection in immunocompromised hosts. *Mayo Clin. Proc. 64* (7): 770–775.

Holland, G.N. 1989. Ocular toxoplasmosis in the immunocompromised host. *International Opth. 13* (6): 399–402.

Humphrey, G.B. et al. 1979. Treatment of overt CNS leukemia. *Am. J. Pediatr. Hematol./Oncol. (1):* 37–47.

Iacobini, S.H. et al. 1986. High-dose cytosine arabinoside: Treatment and cellular pharmacology of chronic myelogenous leukemia blast crisis. *J. Clin. Oncol. 4:* 1079–1088.

Janssens, S., and Decramer, M. 1989. Corticosteriod-induced myopathy and the respiratory muscles. Report of two cases. *Chest 95* (5): 1160–1162.

Jerman, M.R., and Fick, R.B. 1986. Nonbacterial thrombotic endocarditis associated with bone marrow transplantation. *Chest 90* (6): 919–922.

Johnson, N.T. et al. 1987. Acute acquired demyelinating polyneuropathy with respiratory failure following high-dose systemic cytosine arabinoside and marrow transplantation. *B.M.T. 2:* 203–207.

June, C.H. et al. 1985. Profound hypomagnesemia and renal magnesium wasting associated with the use of cyclosporine for marrow transplantation. *Transplantation 39:* 620–624.

June, C.H. et al. 1986. Correlation of hypomagnesemia with the onset of cyclosporine-associated hypertension in marrow transplant patients. *Transplantation 41:* 47–51.

Katirji, M.B. 1987. Visual hallucinations and cyclosporine. *Transplantation 43:* 768–769.

Kelch, B.P. et al. 1990. An unusual extramedullary relapse of acute nonlymphocytic leukemia after allogeneic bone marrow transplantation. *Am. J. Clin. Oncol. 13* (3): 238–243.

Lefvert, A.K., and Bjorkholm, M. 1987. Antibodies against the acetylcholine receptor in hematologic disorders: Implications for the development of myasthenia gravis after bone marrow grafting. *N. Engl. J. Med. 316:* 170–171.

Lew, M.A. 1989. Diagnosis of systemic Candida infections. *Annu. Rev. Med. 40:* 87–97.

Lishner, M. et al. 1990. Cutaneous and mucosal neoplasms in bone marrow transplant recipients. *Cancer 65* (3): 473–476.

Locksley, R.M. et al. 1985. Infection with varicella-zoster virus after bone marrow transplantation. *J. Infect. Dis. 152:* 1172–1181.

Luddy, R.E., and Gilman, P.A. 1973. Paraplegia following intrathecal methotrexate. *J. Pediatr. 83:* 988–992.

Lums, S.R. 1973. The minerals. In Lums, S.R. (ed.). *Nutrition and diet therapy.* St. Louis: The CV Mosby Co.: 132–133.

Luque, F.A. et al. 1987. Parkinsonism induced by high-dose cytosine arabinoside. *Movement Disorders 2:* 219–222.

Malilay, G.P. et al. 1989. Prevention of graft rejection in allogeneic bone marrow transplantation: I. Preclinical studies with antithymocyte globulins. *B.M.T. 4:* 107–112.

McCabe, R.E., and Oster, S. 1989. Current recommendations and future prospects in the treatment of toxoplasmosis. *Drugs 38* (6): 973–987.

McGuire, T.R. et al. 1988. Influence of infusion duration on the efficacy and toxicity of intravenous cyclosporine in bone marrow transplant patients. *Transplantation Proc. 3:* 501–504 (suppl. 3).

McIntosh, S. et al. 1977. Intracranial calcifications in childhood leukemia; an association with systemic chemotherapy. *J. Pediatr. 91:* 909–913.

Meredith, J.T. 1987. Toxoplasmosis of the central nervous system. *Am. Fam. Physician 35* (5): 113–116.

Meyers, J.D. 1988. Management of Cytomegalovirus infection. *Am. J. Med. 85:* 102–106 (suppl. 2A).

Meyers, J.D. 1990. Fungal infections in bone marrow transplant patients. *Sem. Oncol. 17* (3): 10–13 (suppl. 6).

Milliken, S.T., and Powles, R.L. 1990. Antifungal prophylaxis in bone marrow transplantation. *Rev. Infect. Dis. 12:* S374–379 (suppl. 3).

Mitchell, P.H. et al. 1984. *Neurological Assessment for Nursing Practice.* Reston, VA: Reston Publishing Co.

Mitchell, R.B. et al. 1988. Syndrome of idiopathic hyperammonemia after high-dose chemotherapy: Review of nine cases. *Am. J. Med. 85:* 662–667.

Mohrmann, R.L. et al. 1987. Neuropathologic findings after bone marrow transplantation: An autopsy study. *J. Neuropathol. Exp. Neurol. 46:* Abst. #113, 369.

Mohrmann, R.L. et al. 1990. Neuropathologic findings after bone marrow transplantation: An autopsy study. *Human Pathol. 21* (6): 630–639.

Morris, P.J. 1981. Cyclosporin A. *Transplantation 32:* 349–354.

Nand, S. et al. 1986. Neurotoxicity associated with systemic high-dose cytosine arabinoside. *J. Clin. Oncol. 4:* 571–575.

Nelson, K.R., and McQuillen M.P. 1988. Neurologic complications of graft-versus-host disease. *Neurologic Clinics 6* (2): 389–403.

Ochs, J.J. 1989. Neurotoxicity due to central nervous system therapy for childhood leukemia. *Am. J. Pediatr. Hematol./Oncol. 11:* 93–105.

Packer, R.J. et al. 1987. Long-term sequelae of cancer treatment on the central nervous system in childhood. *Med. and Pediatric Oncol. 15* (5): 241–253.

Patchell, R.A. et al. 1985. Neurologic complications of bone marrow transplantation. *Neurology 35:* 300–306.

Patchell, R.A. 1985. Nonbacterial thrombotic endocarditis in bone marrow transplant patients. *Cancer 55:* 631–635.

Peeters, A. et al. 1989. Listeria monocytogenes meningitis. *Clin. Neurol. and Neurosurg. 91* (1): 29–36.

Perren, T.J. et al. 1988. Prevention of herpes zoster in patients by long-term oral acyclovir after allogeneic bone marrow transplantation. *Am. J. Med. 85:* 99–101 (suppl. 2A).

Peters, W.G. et al. 1988. High dose cytosine arabinoside: Pharmacological and clinical aspects. *Blut 56:* 1–11.

Pies, R. 1981. Persistent bipolar illness after steroid administration. *Arch. Int. Med. 141:* 1087.

Pizzo, P.A. et al. 1979. Neurotoxicities of current leukemia therapy. *Am. J. Ped. Hematol./Oncol. 1:* 127–139.

Polson, R.J. et al. 1985. Convulsions associated with cyclosporine A in transplant recipients. Letter. *Br. Med. J. 290:* 1003.

Price, R.A. 1979. Histopathology of CNS leukemia and complications of therapy. *Am. J. Pediatr. Hematol./Oncol. 1:* 21–30.

Price, R.A., and Jamieson, P.A. 1975. The central nervous system in childhood leukemia. II. Subacute leukoencephalopathy. *Cancer 35:* 306–318.

Reyes, M.G. et al. 1983. Myosistis of chronic graft-versus-host disease. *Neurology 33:* 1222–1226.

Roden, J. et al. 1987. Cerebrospinal fluid inflammation during OKT3 therapy. Letter. *Lancet 2:* 272.

Rogers, T.R. 1985. Prevention of infection in neutropenic bone marrow transplant patients. *Antibiotic Chemother. 33:* 90–113.

Rosen, P., and Armstrong, D. 1973. Nonbacterial thrombotic endocarditis in patients with malignant neoplastic diseases. *Am. J. Med. 54:* 23–29.

Rubenstein, L.J. et al. 1975. Disseminated necrotizing leukoencephalopathy: A complication of treated central nervous system leukemia and lymphoma. *Cancer 35:* 291–305.

Rubin, A.M., and Kang, H. 1987. Cerebral blindness and encephalopathy with cyclosporine A toxicity. *Neurology 37:* 1072–1076.

Serota, F.T. et al. 1983. Total body irradiation: Single vs. fractionated exposure as preparation for bone marrow transplantation in treatment of acute leukemia and aplastic anemia. *Int. J. Radiation Oncology Biol. Phys. 9:* 1941–1949.

Skullerud, K., and Halvorsen, K. 1978. Encephalomyelopathy following intrathecal methotrexate treatment in a child with acute leukemia. *Cancer 42:* 1211–1215.

Slatkin, N.F. et al. 1987. Myosistis as the major manifestation of chronic graft versus host disease (GVHD). *Neurology 37:* 205–211 (suppl. 1).

Spriggs, D.R. et al. 1988. Prolonged high dose ARA-C infusions in acute leukemia. *Leukemia 2:* 304–306.

Sullivan, K.M., and Parkman, R. 1983. The pathophysiology and treatment of graft-versus-host disease. *Clinical Haematology 12:* 775–789.

Sylvester, R.K. et al. 1987. Cytarabine-induced cerebellar syndrome: Case report and literature review. *Drug Intell. Clin. Pharm. 21:* 177–180.

Thistlethwaite, J.R. et al. 1987. OKT3 treatment of steroid-resistant renal allograft rejection. *Transplantation 43:* 176–184.

Thomas, E.D. et al. 1975. Bone marrow transplantation. *N. Engl. J. Med. 292:* 832–843.

Thompson, C.B. et al. 1984. Association between cyclosporin neurotoxicity and hypomagnesemia. *Lancet 2:* 1116–1120.

Thompson, C.B. et al. 1986. The risks of central nervous system relapse and leukoencephalopathy in pateints receiving marrow transplants for acute leukemia. *Blood 67* (1): 195–199.

Urbano-Marquez, A. et al. 1986. Inflammatory myopathy associated with chronic graft-versus-host disease. *Neurology 36:* 1091–1093.

van den Broek, P.J. 1988. Infection during neutropenia. *J. Hosp. Infect. 11:* 7–14 (suppl. A).

Wacker, P. et al. 1989. Varicella-zoster virus infections after autologous bone marrow transplantation in children. *B.M.T. 4:* 191–194.

Walker, R.W. et al. 1986. Transient cerebral dysfunction secondary to high-dose methotrexate. *J. Clin. Oncol. 4:* 1845–1850.

Walker, R.W., and Brochstein, J.A. 1988. Neurologic complications of immunosuppressive agents. *Neurol. Clinics 6* (2): 261–278.

Wiesner, R.H. et al. 1988. Selective bowel decontamination to decrease gram-negative aerobic bacterial and Candida colonization and prevent infection after orthotopic liver transplantation. *Transplantation 45* (3): 570–574.

Wingard, J.R. et al. 1987. Aspergillus infections in bone marrow transplant recipients. *B.M.T. 2:* 175–181.

Winston, D.J. et al. 1988. Prophylaxis of infection in bone marrow transplants. *Eur. J. Cancer and Clin. Oncol. 24:* S15–23 (suppl. 1).

Wiznitzer, M. et al. 1984. Neurologic complications of bone marrow transplantation in childhood. *Ann. Neurol. 16:* 569–576.

Zaia, J.A. 1990. Viral infections associated with bone marrow transplantation. *Hematol./Oncol. Clin. N. Am. 4* (3): 603–623.

Chapter 12

Psychosocial Impact of Bone Marrow Transplantation in Adult Patients:

Prehospitalization and Hospitalization Phases

Tim A. Ahles and Peggy Shedd

The psychosocial aspects of bone marrow transplantation (BMT) represent a wide variety of issues, some of which emerged long before the idea of BMT was contemplated by the patient. For the most part, BMT candidates have: (1) coped with the diagnosis of cancer for a significant period of time, (2) experienced chemotherapy and/or radiation and the side effects associated with these treatments, (3) experienced the emotional turmoil associated with relapse, and (4) dealt with the disruption of family, work, school, etc. Therefore, BMT is not a completely unique experience for the patient, but must be viewed within the larger context of living with cancer and its treatment. Unfortunately, to date, no longitudinal research exists examining the impact of previous experience with cancer on coping with BMT. The focus of the present chapter will be on adult BMT patients and their families and the psychosocial issues associated with the period prior to and dur-

ing hospitalization. A variety of psychosocial issues will be discussed. The major issues are further described in a nursing care plan format in Chapter 13. Psychosocial issues for the pediatric population are addressed in Chapter 5, and long-term effects are addressed in Chapter 15.

Prehospitalization

Numerous issues arise during the prehospitalization period, many of which were described in an early paper by Brown and Kelly (1976). First and foremost is the decision to enter a BMT program. This decision is often made at some distance from the transplant center, perhaps after making one visit for a screening evaluation. Consequently, patients are often unfamiliar with the caregivers, facilities, procedures, etc., and will undergo treatment while away from their typical social support network.

Integral to this decision making process is the hope for cure that BMT raises in some patients. Unfortunately, this hope is balanced against a rather frightening set of statistics regarding coping with the physical symptoms and prolonged hospitalization, and the high probability of mortality, morbidity, and relapse (see Part II). The decision making process is further complicated by several additional factors. Patients typically begin considering BMT while they are undergoing a fairly intense medical workup to determine whether or not they are BMT candidates. Therefore, an air of ambiguity surrounds the decision since it is often unclear whether they are BMT candidates at all or whether they will be accepted by a particular transplant center. The ambiguity is compounded by attempting to understand all of the information describing the BMT procedure. Patients are often given a research protocol to read which, for many, is very difficult to understand. Brown and Kelly (1976) describe the time pressure felt by many patients once the process of considering BMT has begun. For some, this is a realistic concern since the window of opportunity for performing BMT is narrow, while for others this is more a perceived time pressure.

This situation is also difficult because at this period, many patients are in remission (e.g., AML patients) or feel relatively healthy. For healthy patients, feeling better than they have for, perhaps, many months further complicates the contemplation of a dramatic procedure such as BMT.

Patients approach the decision to enter a BMT program differently. Some feel that they have no alternatives and are pleased that they have one more option. Others latch on to the chance for cure and become convinced that they will be one of the long-term survivors. Another subset of patients assiduously weigh the pros and cons of conventional treatment alternatives versus BMT. The latter group may be growing in number as BMT is offered earlier in the disease process (e.g., first

remission BMT for acute myelogenous leukemia patients). Here the question of the efficacy of BMT versus conventional treatments is particularly unknown since few randomized trials comparing chemotherapy with BMT have been conducted. However, most patients know that if conventional treatments fail, they may have decreased the probability of a successful BMT because of disease progression or toxicity associated with chemotherapy and radiation.

Two studies have examined the psychosocial status of patients pretransplantation (Magid et al. submitted; Syrjala et al. 1988). Magid et al. (submitted) interviewed 40 patients and matched significant others prior to the initiation of an autologous BMT procedure. Patients expressed concerns regarding fear of death from the procedure and side effects of treatment including nausea, infections and hair loss. Interestingly, level of distress (as measured by the Profile of Mood States) was similar between patients and significant others except that the patients reported a higher level of fatigue. The Manitoba Functional Living Index (FLIC) revealed that patients scored lower than significant others on two scales: (1) physical well-being and activities and (2) family/personal hardships. Thus, patients perceived their physical status as affecting their activity level and personal relationships.

Syrjala and colleagues (1988) obtained a number of psychosocial measures pretransplant including the Beck Depression Inventory and the Brief Symptom Inventory. In general, BMT patients reported scores similar to population norms. However, 41% of BMT patients had anxiety scores of at least one standard deviation above the norm and 35% had depression scores at least one standard deviation above normal.

Clearly, additional research examining psychosocial issues before hospitalization is necessary. However, the above cited studies appear to indicate that BMT patients are coping quite well pretransplant, although a subset may be experiencing significant distress. Below is a case vignette that illustrates several of the issues described above.

Case Vignette

E.D. was a 42-year-old male diagnosed with Hodgkin's disease in 1984. He had been treated with chemotherapy and radiation with good results until two months prior to referral to the Behavioral Medicine section, when his relapse was diagnosed. Evaluation revealed that E.D. had three major areas of concern:

1. He was having difficulty weighing the pros and cons of BMT versus additional radiation therapy. As described above, he was aware that additional radiation might decrease his chance of a successful BMT in the future.

2. However, E.D. had a history of pneumonia related to previous chemotherapy. Therefore, he feared that he would contract pneumonia during the BMT and die.

3. Finally, he was concerned about the prolonged hospitalization and the need to rely on others to care for him.

Further evaluation revealed that E.D. had a long history of difficulty with anxiety, which interfered with decision making. Additionally, it appeared that his anxiety prevented him from conceptualizing questions to ask his oncologist. Consequently, he lacked important information necessary to guide his decision.

The Behavioral Medicine intervention began with basic anxiety management skills, including relaxation and biofeedback, which E.D. quickly mastered. A problem-solving approach was then developed to aid E.D. in conceptualizing questions, which he then wrote down and gave to his oncologist. This approach allowed E.D. to reduce his anxiety and obtain the information necessary to make a decision regarding BMT. He eventually decided to enter the BMT program and is ten months post-transplant at the time of this writing.

This case illustrates several of the issues potentially raised pretransplant and describes a successful intervention, a topic which will be discussed in greater length later in this chapter.

Psychosocial Measures as Eligibility Criteria in BMT

An issue that arises occasionally when considering a new patient for BMT is the patient's ability to handle the procedure emotionally. These discussions typically revolve around the patient's ability to comply with the requirements of BMT (e.g., exercise, mouth care, etc.) and *not* behave in ways that would be potentially detrimental (e.g., pull out IVs or catheters, sign out A.M.A., etc.).

One study from West Germany (Neuser 1988) investigated the issue of personality characteristics and survival time post-BMT. Thirty-five patients with acute leukemia, chronic myelogenous leukemia, or severe aplastic anemia were administered the Personality Research Form (PRF) (Stumpf et al. 1985) prior to BMT. Neuser reported that patients who scored high on the "strive for recognition and help" dimension had a higher survival probability one year post-BMT. He suggested that compliance behavior is the factor mediating between personality and survival. These are interesting results; however, the study requires replication with a larger sample size, additional psychosocial measures, and direct measures of compliance behavior.

These results also need to be balanced against two case reports of patients with significant psychiatric risk factors who underwent BMT. The first report (Kaehler et al. 1989) described a woman with chronic myelogenous leukemia who required an abortion prior to BMT and had a significant family psychiatric history; her mother had bipolar disorder and her sister was schizophrenic. Despite the emotional trauma of the abortion and the high genetic tendency for psychiatric problems, the patient coped well medically and psychologically with BMT.

In the second case (Rappaport 1988), a 32-year-old male with chronic granulocytic leukemia underwent BMT. His psychiatric history was significant in that he was thought to have schizoid or schizotypal personality disorder. Despite a brief psychotic episode during BMT, the patient did very well medically and his psychotic symptoms resolved postdischarge.

The basic problem with this area of study is that health care providers are trying to make predictions about the patient's future behavior based upon current functioning and/or responses to psychosocial measures. The history of research in mental health areas is replete with attempts to predict future behavior. The consensus view is that the ability to predict behavior based upon psychosocial factors is very poor. Anecdotally, transplant centers have reported situations in which patients seemed psychologically healthy pretransplant who had major compliance problems, as well as patients with poor premorbid psychosocial histories who coped well with BMT.

As one can see, this is a complex area with no easy answers. Therefore, although the utilization of psychosocial measures as eligibility criteria for BMT deserves further research, no clear guidelines exist thus far.

Hospitalization

Numerous, significant psychosocial concerns are raised during the hospitalization phase of BMT. This section will focus on several aspects of the BMT during the hospitalization phase including coping with side effects (e.g., nausea, vomiting and pain), the neuropsychological effects of BMT, coping with prolonged hospitalization and isolation, and the impact of BMT on the family.

The Relationship of Psychological Factors to the Occurrence of Physical Symptoms

Chapko and colleagues (1989) examined the time course and variation in pain and nausea in patients with hematologic malignancies and aplastic anemia undergoing allogeneic bone marrow transplantation. Their results demonstrated variation due to diagnosis (patients with hematologic malignancies experienced more pain, whereas

patients with aplastic anemia experienced more nausea) and treatment (patients treated with 1575cGy TBI experienced higher levels of nausea and pain than patients receiving 1200cGy TBI). An additional abstract (Sullivan et al. 1984) examined the occurrence of pain in BMT patients. These investigators reported that 82% of patients with hematologic malignancies and 42% with aplastic anemia experienced pain. The most frequent source of pain for BMT patients was related to oral mucositis. Anecdotally, the severity and frequency of pain problems varies across transplant centers, with the most severe problems occuring in centers that used allogeneic BMT protocols primarily, presumably due to GVHD. These data are important since they describe variables that may influence the occurrence of physical symptoms. Unfortunately, no attempt was made to examine the correlation between psychological factors and the experience of pain, nausea, and vomiting.

However, investigators of other cancer treatment approaches have examined the relationship of psychological factors to the development and exacerbation of nausea, vomiting, and pain. A recent review of the nausea and vomiting literature (Burish and Carey 1986) concludes that, (1) anticipatory nausea and vomiting appears to be a conditioned aversive response, (2) anxiety or general distress exacerbates both pre- and post- treatment nausea and vomiting, and (3) nausea and vomiting can be reduced by psychologically based treatments such as relaxation training, biofeedback, and systematic desensitization.

Similarly, researchers have recognized the importance of psychological factors in pain perception (Melzack and Wall 1965; Turk et al. 1983). In general, theorists believe that factors like anxiety and depression serve to amplify painful sensations. Studies of cancer pain have supported the association between psychological factors and pain (Ahles et al. 1983; Spiegel and Bloom 1983). Additionally, several studies have supported the efficacy of psychologically based approaches to the management of cancer pain (Ahles 1985 and 1987).

The research on nausea and vomiting and pain has demonstrated a clear relationship between psychological variables and the severity of these symptoms. Consequently, it is reasonable to hypothesize that a similar relationship will be found for patients undergoing BMT. Clinically this relationship appears valid and has led to a formal study at various centers looking at the relationship between anxiety and depression and physical symptoms in a BMT population.

Neuropsychological/Cognitive Effects of Chemotherapy and Radiation

Several studies have reported that survivors of childhood acute lymphocytic leukemia treated with chemotherapy and CNS radiation experienced long-term deficits on measures of neuropsychological functioning, IQ, and school achievement (Mulhern et al. 1988; Peckham et al. 1988; Brouwers et al. 1985). More specifically, investigators have reported that this group has difficulty with memory, attention/concentration, and sequencing and comprehension while performing school work.

Relatively little systematic research has been done examining the neuropsychological effects of cancer treatments in adults. However, potential cognitive impairment due to chemotherapy, the cancer itself, and concurrently administered medications have been recognized (Silberfarb 1983). Additionally, delirium has been found to be the most frequently missed diagnosis in psychiatric consultation referrals of 100 consecutive cancer patients (Levine et al. 1978). Two studies (Silberfarb et al. 1980; Oxman and Silberfarb 1980) have systematically evaluated the neuropsychological functioning of adult cancer patients. Silberfarb et al. (1980) reported that patients currently receiving chemotherapy scored significantly lower on the Trails B, Digit Symbol Test, and Cognitive Capacity Screening Test when compared to patients not receiving treatment. In the second study, Oxman and Silberfarb (1980) administered a similar battery prior to the onset of chemotherapy, 24 hours after the onset of chemotherapy, and at a one-month follow-up visit. No significant changes were found. However, the sample size was small (N = 10), the patients had a variety of diagnoses, and different chemotherapeutic regimens were employed. As the authors point out, serial cognitive testing should be employed with "patients who have the same cell type, stage and site of disease, treatment, and premorbid cognitive status" (Oxman and Silberfarb 1980).

The bulk of the data support the hypothesis that chemotherapy and central nervous system radiation regimens cause long-term neuropsychological deficits in childhood leukemia. This issue has been less intensively studied in adult patients, and no studies of the neuropsychological effects of BMT were found. Because of the intensive nature of BMT, it is logical to hypothesize that if neuropsychological deficits occur in adult cancer patients, these deficits should be seen with BMT protocols.

Clinically, patients report difficulty with concentration and memory. Cases of delirium are seen. Fortunately, these major symptoms usually clear by the time the patient is ready for discharge. Anecdotally, however, we have had patients report difficulties in ability to concentrate and learn new information. At this point, it is unclear whether these problems are true cognitive deficits or related to psychological issues such as depression, anxiety, or reintegration into a normal lifestyle.

Research into the neuropsychological effects of BMT is important for several reasons. Understanding the type and extent of cognitive deficits may help to explain why some patients have difficulty understanding information and complying with instructions during hospitalization. Additionally, if long-term neuropsychological deficits are a consequence of BMT, patients need to be aware of this possibility in order to make a truly informed decision regarding entry into a BMT program. Finally, since BMT protocols continue to be developed, knowing the neuropsychological effects of one protocol compared to another may provide valuable data in deciding which treatment approach to pursue. Ideally, treatment regimens could be developed that are effective yet minimize the probability of producing cognitive deficits.

Coping with Prolonged Hospitalization and Isolation

Another major stressor confronting the patient is prolonged hospitalization (Brown and Kelly 1976; Magid et al. submitted). Multiple aspects of the hospitalization are stressful, with the length of stay and the prolonged dependency on others for care identified as major sources of stress. Certainly, the multiple physical symptoms of a medical crisis and confrontation with the possibility of death exacerbate the stress associated with hospitalization. Isolation from friends and family (particularly for patients living a distance from the transplant center) and isolation in an LAF room (particularly for patients undergoing allogeneic BMT procedures) remove many of the means of coping with psychological reactions such as anxiety and depression and feelings of powerlessness and helplessness. Nurses are often the patient's link with the outside world and patients can become overly attached and dependent on transplant nursing staff.

Coping with these multiple stressors may lead to noncompliance with basic requirements such as walking, showering, mouth care, etc. Noncompliance is often a difficult problem to manage, requiring the expertise and coordination of all the members of the BMT team.

Some patients express body image concerns early in the treatment period, i.e., hair loss, weight loss, need for catheters, Hickmans, etc. Acute attention to these issues often fades during the hospitalization, then reemerge post hospitalization.

Little systematic research has examined how well BMT patients cope with prolonged hospital-ization or what nursing interventions might help to alleviate the stress associated with prolonged hospitalization. The few papers that have examined this issue (e.g., Brown and Kelly 1976; Popkin and Moldow 1977; Popkin et al. 1977; Rappaport 1988; Kaehler et al. 1989) have been primarily descriptive or case reports. Understandably, these reports have focused on the difficulties patients experience during BMT. However, larger-scale studies are necessary to define the prevalence of psychosocial problems.

Many staff members in BMT programs are impressed at how well patients cope despite the multiple stressors. Patients certainly experience fluctuations in levels of distress, anxiety, depression, boredom, anger, etc. However, these seem to be relatively transient, often clearing as the patient begins to improve medically. This is not to imply that psychosocial issues should be ignored. On the contrary, the assessment of treatment of psychosocial problems should be an integral part of BMT programs to enhance the ability of patients and families cope more effectively with BMT. The integration of mental health professionals into the treatment program for BMT patients will be described below.

Stress on the Family

Very little has been written about stress on the family during the hospital phase of BMT. However, there are several clearly identifiable sources of stress that are experienced by most family members. First is fear of the death of the patient. Families typically attempt to remain optimistic, particularly when interacting with the patient. However, concerns about death often become more acute as the patient becomes more ill and medical care requirements escalate (e.g., transfer to the intensive care unit).

An associated experience is the feeling of helplessness. Family members often report feeling that they can do nothing but watch a whole myriad of health professionals care for their loved one. The feelings of helplessness, fear, depression, and anxiety are often experienced alone, since the transplant center is a significant distance from their home. Not uncommonly, one family member (usually a spouse or parent) stays with the patient while other family members may only be able to visit for brief periods.

Another source of stress is associated with the potential shift in roles for the spouse of the patient. The spouse may need to take on responsibilities to which they are unaccustomed, e.g., making financial decisions, assuming parenting roles such as disciplinarian, etc. For some, there may be a near role reversal where the spouse becomes the major source of psychological and financial support in the family. This may be stressful for a spouse who feels uncomfortable in some of these roles or overwhelmed with the amount of responsibility when they are accustomed to sharing responsibilities with the patient.

Treatment

Neuser et al. (1990), Patenaude and Rappeport (1984) and Rappaport (1988) have advocated collaboration between hematologists and mental health professionals in caring for BMT patients. In this section we will discuss four areas of treatment: (1) psychological support, (2) specific behavioral interventions, (3) support groups for family members, and (4) psychopharmacologic support.

Psychological Support

At many centers, BMT patients are evaluated and followed, as necessary, by a variety of mental health specialists such as psychiatrists, psychologists, and/or psychiatric clinical nurse specialists. The initial evaluation, ideally occuring prehospitalization, serves to identify preexisting problems (e.g., psychiatric history) that may have an impact upon the patient's treatment course and nursing interventions. More commonly, however, the mental health professionals are available to provide psychological support to the patient

and family as the need arises during hospitalization. Patients and family members often report feeling uncomfortable using the time with physicians and nurses to discuss psychosocial issues since they have so many medical questions. Therefore, they appreciate the opportunity to have time available exclusively for discussing feelings and emotions.

The staff of mental health professionals involved in BMT programs varies considerably, but will ideally include psychologists, psychiatrists, social workers, psychiatric nurses, and consult-liaison services in various combinations to provide support for patients. These resources, however, need to be integrated with the daily support and encouragement offered by the nurses and other members of the BMT team. A team approach in which there is active communication among all professionals caring for the patients is ideal.

Behavioral Interventions

Behavioral techniques are being utilized increasingly in the management of symptoms associated with cancer and cancer treatments, particularly pain (Ahles 1985 and 1987) and nausea and vomiting (Burish and Carey 1986). Three specific interventions will be described that may have relevance for managing mucositis pain and nausea and vomiting: (1) hypnosis, (2) relaxation, and (3) biofeedback.

Hypnosis

Hypnosis has a long history of use as a pain control technique. Several hypnotic strategies for pain reduction have been described (Barber and Gitelson 1980): (1) direct blocking of pain from awareness through the suggestion of anesthesia or analgesia, (2) substitution of another sensation (e.g., pressure) for pain, (3) moving the pain to a smaller or less important part of the body, (4) changing the meaning of the pain so that it becomes less threatening, (5) increasing pain tolerance, and (6) dissociating part of the body from the patient's awareness.

Spiegel (1985) described three basic principles for teaching any hypnotic technique:

1. "Filter the hurt out of the pain." Patients are taught that there is not a one-to-one correlation between the amount of physical damage and the perceived intensity of the pain. By separating the affective component (which amplifies the pain) from the somatic component of the pain, the suffering experienced can be reduced.

2. "Do not fight the pain." Patients are taught that struggling with the pain can cause an exacerbation of it either through increasing reactive muscle tension or the affective component of the pain.

3. "Use self-hypnosis." Finally, the patients are taught self-hypnosis so that they can utilize the techniques apart from the therapist.

In a control-group outcome study, Spiegel and Bloom (1983) demonstrated that hypnosis significantly reduced pain and improved mood in women with metastatic breast cancer. Similarly, research has supported the efficacy of hypnosis in reducing nausea and vomiting associated with traditional chemotherapy approaches (Redd et al. 1982). Anecdotally, we have utilized hypnotic techniques with BMT patients with good success in symptom management. However, no systematic research investigating the use of hypnosis in a BMT population has yet been reported.

Relaxation Training

Relaxation training consists of a set of techniques designed to produce physiological and mental relaxation (Taylor 1978). Two commonly used relaxation procedures are progressive muscle and autogenic relaxation. Progressive muscle relaxation (Bernstein and Borkovec 1973) consists of systematically tensing and relaxing various muscle groups. Additionally, patients are instructed in diaphragmatic breathing exercises and taught to associate expiration with calming words such as "relax." Autogenic relaxation (Schultz 1959), on the other hand, is a relatively passive technique. Patients adopt a quiet attitude and repeat autogenic phrases such as "my arms are warm and heavy" and "my legs feel heavy and relaxed."

Relaxation techniques have been used successfully to control chemotherapy-related nausea and vomiting (Burish and Lyles 1981; Lyles et al. 1982; Redd and Andrykowski 1982) and have been suggested but less well studied for the control of cancer pain (Copley and Cobb 1984; Fleming 1985; Noyes 1981; Payne and Foley 1984). The use of relaxation for symptom management in BMT patients is currently being studied by the Seattle group and has been described by Bayuk (1985).

Biofeedback

Biofeedback has been defined as "a process in which a person learns to reliably influence physiological responses of two kinds: either responses that are not ordinarily under voluntary control or responses that ordinarily are easy to regulate but regulation has broken down because of trauma or disease" (Blanchard and Epstein 1978). Biofeedback training entails the use of special electronic devices that detect and amplify biological responses and convert these amplified responses to signals that are easily understood by the patient. For example, a common signal is a tone where the pitch varies proportionately with the level of the biological response.

One of the most common types of biofeedback is electromyographic (EMG) biofeedback. EMG electrodes are attached to major muscles, e.g., frontalis or trapezius muscles. Patients are taught to reduce EMG activity, which is indicated by a reduction in the biofeedback signal (e.g., the pitch of the tone). Other types of biofeedback include: (1) temperature biofeedback (teaching patients to raise hand temperature); (2) skin conductance level (SCL) biofeedback (teaching patients to reduce SCL); and (3) electroencephalographic (EEG) biofeedback (theta, teaching a person to produce 4–8Hz activity, and alpha, teaching the person to produce 9–13Hz activity).

Biofeedback has been used to control nausea and vomiting (Burish et al. 1981) and pain (Fotopoulos et al. 1979; Fotopoulos et al. 1983). In cancer patients' direct application of biofeedback

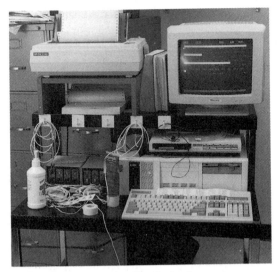

Figure 12.1. Biofeedback Equipment

with BMT patients has not yet been reported. However, portable EMG and GSR units have been utilized for hospitalized BMT patients to enhance relaxation.

Support Groups

Patenaude and colleagues (1986) described a support group for parents and spouses of BMT patients. The issues discussed include: (1) introduction to the BMT unit, (2) helplessness, (3) empathy versus discipline, (4) family relations, (5) religion and money, (6) relation to the medical team, and (7) preparation for discharge.

Because of the isolation requirements at certain institutions, a support group for patients is not possible during their hospital stay. However, in institutions conducting primarily autologous BMT, a patient support group may be considered.

Psychopharmacologic Support

There are some situations and some patients for whom pharmacologic treatment of their psychological distress is necessary. The two most common situations are those of extreme anxiety and moderate to severe delirium, with depression occasionally treated.

Pharmacologic treatment of anxiety for BMT patients is a cost/benefit question. The distress that the anxiety causes the patient must be weighed against the CNS depressant effects of anxiolytics. BMT patients are often sedated from antiemetics, narcotics, and hypnotics as well as fatigued from fevers, fluid and electrolyte disturbances, hematologic derangements, and respiratory problems. Caregivers must carefully weigh the addition of any sedating medication to such a clinical picture. An added consideration is that BMT patients are chronic patients; their long-term use of benzodiazepine anxiolytics should be carefully monitored to minimize physical or psychological dependence.

However, in spite of these obvious concerns, there are times when benzodiazepines are indicated for the treatment of anxiety. Most clinicians advocate using the shorter acting benzodiazepines to minimize the build-up of sedation that can occur with longer acting agents. Accompanying this regimen with behavioral techniques to assist the patient in coping with their understandable anxiety can help to decrease the use of medications as well as assist the patient to regain a sense of control and accomplishment. Reevaluating the use of and necessity for anxiolytics periodically throughout the hospitalization can also help to keep their use at an acceptable minimum.

Delirium poses an obvious risk to this medically ill, frail population. If delirium is kept to a minimum, basic reorientation methods as well as repetition of information and directions can often suffice to manage the patient adequately. However, if the cause is not determined and treated, a mild delirium can progress to a more severe problem. An agitated patient can inadvertently cause himself a tragedy by struggling with a caregiver who is attempting to keep him in bed or away from whatever tubing he is attempting to pull out. The physical damage such action can cause a BMT patient with thrombocytopenia is of concern. In these situations, it may be necessary to sedate and treat the patient with one of the neuroleptic medications.

The choice of neuroleptic is usually determined by evaluating the potential side effects of the specific agent. However, patients that are already using a neuroleptic successfully as part of their antiemetic regimen can often easily tolerate an increase in dose, rather than complicating the picture with a different neuroleptic. The extrapyramidal system (EPS) side effects associated with the neuroleptics must be carefully monitored to minimize their distressing occurrence. Sometimes switching to a different neuroleptic is possible, but there are some unfortunate patients who react to all of the neuroleptics. In this case, clinicians must weigh the use of additional medications to treat these side effects against the necessity of using the neuroleptic.

There are also rare instances where a BMT patient's discouragement and demoralization progresses to an actual psychiatric, major depression where the use of antidepressant medications may be indicated. This use must be weighed against the potential deliriogenic actions: dry mouth problems, constipation, postural hypotension, and other side effects of the tricyclic antidepressant medications. In this medically ill, frail population, the choice of antidepressant should be heavily determined by the specific medication's side effects. Another major problem with the tricyclic antidepressants is the period of time that most BMT patients are NPO due to oral infections. Parenteral use of these medications is not common, so clinicians should treat them cautiously. Intramuscular dosing, the most common parenteral route of administration, is contraindicated in this thrombocytopenic population. This leaves only intravenous administration, which has been done only rarely.

These major drawbacks of antidepressant medications, added to the necessity of starting the patient on a low dose and building up slowly in order to minimize side effects, reinforces the position that antidepressant medications are not a rapid solution to the depressed patient problem.

These are clearly not appropriate for the temporarily discouraged patient who will feel better in the near future when his counts come up and his physical status improves. These medications should be reserved for the severely depressed patient who has consistently shown significant depressive symptoms for several weeks and/or has a significant past history of major affective disorder.

Dependence and Addiction

The use of potentially addictive medications, particularly the benzodiazepines, for control of anxiety and nausea and narcotics for the control of pain and rigors, typically raises concerns regarding the potential for the development of dependence and addiction. This issue has not been systematically studied in BMT patients. However, data from other medical populations suggests that the risk of developing problems of dependency and addiction are quite low when these medications are used in a medically appropriate manner to treat relatively acute problems (Porter and Jick 1980; Angell 1982).

Measurement of Psychological and Somatic Symptoms

Below is a description of measures commonly used in psychosocial oncology research. The focus of this review is on measures that are brief and practical, but have evidence supporting their reliability and validity. These instruments have potential for use clinically, in addition to their role in research projects designed to evaluate psychosocial issues of BMT patients prior to and during hospitalization.

Psychological Measures

There are a variety of measures for psychological symptoms. However, the most common measures used in cancer research include the Beck Depression Inventory (Beck et al. 1961), Zung Depression Scale (Zung 1965), Spielberger State-Trait Anxiety Inventory (Spielberger, Gorsuch, and Lushene 1970), Profile of Mood States (POMS) (McNair, Lorr, and Droppleman 1971), Brief POMS (Cella et al. 1987), Symptom Checklist-90 (Derogatis 1977), the shorter version of the SCL-90, the Brief Symptom Inventory (Derogatis and Meyer 1979), and the Manitoba Functional Living Index (Schipper et al. 1984). These measures have evidence supporting their reliability and validity and have been shown to be practical for use with a cancer population.

In addition to standardized questionnaires, investigators have utilized visual analogue scales (VAS) of depression, anxiety, and distress (Ahles et al. 1984; Aitken 1974). These scales typically take the form of 10cm lines anchored at the left end with "No distress" (anxiety, depression) and on the right with "Extreme distress" (anxiety, depression). The patient simply places a slash along the line indicating the level of distress. The major advantage of a VAS is its simplicity and consequently the possibility of asking patients to complete these on a daily basis.

Somatic Symptoms

The two most commonly used pain assessment instruments in the cancer pain area are the McGill (Melzack 1975) and the Dartmouth McGill Pain Questionnaires (Corson and Schneider 1984). Additionally, self-report measures of pain include VAS, numerical rating scales (0–10 or 0–100), and adjective measures (i.e., choosing the adjective that most closely describes the pain). The Memorial Pain Card (Fishman et al. 1987) combines several scales into one convenient rating card: (1) VAS mood, pain, and pain relief and (2) an adjective measure of pain.

Finally, measures of nausea and vomiting include VAS-nausea, the frequency of vomiting, or the number of days on which vomiting has occured and the Morrow Assessment of Nausea and Emesis (Morrow 1984).

Conclusion

Multiple psychosocial issues exist for patients undergoing BMT and their families. Some of these issues may be unique to BMT, while others are similar to those experienced by cancer patients in general who are involved in active treatment. On the positive side, many potential psychosocial interventions have been developed for cancer populations. However, the most effective and efficient approach for integrating these strategies into BMT programs has yet to be established.

References

Ahles, T.A. 1985. Psychological approaches to the treatment of cancer-related pain. *Seminars in Oncology Nursing 1*: 141–146.

Ahles, T.A. 1987. Psychological techniques for the management of cancer pain. In McGuire, D.B., and Yarbro, C.H. (eds.). *Cancer Pain Management*. Orlando: Grune & Stratton.

Ahles, T.A., Blanchard, E.B., and Ruckdeschel, J.C. 1983. The multidimensional nature of cancer related pain. *Pain 17*: 272–278.

Ahles, T.A., Ruckdeschel, J.C., and Blanchard, G.B. 1984. Cancer-related pain: II. Assessment with visual analogue scales. *Journal of Psychosomatic Research 28*: 121–124.

Aitken, R.C.B. 1974. Assessment of mood by analogue. In Beck, A.T., Resnick, H.L.P., and Lettier, D.J. (eds.). *The Prediction of Suicide*. Bowie, MD: Charles Press.

Angell, M. 1982. The quality of mercy. *N. Engl. J. Med. 306*: 98–99.

Barber, J., and Gitelson, J. 1980. Cancer pain: Psychological management of using hypnosis. *CA 30*: 130–136.

Bayuk, L. 1985. Relaxation techniques: An adjunct therapy for cancer patients. *Seminars in Oncology Nursing 1*: 147–150.

Beck, A.T. et al. 1961. An inventory for measuring depression. *Arch. Gen. Psychiatry 4*: 561–571.

Bernstein, D.A., and Borkovec, T.D. 1973. *Progressive Relaxation Training*. Champaign, IL: Research Press.

Blanchard, E.B., and Epstein, L.H. 1978. *A Biofeedback Primer*. Reading, MA: Addison-Wesley.

Brouwers, P. et al. 1985. Long-term neuropsychological sequelae of childhood leukemia: Correlation with CT scan abnormalities. *J. Pediatr. 106*: 723–728.

Brown, H.N., and Kelly M.J. 1976. Stages of bone marrow transplantation: A psychiatric perspective. *Psychosomatic Medicine 38*: 439–446.

Burish, T.G., and Carey, M.P. 1986. Conditioned aversive responses in cancer chemotherapy patients: Theoretical and developmental aspects. *Journal of Consulting and Clinical Psychology* 54: 593–600.

Burish, T.G., and Lyles, J.N. 1981. Effectiveness of relaxation training in reducing adverse reactions to cancer chemotherapy. *Journal of Behavioral Medicine* 4: 65–78.

Burish, T.G., Shartner, C.D., and Lyles, J.N. 1981. Effectiveness of multiple-site EMG biofeedback and relaxation in reducing the aversiveness of cancer chemotherapy. *Biofeedback and Self-Regulation* 6: 523–535.

Cella, D.F. et al. 1987. A brief POMS measure of distress for cancer patients. *Journal of Chronic Disease* 40: 939–942.

Chapko, M.K. et al. 1989. Chemoradiotherapy toxicity during bone marrow transplantation: Time course and variation in pain and nausea. *B.M.T.* 4: 181–186.

Copley Cobb, S. 1984. Teaching relaxation techniques to cancer patients. *Cancer Nursing* 7: 157–164.

Corson, J.A., and Schneider, M.J. 1984. The Dartmouth Pain Questionnaire: An adjunct to the McGill Pain Questionnaire. *Pain* 19: 59–69.

Derogatis, L.R. 1977. *Administration, Scoring and Procedures Manual for the SCL-90-R.* Baltimore: Clinical Psychometric Research.

Derogatis, L.R., and Meyer, J.K. 1979. A psychological profile of the sexual dysfunctions. *Archives of Sexual Behavior* 8: 201–223.

Fleming, U. 1985. Relaxation training for far advanced cancer. *The Practitioner* 229: 471–475.

Fotopoulos, S.S., Graham, C., and Cook, M.R. 1979. Psychophysiologic control of cancer pain. In Bonica, J.J., and Ventafridda, V. (eds.). *Advances in Pain Research and Therapy*, Vol. 2. New York: Raven Press.

Fotopoulos, S.S. et al. 1983. Cancer pain: Evaluation of electromyographic and electrodermal feedback. *Progress in Clinical Biological Research* 132D: 33–53.

Fishman, B. et al. 1987. The Memorial Pain Assessment Card: A valid instrument for the evaluation of cancer pain. *Cancer* 60: 1151–1158.

Kaehler, S.L., Goodwin, J.M., and Young, L.D. 1989. Bone marrow transplantation: Mastering the experience despite psychological risk factors. *Psychosomatics* 30: 337–341.

Levine, P., Silberfarb, P.M., and Lipowski, Z.J. 1978. Mental disorders in cancer patients: A study of 100 psychiatric referrals. *Cancer* 42: 1385–1391.

Lyles, J.N. et al. 1982. Efficacy of relaxation training and guided imagery in reducing the aversiveness of cancer chemotherapy. *Journal of Consulting and Clinical Psychology* 50: 509–524.

Magid, D.M. et al. In preparation. A longitudinal psychosocial assessment of high dose chemotherapy and autologous bone marrow reinfusion for patients and their significant other.

McNair, D.M., Lorr, M., and Droppleman, L.F. 1971. *Profile of Mood States.* San Diego: Educational and Industrial Testing Service.

Melzack, R. 1975. The McGill Pain Questionnaire: Major properties and scoring methods. *Pain 1*: 277–299.

Melzack, R., and Wall, P. 1965. Pain mechanisms: A theory. *Science* 150: 971–979.

Morrow, G.R. 1984. Clinical characteristics associated with the development of anticipatory nausea and vomiting in cancer patients undergoing chemotherapy treatment. *J. Clin. Oncol.* 2: 1170–1176.

Mulhern, R.K. et al. 1988. Memory function in disease-free survivors of childhood acute lymphocytic leukemia given CNS prophylaxis with or without 1800 cGy cranial irradiation. *J. Clin. Oncol.* 6: 315–320.

Neuser, J. 1988. Personality and survival time after bone marrow transplantation. *Journal of Psychosomatic Research 32*: 451–455.

Neuser, J. et al. 1990. Principles of supportive psychological care for patients undergoing bone marrow transplantation. *Haematology and Blood Transfusion 33*: 583–586.

Noyes, R. 1981. Treatment of cancer pain. *Psychosomatic Medicine 43*: 57–70.

Oxman, T.E., and Silberfarb, P.M. 1980. Serial cognitive testing in cancer patients receiving chemotherapy. *Am. J. Psychiatry 137*: 1263–1265.

Patenaude, A.F., Levinger, L., and Baker, K. 1986. Group meetings for parents and spouses of bone marrow transplant patients. *Social Work in Health Care 12*: 51–65.

Patenaude, A.F., and Rappeport, J.M. 1984. Collaboration between hematologists and mental health professionals on a bone marrow transplant team. *Journal of Psychosocial Oncology* 2: 81–92.

Payne, R., and Foley, K.M. 1984. Advance in management of cancer pain. *Cancer Treatment Reports* 68: 173–183.

Peckham, V.C. et al. 1988. Educational late effects in long-term survivors of childhood acute lymphocytic leukemia. *Pediatrics 81*: 127–133.

Popkin, M.K., and Moldow, C.F. 1977. Stressors and responses during bone marrow transplantation. *Arch. Intern. Med. 137*: 725.

Popkin, M.K. et al. 1977. Psychiatric aspects of allogeneic bone marrow transplantation for aplastic anemia. *Diseases of the Nervous System 38*: 925–927.

Porter, J., and Jick, H. 1980. Addiction rare in patients treated with narcotics. *N. Engl. J. Med. 302*: 123.

Rappaport, B.S. 1988. Evolution of consultation-liaison services in bone marrow transplantation. *General Hospital Psychiatry 10*: 346–351.

Redd, W.H., Andresen, G.V., and Minagawa, R.Y. 1982. Hypnotic control of anticipatory emesis in patients receiving cancer chemotherapy. *Journal of Consulting and Clinical Psychology* 50: 14–19.

Redd, W.H., and Andrykowski M.A. 1982. Behavioral intervention in cancer treatment: Controlling aversion reactions to chemotherapy. *Journal of Consulting and Clinical Psychology* 50: 1018–1029.

Schipper, H. et al. 1984. Measuring the quality of life of cancer patients: The functional living index: Development and validation. *J. Clin. Oncol.* 2: 472–483.

Schultz, J.H. and Luthe, W. 1959. *Autogenic Training.* NY: Grune and Stratton.

Silberfarb, P.M. 1983. Chemotherapy and cognitive defects in cancer patients. *Annu. Rev. Med.* 34: 35–46.

Silberfarb, P.M., Philbert, D., and Levine, P.M. 1980. Psychological aspects of neoplastic disease: II. Affective and cognitive effects of chemotherapy in cancer patients. *Am. J. Psychiatry* 137: 597–601.

Spiegel, D. 1985. The use of hypnosis in controlling cancer pain. *CA* 35: 221–231.

Spiegel, D., and Bloom, J.R. 1983. Pain in metastatic cancer. *Cancer* 52: 341–345.

Spielberger, C.D., Gorsuch, R.L., and Lushene, R.G. 1970. *Manual for the State-Trait Anxiety Inventory.* Palo Alto: Consulting Psychologist Press.

Stumpf, H. et al. 1985. *Deutsche Personality Research Form (PRF).* Göttingen: Hogrefe.

Sullivan, K.M. et al. 1984. Pain following intensive chemo-radiotherapy and bone marrow transplantation (BMT). *Pain 2:* 5215 (suppl.).

Syrjala, K.L. et al. 1988. Physical and psychosocial functioning in the first year after bone marrow transplantation: A prospective study. *Presented at the Society of Behavioral Medicine.*

Taylor, B.C. 1978. Relaxation training and related techniques. In Agras, S. (ed.). *Behavior Modification: Principles and Clinical Applications.* Boston: Little, Brown, and Co.

Turk, D.C., Meichenbaum, D., and Genest, M. 1983. *Pain and Behavioral Medicine.* New York: Guilford Press.

Zung, W.W. 1965. A self-rating depression scale. *Arch. Gen. Psychiatry* 12: 63–70.

PART III

Issues of Survivorship

Chapter 13

Ambulatory Care: Before and After BMT

Patricia Corcoran Buchsel

Bone marrow transplant (BMT) has evolved from an experimental therapy for end-stage leukemic patients to a recommended treatment for patients with certain malignant and nonmalignant disorders (Thomas 1988; Storb and Thomas 1983). Expanding unrelated marrow donor pools (Beatty et al. 1989), advances in supportive care, and the development of less toxic preparative regimens have most currently contributed to the success of this procedure. In addition, recent isolation and production of several naturally occurring molecules, called growth factors, has dramatically hastened the recovery of transplanted marrow (Andreeff and Welte 1989). As the effectiveness and availability of this treatment modality improves, both the demand and application of this procedure will increase. There are currently more than 200 transplant units in the world and over 12,000 transplants have been performed worldwide. All of these advancements combined with the shift of more acute, high-tech care to patients in the outpatient setting has caused a continued and sig-

nificant growth in the number and types of ambulatory care and transitional units available for bone marrow transplant patients.

Concurrent with advances in medical management of marrow and organ transplant, costs of this procedure have increased significantly. Rising costs of technology and out-of-pocket expenses incurred by patients and families while undergoing BMT have escalated the cost of marrow transplant up to $200,000. Consequently, issues of cost-benefit ratios for transplantation have received much attention (Durbin 1988).

One of the greatest challenges to marrow transplant teams is to seek alternative methods for delivery of cost-effective care to the marrow recipient and family. A major solution to reducing costs of hospitalization is to reduce the length of stay in the hospital. This can often be acheived by offering selected services in ambulatory care units that were traditionally provided only in the hospital setting (Stream 1983). This model of care has been pioneered successfully in marrow transplantation (Buchsel and Kelleher 1989) and other populations (Brooten et al. 1986). In addition, patients and their families often prefer the quality of life that can be offered in a clinic or home care setting (Buchsel and Parchem 1988).

Management Considerations

Ambulatory Care Design

Comprehensive evaluation of marrow transplant candidates and their donors pretransplant, and a significant amount of supportive care for recipients post-transplant, can be successfully provided in ambulatory care units. Outpatient areas may be located within or near inpatient units or incorporated into hematology and oncology ambulatory clinics associated with inpatient transplant units. Important considerations in determining clinic location are proximity to other specialty clinics, availability of emergency support, as well as, well-established links with community resources for home health care (Buchsel and Parchem 1988).

Patient Traffic Flow

Particular attention must be focused on management strategies for efficient patient traffic flow patterns, easy access to medical records and patient account representatives, acquisition of medical supplies, and access to ancillary support services. Examination rooms are placed in areas that provide convenience and confidentiality for patients and physicians. A major consideration is to avoid crowded conditions for immunosuppressed patients especially in waiting and treatment room areas. Figure 13.1 illustrates an efficient clinic design that has been effectively instituted in a major BMT center.

Spaces for consultation with medical, nursing, pharmacy, social work, and other supportive services need to be identified. Special attention

should be focused on the distances that patients will need to travel from one service to another. Fatigue is a classic and persistent symptom of transplant patients and must be considered in relation to proximity of ancillary and support services (Ford and Ballard 1988).

Administrative Issues

Nursing administrators must address patient/nurse ratios, staffing patterns, staff development, risk management, and quality assurance program evaluations. Direct and frequent communication patterns among key personnel across disciplines can establish and maintain the smooth transition of patients from inpatient to outpatient services. Consistency between inpatient and outpatient care procedures and routines is particularly important in ensuring continuity of care.

Due to the recent trend of attempting to reduce the cost of marrow transplantation by shortening inpatient stays (Welch and Larson 1989), outpatient acuity levels are rising. There is an urgent need for ambulatory care nurse managers to identify patient classification systems to capture this rising acuity in order to appropriately match the required numbers and types of personnel to meet the patient service demand. Little is written in the nursing literature regarding nursing care models for ambulatory oncology patients. Some traditional patient care models for physicians offices, clinics, and ambulatory centers for oncology patients have been described (Tigne and Fisher 1988). The marrow transplant patient, however, requires complex medical care and the concept of the nurse as the case manager for patient, donors, and family members is receiving attention as an important health care delivery system. Instituting billing procedures to facilitate appropriate reimbursement for these high-acuity services is an additional major concern for the ambulatory care nurse manager.

Paramount to the care of these patients and families is an experienced marrow transplant team that can expertly care for this patient pop-

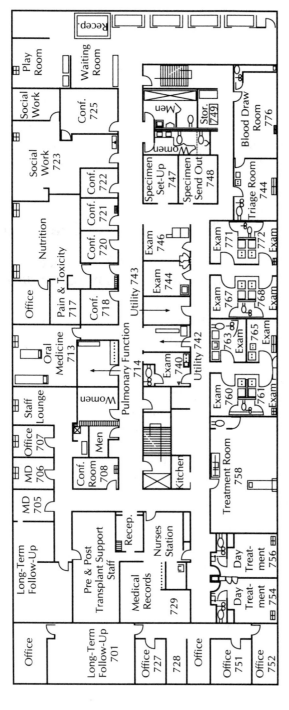

Figure 13.1. A Sample Floor Plan for an Ambulatory BMT Clinic

ulation (ASCO/ASH 1990). The wide variety of medical, nursing, and ancillary personnel required for the outpatient management of marrow recipients is outlined in Table 13.1.

Clinic Function

The function of the ambulatory care clinic is to provide care for transplant candidates in the preevaluation phase prior to admission to the BMT unit and after discharge from the hospital. A comprehensive ambulatory care unit will provide staff and facilities for the evaluation of five distinct patient populations: (1) consult patients, (2) marrow transplant candidates, (3) post-transplant patients, (4) family members, and (5) long-term follow-up patients (see Figure 13.2).

BMT involves not only the patient but the family members as well. The success of BMT is largely dependent on the availability of healthy, histocompatible donors for marrow donation and for blood component support after BMT. Health care may need to be provided for family members who are either marrow, platelet, or granulocyte donors. Donors will undergo general or spinal anesthesia for marrow harvest and require follow-up monitoring of harvest sites and for any ill effects of anesthesia (Buckner et al. 1984). Health problems of donors require immediate attention so that they can be available for platelet phereses to support the patient during thrombocytopenia.

Pretransplant Evaluation

Ambulatory Patient Care for the Marrow Transplant Candidate

Evaluation of potential marrow recipients and their families is performed in an ambulatory care setting unless patients are acutely ill. Patients are

Table 13.1. Medical, Nursing, and Support Services for BMT Ambulatory Care

Medical	Nursing	Support Services	Ancillary
Medical Director/Administrator	Staff Nurses	Physical therapy	Virology lab
BMT Physician	Nurse Manager	Day surgery	Microbiology lab
Oncologist/Hematologist	Nurse Clinicians/Case Managers	Nutritionist	Blood bank
Infectious Disease Specialist	Discharge Planner	Social services	Central supply
Pulmonary Medicine	Research Nurse	Pharmacy	Housekeeping
Gastroenterology	Home Health Nurses		Secretarial
Renal	Clinical Nurse Specialist		Medical records
Urology	Licenced Practical Nurses		Administrative
Dental	Certified Nursing Assistants		Pulmonary function
Radiology			Billing office
Neurology			personnel
Cardiology			Laundry
Reproductive Medicine			
Ophthalmology			
Allergy			
Immunology			
Emergency Service			
Rheumatology			
Psychiatry			
Behavioral Medicine			

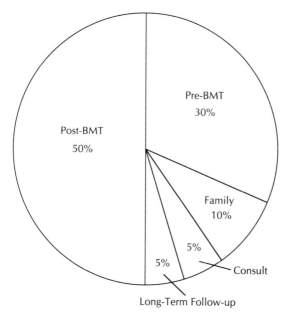

Figure 13.2. A Typical BMT Outpatient Population Mix

referred for marrow transplant by their community hematologist or oncologist and clear communication and expectations provide continuity and consistency of care. Marrow transplant physicians and referring physicians need to agree on the expected outcomes of BMT for their patients and discussion of disease and survival statistics should be consistent between these physician groups (Levine 1986).

BMT is a highly toxic procedure due to the high doses of chemotherapy and radiation required to ablate the patient's immune system and/or eradicate any underlying residual malignant disease. Consequently, transplant candidates are screened for organ dysfunction that may place them at high risk for the development of a fatal complication from the highly toxic immunosuppressive and conditioning therapy (Press et al. 1986). The purpose of the pretransplant evaluation is to:

1. Determine the appropriate type of the transplant: autologous, allogeneic, syngeneic, or unrelated;

2. Select the most appropriate donor for allogeneic patients;

3. Assess the candidate's physical ability to have a BMT;

4. Identify potential medical complications that may compromise the candidate's prognosis (see Table 13.2), e.g., underlying infectious disease, cardiac toxicity, elevated liver function tests;

5. Treat any compromising medical problems that place the patient at high risk for toxicities associated with BMT;

6. Identify appropriate conditioning protocols for BMT;

7. Educate the patient and family about all aspects of the BMT process and recovery.

Additional information regarding preevaluation testing and staging to determine the appropriateness of a candidate for marrow transplantation and donor preevaluation has been reviewed in Part I of the text.

The risks of marrow transplant must be cautiously weighed against the possible "cure" of transplant. As sicker and older patients are considered eligible for transplantation, difficult ethical considerations will emerge in choosing the most eligible candidate in terms of resource allocation and shared resources.

Nursing Implications

It is important that nurses recognize and address the special needs of prospective transplant candidates and their families. Patients leave behind familiar support systems of home, close relatives, and their primary health care team. They may arrive fatigued from transcontinental or international air travel and some speak little or no English. Some patients arrive ill from previous chemotherapy or hospitalization and require immediate medical and nursing care. Nursing assessment includes triage skills with sensitivity to ethnic and cultural variations. Nurses caring for these patients require a broad education in malignant disease and its treatment so that they can better understand the past history of the patient

Table 13.2. Evaluation of Pre-Bone Marrow Transplant Organ Toxicity

Medical Evaluation	Clinical Evaluation	Rationale
Confirm "reported" diagnosis	Repeat marrow aspiration & biopsy	Evaluates appropriateness for BMT Makes unequivocal diagnosis Determines conditioning protocol
Identify previous treatments to estimate level of response to conventional (antileukemic) therapy	History and physical; Review pre-transplant medical records	Provides vital information about prognosis for BMT Identifies potential cumulative toxicity (especially related to prior treatment with anthracyclines, cisplatin, bleomycin, and radiation)
Identify active disease	MRI, CT scan, biopsy node Tumor staging studies for malignant diseases 1. Bone marrow biopsy 2. Central nervous system 3. Sanctuary sites 4. Others as required	Identifies bearing on diagnosis or need for adjunctive therapy (local radiation, intrathecal chemotherapy)
Identify comorbid medical problems	Toxicity Screening 1. Pertinent history 2. Serum tests of renal, hepatic, and endocrine function 3. Pulmonary function tests including arterial blood gases and diffusing capacity of carbon monoxide (DLCO) 4. Left ventricular cardiac function evaluation 5. Creatinine clearance 6. Human immunodeficiency virus (HIV)	Identifies possible complicating organ toxicity
Transfusion history	History of number, type, results, and relation ABO typing	May influence type of conditioning or indicate desirability of one type of donor over another
Allergies/Adverse drug reactions	History & physical	Determines that "reported" allergies are real allergies. Determines other adverse effects to medications. Most BMT recipients receive penicillins, trimethoprimsulfomethoxazole, amphotericin
Psychologic assessment	Patient report of psychosocial functioning	Identifies history of psychologic instability or a psychiatric diagnosis
Determine pregnancy in women	History & physical Menstrual history & physical Human chorionic gonadotrophin (HCG)	High toxicity conditioning treatment may cause spontaneous abortion

Table 13.3. Social Service Considerations for BMT Candidates

Prior to Arrival to BMT Center

Discuss economic issues with patient/family (fundraising)

Discuss living arrangements with patient/family

Identify possible community resources

Provide family with relevant printed information about BMT

Discuss impact of protective isolation on patient/family (especially laminar air flow)

Arrange for volunteers for patient/family at BMT unit

Arrange for transportation to transplant unit

Discuss with patient/donor/family time needed away from home for BMT

Provide ongoing psychosocial support for family

as it relates to BMT. Marrow transplantation places significant psychological, physical, and financial burdens on patients. Often marrow transplant is the last hope for these candidates and transplant teams must support patient treatment choices (Buchsel and Parchem1988). The services of social work departments are also critical in preparing and supporting patients and families through this transition. Examples of the types of support provided by social service departments are listed in Table 13.3.

Family Conference

Family conferences prior to admission to the hospital for transplant are an ideal method for introducing the patient and family to the transplant team. The primary function of this meeting is to explain all aspects of the BMT procedure and to obtain informed consent from the patient (and the donor in the case of allogeneic BMT). Patients should be encouraged to take notes, bring a tape recorder, or find another means to assist them in clearly recalling all that is being explained. Obtaining informed consent requires that attending physicians explain the benefits and risks of transplantation, alternatives to BMT, and the statistics

for long-term survival. This initial meeting may be one of the most significant interactions in beginning the development of a trusting relationship between the patient and the transplant team (Carney 1987; Lesko et al. 1989).

Acute and long-term toxicities of BMT are also reviewed and the patient and donor have the opportunity to present their concerns before beginning an extensive physical evaluation (Patenaude and Rappeport 1982; Wolcott 1986). The nurse is an active participant in this conference and acts as a patient advocate and coordinator for the transplant team (Carney 1987).

Once informed consent is obtained, the patient, donor, and other family proceed through evaluation. If the patient is going to have an unrelated donor BMT, arrangements for obtaining marrow from the volunteer donor are made. For reasons of confidentiality, unrelated donors are usually evaluated and harvested in an institution apart from the BMT unit. (Donor issues are discussed in detail in Chapter 5.)

Patient Education

Intensive patient and family education is imperative to provide an adequate understanding of the transplant process. It is often the nurse who provides in-depth teaching about the toxicities resulting from conditioning regimens (Ford and Ballard 1988). Patient and family education usually begins prior to the patient's arrival at the transplant center. Nurses in general oncology units can offer valuable information to patients before they make the transition to the bone marrow transplant center. For example, it is important that both female and male patients who have reached puberty understand that they may be sterile as a result of previous chemotherapy or may become sterile due to the high-dose radiation or chemotherapy used in preparative regimens. Sperm banking prior to transplant may be an option for males with viable sperm. Women can be reassured that cyclic hormone replacement may prevent or temper the symptoms of premature menopause. Options for post-transplant in vitro fertilization and artificial insemination have not been fully explored for these patients (Buchsel 1990). See Chapter 14 for a complete discussion of reproductive and fertility considerations in BMT.

Teaching can be facilitated by the use of videos to explain basic but essential concepts of care, such as, right atrial catheter care, protective isolation, total body irradiation, and hospital routines. If possible, tours of the inpatient setting are an excellent way to prepare patients and families. Occasionally, patients may request to speak with other patients or family members of current or discharged patients to get a sense of what a BMT is "really like." Discretion is important in arranging such interactions, but these meetings can be very important to the prospective transplant candidate.

Right Atrial Catheter Placement

Placement of a right atrial catheter is a prerequisite with BMT to provide accessibility to the patient's circulatory system. ABO blood types are identified at the time of tissue typing. If blood types are different (allogeneic), and patients and donors are mismatched at one or two antigens, a large lumen central catheter will be placed so that the patient can undergo a plasma exchange to eliminate antibodies against the ABO group of the donor. After transplant, the recipient will often have the same blood type as the donor (Bensinger et al. 1982; Ford and Ballard 1988). These catheters can be placed in outpatient surgical areas and patients and families are taught clean and sterile technique for catheter management.

Marrow Donor

Risks to marrow donors are minimal but donors are carefully evaluated for general or spinal anesthesia for marrow harvest. This evaluation is addressed in Part 1 of the text.

Emotional as well as physical preparation of the donor is critical and done weeks prior to marrow harvest. Several factors influence the

amount of counseling and education a donor needs prior to marrow harvest (Ruggiero 1988). These factors include not only the relationship the donor has with the patient and family, but the donor's own life responsibilities as well. Family donors may be required for platelet support for up to three months after marrow transfusion and this availability requirement can be a burden to the family.

Numerous studies have confirmed some long-term psychologic effects on marrow donors of patients who have died as a result of BMT. Mood changes, lack of self-esteem, altered relationships, and guilt have been identified as long-term sequelae based on the donor's perception of the success or failure of the marrow transplant (Lesko and Hawkins1983; Lesko 1989).

Marrow donors are usually admitted to the hospital for marrow harvest on the day of surgery and discharged 24 to 48 hours after surgery. Postoperative follow-up care for assessment of donors includes examination of aspiration sites for possible infection. In addition, the donor will need to be evaluated for possible postoperative nausea and vomiting, pain, and any adverse emotional or psychologic problems (Holcombe 1987).

Although there have been almost 1,000 unrelated marrow donor transplants, research is lacking that defines the long-term or adverse effects of marrow donation in this donor population. As these transplants increase long-term studies may become available to define the counseling needs of this group.

Once these important outpatient procedures are complete the marrow transplant patient is admitted to the hospital for marrow transplant.

Hospital to Outpatient

Marrow recipients are being discharged from the hospital earlier in their recovery phase than in the past because of (1) issues of cost containment, (2) less toxic pharmacologic agents, and (3) advancements in the supportive management of transplant recipients. As mentioned previously, immunomodulators and growth factors have enhanced early engraftment and it is not unusual for those patients receiving growth factors to be discharged from the hospital as early as fifteen to twenty days after BMT (Nemunaitis et al. in press; Andreeff and Welte 1989). Although circumstances and data differ throughout the world, a major transplant center reports an average length of hospital stay of 35 days after BMT and readmission rates of 50%. The major cause of readmission is for sepsis requiring antibiotic therapy (Buchsel and Parchem 1988).

Discharge from Hospital

Preparation for discharge begins well before patients are actually discharged from the hospital. The role of a discharge planner can be essential in facilitating the transition from twenty-four hour monitoring to an outpatient setting (Chielens and Herrick 1990). The discharge planner acts as a liaison between inpatient units and outpatient care and collaboration between units is a key to successful discharge. Patient and family teaching highlights prevention of complications based on basic hygiene. Hand washing is stressed. Families give return demonstrations in delivering parenteral infusions and care of the central catheters. Instructions include reportable symptoms (see Table 13.4) that require emergency care after clinic hours. Prolonged impairment of normal immune function from high-dose conditioning regimens, immunosuppressive medications, and the presence of graft-versus-host disease (GVHD) place the BMT patient at risk for life-threatening infections (Buchsel 1990). Consequently, close medical monitoring is required until at least 100 days after BMT and can be provided through the ambulatory care clinic.

Feelings of insecurity and dependency have been reported in marrow transplant patients at time of discharge (Haberman 1988). Nurses involved in discharge planning can help to allay patient fears by reinforcing the idea that their care

Table 13.4. Reportable Symptoms

1. a) Temperatures > 38°C, shaking chills, or dizziness without steroids
   b) Temperatures > 37.5°C with steroid therapy
2. Changes in the appearance of right atrial catheter insertion site (redness, pain, drainage, swelling)
3. Changes in the color or consistency of bowel movements (increasing volume or frequency)
4. Changes in the color of urine
5. Appearance of a skin rash
6. Cough or shortness of breath
7. Nausea or vomiting
8. Anorexia
9. Inability to take prescribed medications
10. New onset of pain
11. Any noticeable bleeding, e.g., bleeding gums, nosebleed
12. Decreasing energy level
13. Mouth sores or "cold sores"

will not be compromised in the ambulatory setting. This phase of BMT is an excellent time for patients to view themselves as progressing through the continuum of recovery and wellness (Haberman 1988).

It is important for transplant teams to have discharge protocols for continuity and efficacy of care. Established discharge criteria are outlined in Table 13.5. Discharge parameters will become more liberal as more sophisticated and less toxic parenteral therapy is managed safely in outpatient and home care settings.

Post-Transplant Care (Discharge to day 100)

Key aspects of outpatient care are prevention and symptom management of complications from BMT during the early recovery phase (Sullivan et al. 1984; Stream 1983). Symptoms of various transplant complications and drug toxicities are outlined in Table 13.6. BMT can cause multi organ toxicities, and complications can cloud the major cause of symptoms. Nursing care is based on com-

Table 13.5. Established Discharge Criteria for Bone Marrow Transplantation Patients

1. Oral intake > 50% of baseline nutrient requirments
2. No more than 1500ml of parenteral fluid within 24 hours is required
3. Nausea and vomiting controlled with oral medication
4. Diarrhea controlled at < 500ml/d
5. Afebrile and off intravenous antibiotics for 48 hours
6. Platelet count > 15,000mm^3
7. Granulocytes > 500mm^3
8. Hematocrit > 30% for adults, > 25% for children
9. PO medications, for example, narcotics, antihypertensives, cyclosporine, and prednisone, are tolerated for 48 hours
10. Family support within home

prehensive organ system assessment. Nursing responsibilities include monitoring vital signs, including postural blood pressures, excellent triage skills, and prompt recognition and reporting of symptoms (Buchsel and Parchem 1988). Standardized assessment tools that outline the patient's status upon discharge and summarize problems requiring follow-up in the outpatient setting can provide essential information and promote continuity of care between settings (Chielens and Herrick 1990) (see Figure 13.3).

Management of these symptoms can be enhanced by incorporating protocols that allow nurses to evaluate initial classic symptoms of post-transplant problems. For instance standing orders that include obtaining a chest x-ray and blood, sputum, urine, and other body fluid cultures can be developed to assess the patient who presents with fever. Nausea and vomiting can be initially managed with standing orders for antiemetics and hydration until the precise etiology can be determined. Initiation of protocols for management of occluded central catheters can expedite safe patient care and avoid undue patient waiting time if blood transfusions, medication infusions, or

blood work are needed. Dietary consultations can be initiated at the first sign of excess weight loss or other nutritional deficits.

Nursing Implications of Ambulatory Care for the Post-BMT Patient

Supportive care from a multidisciplinary transplant team is imperative for successful recovery of BMT recipients. Daily to weekly examination of the marrow recipient is required in the early post-transplant phase. Emphasis is placed on infection prevention. Patients and family members are given basic instructions that can apply to most living situations. Nursing responsibilities are to allay patient anxieties and carefully and patiently reinforce rationales for prevention behaviors (see Table 13.7).

Initially, patients may require blood tests three to seven times per week to monitor blood chemistries and hematologic parameters. Weekly chest x-rays, serial bone marrow aspiration and biopsies, lumbar punctures, and intrathecal medications are also necessary for most patients. In addition red blood cells and platelet transfusions, immunosuppressive medications, immunoglobulin therapy, and total parenteral nutrition (Aker et al. 1983) may need to be incorporated into the patient's daily ambulatory care routine. Fluid balance is a challenge to maintain in the ambulatory care or home care setting and can be further complicated by the numerous treatment or symptom management intravenous medications. Portable ambulatory infusion pumps are almost mandatory to allow patients who receive a high number of infusions to be truly ambulatory.

Chronic Graft-Versus-Host Disease Evaluation

At approximately day 80 after marrow transplant patients are prepared for discharge home. A battery of tests are initiated to evaluate the patient for chronic GVHD (see Table 13.8). Protocols designed to prevent or treat chronic graft-versus-host disease and other potential transplant-re-

Table 13.6. Symptoms Managed in the Bone Marrow Transplant Ambulatory Care Setting

Symptoms	Possible Causes
Fever	Bacterial, (Gram-negative, Gram-positive sepsis) fungal infection (*Candida, Aspergillus*)
	Interstitial pneumonia, (bacterial, viral, idiopathic)
	Herpes simplex virus, varicella zoster
	GVHD
	Hepatitis
	Granulocytopenia
	Blood product transfusions/Drug toxicity
	Recurrent disease
Nausea	GVHD
Vomiting	Gastrointestinal infection (CMV, *Salmonella, Shigella, C. difficile*)
Diarrhea	Mucositis
	Leukoencephalopathy, encephalitis, subdural hematoma
	Septicemia
	Adrenal insufficiency
	Liver disease
	Cholecystitis, pancreatitis
	Hyperalimentation withdrawal
	Psychological
	Drug toxicity
Bleeding	Thrombocytopenia
	GVHD, gut
	Hemmorhagic cystitis
	Drug-related (prednisone)
	Herpes simplex virus infection
Pruritus	Acute & chronic GVHD
	Herpes varicella zoster
	Drug toxicity
	Blood product transfusions
Rash	GVHD, HSV, drug toxicity
Fatigue	Drug related (interferon)
	Altered sleep patterns
	Premature menopause
	Psychological stress
Dyspnea	Sinopulmonary infection; restrictive, obstructive lung disease; CMV pneumonia
Pain	Herpes zoster, relapse, GVHD, peptic ulcer disease, mucositis, gastritis
Weight loss	Dehydration, mucositis, GVHD, drug-related therapy, depression, malabsorption, body image
Vasomotor instability	Leukoencephalopathy
a. nervousness	Premature menopause, drug toxicity
b. anxiety	Hypomagnesemia
c. irritability	
d. depression	

(continued)

Table 13.6.   *Continued*

Symptoms	Possible Causes
Jaundice	GVHD, infection, drug toxicity, hepatitis
Body image changes	Alopecia Wearing a mask Drug-related (cyclosporine/prednisone) Hyperalimentation High-dose chemotherapy, TBI Presence of venous access catheter Early menopause/sterility Growth and development problems
Psychological: role changes, adaptation/ integration into community	Issues of survival Feelings of taking "advantage" of donor Rehabilitation needs Rebirth or Lazarus syndrome Survival syndrome Role changes within family

lated problems are initiated (Sullivan et al. 1984; Sullivan 1986). The primary purpose of this evaluation is to assure that patients return to their primary care physicians in an optimal level of health and that these primary care physicians have the ability and facilities to care for their patients. In addition, the evaluation for presence of GVHD and other valuable data is gathered to be used by long-term follow-up teams. This phase of transplant is an anxious time for patients and is viewed as the last major hurdle toward recovery. Long-term follow-up teams play an important role in the transition of care to home. Discharge conferences that include a member of the long-term team supports continuity of care and facilitates the transition to wellness (Nims and Strom 1988).

Patients are requested to remain in the care of the outpatient BMT teams until approximately day 100 after BMT. It is at this time that most acute transplantation-related complications have been resolved and most patients can return to the care of their hometown physicians.

Long-Term Care (Day l00 after BMT)

The importance of a long-term follow-up team to aid primary care physicians and patients after they have returned to their communities cannot

be underestimated. Intensive research in recognizing, treating, and preventing the late and adverse effects of BMT has been directly responsible for the growing number of marrow recipients living normal lives. Nurses involved in long-term follow-up of patients are an integral part of the ambulatory care BMT team (Buchsel 1986; Nims and Strom 1988). Knowledge of nursing interventions and prevention of potential long-term complications are discussed in Chapter 15.

Long-term complications are those complications that occur about 100 days after BMT and are reviewed in Chapter 15 (Sullivan 1984). As less toxic conditioning regimens emerge, potential adverse reactions will decrease. Conversely, newer toxicities may reveal themselves as patients survive longer.

Future Trends

Medical teams in ambulatory BMT units will continue to become even more innovative in expanding the delivery of care and procedures that can be safely managed in outpatient settings. Advances made in recombinant DNA and hematopoietic growth factors hold promise for stimulating rapid recovery after marrow grafting. As a

Anticipated discharge date _____

Name_____

Age_____   Allergies _____

Diagnosis_____   HA line _____

Date of transplant _____/_____/_____   Type _____

Type of transplant_____   Problems _____

Protocols _____

GVHD prophylaxis: MTX CSP MTX+CSP GVHD treatment: _____

CMV prophylaxis: (CMV-): _____ screened blood   CMV-1g (CMV+): _____   CMV titer: _____

Infection prophylaxis: LAF PSA Immunoglobulin

IT MTX_____   Last CXR _____

Assessment of Home Environment

Location _____   Phone _____

_____

   Will this change during patient's stay? _____

Physical setup_____

Safety factors _____

Problems:

Assessment of Home Care Providers

Who_____

   Will this change during patient's stay? _____

Figure 13.3. Discharge Information Sheet

Ability to provide HA care and HA infusion:

Home health care referral?

Family and patient profile:

Capabilities and Needs While an Outpatient

Special Needs

Blood products:

Antibiotics:

Amphotericin:

HA and/or hydration:

_____ Day Post-transplant

Inpatient Problems

Graft: _____

Infection: _____

GVHD: _____

Other: _____

Ongoing Problems

Reprinted with permission: Chielens and Herrick 1990.

Figure 13.3.   *Continued*

Table 13.7. Basic Instructions for Bone Marrow Transplant Patients

- Wear a mask until six months after transplant
- Practice good hand washing techniques
- Limit number of sexual partners
- Practice "safe sex"
- Avoid infectious persons
- Avoid school/work for six months
- Avoid hot tubs, public swimming pools
- Avoid live viral vaccines for one year post-BMT

result, hospital stays will be shorter and patients will more easily make the transition to outpatient centers. Visionary administrators will continue to support the care of patients in less traditional models of care, e.g. infusion centers. Research on day hospital programs have been initiated for oncology patients who have undergone aggressive diagnostic and therapeutic procedures.

When compared to intensive inpatient treatment, day hospital care in certain circumstances has proved more cost-effective without any ad-verse effect on the patient's physical or functional outcome. Research in non-oncologic areas has compared early discharge with home health support to traditional care with similar results (Brooten et al. 1986). Current research is aimed at reducing the cost of BMT with early discharge patients receiving home health care support.

The projected increase in the number of marrow transplants will demand cost-effective health care delivery systems. Models of care that can support the increasing number of patients receiving intravenous antibiotics, growth factors, and blood products in the home setting (Rutman et al. 1990) will continue to be developed. Consequently, there is a growing need for oncology nurses with marrow transplant knowledge to enter home health care.

Newer techniques of marrow harvesting may soon allow donors to be regularly harvested in outpatient settings (Thomas 1988). New research indicates that peripheral blood stem cell harvests performed in outpatient settings may become a common practice in the near future (Applebaum 1989).

Table 13.8. Tests to Diagnose Chronic Graft-Versus-Host Disease

Systems affected by GVHD	Signs and Symptoms	Clinical Evaluation
Skin	Dry, flaky skin, scleroderma	Physical exam and skin biopsy
Oral	"White" patchy lichen planus lesions	Physical exam and lip biopsy
	Taste changes	
Eyes	Dry, scratchy eyes	Schirmer's tear test OS/OD
Liver	Lab values above > 292, > 41, > 1.2	Alkaline phosphatase/SGOT/total bilirubin
Lungs	Obstructive/Restrictive lung disease: abnormal PFTs	Pulmonary function tests
Immune system	Serological indicators of return of immune function	ANA, AMA, ASMA, RA, GGT IgA, IgM, IgE, C_3, C_4 (complement studies) Immunoglobulin subclasses Immunoglobulin titers Direct Coombs' test
Vaginal	Dry, constricted, striated vaginal tract	Gynecological exam
	Difficult intercourse	

Nursing Implications

The high cost of marrow transplant can be reduced by providing a health care delivery system that offers sophisticated and coordinated ambulatory care. Current and future marrow transplant teams will require vision to anticipate and develop safe, cost-effective alternative care settings. Patient acuity levels in the ambulatory care setting are increasing as the number of procedures and treatments that can be safely performed as an outpatient continue to escalate. Undoubtedly, new models of ambulatory care will emerge. Effective patient care of marrow candidates and survivors can be enhanced by nurses preparing to meet this challenge of offering safe, cost-effective ambulatory care for the BMT population.

Acknowledgement: Supported in part by grant numbers CA188221 and CA15704, awarded by The National Cancer Institute.

References

Aker, S.N. et al. 1983. Nutritional assessment in the marrow transplant patient. *Nutr. Supp. Serv. 3:* 22–37.

Andreeff, M., and Welte, K. 1989. Hematopoietic colony-stimulating factors. *Seminars in Oncology 16* (3): 211–229.

Applebaum F.R. 1989. Allogeneic marrow transplantation for malignancy: Current problems and prospects for improvement. In Magrath, I.T. (ed.). *New Directions in Cancer Treatment.* Heidelberg: Springer-Verlag, pp. 143–165.

ASCO/ASH Special Announcement. 1990. ASCO/ASH recommended criteria for the performance of bone marrow transplantation. *Blood 75* (5): 1209.

Beatty, P.G. et al. 1989. Marrow grafting from HLA-matched unrelated donors. *Blood 74* (7) (suppl. 1): 122A.

Bensinger, W. I. et al. 1982. ABO-incompatible marrow transplants. *Transplantation 33:* 427–429.

Bortin M.M., and Rimm, A.A. 1986. Increasing utilization of bone marrow transplantation. *Transplantation 42:* 229–234.

Brooten, D. et al. 1986. A randomized clinical trial of early hospital discharge and home follow-up of very-low-birth-weight infants. *N. Eng. J. Med. 315:* 934–939.

Buchsel, P. 1986. Long-term complications of allogeneic bone marrow transplantation: Nursing implications. *O.N.F. 13:* 61–70.

Buchsel, P. 1989. Ambulatory care of the bone marrow recipient: pre- and post-transplant considerations. *Puget Sound Quarterly 12:* 1.

Buchsel, P. 1990. Bone marrow transplantation. In Groenwald, C. et al. (eds.). *Cancer Nursing: Principles and Practice,* Second Edition. Boston: Jones and Bartlett, pp. 307–337.

Buchsel, P., and Kelleher, J. 1989. Bone marrow transplantation. *Nurs. Clin. North Am. 24* (4): 907–938.

Buchsel, P., and Parchem, C. 1988. Ambulatory care of the bone marrow transplant patient. *Semin. Oncol. Nurs. 4:* 41–46.

Buckner, C.C. et al. 1984. Marrow harvesting from normal donors. *Blood 64:* 630–634.

Carney, B. 1987. Bone marrow transplantation: Nurses' and physicians' perceptions of informed consent. *Cancer Nursing 10* (5): 252–259.

Chielens, D., and Herrick, E. 1990. Recipients of bone marrow transplants: Making a smooth transition to an ambulatory care setting. *O.N.F. 17* (6): 857–862.

Durbin, M. 1988. Bone marrow transplantation: Economic, ethical, and social issues. *Pediatrics 82* (5): 774–782.

Ford, R., and Ballard, B. 1988. Acute complications after bone marrow transplantation. *Semin. Oncol. Nurs. 4* (1): 15–24.

Haberman, M.R. 1988. Psychosocial aspects of bone marrow transplantation. *Semin. Oncol. Nurs. 4* (1): 55–59.

Holcombe, A. 1987. Bone marrow harvest. *Patient Education 14:* 63–65.

Lesko, L.M. 1989. Bone marrow transplantation. In Holland, J.C. and Rowland, J.H. (eds.). *Handbook of Psychooncology: Psychological care of the patient with cancer.* NY: Oxford University Press, pp. 163–173.

Lesko, L.M., and Hawkins, D.R. 1983. Psychological aspects of transplantation medicine. In Akhtar, S. (ed.). *New Psychiatric Syndromes: DSM-III and Beyond.* New York: Aronson, pp. 265–309.

Lesko, L.M. et al. 1989. Patients', parents', and oncologists' perceptions of informed consent for bone marrow transplantation. *Medical and Pediatric Oncology 17:* 181–187.

Levine, R.J. 1986. Referral of patients with cancer for participation in randomized clinical trials: Ethical considerations. *CA 36* (2): 95–99.

Nemunaitis, J. et al. in press. Phase I/II trial of recombinant human granulocyte-macrophage colony stimulating factor following allogeneic bone marrow transplantation. *N. Eng. J. Med.*

Nims, J.W., and Strom, S. 1988. Late complications of bone marrow transplant recipients: Nursing care issues. *Semin. Oncol. Nurs. 4* (1): 47–54.

Patenaude, A.F., and Rappeport, J.M. 1982. Surviving bone marrow transplantation: The patient in the other bed. *Ann. Intern. Med. 9* (7): 915–918.

Press O.W., Schaller, R.T., and Thomas, E.D. 1986. Bone marrow transplant complications. In Toledo-Pereyra, L.H. (ed.).

Complications of Organ Transplantation. NY: Marcel Dekker, pp. 399–424.

Ruggiero, M.R. 1988. The donor in bone marrow transplantation. *Semin. Oncol. Nurs. 4* (1): 9–14.

Rutman, R. et al. 1990. Home transfusion for the cancer patient. *Semin. Oncol. Nurs. 6* (2): 163–167.

Storb, R., and Thomas, E.D. 1983. Allogeneic bone marrow transplantation. *Immunol. Rev. 71*: 78–102.

Stream, P. 1983. Functions of the outpatient clinic. *Nurs. Clin. North Am. 18*: 603–610.

Sullivan, K.M. 1986. Acute and chronic graft-versus-host disease in man. *Int. J. Cell Cloning 4* (suppl. 1): 42–93.

Sullivan, K.M. et al. 1984. Late complications after marrow transplantation. *Semin. Hematol. 21*: 53–63.

Thomas, E.D. 1988. The future of marrow transplantation. *Semin. Oncol. Nurs. 40*: 74–78.

Tigne, M., and Fisher, S. 1988. A study of the oncology nurse role in ambulatory care. *O.N.F. 12*: 23–27.

Welch, H.G., and Larson, E.B. 1989. Cost effectiveness of bone marrow transplantation in acute nonlymphocytic leukemia. *N. Eng. J. Med. 321* (12): 807–812.

Wolcott, D.L. et al. 1986. Adaptation of adult bone marrow transplant recipient long-term survivors. *Transplantation 41*: 478–488.

Chapter 14

Psychosexual Adjustment and Fertility Issues

Jamie S. Ostroff and Lynna M. Lesko

Introduction

During the past twenty years, there have been major advances in transplantation medicine. As a result of progress in the fields of supportive and intensive care, histocompatability typing, and immunosuppressive drugs, bone marrow transplantation (BMT) is rapidly changing from a controversial research procedure with high morbidity and mortality to a widely used treatment modality offering potential cure for a growing number of patients with neoplastic disease (Lesko and Hawkins 1983; Lesko 1989). Increases in the likelihood of long-term survival for many patients diagnosed with neoplastic diseases that were previously resistant to conventional therapies has led to greater attention to the long-term adaptation of BMT patients.

Recent research has focused on the numerous medical and psychosocial consequences of children and young adults successfully treated for cancer (Meadows and Hobbie 1986; Cella and Tross 1986; Tross and Holland 1989; Welch-McCaffrey et al. 1989) (see Table 14.1). Much attention has been given to the medical late effects of cancer survivors. Conventional antineoplastic therapy can adversely affect virtually all major body systems as is evident from heightened risk of secondary malignancies, persistent immunosuppression, cardiomyopathy, pulmonary fibrosis, renal failure, cognitive impairment, endocrine abnormalities, and infertility (Byrd 1985; Li 1977; Meadows and Hobbie 1986; Thompson et al. 1987). In addition, several studies have documented the psychosocial sequelae of cancer survivors. Most notable among these psychological late effects are fear of recurrence, uncertainty about the future, heightened anxiety and depression, sense of personal inadequacy and diminished sense of personal control, and difficulty reentering family, vocational, school and friendship networks (Cella and Tross 1986; Fobair et al. 1986; Koocher and O'Malley 1981; Teta et al.

Table 14.1. Late Effects of Cancer Treatment

System	Late Effects
Cardiovascular	Cardiomyopathy
	Congestive heart failure
	Pericarditis
Endocrine	Hypothalamic-pituitary axis dysfunction
	Hypo/Hyperthyroidism
	Gonadal dysfunction
	Growth retardation
	Infertility
Gastrointestinal	Hepatic injury
	Chronic enteritis (GVHD)
Musculo-skeletal	Osteoporosis
	Growth retardation
Neurological	Encephalopathy
	Peripheral neuropathy
	Cognitive impairment
Pulmonary	Interstitial pneumonitis
	Pulmonary fibrosis
Urological/ Nephrological	Nephritis
	Chronic cystitis
	Renal failure
Oncological	Second malignancies
Dental	Tooth decay
Ophthalmologic	Cataracts
Immunologic	Persistent immunosuppression
	Chronic fatigue
Psychological	Fear of relapse
	Anxiety/Depression
	Somatic preoccupation
	Body image concerns
	Low self-esteem
	Family disruption
	Reentry issues: school, peers, vocation
	Transition from "sick role" to "well role"
	Social isolation and withdrawal

1986; Ostroff et al. 1989; Rieker et al. 1985). In aggregate, these findings suggest that childhood and young adult cancer survivors experience increased levels of psychological distress but that this distress neither reaches the magnitude associated with clinical psychopathology nor results in global psychosocial impairment.

Given the toxicity and psychological demands of the BMT regimen, BMT patients may experience additional short- and long-term sequelae that may adversely affect their physical, psychological, and interpersonal functioning (Lesko and Hawkins 1983; Lesko 1989). Wolcott and colleagues (1986) found that the majority of patients, who were at least one year post-BMT, experienced good psychological and medical outcomes. However, approximately 25% of their sample of long-term BMT survivors reported heightened emotional distress, chronic fatigue, low self-esteem, and global life dissatisfaction (Wolcott et al. 1986). Andrykowski and colleagues (1987) found that patients who were younger at the time of transplant (less than 30 years old) experienced better functioning in psychological and physical domains. In addition, they found that current functioning was not associated with the duration of time since transplant, diagnosis of acute or chronic graft-versus-host disease, or total radiation dose. Lesko and her colleagues (1989) compared young adult, acute leukemia survivors treated with either conventional chemotherapy alone or with conventional chemotherapy followed by BMT. They found no differences in global or illness-specific psychological distress, death anxiety, and social adjustment between these two subgroups of leukemia survivors. Thus, they concluded that BMT survivors experienced no greater psychosocial difficulties than leukemia survivors treated with conventional chemotherapy. In summary, these studies suggest wide variability in patients' post-BMT adjustment.

In this chapter, we will highlight clinical and research findings addressing the impact of BMT on patients' reproductive and sexual functioning. First, we will outline the effect of cancer treatment, and more specifically BMT, on gonadal function. Second, we will describe the more commonly seen psychosexual difficulties presented by BMT patients. Third, techniques for conducting a sexual assessment and clinical interventions in the transplant setting will be explained. Finally, recommendations for future research will be provided.

Cancer Treatment and Gonadal Function

To quote Sherins and Mulvihill (1989), "neoplastic disease and its treatment can potentially interfere with any cellular, anatomical, physiological, behavioral, or social processes that contributes to normal sexual and reproductive function." The reader should review this excellent and comprehensive chapter as background to material presented here. Other excellent reviews include papers by Maguire (1979), Ash (1980), Schilsky et al. (1980), Bajorunas et al. (1986a and 1986b), Gradishar and Schilsky (1989), Von Eschenbach and Schover (1984a and 1984b), and Auchincloss (1989), who have expertly synthesized the medical and physiological issues of gonadal dysfunction secondary to cancer and its treatment and recommend effective psychosexual rehabilitation interventions. Surgery, radiotherapy, and chemotherapy treatments can all affect gonadal and sexual functioning.

Chemotherapy-Related Dysfunction

Chemotherapeutic agents, singly or in combination, have a profound impact on male and female gonadal function. For men, several agents produce a dose-related depletion of the germinal epithelium lining resulting in decreased testicular volume, oligospermia, azoospermia, and possible infertility. Low sperm count and elevated FSH levels are physiological indicators of such germinal aplasia. The Stertoli cells, which produce testosterone,

are more resistant to chemotherapeutic agents, and subsequently, testosterone levels remain within normal range (Sherins and Mulvihill 1989). The chemotherapeutic agents most associated with testicular germ cell aplasia and infertility are listed in Table 14.2. Combination chemotherapy has an even more profound effect on the germ cell epithelium. While MOPP (nitrogen mustard, vincristine [Oncovin], procarbazine, and prednisone) treatment for lymphoma clearly produces irreversible germinal dysfunction (germinal aplasia, azoospermia, testicular atrophy, and elevated FSH), other regimens such as ABVD (Adriamycin, bleomycin, vinblastine, and DTIC) are equally as efficacious and cause less gonadal toxicity. Thirty-five percent of such patients develop germ cell aplasia but spermatogenesis usually always recovers (Sherins and Mulvihill 1989; Loescher et al. 1989). Chemotherapy-induced germinal cell aplasia is common with vinblastine, bleomycin, and cisplatin regimens for testicular cancer patients. Azoospermia appears to be reversible within two to three years in approximately half of such patients. However, 75% of such men may have low sperm counts prior to chemotherapy (Sherins and Mulvihill 1989). Additional chemotherapy during autologous BMT severely complicates gonadal recovery, as does retroperitoneal lymph node dissections. Chemotherapeutic agents are not known to directly affect the sexual response cycle (desire, arousal, ejaculation/orgasm) of men.

Ovarian failure has been documented in women receiving single agent and combination chemotherapy; such agents and their gonadal toxicity are listed in Table 14.2. Ovarian failure is evident by dysfunction of the ova and follicles, ovarian fibrosis, low estradiol levels, and elevated serum FSH and LH, resulting in amenorrhea and menopausal symptoms of estrogen deficiency (e.g., hot flashes, vaginal dryness, vaginitis, dyspareunia, irritability, decreased libido, vaginal epithelium atrophy and endometrial hypoplasia). (Normal oogenesis and hormonal ovarian plu-

Table 14.2. Chemotherapeutic Agents Associated with Infertility

Risk of Infertility	Drug	
	Male	Female
High-Definite	Chlorambucil	Chlorambucil
	Cyclophosphamide	Cyclophosphamide
	Nitrogen mustard	Nitrogen mustard
	Busulfan	Busulfan
	Procarbazine	Procarbazine
	Nitrosoureas	L-Phenylalamine mustard
Probable	Doxorubicin	
	Vinblastine	
	Cytosine arabinoside	
	Cisplatin	
Unlikely-Low	Methotrexate	Methotrexate
	5-Fluorouracil	5-Fluorouracil
	6-Mercaptopurine	6-Mercaptopurine
	Vincristine	
Unknown	Bleomycin	Doxorubicin
		Bleomycin
		Vinca alkaloids
		Cisplatin
		Nitrosoureas
		Cytosine arabinoside

Adapted from: Sherins, R.J., Mulvihill, J.J., (1989) Gonadal Dysfunction. In Devita, V., Hellman, S., and Rosenberg S.A. (eds.). *Cancer: Principles and Practice of Oncology.* Philadelphia: J.B. Lippincott Company: p. 2172–2173.

prology is expertly reviewed by Gradishar and Schilsky [1989].) The cumulative dose of the chemotherapeutic agent and the age of the patient influence the frequency and duration of amenorrheic symptomatology. It appears that older women are less able to tolerate larger cumulative drug doses before amenorrhea develops and have a greater likelihood of permanent dysfunction when treatment is stopped.

Alkylating agents appear to be the most notorious cause of ovarian failure, particularly in the older patient. Combination chemotherapy, as in the male patient, can cause gonadal dysfunction in women. MOPP treatment for Hodgkin's disease produces ovarian dysfunction in 40–50% of women (gonadal dysfunction is much lower than for men). However, long-term follow-up is necessary to determine whether the women who experience little ovarian failure are at risk for early

menopause and premature ovarian failure five to ten years after therapy (Sherins and Mulvihill 1989).

Unlike gonadal dysfunction in men, ovarian failure and subsequent low estradiol levels can directly and indirectly affect the sexual response cycle in woman. Low estrogen levels can result in decreased libido, vaginal atrophy, decreased vaginal secretions, and dyspareunia; all of which can have deleterious effects on desire, arousal, and orgasm.

Surgery and Gonadal Dysfunction

Very few patients who undergo BMT will have had previous surgery for pelvic or genital cancer that could affect gonadal function. Retroperitoneal lymph node dissection for testicular cancer staging may injure sympathetic innervation of the pelvic viscera and result in retrograde ejaculation and inadequate emission of sperm. However, capacity for libido, erection, and sensation of orgasm are usually not impaired (Sherins 1987; Shalet 1987; Sherins and Mulvihill 1989; Schover and Jensen 1988; Loescher et al. 1989).

Radiotherapy-Related Dysfunction

Although research has been done on the gonadal toxicity of chemotherapeutic agents, little is known about the adverse effects of radiotherapy (Sherins and Mulvihill 1989; Barrett et al. 1987). The testes are very radiosensitive; damage (both to the germinal epithelium and to Leydig cells) and recovery appear to be dose-dependent. Temporary azoospermia develops after 150–2000 cGy, and men who receive 2000–3000cGy require at least three years to recover normal production. Permanent sterility is achieved at 6000cGy. Unfortunately, adolescents and young men receiving higher doses of radiation (2400cGy) to the testes as prophylaxis (for gonadal relapse of ALL) demonstrate not only germinal aplasia but Leydig cell dysfunction resulting in testosterone deficiencies. Radiotherapy may also cause erectile and ejaculatory difficulties, thereby affecting the male sexual response cycle.

Similarly for women, gonadal dysfunction and infertility after radiotherapy is dose-related, and unlike men, is also age dependent. To quote Loescher et al. (1989), "Permanent infertility occurred in 60% of women aged 15–40 and in 100% over age 40, after 25–500GY treatments." Permanent infertility in women aged 15–40 occurred 70% of the time after receiving 500 to 800cGy (Gradishar and Schilsky 1989). Particularly in lymphoma therapy, the ovary may be shielded from radiation by surgically placing the ovaries midline behind the uterus. This procedure appears to lower the risk of ovarian failure to 50% of women receiving pelvic radiation (Sherins and Mulvihill 1989).

Radiation may also alter vaso-congestive mechanisms of female genital arousal, decrease

vaginal lubrication during the excitement phase, and result in dyspareunia due to vaginal stenosis, atrophy, fibrosis, and vaginitis. Thus, radiation may adversely affect all phases of the female sexual cycle.

Bone Marrow Transplantation

To date there has been little or nothing written about the ovarian and testicular function of patients undergoing autologous BMT. For now, we will need to extrapolate crucial information on endocrine/gonadal function, fertility/pregnancy, and psychosexual functions from the few allogeneic transplant studies (Card et al. 1980; Jacobs and Dubousky 1981; Deeg et al. 1983; Sanders et al. 1983; Sanders 1987; Barrett 1987; Sanders et al. 1988; Benker et al. 1989; Mumma et al. 1989).

The reader should review several reports by Sanders and colleagues examining gonadal function following allogeneic marrow transplantation (Sanders et al. 1983; Sanders 1987; Sanders et al. 1988). However, we need to be cautious in extrapolating these data to all autologous patients, particularly those patients who have undergone treatment for testicular cancer. Sanders reports data on pre- and post-pubertal men and women who have undergone BMT for aplastic anemia (cyclophosphamide [CY] 200mg/kg) and acute leukemia (CY 120mg/kg and 9.2–15.8cGy total body irradiation [TBI]). Both CY and TBI may produce gonadal dysfunction and germ cell destruction, from which total recovery may be possible in a select few.

In summary, Sanders' extensive follow-up of patients reveals the following: (1) After receiving a high-dose alkylating agent such as CY alone for BMT, most prepubertal children develop normally through puberty and have normal gonadotropin levels (LH: luteinizing hormone, FSH: follicle stimulating hormone). Of course those children diagnosed with aplastic anemia received no prior gonadal toxic treatments prior to BMT. (2) The majority of prepubertal children with acute leukemia who received CY and TBI as a preconditioning regimen have delayed puberty and abnormal gonadotropin levels. However, a few girls did achieve menarche, which suggests that radiation to the ovary of a prepubertal girl may not result in permanent damage. Testosterone or estrogen/progesterone supplementation may be necessary in that case. (3) The majority of adults who received CY-only regimen regained normal gonadal function. Approximately 50% of women had return of their menstrual cycles 6–18 months post-BMT, however recovery was transient for some (two to six years), with development of menopausal symptoms, low estradiol, and elevated gonadotropin levels (Sanders et al. 1988). All men had normal testosterone levels after BMT and most regained normal gonadotropin levels. Limited data was available on semen analysis. Sixty-seven percent of the patients appeared to have detectable sperm counts. (4) Primary gonadal dysfunction appears to occur in all patients who are postpubertal at transplant following a combination of CY and TBI. All of these patients had leukemia and received prior cytoreductive therapy. Women had primary ovarian failure, amenorrhea, and elevated gonadotropin levels. Recovery of ovarian function occurred in less than 10% of women between three and seven years after transplantation; all were 26 years and younger at BMT. Menopausal symptomatology (i.e., amenorrhea, vaginitis, decreased vaginal lubrication, osteoporosis, vasomotor instability, and dysphoria) was evident in at least 75% of the women who were greater than 26 years at BMT. All men had normal testosterone levels, and a majority (88%) had normal LH levels. FSH was elevated in 76% of the patients with azoospermia in 94% of the patients. Hormonal replacement in women appeared efficacious in relieving menopausal symptoms. Sanders and colleagues (1988) estimated that the probability of developing ovarian failure after receiving CY and TBI was 0.35 by seven years for women receiving CY alone, and 1.00 at one year. Women receiving CY only, had a 0.92 probability of ovarian recovery at seven

years and those receiving both CY and TBI had a 0.24 probability of recovery. They concluded that both greater patient age and TBI were significantly correlated with a greater probability of ovarian failure.

Bone Marrow Transplantation and Pregnancy

There have been a few reports of pregnancies and deliveries of normal children in women with severe aplastic anemia treated with allogeneic bone marrow transplantation (Card et al. 1980; Jacobs and Dubousky 1981; Deeg et al. 1983; Sanders et al. 1988). Even though normal infants were delivered 15–24+ months post-transplantation, success must be tempered by the fact that these female patients, unlike other patients undergoing BMT, (1) had no previous induction or conditioning chemotherapy regimens, and (2) received only high dose cyclophosphamide as a preparatory regimen for their BMT (i.e., no radiation), and (3) in general, the majority were young at time of transplant. All these conditions probably lead to less gonadal dysfunction. Unfortunately, not all such patients with aplastic anemia become pregnant, or successfully deliver a normal infant. Moreover, these results cannot be inferred for autologous BMT patients due to differences in therapeutic regimen prior to transplant and preconditioning regimens. There are limited accounts of men who have undergone BMT for aplastic anemia or leukemia and fathered normal children (Sanders et al. 1983). See Table 14.3 for those results.

Specific Sexual Disorders Associated with BMT

Human sexuality is usually categorized by sex therapists and researchers according to a multiphasic sexual response cycle divided into the phases of desire, arousal, orgasm, and resolution (Kaplan 1974 and 1983). According to this model

Table 14.3. Pregnancy and Allogeneic BMT

Study	Patient/Disease/TX	Results
Card et al. 1980	Female/aplastic anemia 29 years old at BMT chemotherapy	Case report delivered normal infant 24 months post-BMT
Jacobs and Dubousky 1981	Female/aplastic anemia 36 years old at BMT chemotherapy	Case report delivered normal infant 21 months post-BMT
Deeg et al. 1983	Female/aplastic anemia 25 years old at BMT chemotherapy	Case report delivered normal infant 23 months post BMT
Sanders et al. 1983	31 males/aplastic anemia chemotherapy	3 pts fathered 4 children
	41 males/leukemia chemotherapy and TBI	1 pt fathered 2 children
Sanders et al. 1988	43 females/aplastic anemia chemotheraphy	
	27 age < 26 yrs at BMT	6 pts/8 pregnancies 5 pts delivered 7 normal infants 1 pt had elective abortion
	16 age > 26 yrs at BMT	3 pts/4 pregnancies 1 normal delivery
	144 females/leukemia chemotherapy and TBI	9/144 ovarian recovery all 13–25 years old at BMT 3 pregnancies in 2 women at 3,5,6 years no live births

of the normal human sexual response, the desire phase is characterized by sexual thoughts and fantasies as well as interest in having sexual activity. The arousal phase consists of a subjective sense of sexual pleasure and accompanying physiologic changes. For men, penile tumescence leading to erection and the appearance of glandular secretions characterize the arousal phase. For women, pelvic vasocongestion, vaginal lubrication, and swelling of the external genitalia are signs of female arousal. Orgasm is a period of peak sexual pleasure, with release of sexual tension and rhythmic muscular contractions. In the male, there is the sensation of ejaculatory inevitability, which is followed by emission of semen. Finally, during the resolution phase there is a sense of relaxation. Sexual disorders can occur at one or more phases

of the sexual response cycle and are categorized by the *Diagnostic and Statistical Manual of Mental Disorders,* (American Psychiatric Association 1987) into sexual desire disorders, sexual arousal disorders, orgasm disorders, and sexual pain disorders.

In the following section, we will describe the impact of BMT on the sexual response cycle according to the diagnostic categories listed in the *Diagnostic and Statistical Manual of Mental Disorders* (American Psychiatric Association 1987) which are summarized in Table 14.4. Attention will also be given to plausible physical and psychological mechanisms for understanding sexual difficulties in this special population. Given the paucity of controlled research on the sexual adjustment of BMT patients, much of the material

Table 14.4. Sexual Disorders with Bone Marrow Transplantation

Phase	Sexual Dysfunction	Relevance to BMT Patients and Survivors
Desire Sexual thoughts, daydreaming fantasies; finding potential partner attractive	Inhibited sexual desire disorder Loss of interest in sex: few or no thoughts about sex, negative ("antisexual") attitudes about sex Anxious, panicky feeling about sex avoidance of sexual situations	Not unusual when patient is in active treatment. Prolonged separation due to lengthy hospitalization, reverse isolation. After treatment, loss of desire may be related to treatment side effects, psychological factors (depression, anxiety) and partner issues, fear of infections, body image concerns, pain, GVHD, fatigue. Often requires longer treatment of couple by sex therapist because of prominent psychological component.
Arousal Subjective sense of excitement and pleasure; penile erection	Inhibited sexual arousal disorder Erectile impotence in men: difficulty attaining or maintaining an erection	No direct physiological link between BMT and erectile function. Treatment depends on cause. Counseling to decrease anxiety and decrease focus on performance. Rare complaint in BMT patients, unless preexisting.
Vaginal lubrication and engorgement in women	Impaired vaginal lubrication and engorgement in women	Common after pelvic irradiation, or any treatment that causes women ovarian loss or failure. Patient may complain of dry, sore vagina or painful intercourse. Treatment: estrogens, (local or systemic), lubricant, taking more time for foreplay, communication issues.
Orgasm Reflex muscle contractions, associated with pleasure, ejaculation and emission in men, pleasurable sensation in women	Inhibited female orgasm: anorgasmia	May be related to fatigue, depression, stress, medication, anxiety, inadequate arousal phase. Need longer or more direct stimulation of clitoris. Address need for time and relaxation, communication issues with partner.
	Inhibited male orgasm: retarded ejaculation Premature ejaculation: inability to control timing of orgasm	May be related to fatigue, depression, stress, medication, anxiety. Rare complaint in BMT patients, unless pre-exisitng. More common in young BMT patients and after prolonged period of abstinence.
	Retrograde ejaculation	May occur after pretransplant surgical staging of testicular cancer patients

(continued)

Table 14.4. *Continued*

Phase	Sexual Dysfunction	Relevance to BMT Patients and Survivors
Other	Dyspareunia: pain with intercourse	Often leads to sexual avoidance unless treated promptly.
		Requires thorough gynecological evaluation and treatment of cause (irradiation changes, estrogen deficiency). Practice "no painful sex" rule (i.e., no intercourse unless medical cause is adequately treated)
	Vaginismus: vaginal muscle spasm, penetration painful or impossible	Reponse to pain or fear of pain with penetration.
		Good prognosis with combined relaxation and sequenced penetration treatment, done by patient herself, then with partner.

With permission. *Handbook of Psychooncology*, edited by Holland, J.C. and Rowland, J.H. Oxford University Press. 1989.

presented will be based on the authors' clinical experience as psychiatric consultants to the allogeneic and autologous BMT services at Memorial Sloan-Kettering Cancer Center and research comparing the psychosexual adjustment of cancer survivors treated with either BMT or conventional chemotherapy.

Generally speaking, patients rarely express sexual concerns prior to or during the acute hospitalization for their BMT. This is not terribly surprising since patients are quite debilitated by the preparatory conditioning regimen and almost uniformly preoccupied with more life and death issues such as, separation from family, "surviving the transplant," marrow engraftment, and their "counts." While sexual functioning is not a primary concern for hospitalized BMT patients, standard requirements for a sterile, germ-free environment during periods of bone marrow suppression and the lengthy hospitalization (approximately one to two months) associated with the transplant impose severe restrictions on couples' intimacy and sexuality. In addition, acute and chronic GVHD and scars from Hickman and Broviac catheters may increase body image concerns, which may subsequently impair sexuality. For most patients and their partners, the transplant and immediate, post-hospitalization convalescence represent periods of sexual abstinence due to fatigue, pain, skin rashes, and other complications secondary to the transplant as well as the acute stress of the transplant on patients and their partners.

Post-BMT convalescence is quite lengthy since physical and psychological rehabilitation may last for six to twelve months. Up until this point, patients often complain of persistent fatigue, anxiety about infections, depression, and difficulty reentering their normal home and work activities (Lesko et al. 1989). Generally, BMT patients become more concerned about their sexual health as their physical health status improves. Sexual interest and activity generally are not resumed until at least six months post-transplant. Thus, sexual concerns and disorders usually will be presented to the transplant team relatively late in the BMT rehabilitation period.

The most common sexual disorder presented by male and female BMT patients is hypoactive *sexual desire disorder*. When compared to healthy nonpatients, female acute leukemia patients treated with BMT reported significantly lower sexual drive (Mumma et al. 1989). Low sexual desire (American Psychiatric Association 1987) consists of persistently deficient or absent sexual thoughts, fantasies, and desire for sexual activity. This diagnosis should always be made in the context of the patient's precancer sexual desire, age, sex and physical health status. The sexual desire of BMT patients may be diminished for several direct reasons such as persistent fatigue, body image concerns (e.g., skin lesions caused by GVHD, catheter insertion), depression, and reluctance to resume sexual activity following prolonged abstinence. In addition, among female BMT patients, low estrogen levels secondary to cancer treatment also contribute to decreased sexual desire. Other indirect reasons for decreased sexual desire include patients' avoidance of sexual activity secondary to painful intercourse or decreased sexual satisfaction. Partners may inadvertently contribute to patients' low sexual desire by being reluctant to initiate sex until reassured by the medical staff that sexual activity will not interfere with the rehabilitation process or endanger the convalescence of the patient. In addition, low sexual desire is positively correlated with shorter time since diagnosis, being more psychologically distressed, having more illness-related problems, and poorer body image and sexual satisfaction (Mumma et al. 1989).

Male and female *sexual arousal disorder* (American Psychiatric Association 1987) consists of a persistent or recurrent lack of a subjective sense of sexual excitement and pleasure during sexual activity. For men, sexual arousal is also characterized by persistent or recurrent partial failure to attain or maintain erection during sexual activity. As stated earlier, no studies have documented adverse direct physiological effects of BMT on male erectile functioning. However, pretransplant surgical staging of testicular cancer prior to autologous BMT may result in retrograde ejaculation and erectile dysfunction. Therefore, most cases of male arousal disorder will have a

psychogenic etiology. For instance, high levels of anxiety may interfere with sexual arousal and erectile functioning. In contrast, female BMT patients are likely to experience several physiological changes that may impair female arousal. As stated earlier, ovarian failure and concomitant low estradiol levels secondary to chemotherapy and radiation, are associated with decreased vaginal blood flow and secretions that have a direct impact on female arousal. In addition, without these physical signs of sexual excitement, many women may not subjectively experience sexual pleasure.

Inhibited male and female *orgasm disorder* (American Psychiatric Association 1987) is characterized by a persistent or recurrent delay in, or absence of orgasm following a normal sexual excitement phase that is adequate in focus, intensity, and duration as judged by the clinician. Assuming no preexisting orgasm disorder, male BMT patients are not likely to complain of orgasm problems (however testicular cancer patients who have undergone retroperitoneal node dissection may have some orgasmic dysfunction). After a prolonged period of abstinence or in cases of heightened anxiety, male BMT patients may ejaculate prematurely; however, this problem is usually short-lived with reassurance and resumption of sexual activity. Another reason that male BMT patients rarely present with orgasm disorders is that the preceding sexual response phase of arousal is generally intact. On the other hand, women may complain of anorgasmia secondary to diminished sexual arousal. It should be evident that impairment in one sexual response phase may adversely affect another aspect of sexuality such that a more complex sexual problem develops.

Finally, *sexual pain disorders* are relatively common among female BMT patients. Given the increased likelihood of ovarian failure secondary to chemotherapy and radiation, the experience or fear of sexual pain is somewhat common for female BMT patients. Insufficient lubrication and vaginal atrophy are linked to dyspareunia (American Psychiatric Association 1987), recurrent or consistent genital pain before, during or after sexual intercourse. Vaginismus (American Psychiatric Association 1987) is characterized by involuntary spasm of the musculature of the outer third of the vagina. In addition, heightened anxiety or "spectatoring," being preoccupied with extraneous thoughts, during sex also reduces arousal, which in turn may lead to painful intercourse. In our clinical experience, sexual pain disorders are rare among male BMT patients (see Table 14.5).

Assessment of Sexual Functioning

The following section will outline the fundamental aspects of conducting an evaluation of sexual functioning in the transplant setting. A comprehensive sexual history is the cornerstone of a thorough evaluation of sexual functioning. Sexual problems among cancer survivors are usually the result of both the emotional and psychological distress evoked by the illness and its treatment, and the physiologic consequences of the type of cancer and the treatments utilized (Von Eschenbach and Schover 1984a and 1984b). Certainly, this multidimensional etiology is also true for BMT patients for whom sexual difficulties are often the blending of both physical and psychological factors. Given that the cause of sexual difficulties is usually due to a number of psychogenic *and* organic insults to one's sexual health, it is imperative to place assessment of sexual functioning in the broader context of BMT patients' past and current physical, psychological, and interpersonal domains. Therefore, assessment must include the physical, emotional, and relationship aspects of sexuality.

Table 14.5. Summary of Treatment Effects on Gonadal Dysfunction

		Female				
	Hormones	Fertility	Desire	Arousal	Orgasm	Dyspareunia
Chemotherapy*	↓Estradiol ↑LH ↑FSH	↓ova	↓	↓	↓	↑
Surgery	Excluding hysterectomy oophorectomy	nl	nl	nl	nl	—
Radiation*	↓Estradiol ↑LH ↑FSH	↓ova	↓	↓	↓	↑

*Age and dose dependent

		Male				
	Hormones	Fertility	Desire	Arousal	Orgasm	Dyspareunia
Chemotheraphy*	nl LH ↓ FSH nl testosterone	↓ sperm	nl	nl	nl	—
Surgery	possible ↓ testosterone	↓ sperm	nl	nl	↓	↑
Radiation*	nl LH ↓ FSH nl testosterone	↓ sperm nl	nl	nl	nl	nl

*Dose dependent

Many staff consider dealing with the sexuality of their patients to be quite challenging and they often perceive many barriers to addressing sexual issues (Auchincloss 1989). The initial challenge in conducting an assessment of sexual functioning is one of "communication comfort." BMT patients rarely ask for help with a sexual problem, even though research conducted with anonymous cancer patients suggests that up to 90% of these patients experience sexual concerns and difficulties (Andersen 1985). This paradox points to the need for primary care clinicians to encourage patients to ask questions and voice concerns of a sexual nature. However, few oncologists and oncology nurse clinicians have been trained to assess and treat sexual disorders secondary to cancer or its treatment. Given that BMT patients may be at particular risk for sexual dysfunction and, like most cancer patients, they may be reluctant to initiate discussions about sexual concerns, it is crucial that clinicians on the transplant team develop skill and competence in assessing the nature of patients' sexuality and making appropriate interventions or referrals, when warranted.

An important preliminary issue is when the topic of sexuality should be raised. Some patients may ask questions or raise sexual concerns during the pretransplant period. These patients are clearly indicating their interest in understanding how the transplant will affect their sexuality and want to know how they can best prepare to preserve their sexual intimacy. However, it should not be assumed that patients who do not directly ask about sexual issues are not interested in the effects of BMT on sexual functioning. In contrast, research has shown that a wide variety of sexual concerns are almost universal among cancer patients even though very few patients raise these issues directly (Vincent et al. 1975). Health professionals who address sexual issues early in the transplant process convey a willingness to discuss these topics, provide a legitimacy to sexual health as an important aspect of the quality of life, and promote sexual health as a realistic expectation for post-BMT survivors. Patients who

are encouraged to discuss sexual concerns during the pretransplant interview most likely will feel more comfortable raising concerns during the post-transplant rehabilitation period. Therefore, we recommend asking general questions about sexuality as a routine part of the pretransplant psychosocial assessment. Open-ended questions such as "How has your sexuality been affected by your illness and its treatment?" and "What concerns do you have about the effects of the BMT procedure on your sexual or reproductive functioning?" provide an invaluable baseline for comparing post-treatment sexual functioning. Questions about sexual functioning should also be included as a routine part of follow-up care since patients often resume interest in sexual activity approximately three to six months post-transplant.

In those cases when a particular sexual problem is noted, a more extensive assessment is needed. This evaluation may be done by a trained member of the transplant team or referred to a mental health professional who specializes in evaluating the sexual functioning of medically ill patients. The following description of the nuts-and-bolts of a sexual history is based on work conducted by Auchincloss (1989) and Schover and Jensen (1988) in adapting the evaluation model, originally proposed by Kaplan (1983), for cancer patients.

It is important to assess each phase of the sexual response cycle (desire, arousal, orgasm) so as to identify the extent of the problem. As stated earlier, loss of desire is a common complaint among male and female BMT patients. It is important to ask patients "How often do you have sexual intercourse?", "How often do you have sexual thoughts or fantasies?", "Have there been any changes in your sexual desire?", and "What factors contribute to your loss of sexual interest?" In terms of arousal disorders (e.g., difficulty attaining or maintaining an erection, lack of vaginal lubrication and swelling), it is important to ask patients whether they feel excited and aroused during sex. Male BMT patients should be asked whether if, given adequate stimulation, they develop and maintain an erection during sex, while females should be asked whether they notice signs of arousal, such as vaginal swelling and wetness. Impairments in female sexual arousal often lead to painful intercourse and subsequent avoidance of sex. Painful intercourse should be thoroughly assessed. Finally, an inability to have an orgasm or changes in orgasm can result from the psychological or physical effects of cancer treatment. Patients need to be asked whether they experience orgasms during sex.

In addition to identifying the nature of the sexual problem, it is critical to get a detailed description of the onset, severity, and frequency of any sexual complaints. A careful history highlighting "When did the problem begin?", "How often is it a problem?", "How much does it interfere with either you or your partner's sexual enjoyment?", and "What do you and your partner do when this problem arises?" should be obtained. It is important to explore nonsexual aspects of the patient's intimate relationship and whether they have ever experienced sexual problems before.

Although many professionals and patients may be unaccustomed to the private nature and explicitness of the sexual history, several techniques can facilitate the clinician's and the patient's comfort in discussing sexual issues. Conducting a sexual history in a private, professional setting after explaining the rationale of the sexual evaluation, and assuring patient confidentiality are instrumental in establishing initial rapport and decreasing anxiety. Similarly, starting with less sensitive material and then moving to more sensitive areas is a good way to gradually increase nurse and patient comfort. In addition, "normalizing" sexual questions by prefacing them with explanations of wide variation in normal sexual practices and how common these concerns are among BMT patients will help patients feel less threatened by their fears of being perceived as aberrant. For example, it may be helpful to preface a question about frequency of sexual in-

tercourse by stating that there is obviously no right or wrong answer and that most couples find that sexual activity is dependent on many factors such as energy level and the availability of a private place. As with other counseling situations, a nonjudgemental stance and a tolerance for the wide variation in expression of normal sexual functioning, are critical in eliciting an honest account of sexual practices as well as in establishing a solid foundation for a therapeutic relationship. Likewise, empathy and sensitivity provide a supportive context for the exploration of sexual issues. With practice, most nurse clinicians find that they can conduct an initial sexual functioning evaluation with comfort and confidence.

In addition to the sexual history, a complete assessment of a sexual complaint should include a medical evaluation. Since it is certainly plausible that BMT patients could experience sexual difficulties that are not secondary to their transplantation, the medical evaluation should be broad-based and targeted to the full array of organic factors that are associated with sexual dysfunction. This medical assessment should include a history of general health, cancer disease and treatment, and current medications. A physical examination is particularly helpful for working up dyspareunia in that a pelvic examination provides information about the extent of vaginal atrophy, stenosis, and fibrosis, which are relatively common late effects of treatment-induced menopause. Finally, in addition to serum blood levels of hormones, several laboratory procedures have been developed for the specific evaluation of male and female sexual disorders. Readers interested in a more thorough discussion of the medical assessment of sexual disorders among the medically ill should see Schover and Jensen (1988) for an excellent review of this area.

In summary, the goal of the sexual assessment is to gather information that enables the clinician (1) to determine the extent to which the patient's sexual functioning has been preserved, (2) to identify potential sexual problems that the patient and his or her partner may be experiencing, (3) to better understand the factors related to the onset and maintenance of the sexual problem, and (4) to develop an appropriate treatment plan that addresses the patient's particular needs. Most important, early identification of sexual concerns and difficulties is crucial in the prevention of sexual dysfunction secondary to bone marrow transplantation. By identifying potential problems early in the transplant, it is more likely that sexual health will be well-preserved following the transplant. Implicitly, conducting a sexual assessment conveys a sense of importance to the goal of preserving the sexual health of BMT patients. This goal is in accordance with the more global effort to improve the quality of life for all cancer patients.

Interventions Aimed at Improving Sexual Functioning

The PLISSIT Model

Once the assessment has been completed and a particular sexual problem has been identified, the nurse clincian's next step is to formulate a treatment plan that specifically addresses the patient's individual needs. According to Annon's (1976) PLISSIT model of progressive intervention, clinical interventions should be utilized in a sequential manner, depending on the severity of the problem. The process begins with permission (P), then limited information (LI), and proceeding to specific suggestions (SS), and intensive therapy (IT), if warranted. Each level requires a greater degree of therapist skill and competence. The necessary level of treatment should be determined during the sexual assessment. The PLISSIT treatment model has been found useful in oncology nursing settings (Cooley et al. 1986), as summarized in Table 14.6.

Permission (P)

Permission encourages a patient to discuss a sexual concern. Giving permission to discuss sexuality often reassures patients of the normalcy of their concerns and of the appropriateness of monitoring sexual health as an important part of comprehensive cancer rehabilitation. In and of itself, permission to discuss sexual concerns with the transplant team members often reduces fear and anxiety about sexual impairment. By initiating discussions about sexual functioning, clinicians encourage BMT patients and their partners to further discuss sexual concerns with each other and with members of the transplant team. When sexual issues are raised during an evaluation, nurses provide a useful first step in clinical intervention toward preserving the sexual health of their BMT patients. When viewed in this manner, P is seen as primary prevention of sexual disorders secondary to BMT. Giving permission to discuss sexuality sets the stage for the next level of clinical intervention: limited information.

Limited Information (LI)

Limited information includes the full range of patient education services. Several informative pamphlets on male and female sexuality are available from the American Cancer Society and often each transplant service has materials developed for their own patients. These guidebooks include diagrams of male and female genital/reproductive organs, explanations of the sexual side effects of cancer treatment, and basic advice on sexual rehabilitation. Obviously, information about the possible sexual and reproductive sequelae of BMT should be a standard part of the informed consent procedure. Accurate information about sexuality enhances patients' ability to make sound decisions and choices about methods of preserving sexual health. In addition, patient education helps to dispel misconceptions regarding sexual activity. Patients are often reluctant to engage in sexual activity after there has been a period of abstinence due to medical treatment. Reassurances about the safety of resuming sexual functioning are often viewed as helpful to patients and their partners.

Table 14.6. Treatment Strategies for Sexual Disorders

Sexual Disorder	P	LI	SS	IT	Comment
Desire disorder	Assess and encourage discussion about treatment with staff and partner	Patient and partner education about common causes of low desire; explain reproductive sexual side effects of BMT Reassure patients and partners of safety of sex post-BMT	Plan "romantic" evening with partner; plan sexual activity when rested and relaxed; make time for sexual activity	Refer to sex therapist	May require more intensive treatment by sex therapist due to prominence of illness-related and global psychological factors
Female arousal disorder	Same	Patient education about radiation and chemotherapy impact on sexual arousal	Water-based genital lubricant; increase time and intensity of clitoral vaginal stimulation	Relaxation techniques; refer for hormone replacement therapy	
Male arousal disorder	Same	Same	Encourage prolonged non-demand penile stimulation; discourage performance anxiety	Refer to sex therapist and refer to urologist for thorough work-up of possible organic cases	
Pain disorders: dyspareunia	Same	Patient/Partner education	Alter position during sexual intercourse: water-based lubricant; encourage adequate arousal prior to penile penetration, discourage sexual intercourse until cause of painful intercourse has been treated	Refer to sex therapist and gynecologist; hormone replacement therapy	Needs to be treated promptly in order to prevent impairment in all sexual phases

Table 14.6. *Continued*

Sexual Disorder	P	LI	SS	IT	Comment
Vaginismus	Same	Same	Alter position during sexual intercourse	Relaxation techniques combined with vaginal dilation exercises	
Female orgasm disorder	Same	Patient/Partner education about impact of BMT on orgasm	Recommend longer or more direct clitoral stimulation, encourage communication with partner; plan sex when rested and relaxed	Refer to sex therapist or gynecologist	
Male orgasm disorder	Same	Same	Encourage adequate penile stimulation, plan sexual activity accordingly during time of maximum relaxation and energy	Refer to sex therapist or urologist	

Specific Suggestions (SS)

The next level of intervention involves making specific suggestions about sexuality. At this stage of intervention, a specific sexual concern or disorder has been identified during the sexual assessment. These specific suggestions may involve a combination of medical and psychosexual recommendations.

For instance, as stated earlier, radiation-induced vaginal changes (e.g., stenosis, fibrosis, and decreased lubrication) may diminish arousal and excitement, thereby leading to increased likelihood for dyspareunia and decreased orgasmic response. Hormonal imbalance may further reduce vaginal secretions and lead to painful intercourse. These impairments, in turn, may lead to a per-

nicious cycle of patient and/or partner avoidance of sexual activity and lowered desire. Treatment for radiation-induced vaginal changes should include support and education. Specific suggestions such as trying different positions for sexual intercourse and using an external, water-based lubricant along with finger dilation of the vagina can be helpful during foreplay to assist in easier entry of the penis. Many women find that the female superior position offers greater control over the rate of thrusting and the depth of penetration and therefore they feel less anxious about experiencing pain and respond more easily during intercourse. Given that radiation-induced vaginal changes often slow a female's excitement response, couples should be encouraged to engage in adequate foreplay prior to intercourse so as to enable the female BMT patient to be fully aroused.

For most BMT patients, separations due to prolonged hospitalization, preoccupation with medical decisions, and fatigue often diminish sexual desire. Some patients complaining of diminished sexual desire respond to specific suggestions to plan a "date" with their partner, which often promotes sexual intimacy.

Intensive Treatment (IT)

It is important to remember that the etiology of sexual complaints is often complex and that more intensive psychological and/or medical treatment may be necessary for some patients. Intensive therapy requires a highly trained and competent professional who specializes in treating sexual disorders among medically ill patients. There is a growing cadre of mental health professionals with advanced training in sexual and marital therapy. While many hospitals have identified appropriate referrals in their area, an additional source for identifying a competent sex therapist is the American Association of Sex Educators, Counselors and Teachers (AASECT).*

In recent years, the subspecialty of sex therapy has established itself as a well-researched and highly effective treatment for many sexual disorders. Readers interested in gaining detailed information about the principles and practices of sex therapy should see recent books by LoPiccolo and LoPiccolo (1978), Kaplan (1974, 1979, and 1983) and Leiblum and Pervin (1989).

The following two clinical vignettes illustrate many of the psychosexual issues that patients undergoing BMT express. Both cases happen to be women, who express such issues more often than their male counterparts, but who may actually exhibit more problems, based on our clinical and research experiences. Both cases reveal that patients never exhibit just one complaint nor are the issues as clear-cut as in the *Diagnostic and Statistical Manual of Mental Disorders* criteria; many issues multiply and are compounds of sexual and psychosocial functioning.

Case Vignette I

A 37-year-old married woman who was post-BMT for nine months with no evidence of Hodgkin's disease was referred to the sex counseling clinic for treatment of low sexual desire. She complained of being too tired for sex and not experiencing sexual pleasure with her husband during sexual intercourse. She wondered whether she was normal and worried that her husband was angry, sexually frustrated, and found her less attractive. She also stated that she often experienced pain during sexual intercourse and added that it was worse during prolonged and deep penile penetration. When interviewed, her husband stated that he was not comfortable with sexual activity due to his concerns about hurting his wife, not wanting to tire her, and feeling that sex was less of a priority following her cancer treatment. He stated that he initiated sex much less than he used to and that when he did he tried to get it over with as soon as possible. Neither of them had discussed current preferences for sexual activity with each other. The first step in the treatment plan involved providing information about the causes of their multiphase sexual difficulties. This patient was referred for a thorough endocrine workup, which revealed ovarian failure secondary to chemotherapy and radiation treatment. She was started on estrogen replacement therapy and encouraged to use a water-based vaginal lubricant prior to sexual intercourse and experiment with various positions that would reduce discomfort during intercourse. She found that the female superior position afforded her maximum comfort and control over the rate and depth of penile penetration. She and her husband were encouraged to plan at least one evening per week when they did something enjoyable together. This particular suggestion was initially quite difficult for them and it became apparent that they were out of practice

---

* AASECT: 11 Dupont Circle. N. W. Suite 220, Washington, D. C. 20036.

discussing and doing non-cancer-related activities. At one year follow-up, this patient and her partner reported improved sexual relations.

Case Vignette II

A 22-year-old single woman was referred to the psychiatry service during her autologous bone marrow transplant for lymphoma. A psychiatric consultation at that time was requested to rule out depression during her convalescence in the hospital. She was followed weekly as an outpatient for the first six months after discharge. During this time, she was living by herself and complained of extreme fatigue, malaise, and difficulty adjusting to being outside of the hospital because of these physical problems. After six months she obtained her first job as an architect in a small firm. Since she had gone to school previous to her cancer diagnosis, this was her first "real" job after graduating with her degree. During this time she continued in psychotherapy and related many adjustment problems concerning "Who she should tell at work about her illness," "What would happen if she became ill again," "How much time would she have to take off," "How would she manage her numerous outpatient visits," and "Would her supervisor at work allow her such time." During subsequent psychotherapy sessions she revealed that she felt quite uncomfortable about her body. She had many visible minor scars from broviac catheters, an episode of herpes zoster, and also had lost a considerable amount of weight. She felt extremely uncomfortable about her body and felt that it was damaged in some way by her illness and her transplant. Many of her sessions revolved around how she could ever meet any young men her own age and if she did how would she tell them about her illness, let alone her issues of infertility. Over the several months, she subsequently was very successful at work, began to go on several blind dates, and dated several young men. One she became particularly interested in was approximately three years younger than herself and was very sexually

naive. Prior to the patient's illnesses, in college, she had been engaged to a fellow student. They were living together and she was sexually active. Upon meeting this new gentleman, she had many worries concerning telling him about her cancer diagnosis, the transplant itself, the physical sequelae that she experienced, and also her inability to have children. "Who would have someone like me who is half a woman?" It became evident the patient was extremely anxious about initiating any long-term relationship, let alone engaging in a physical relationship. She finally became comfortable with this boyfriend only after he told her that both his parents had had episodes of cancer and they were doing quite well. With that she felt more comfortable in revealing much of her past history. Slowly, as she became psychologically more comfortable in this relationship, she began to develop a sexual relationship with him. He was extremely naive and due to both of their anxieties, his because of the newness of initiating intercourse and hers because of feeling uncomfortable about her body and not having engaged in any sexual activity in approximately four years, their whole physical relationship was shrouded and surrounded in psychological turmoil and anxiety. It also became evident that the anxiety contributed to a problem with sexual desire and also arousal. However, it became much more apparent that arousal and actual orgasm were inhibited due to decreased vaginal secretions and most likely low estrogen levels secondary to the radiation and chemotherapy both from her original Hodgkin's treatment and the bone marrow transplant procedure. She was referred for a thorough endocrine workup, which revealed ovarian failure secondary to radiation treatment. She started estrogen replacement therapy, and was encouraged to use water-based vaginal lubricants prior to sexual intercourse and also experiment with various positions that would reduce discomfort during intercourse. She subsequently discontinued her endocrine replacement because of weight gain and headaches. She continued a physical relationship with this young man, and because the relationship deepened, he became more experienced and her anxiety decreased because she felt comfortable with him. Issues of lack of sexual desire and arousal disappeared over the next couple of months. She subsequently broke up with this young man six months into the relationship, but has continued to meet other gentlemen through work associates and has felt extremely comfortable engaging with them in various relationships. She has continued to be quite successful at work and is in the process of changing jobs so that she will have better health benefits and vacation leave. She is considering pursuing adopting a child as a single parent.

Combining Sexual Counseling with Medical Treatments

Given the complex etiology and manifestations of sexual and reproductive problems, a multidisciplinary approach is often necessary. Hormone replacement therapy, sperm banking, and pharmacologic and surgical means of protecting fertility during treatment will be discussed.

Hormonal Replacement Therapy

Hormone replacement may be effective in several situations with patients undergoing BMT. For example, some adolescent or prepubertal boys receiving radiation may need testosterone replacement in order to promote the development of secondary sexual characteristics, and all women who have undergone premature menopause after treatment for BMT need hormonal replacement. Low-dose estrogen and progesterone combinations and topical estrogen ameliorate most of the menopausal symptomatology. Nonhormonal drug therapies (e.g., clonidine) may be helpful in relieving menopausal symptoms in women who refuse initial estrogen replacement.

It has been suggested that hormone replacement during chemotherapy may suppress germ cell proliferation, thereby preventing antineoplastic therapy–associated gonadal toxicity (Redman and Bajorunas 1987; Redman et al. 1986; Chapman and Sutcliffe 1981). Gonadal protection during chemotherapy has included administering testosterone in men, oral contraceptives in women, and gonadotropin releasing hormone (GnRH) analogues in both sexes. Unfortunately, results from preliminary studies have not proved efficacious (Schover and Jensen 1988).

Sperm Banking

An appropriate and relatively effective method of protecting fertility in men undergoing BMT is sperm banking. Unfortunately, semen from pretreated cancer patients and treated patients about to undergo BMT may reveal low sperm count and poor or inadequate sperm mobility. Approximately half of the men with testicular cancer or lymphoma have abnormal sperm specimens that prevent sperm banking prior to any cancer treatment. However, cryobanking should be encouraged for all male patients; even if sperm counts are low. Multiple ejaculates can increase the total number of viable sperm for storage. In summary, this procedure involves sensitive encouragement by BMT staff for patients to bank sperm, a receptive patient who has undergone little or relatively nontoxic cancer treatment, the availability of a local sperm banking facility, and enough time for travel and banking. These last factors are critical and often unavailable. Many insurance companies do not currently reimburse the costs associated with this procedure and financial constraints may present a barrier for some men who wish to take advantage of this technique.

Other Fertility Options

An experimental option available to women prior to bone marrow transplantation is in vitro fertilization (IVF). Several fertility centers have developed highly innovative programs where women ending chemotherapy for their cancers are stimulated with hormonal therapy in order to collect ovum for fertilization and then storage. Possible use of these fertilized ovum after transplantation is a new and highly ethically and emotionally charged area of patient concern particularly for the potential father of a woman who has unsuccessfully proceeded through the transplant procedure.

Recommendations for Future Research

A thorough review of the literature reveals a relative absence of empirical studies examining the impact of bone marrow transplantation on sexual functioning. Clinical experience and research findings borrowed from the general literature of cancer survivors serves as a foundation for current clinical practice. However, further clarification of the incidence, nature, and risk factors associated with sexual dysfunction among BMT patients is needed in order to develop and refine prevention and rehabilitation efforts geared toward maintenance of sexual health among cancer survivors treated with BMT. This call for further specificity in our research efforts is reflected in Andersen's (1985) overall recommendation that we need to answer the question "What disease/treatment contexts produce what kind of sexual difficulties for which subgroups of cancer patients over what time course, and what are the etiologic components?"

Considering the growing use of BMT as a curative treatment for many neoplastic disorders, it is important to consider whether the addition of BMT to the treatment protocol for a specific disease produces effects different from those found in patients who had been treated with conventional treatment only. For instance, Lesko and her colleagues (1989) compared the sexual functioning of acute leukemia survivors treated with either conventional chemotherapy alone or conventional chemotherapy followed by allogeneic bone marrow transplantation. They found that there were no significant differences in sexual desire, satisfaction, and body image between these two subgroups of long-term leukemia survivors. They concluded that leukemia survivors treated with BMT experienced no greater psychosexual sequelae than their conventional treatment counterparts, who noted significant decline in sexual satisfaction. This research protocol was also conducted with chronic leukemia patients treated with either conventional chemotherapy alone or followed by allogeneic BMT and the results were similar in that BMT patients fared no worse in terms of their sexual health.

There are several methodological suggestions that would help researchers in the field develop a data base for expanding our knowledge of the sexual functioning of BMT patients. Prospective studies of patients with the various diagnoses (e.g., acute leukemia, Hodgkin's disease, testicular and breast cancer) currently treated with BMT must be conducted. Careful attention needs to be paid to subject selection criteria to ensure treatment-group comparability. Given the multiplicity of disease and treatment-related factors that are related to sexual functioning, it is important for investigators to accrue patients that are homogeneous with regard to disease site, treatment regimen, phase of treatment (e.g., active treatment, post-treatment) and prognosis. The issue of differences in sexual morbidity among male and female BMT patients must also be addressed, in light of the differential effects of BMT on gonadal function.

In addition, research findings based on psychometrically robust questionnaires developed to study sexual functioning and physiological indices of sexual response (e.g., estrogen and gonadotropin levels) will advance our knowledge in this area. For instance, Derogatis' Sexual Functioning Inventory (Derogatis 1975) measures three dimensions of sexual functioning: degree of sexual interest, sexual satisfaction, and body image. Several semistructured interviews have been developed to assess sexual functioning (Schover and Jensen 1988). It is quite helpful to include both self-report questionnaires and clinical interviews in an assessment battery to account for patient preferences in disclosing sensitive information. Including patients' spouses in data collection will enable a more dyadic perspective of how couples maintain sexual and global relationship satisfaction. Longitudinal studies will allow researchers to observe when, during the course of treatment, patients experience sexual dysfunction as well as the process of sexual readjustment post-BMT. Finally, research that assesses multidimensional indices of quality of life, including sexual functioning, will help professionals to understand factors necessary for optimal adjustment among post-BMT cancer survivors.

Acknowledgments: This work has been supported in part by a Leukemia Society of America Scholars' Grant awarded to Dr. Lesko as well as the Rudin Foundation in New York and the National Cancer Institute.

References

American Psychiatric Association. 1987. *Diagnostic and Statistical Manual of Mental Disorders,* Third Edition, Revised. Washington, DC.: American Psychiatric Association.

Andersen, B. 1985. Sexual functioning morbidity among cancer survivors: Current status and future directions. *Cancer 55:* 1835–1842.

Andrykowski, M., Henslee, P., and Farrall, M. 1987. Physical and psychosocial functioning of adult survivors of allogeneic bone marrow transplantation. *B.M.T. 4:* 75–81.

Annon, J. 1976. *Behavioral Treatment of Sexual Problems,* Vol. 1, *Brief Therapy.* Honolulu: Enabling Systems.

Ash, P. 1980. The influence of radiation on fertility in man. *The Br. J. Radiol. 53:* 628; 271–278.

Auchincloss, S. 1989. Sexual dysfunction in cancer patients: Issues in evaluation and treatment. In J. Holland and J. Rowland (eds.). *Handbook of Psychooncology: Psychological Care of the Patient with Cancer.* New York: Oxford Press.

Bajorunas, D.R., and Redman, J.R. June, 1986a. Effects of cancer therapy on endocrine function. *Primary Care and Cancer:* 90R–210R.

Bajorunas, D.R., and Redman, J.R. July, 1986b. Effects of cancer therapy Part 2—Male and Female. *Primary Care and Cancer:* 520R–590R.

Barrett, A. et al. 1987. Late effects of total body radiation. *Radiotherapy and Oncology 9:* 131–135.

Benker, G. et al. 1989. Allogeneic bone marrow transplantation in adults: Endocrine sequelae after 1–6 years. *Acta Endocrinologic* (Copenh.) *120:* 37–42.

Byrd, R. 1985. Late effects of treatment of cancer in children. *Pediatr. Clin. North Am. 32:* 835–857.

Card, R.T. et al. 1980. Successful pregnancy after high dose chemotherapy and marrow transplantation for treatment of aplastic anemia. *Exp. Hematol. 8* (1): 57–60.

Cella, D., and Tross, S. 1986. Psychological adjustment to survival from Hodgkin's disease. *Journal of Consulting and Clinical Psychology 54:* 616–622.

Chapman, R., and Sutcliffe, S. 1981. Prediction of ovarian function by oral contraception in women receiving chemotherapy for Hodgkin's disease. *Blood 58:* 849–851.

Cooley, M., Yeomans, A., and Cobb, S. 1986. Sexual and reproductive issues for women with Hodgkin's Disease: Application of PLISSIT model. *Cancer Nursing 9:* 248–255.

Deeg, H.J. et al. 1983. Successful pregnancy after marrow transplantation for severe aplastic anemia and immunosuppression with cyclosporine. *JAMA 250* (5): 647.

Derogatis, L. 1975. *Derogatis Sexual Functioning Inventory.* Baltimore, MD: Clinical Psychometric Research.

Fobair, P. et al. 1986. Psychosocial problems among survivors of Hodgkin's disease. *J. Clin. Oncol. 4:* 805–814.

Gradishar, W.J., and Schilsky, R.L. 1989. Ovarian function following radiation and chemotherapy for cancer. *Seminars in Oncology 16* (5): 425–436.

Jacobs, P., and Dubousky, D.W. 1981. Bone marrow transplantation followed by normal pregnancy. *American Journal of Hematology 11:* 209–212.

Kaplan, H. 1974. *The New Sex Therapy: Active Treatment of Sexual Dysfunctions.* New York: Brunner/Mazel.

Kaplan, H. 1979. *Problems of Sexual Desire.* New York: Brunner/Mazel.

Kaplan. H. 1983. *The Evaluation of Sexual Disorders.* New York: Brunner/Mazel.

Koocher, G., and O'Malley, J. 1981. *The Damocles Syndrome: Psychosocial Consequences of Surviving Childhood Cancer.* New York: McGraw-Hill.

Leiblum, S., and Pervin, L. 1989. *Principles and Practice of Sex Therapy.* New York: Guilford Press.

Lesko, L. 1989. Bone marrow transplantation. In J. Holland and J. Rowland (eds.). *Handbook of psychooncology. Psychological care of the patient with cancer.* New York: Oxford Press.

Lesko, L., and Hawkins, D. 1983. Psychological aspects of transplantation medicine. In S. Akhtar (ed.). *New Psychiatric Syndromes: DSMIII and Beyond.* New York: Aronson.

Lesko, L. et al. 1989. Long-term psychological adjustment of acute leukemia survivors: Impact of bone marrow transplantation vs. conventional chemotherapy. Manuscript submitted for publication.

Li, F. 1977. Follow-up of childhood cancer survivors. *Cancer 84:* 1776–1778.

Loescher, L. et al. 1989. Surviving adult cancers. Part 1: Physiological effects. *Ann. Intern. Med. III:* 411–432.

LoPiccolo, J., and LoPiccolo, L. 1978. *Handbook of sex therapy.* New York: Plenum Press.

Maguire, L.C. 1979. Fertility and cancer therapy. *Postgrad. Med. 65:* 293–299.

Meadows, A., and Hobbie, W. 1986. The medical consequences of cure. *Cancer 58:* 524–528.

Mumma, G., Lesko, L., and Mashberg, D. 1989. Psychosexual adjustment of acute leukemia survivors treated with bone marrow transplantation and conventional chemotherapy. Manuscript submitted for publication.

Ostroff, J., Smith, K., and Lesko, L. 1989. Promotion of mental health among adolescent cancer survivors and their families. *Proceedings of the Mental Health Services for Children and Adolescents in Primary Care Settings: An NIMH Research Conference.*

Redman, J.R., and Bajorunas, D.R. 1987. Suppression of germ cell proliferation to prevent gonadal toxicity associated with cancer treatment. In *Proceedings of the workshop on psychosexual and reproductive issues affecting patients with cancer.* American Cancer Society Publication #87-5M-4515, p. 90–94.

Redman, J. et al. 1986. Prospective, randomized trial of testosterone cypionate to prevent sterility in men treated with chemotherapy for Hodgkin's disease: Preliminary results. In *Proceedings of the 14th International Cancer Congress.* Budapest, Basel: S. Kargen, p. 440.

Rieker, P., Edbril, S., and Garnick, M. 1985. Curative testis cancer therapy: Psychosocial sequelae. *J. Clin. Oncol. 3:* 1117–1126.

Sanders, J.E. et al. 1983. Late effects of gonadal function of cyclophosphamide, total body radiation, and marrow transplantation. *Transplantation 36* (3): 252–255.

Sanders, J.E. 1987. Ovarian and testicular function following marrow transplantation. *International Conference on Reproduction and Human Cancer.* Bethesda, MD: National Cancer Institute.

Sanders, J.E. et al. 1988. Ovarian function following marrow transplantation for aplastic anemia or leukemia. *J. Clin. Oncol. 6:* 813–818.

Schilsky, R.L. et al. 1980. Gonadal dysfunction in patients receiving chemotherapy for cancer. *Arch. Intern. Med. 93:* 109–114.

Schover L., and Jensen, S. 1988. *Sexuality and chronic illness: A comprehensive approach.* New York: Guilford Press.

Shalet, S. 1987. Reproductive hazards of radio- and chemotherapy in children. *International Conference on Reproduction and Human Cancer.* Bethesda, MD: National Cancer Institute.

Sherins, R.J. 1987. Reproductive hazards of radiotherapy and chemotherapy in adult males. *International Conference on Reproduction and Human Cancer.* Bethesda, MD: National Cancer Institute.

Sherins, R.J., and Mulvihill, J.J. 1989. Gonadal dysfunction. In DeVita, V.T., Jr., Nellman, S., and Rosenberg, S.A. (eds.). *Cancer: Principles and practice of oncology.* Philadelphia: Lippincott, pp. 2170–2181.

Teta, M. et al. 1986. Psychosocial consequences of childhood and adolescent cancer survivors. *Journal of Chronic Disease 39:* 751–759.

Thompson, E. et al. 1987. Normal physical and psychosocial function in the majority of childhood cancer patients surviving 10 years or more from diagnosis. *Proceedings of the American Society of Clinical Oncology 6:* 258.

Tross, S., and Holland, J. 1989. Psychological sequelae in cancer survivors. In J. Holland and J. Rowland (eds.). *Handbook of psychooncology: Psychological care of the patient with cancer.* New York: Oxford Press.

Vincent, C. et al. 1975. Some sexual and marital concomitants of carcinoma of the cervix. *Southern Med. J.* 68:552–558.

Von Eschenbach, A., and Schover, L. 1984a. The role of sexual rehabilitation in the treatment of patients with cancer. *Cancer* 54:2662–2667.

Von Eschenbach, A.C., and Schover, L.R. 1984b. Sexual rehabilitation of cancer patients. In A.E. Gunn (ed.). *Cancer Rehabilitation.* New York: Raven Press, pp. 155–173.

Welch-McCaffrey, D. et al. 1989. Surviving adult cancers. Part 2: Psychosocial implications. *Ann. Intern. Med. 111:* 517–524.

Wolcott, D. et al. 1986. Adaptation of adult bone marrow transplant recipient long-term survivors. *Transplantation 41:* 478–484.

Chapter 15

Survivorship and Rehabilitation

Janet W. Nims

In the late 1950s, when marrow grafts were first attempted in humans, little was known about transplant antigens. Supportive care techniques, such as granulocyte transfusions and platelet transfusions, were in their infancy, and only a few antibiotics were effective. Despite these problems, investigators in North America and Europe worked with murine, canine, and primate models in an attempt to induce tolerance and graft acceptance (Van Bekkum and DeVries 1967; Thomas et al. 1975). A few clinical studies were done successfully with identical twins (Thomas et al. 1959). However, since the results of the early trials of allogeneic transplants were disappointing, no further such transplants were undertaken for almost a decade (Mathe et al. 1965). Since 1968, approximately 10,000 to 15,000 patients have been transplanted with a 45–50% survival rate. A good number of these patients have been transplanted since the mid-1980s and are therefore less than five years from transplant (Thomas 1988). This relatively small but growing number of patients has significant physiologic, psychosocial, and life style adjustments to make following the transplant process.

There has been little research on issues of survivorship in cancer patients in general and in marrow recipients in particular (Wolcott et al. 1986; Smith and Lesko 1988; Hoffman 1989). Marrow transplantation research emphasis has focused primarily on treatments for sustaining remission as well as alleviating short- and long-term physiologic effects. This emphasis has contributed to the increasing number of patient survivor days after marrow transplantation. However, there is a growing realization of the need and importance of research on the more holistic effects of this treatment on the growing population of long-term survivors.

Concepts of sickness and cure are insufficient to fully describe the series of events that occurs in patients and families involved in the marrow transplantation process. Survival is a more useful concept because it is a broader idea that characterizes everyone from the onset of their disease through the remainder of their life regardless of course (Mullan 1985).

Although outcomes and circumstances vary widely from person to person, most patients and families go through very similar and predictable phases of survival. These are not necessarily formal stages, but rather a progression of events—the seasons of survival (Mullan 1985). As described by Mullan (1985) these seasons are called acute, extended, and permanent survival.

In bone marrow transplantation, more is known about early reactions to survival in the acute and extended survival periods; however, information on extended and permanent phases is less accessible when patients are followed far from the original transplant center. This has limited the empirical data on typical responses of long-term marrow transplant survivors. However, as the number of patients increases and more is known about the quality of long-term survival, information of this type may assist patients deciding on transplantation as a treatment option and in accurately determining rehabilitation needs.

Acute Survival

The acute survival period is primarily a medical stage that includes the first year following bone marrow transplantation and is often emotionally dominated by fear. Coping with the effects of therapy and the inherent long-term sequelae occupies all of the adaptive energies of most patients. These complications (described below) are generally related to the effects of the intensive cytoreductive treatment before transplantation, delay in recovery of the immune system, graft-versus-host disease, prolonged immunosuppressive therapy (Sullivan et al. 1984) and, for some patients, relapse of their initial disease.

Some patients with chronic graft-versus-host disease (see Chapter 7) find the symptoms of this complication harder to live with than their initial potentially terminal illness. Dry and light-sensitive eyes, as well as a wide variety of skin changes, can require intensive medical management and be a constant irritation causing continued discomfort. Changes in body image, defined in Chapter 14, can be a significant factor in coping with manifestations of chronic GVHD. Low-grade gastrointestinal discomfort (weight loss, generalized malaise, and risk of opportunistic infection) can persist beyond discharge from the hospital and can be a source of constant concern.

Medications to control chronic graft-versus-host disease have side effects that can cause further debilitation. Corticosteroids may cause mood swings with high levels of irritability and anxiety. Long-term use might result in muscle wasting, weakness, osteoporosis, aseptic necrosis, or adrenal insufficiency (Sullivan et al. 1984), as well as an increase in the growth rate of cataracts (Deeg et al. 1984). Cyclosporine may cause nausea, hirsutism, tremors, and somnolence (Kahan 1989). A higher risk of infection in this subpopulation due to the delayed return of immune function can cause further anxiety for the patient and family.

Lack of compliance with the complex and protracted treatment regimens may be the cause of some physical manifestations of chronic GVHD, rather than refractoriness to treatment (Sullivan et al. 1988; Given and Given 1989). If undetected, the resulting untreated chronic GVHD may result in permanent disabilities, which could include contractures and scleroderma with resultant poor pulmonary function and occasionally, blindness. Patients undergoing treatment for chronic GVHD who appear to have an intractable disease might benefit from interventions to enhance compliance (Given and Given 1984 and 1989; Richardson et al. 1988). For instance, nurses may attempt to enter into a partnership relationship or contract with patients regarding this difficult aspect of treatment, thereby potentially facilitating compliance.

Numerous emotional and psychological reactions are common during the stage of acute survival. Although not classified as major psychiatric disorders, these problems can cause significant distress, which may interfere with daily functioning (Smith and Lesko 1988). Fear of recurrences after a very rigorous treatment begins as watchful waiting and may escalate to panic with every small change or twinge of pain. Depression and guilt overcome some recipients and may require professional intervention (Wolcott et al. 1986). Depression may be caused by a wide variety of situations such as isolation, spiraling fatigue, changes in familial roles, and changes in relationships. Guilt may be caused by the simple fact that the patient is alive while other "classmates" are not (Patenaude and Rappeport 1982).

Marrow transplantation can also have an impact on family relationships. Sometimes the patient perceives that he or she is an emotional and financial burden on the family (Nims and Strom 1988). Donors may experience changes in relationships with recipients (Gardner et al. 1977; Brown and Kelly 1976), ranging from strained to overwhelming intrusion (Lesko and Hawkins 1983). Family members may feel the burden of delivering adequate medical and personal care. They too may feel emotional and physical fatigue. Some care givers become angry and frustrated with the chronicity of transplant sequelae.

During this season, the effect of the transplantation process may also cause changes in the relationships between recipients and friends. It is often not until the patient has undergone significant physical recovery that they are able to attend to personal emotional needs and family and social relationships (Frymark 1990). When that does occur, patients often have made subtle changes in their life priorities and perspectives, whereas friends, and even perhaps family, have not. Accepting these changes is often difficult for those close to the patient (Lesko and Hawkins 1983).

In general, when the patient has successfully completed the first year after transplantation, the acute phase is over and the next season has begun.

Extended Survival

Extended survival extends from the subsequent post-transplant period to approximately the end of year five, and is primarily a period of adjusting and adapting to home, school, and work situations (Mullan 1985). The experience varies according to the individual's coping skills, physical sequelae, and other factors. For instance, in two studies of long-term survivors the age at which transplant was performed (< 30), rather than the length of time since the transplant procedure, was associated with improved psychosocial functioning and adaptation (Andrykowski et al. 1989a, Wolcott et al. 1986a). This finding could suggest that recovery is not only a function of the passage of time. Furthermore, a longitudinal study of BMT survivors in which long-term difficulties in physical, occupational, emotional, and cognitive functioning persisted in those studied between three to five years post-BMT suggested that a ceiling in recovery may be reached within a few years (Andrykowski et al. 1989b). In that study, after a plateau was reached, no further recovery of function occurred.

Chronic GVHD typically occurs within 3–12 months, but in rare cases may still manifest itself as late as 15 months after transplantation (Sullivan et al. 1984). Some patients with resistant chronic GVHD may require therapy for its attendant changes for as long as five years after transplantation. Although this phenomenon is rare, it does exist (Sullivan et al. 1984), and treatment plans for postacute care rarely address the problems of reentering the active world with this continued disability. In general, however, patients free of chronic GVHD after the first year tend to move toward normalization at a more rapid rate without this continued reminder of illness.

Recognition that 7–20% of long-term survivors have a laboratory decrease in pulmonary function in the form of either restrictive or obstructive disease or bronchiolitis obliterans may be a factor in return to normal activity (Clark et al. 1985). Clinical manifestations of restrictive lung disease are less frequent (7%). Among patients with the extensive form of chronic GVHD, however, 5–10% develop severe obstructive airway disease, which resembles obliterative bronchiolitis and may effect the ability to resume normal activity (Clark et al. 1985).

Issues of sexuality may not arise for one to two years after transplant. If the patient is prepubescent at the time of transplant, this period may be even longer. Sexuality is an important part of everyday life, and is one facet of the human need for closeness, playfulness, touch, caring, and pleasure. "Feelings about sexuality influence our zest for living, our self-image, and our relationships with others" (Schover 1988a; Schover 1988b). Patients and doctors often hesitate to discuss the effects of treatment on sexuality. The important point to remember is that pleasurable, sexual touching is always possible, regardless of circumstances or medical history. Even when sexual activity is impractical, physical expression of affection remains an important way of sharing intimacy. Wide varieties of sexual attitudes and practices prevail and defining "normal" activity is virtually impossible. Using the patient's own norms and helping with adaptations and adjustments, if necessary, may be an important component of facilitating reentry. (See Chapter 14 for a full discussion of psychosexual adjustment and fertility issues.)

Cataracts may develop three to six years after total body irradiation (TBI). About 80% of patients given TBI in a single dose develop cataracts, and about half of them require cataract extraction. This can be safely performed even in the presence of dry eyes. There have been no complications to date of intraocular lens placement. It appears that the use of chronic steroid therapy may also contribute to the development of cataracts. In contrast, the use of fractionated irradiation appears to reduce the risk of cataracts (only 25% incidence at six years). In patients with chronic GVHD, ocular sicca may require punctal ligation to enhance the moistening effect of the remaining tear film (Deeg et al. 1984).

Fear of recurrence continues to be a punishing worry. This worry continues for those who have been treated for malignancies as well as those (although less so) without malignancies. At this point, patients begin to internalize the impact that bone marrow transplantation has had on their lives. Planning for the future may be difficult for some. Depending on the amount of disability, there may be considerable readjustment in lifestyle.

Lack of gonadal function, delayed growth, and the other changes already mentioned resulting from chronic GVHD, may all influence future planning. Despite these complications, extended survival is not predominantly a medical phase, and doctors and nurses have a diminishing role in providing support and counseling; however, patients and families continue to adjust to daily living. Preoccupation with daily survival is less important, and looking to the future takes precedence. The result of the diminishing role of the health care team is a void that leaves many patients and families fending for themselves in a "healthy" world (Hoffman 1989).

Permanent Survival

"Permanent survival has several dimensions. There is no moment of cure, but rather an evolution from the phase of extended survival into a period when the activity of the disease or likelihood of recurrence is minimal" (Mullan 1985). Physically and emotionally, the experience of diagnosis and treatment leaves a lasting impression on the marrow recipient and the family. No matter how long they live, survivors are weary, relieved, proud, and often shy about this accomplishment. Adjusting lifestyles for maximum function and learning to understand the experience often takes many years.

Problems with employment and insurance can occur. In one longitudinal study of BMT survivors, only 50% (8/16 patients) of patients had returned to work nearly four and one-half years after BMT. Almost a third of the nonworking sample cited health-related reasons for their unemployment. Those who were employed stated that they had reduced hours or other limitations in the amount or type of work they performed (Andry-kowski et al. 1989b). Discrimination of various sorts is also experienced as survivors seek employment and advancement (Hoffman 1989). Health and life insurance are difficult issues as many companies are reluctant to insure former patients or they may exclude coverage for anything remotely related to the initial disease. Others not only encounter prejudice but are unable to advance in their career or change their employment for fear of loss of insurance due to their former illness.

Understanding and placing the experience of the initial diagnosis, treatment, and recovery in perspective is often a lifetime task. The degree of concern ebbs and flows over time. Availability of members of the health care team and open communication is often the only intervention required. However, awareness of other sequelae, such as secondary malignancy due to the intensive chemoradiotherapy, may also be a factor in recovery. Although uncommon, secondary malignancy can occur as long as ten to fifteen years after transplantation (Deeg et al. 1988; Witherspoon et al. 1989) (see Table 15.1).

Treatment of reproductive and endocrine functions of young people who have been successfully treated with BMT is a rapidly changing area in which up-to-date information is not always available. As mentioned earlier, these concerns may arise during the extended or permanent survival phases depending on the patient's age at transplant. Greater longevity after transplantation has increased the importance of this aspect of recovery. As new discoveries occur, there may be answers to particular gonadal and growth problems that were not previously available.

Health maintenance and early detection of alterations in normal development are often very important issues to this group of patients (Sanders et al. 1988; Wiley and House 1988). Because denial of past illness and the desire to normalize is strong, patients may not maintain regular oncology or hematologic examinations. An important role of the health care professional in the phase of permanent survival is to help the patient and family live as fully as possible while supplying supportive intervention where appropriate. Long-term chronic problems can seem overwhelming at times and difficult to solve. An interdisciplinary

Table 15.1. Incidence and Rates of Secondary Cancer After Bone Marrow Transplantation at Fred Hutchinson Cancer Research Center 1970–Feb. 1987

Type of Secondary Cancer (35:2145)*	Median Time After BMT	Median Age of BMT
Solid Tumors (13)†	4.3 yrs. (2 mos.–13.9 yrs.)	21 yrs. (6–57 yrs.)
Basal Cell Ca. (1)	5.1 yrs.	38 yrs.
Squamous Cell Ca. (2)	5.1 yrs. & 13.9 yrs.	21 & 34 yrs.
Adenocarcinoma (3)	12.2 yrs. (2.5 mos.–13.4 yrs.)	48 yrs. (28–57 yrs.)
Malignant melanoma (3)	4.6 yrs. (1.8–10.1 yrs.)	16 yrs. (8–18 yrs.)
Glioblastoma multiforme (3)	3.8 yrs. (11.8 mos.–5.4 yrs.)	7 yrs. (6–8 yrs.)
Invasive vulvar carcinoma (1)	3.5 yrs.	31 yrs.
New Leukemia (6)	6.7 mos. (1.9 mos.–6.2 yrs.)	14 yrs. (7–26 yrs.)
ALL (4)	5.2 mos. (1.9 mos.–6.2 yrs.)	12 yrs. (7–16 yrs.)
ANLL (1)	75.9 mos.	25 yrs.
Granulocytic Sarcoma (1)	6.1 mos.	26 yrs.
Non-Hodgkin's Lymphoma (16)	2.5 mos. (2 mos.–4.9 yrs.)	19 yrs. (2 yrs.–58 yrs.)

*Thirty-five cancers in 2145 total patients. †Numbers in parentheses represent the number of cancers of each type. Adapted from Witherspoon 1988.

approach is often necessary. In general, the marrow transplant patient's health depends on delicate interactions of organic, psychological, social, and cultural forces, and is not confined to the results of the treatment-related, biological disturbances. Effective survival involves the whole person and is not limited solely to physiologic repair.

Strategies for Survival and Rehabilitation

An appreciation of the seasons of survival can help both health professionals and patients develop better strategies for dealing with this challenging life event. Creating a supportive and caring climate that promotes a partnership relationship can encourage compliance (see Figure 15.1). The goal of this relationship is to increase the effectiveness of treatment, thereby improving overall survival and the quality of life. Knowledge of Erickson, Piaget, and Kohlberg's life tasks (discussed in

Chapter 4 on pediatric perspectives) will aid in creating a caring, supportive climate that is directed at the age and developmental level of the survivor. Systematic referrals for patients by oncologists, primary care physicians, and nurses to support and counseling services can assist patients in adjustment, relieve suffering, and stimulate further development of the scarce resources available for patient rehabilitation.

Intense supportive care by nursing, dietary, and physical therapy (Decker et al. 1989; James 1987; Holtzman 1988) all play a part in strategies for survivorship (Corcoran-Buchsel and Parchem 1988). (Many of these services were detailed in the other chapters.) Screening studies for evidence of chronic GVHD coupled with in-depth discharge planning are major elements of the intensive evaluation of the patient and family in anticipation of their return to their community and referring health care teams (see Table 15.2).

Once the patient returns to the referring health care team, a designated patient care co-

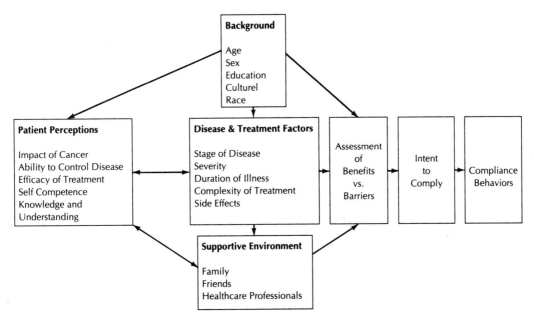

Reprinted with permission, Given and Given *ONF*, Vol. 16, No. 1, 1989.

Figure 15.1. Model Describing Variables Related to Compliance Behaviors

Table 15.2. Discharge Planning

Baseline studies (general)
Screen for C-GVHD
Current status   engraftment   ophthalmology
                  immune system   oral medicine
                  hematological   medications
                  renal
                  hepatic

Disease-related studies
CT, MRI, special blood studies

Discharge conference
Medical implications
Nursing—ADL
            Video and written material
Dietary—written material

Communication
Doctor-Doctor   Verbal and written
Nurse-Nurse   Verbal and written
Availability of resource

---

ordinator can best organize each individual patient's needs. An interdisciplinary team approach seems to be best suited for good results with, of course, the agreement and cooperation of the patient and family (McKenna 1986). Not every patient requires rehabilitation services, but when necessary these services must be effectively coordinated.

Unfortunately, until recently, rehabilitation needs and potential were not routinely assessed, when in fact rehabilitation plans are often most effective when identified at the time of diagnosis (Hoffman 1989) or entry into the transplant program. Some treatment centers include physical and occupational therapy in various regimens while patients are in the early stages after transplantation (James 1987; Holtzman 1988; Decker et al. 1989). However, few acute care treatment facilities are equipped to continue extensive involvement and rehabilitation of survivors over all of the seasons of survival.

A good understanding of the rehabilitation process can assist in determining the best recovery plan. In 1971, Federal legislation gave a boost to cancer rehabilitation efforts by passing the National Cancer Plan. In 1972, a planning conference was sponsored by the National Cancer Institute to explore ways to improve the quality of life of the cancer patient. Four objectives of rehabilitation were identified:

1. Psychological support once cancer has been diagnosed;

2. Optimal physical functioning following cancer treatment;

3. Vocational counseling, when indicated, as early as possible;

4. Optimal social functioning as the ultimate goal of all cancer control treatment (DeLisa et al. 1989).

A great deal of progress has been achieved over the last 15 years in rehabilitation programs for solid tumor patients (Hoffman 1989). Witness, for example, the Ostomy Clubs, Reach for Recovery program, and the National Campaign to Stop Smoking. Similar principles apply to the marrow transplant recipient. As with other cancer patients, rehabilitation is a shared responsibility (DeLisa et al. 1989). Goals should be realistic and consistent with physiological and environmental limitations. While addressing physical rehabilitation factors, psychological and social issues must also be considered for patient motivation (see Table 15.3).

Through the seasons of survival, built-in flexibility and serial evaluations of areas of ability, as well as disability, are noted for future consideration. Knowledge of chemoradiotherapy sequelae, as well as immune system recovery and chronic graft-versus-host disease potential disabilities, are essential for the rehabilitation coordinator of the marrow transplant patient. Those patients without chronic GVHD generally have fewer physical rehabilitation needs, but may require psychosocial interventions involving education, social support, employment discrimination, or insurance and social security.

Patients with chronic GVHD may require more intensive rehabilitation intervention. Should chronic GVHD be intractable for natural or poor

Table 15.3. Marrow Recipient Rehabilitation Team Members: Specialty and Function

Hematologist/Oncologist/Physician's Assistant

Diagnosis and treatment
- functional deficit (mobility, self-care, communication)
- status of immune system
- status of engraftment
- status of chronic GVHD

Prescribe others to treat
- exercise tolerance

Interdisciplinary team management

Oncology-Rehabilitation Nurse

Evaluate
- compliance
- ADL-ROM
- serial assessments

Assist primary care giver in management

Patient/Family education
- support
- disease and medication side effects with appropriate interventions

Psychologist

Problem-solving skills

Memory and perceptual functioning

Adjustments to body image

Counseling involving
- death and dying
- body and lifestyle changes
- behavioral strategies
  sexuality
  stress

Physical Therapist/Physiatrist

Evaluate
- ROM
- muscle strength
- mobility skills
- modifications

Provide exercises to
- maintain and increase ROM
- increase strength, endurance, and coordination

Occupational Therapist

Evaluate and train in
- basic self-care
- ADL skills

Assist with
- vocational and avocational activities
- family education
- maintenance of strength and endurance

Social Worker

Evaluate environment

Counseling involving
- living situations
- community resource utilization
- finances
- patient/family support
- patient/family treatment participation
- employment related problems

Vocational Counselor

Evaluate and counsel regarding
- formulation of goals and action plans
- vocational interest and skills in relation to disease-related factors

Liaison with
- placement and training agencies
- present and/or potential employers
- insurance providers

Other Team Members (per patient's needs)
- Dietician
- Dentist/Dental hygienist
- Chaplain

Adapted from *Cancer Principles and Practice of Oncology*, 3rd edition.

compliance reasons, a more concerted effort toward cultivating a partnership and intervention may be required (Given and Given 1989). As an example, patients who experience scleroderma, whether generalized or localized, require intensive physical therapy. This phenomenon usually occurs as a late effect (more than one year post-transplant). For this chronic GVHD sequela, the physiatrist provides important direction for the entire health care team.

Chronic GVHD-mediated scleroderma, while mimicking naturally occurring scleroderma, may be a self-limiting complication. Therefore, unless constant regular therapy is maintained until the graft-versus-host disease is quiescent, the patient may have permanent disability. Resultant physical sequelae may range from minor inconveniences to radical changes and should be dealt with aggressively as part of the rehabilitation process. The difficulty arises in the unknowns, such as how long GVHD remains active, how long to maintain therapy, and when the full potential has been reached. Frustration on the part of the physical therapist as well as the patient may result from these inconsistencies and cause a breakdown in care. It takes coordination of the entire health care team to make these decisions. The patient is always included in each evaluation and decision-making session.

Prepubescent children may have the additional problem of retarded growth and development. Long-term counseling may be required as they progress through adolescence to adulthood. When these patients are grown, their initial entry into the work world may be discouraging (Durbin 1988). Patients with small stature or runting caused by a combination of long-term steroid use and chemoradiotherapy may require guidance for ultimate independent living.

At diagnosis, increasing awareness of fertility options on the part of primary care physicians can lead male patients to sperm-banking and females to consider storage of fertilized ova (Hamilton 1989). Heightened awareness is contributing to efforts to maximize growth and development in prepubertal treated patients (Sanders et al. 1988). Timing of this intervention is essential for any degree of normalization. Health maintenance should be of primary concern during these years, with semiannual evaluations. In female patients who are postpubertal, gynecological evaluations should be done semiannually. Prior studies have led to recognition of fertility problems and attempts to alleviate them by shielding the reproductive organs, and timing of chemotherapy doses have been attempted (Sanders et al. 1988).

Survivors of transplantation might also benefit from participation in organized support groups as well as self-help groups (NCCS Networker 1988 and 1989). The National Coalition of Cancer Survivors is attempting to gather strength from the ranks of survivors to increase awareness as well as obtain solutions to issues involving the survivor.

Newsletters, networking, and patient reunions all provide opportunities for marrow transplant survivors to become involved and support each other. Integration into the cancer survivor network and legislative lobbying for representation will help all survivors. Increased involvement has an impact across society. Educating people on all levels relieves stigma in the workplace and discrimination in employment and heightens awareness of the problems associated with cancer and its treatments. Just as specific treatment outcomes have support groups and nationally recognized programs, e.g., Reach for Recovery, so too do the specific needs of the marrow transplant patient require an outlet. Small groups and individuals are working hard to support patients undergoing the decision-making process regarding treatment. Memorial Sloan-Kettering and the Fred Hutchinson Cancer Research Center both have groups of volunteers, including expatients, who assist and support patients and families through the transplant process. Nothing seems to bolster the spirits of patients in the acute care setting as much as seeing a former patient a year or more after transplantation. Each center has different and very effective support programs; however, resources for the subsequent seasons of survival are lacking.

Fledgling programs for survivors are scattered throughout the nation. Former patients along with health care professionals interested in assisting might facilitate such programs with the development of educational material, networking between transplant centers, contributions to survivor-mediated publications, and lending expertise to survivor lobbyists (Hoffman 1989).

Research teams are aiming at more effective eradication of malignant cells, stem cell enrichment, improved allogeneic engraftment, and acceleration of immune reconstitution along with graft tolerance (Deeg et al. 1988). Research continues to improve preparative regimens by introducing new drugs and manipulating old ones. Biologic response modifiers such as GM-CSF are used in conjunction with cyclophosphamide to enhance and stimulate cell numbers, increasing the efficiency of the alkylating agent. Early detection and treatment of veno-occlusive disease circumvents death from this cause (Ford and Ballard 1988). Prognostic indicators of GVHD are now noted at the tissue typing level so that those at high risk for GVHD receive more intense prophylaxis regimens (Storb et al. 1983; Wingard et al. 1989). The increasing success of this research, coupled with the known problems of the transplant survivor, evinces the need for a coordinated long-term planning approach for the newly diagnosed patient and family.

Changing attitudes is a good beginning. Oncology rehabilitation nurses can be a compelling force to institute care plans that encompass the life spectrum of a particular patient. Provisions for rehabilitation should be flexible and dependent on preparative regimens and outcomes of treatment. The disease does not always win, and adjustments and interventions may be required throughout a lifetime. Knowledge of available resources, treatments, medications and their side effects, and cultivating a *partnership* relationship appear to be how nursing can best serve the transplant survivor. Studies are now in use on patients at high risk for relapse. The new technology of the biologic response modifiers is being tested as maintenance therapy after transplant in this population.

Along with the improvement of treatment and "good risk" patients leading relatively normal lives is the introduction of "higher risk" patients and their unknown outcomes. Increase in age at time of transplant (> 55 years), resistant disease, and a wider variety of genetic disorders may challenge nursing to a different set of expectations and outcomes. Even so, the basic needs of this patient population may best be served by inclusion in programs already formed. The outcomes and problems are similar. An appendix at the end of the text lists headquarters of several societies and groups that provide information as well as avenues for self-help and self-participation.

It is important for members of the health care team to become involved in survivor issues, and to include patient participation, perhaps beginning with their own particular center. Assembling a "survivor kit" for patients would be a reasonable beginning. The first section could explain the diagnosis, treatment, expected outcomes, and how best to prepare for the seasons to come. There are many isolated brochures on a given pertinent subject, but few materials gathered together and tailor-made for a given individual. New and very complicated treatment regimens can and do confuse patients. These kits might explain the rationale, while also defining methods of coping medically and psychologically after taking the patient through the process and then continuing with methods of permanent survival.

Coordinating such material could be an exciting challenge for the oncology nurse coordinator and lead to increased resources for all marrow transplant survivors.

An analysis of survival is complex but is becoming a major factor in evaluating the success of a treatment outcome for different types of transplantation. Increasing numbers of survivors have compelled the health care team to look at quality of life issues after transplantation. Quality of life studies are being performed via biosocial assessment to help define the life changes and adaptations after transplantation (Andrykowski et al. 1989a and 1989b; Smith and Lesko 1988; Hoffman 1989). Also, small studies have been performed on donor participation and sequelae, medical as well as psychological (Wolcott et al. 1986b; Van der Wal et al. 1988).

Bone marrow transplantation highlights the best and worst aspects of our current medical knowledge; the awesome task of balancing intensive treatments that will effectively eradicate disease while maintaining some semblance of biopsychosocial normalcy for the patient following such treatment challenges the transplant team. The courage of patients and their families and the intensive nature of the treatment often sustains team members and creates lasting relationships. The task now is to further assist and broaden that relationship to a partnership in survival.

Acknowledgement: Supported in part by PHS Grant Nos. CA18029, CA47748, and CA18221, awarded by the National Cancer Institute, and Grant No. HL36444, awarded by the Heart, Lung, and Blood Institute, NIH, DHHS.

References

Andrykowski, M.A. et al. 1989a. Physical and psychosocial functioning of adult survivors of allogeneic bone marrow transplantation. *B.M.T.* 4: 75–81.

Andrykowski, M.A. et al. 1989b. Longitudinal assessment of psychosocial functioning of adult survivors of allogeneic bone marrow transplantation. *B.M.T.* 4: 505–509.

Brown, H.N., and Kelly, M.J. 1976. Stages of bone marrow transplantation: A psychiatric perspective. *Psychosom. Med.* 38: 439–446.

Clark, J. et al. 1985. Obstructive lung disease after allogeneic marrow transplantation. *Ann. Intern. Med.* 111: 368–376.

Corcoran-Buchsel, P., and Parchem, C. 1988. Ambulatory care of the bone marrow transplant patient. In Yarbro, E.H. (ed.). *Seminars in Oncology Nursing.* Philadelphia: Grune & Stratton, pp. 41–46.

Decker, W.A. et al. 1989. Psychosocial aspects and the physiological effects of a cardiopulmonary exercise program in patients undergoing bone marrow transplantation (BMT) for acute lukemia (AL). *Transplantation Proceedings* 21 (1): 3068–3069.

Deeg, H.J. et al. 1984. Cataracts after total body irradiation and marrow transplantation: A sparing effect of dose fractionation. *Int. J. Radiation Oncology Biol. Phys.* 10: 957–964.

Deeg, H.J. et al. (eds.). 1988. *A Guide to Bone Marrow Transplantation.* New York: Springer-Verlag.

DeLisa, J.A. et al. 1989. Rehabilitation of the cancer patient. In DeVita, V.D., Hellman, S., Rosenberg, S.A. (eds.). *Cancer. Principles and Practice of Oncology,* 3rd edition. Philadelphia: J. B. Lippincott, pp. 2333–2367.

Directory of Resources. 1986. In Holleb, A.I., Subak-Sharpe, G.J., White, W.H., Kasofsky, P. (eds.). *The American Cancer Society Cancer Book.* Garden City, NY: Doubleday & Co., pp. 611–622.

Durbin M. 1988. Bone marrow transplantation: Economic, ethic, and social issues. *Pediatrics* 82: 774–782.

Ford, R., and Ballard, B. 1988. Acute complications after bone marrow transplantation. *Seminars in Oncology Nursing* 4 (1): 15–24.

Frymark, S. 1990. Cancer Rehabilitation in the outpatient setting. *Oncology Issues: The Journal of Cancer Program Management* 5 (1): 12–17.

Gardner, G. et al. 1977. Psychological issues in bone marrow transplantation. *Pediatrics* 60: 625–631.

Given, B.A., and Given, C.W. 1984. Creating a climate for compliance. *Cancer Nurs.* 7: 139–147.

Given, B.A., and Given, C.W. 1989. Compliance among patients with cancer. *O.N.F.* 16: 97–103.

Hamilton, P. 1989. Letter to the editor. *The Cancer Journal* 2: 406.

Hengeveld, M.W. et al. 1988. Psychological aspects of bone marrow transplantation: a retrospective study of 17 long-term survivors. *Bone Marrow Transplantation* 3: 69–75.

Hoffman, B. 1989a. Cancer survivors at work: Job problems and illegal discrimination. *O.N.F.* 16: 39–43.

Hoffman, B. 1989b. Current issues of cancer survivorship. *Oncology* 3 (7): 85–95.

Holtzman, L.S. 1988. Physical therapy intervention following bone marrow transplantation. *Clinical Management* 8 (2): 6–9.

James, M.C. 1987. Physical therapy for patients after bone marrow transplantation. *Phys. Ther.* 67 (6): 946–952.

Kahan, B.D. 1989. Drug Therapy. Cyclosporine. *N. Engl. J. Med.* 321: 1725–1738.

Lesko, L.M., and Hawkins, D.R. 1983. Psychological aspects of transplantation medicine. In Akhtar, S. (ed.). *New Psychological Syndromes.* Jason Aronson, pp. 265–309.

Mathe, G. et al. 1965. Adoptive immunotherapy of acute leukemia: Experimental and clinical results. *Cancer Res.* 25: 1525–1531.

McKenna, R.J. 1986. Rehabilitation of the cancer patient. 1986. In Holleb, A.I., Subak-Sharpe, G.J., White, W.H., Kasofsky, P. (eds.). *The American Cancer Society Cancer Book.* Garden City, NY: Doubleday & Co., pp. 201–224.

Mullan F. 1985. Seasons of survival: Reflections of a physician with cancer. *N. Engl. J. Med.* 313: 270–273.

NCCS Networker. 1988. *Vol 2,* Summer.

NCCS Networker. 1989. *Vol 3,* Winter.

Nims, J.W., and Strom, S. 1988. Late complications of bone marrow transplant recipients: Nursing care issues. *Seminars in Oncology Nursing* 4 (1): 47–54.

Patenaude, A.F., and Rappeport, J.M. 1982. Surviving bone marrow transplantation: The patient in the other bed. *Ann. Intern. Med.* 97: 915–918.

Richardson, J.L. et al. 1988. The influence of symptoms of disease and side effects of treatment on compliance with cancer therapy. *J. Clin. Oncol. 6:* 1746–1752.

Sanders, J.E. et al. 1988. Growth and development in children after bone marrow transplantation. *Horm. Res. 30:* 92–97.

Schover, L.R. 1988a. *Sexuality and cancer for the man who has cancer, and his partner.* NY: American Cancer Society.

Schover, L.R. 1988b. *Sexuality and cancer for the woman who has cancer, and her partner.* NY: American Cancer Society.

Smith, K., and Lesko, L.M. 1988. Psychosocial problems in cancer survivors. *Oncology 2* (1): 33–44.

Storb, R. et al. 1983. Predictive factors in chronic graft-versus-host disease in patients with aplastic anemia treated by marrow transplantation from HLA-identical siblings. *Ann. Intern. Med. 98:* 461–466.

Sullivan, K.M. et al. 1984. Late complications after marrow transplantation. *Semin. Hematol. 21:* 53–63.

Sullivan, K.M. et al. 1988. Prednisone and azathioprine compared with prednisone and placebo for treatment of chronic graft-versus-host disease: Prognostic influence of prolonged thrombocytopenia after allogeneic marrow transplantation. *Blood 72:* 546–554.

Thomas, E.D. 1988. The future of marrow transplantation. *Seminars in Oncology Nursing 4* (1): 74–78.

Thomas, E.D. et al. 1959. Supralethal whole body irradiation and isologous marrow transplantation in man. *J. Clin. Oncol. 38:* 1709–1716.

Thomas, E.D. et al. 1975. Bone marrow transplantation. *N. Engl. J. Med. 292:* 832–843, 895–902.

Van Bekkum, D.W., and De Vries, M.J. 1967. *Radiation Chimeras.* London: Logos Press Limited.

van der Wal, R., Nims, J., and Davies, B. 1988. Bone marrow transplantation in children. *Canc. Nurs. 11:* 132–143.

Wiley, F.M., and House, K.U. 1988. Bone marrow transplant in children. in Yarbro, E.H. (ed.). *Seminars in Oncology Nursing.* Philadelphia: Grune & Stratton, pp. 31–40.

Witherspoon, R.P., and Storb, R. 1984. Immunologic aspects of marrow transplantation. *Transplant Immunol. 9:* 187–207.

Witherspoon, R.P. et al. 1989. Secondary malignancies following marrow transplantation for aplastic anemia or leukemia. *N. Engl. J. Med. 321:* 784–789.

Wolcott, D.L. et al. 1986a. Adaptation of adult bone marrow transplant recipient long-term survivors. *Transplantation 41:* 478–483.

Wolcott, D.L. et al. 1986b. Psychological adjustment of adult bone marrow transplant donors whose recipient survives. *Transplantation 41:* 484–488.

PART IV

The Care Environment

Chapter 16

Nursing Staff Stresses and Ethical Dilemmas in Caring for Bone Marrow Transplant Patients

Peggy Shedd

Staff members involved in the care of bone marrow transplant patients are familiar with the stresses of their work. Some of the specific issues facing the staff include relationships with the patients, their families, and other staff, as well as the concerns and ethical dilemmas arising out of such aggressive treatment and its high complication and mortality rates. This chapter explores these issues and also offers some ideas of ways for staff to cope with them.

Staff-Patient/Family Relationships

The relationship that can develop between bone marrow transplant patients and staff can be intense. These patients receive care for a prolonged period of time, by a relatively small number of staff, for a medically intense hospitalization. The care that one unit gives can extend from before

the transplant hospitalization itself to previous episodes of chemotherapy treatment or even back to the time of initial diagnosis. After the transplant hospitalization, patients may return for treatment of complications associated with continuing immunosuppression and thrombocytopenia. Each of these hospitalizations are intense, crisis-laden episodes in a chronic illness experience with high mortality rates. These features contribute to the formation of close, involved staff-patient relationships (Pot-Mees 1987; Brack et al. 1988).

Hospitalization for bone marrow transplantation includes some form of protective isolation for patients. This isolation has varied throughout the years. Initially, in the 1960s and 1970s, isolation involved small tents or bubbles that just enclosed the patient's bed and perhaps a small amount of floor space with a chair. Then, the laminar air flow room was introduced, which provides more room, but staff and visitors are kept from the patient by wearing protective isolation clothing that precludes physical touching. Finally, single rooms with strict reverse isolation precautions are now increasingly being used.

The use of isolation, no matter how strict, reinforces the closeness of the patient-staff relationship. Encounters are limited to those staff who have close enough contact to warrant the extensive cleansing and garbing preparations necessary to enter the patient's space, which intensifies those few encounters. Casual encounters with other patients or staff are minimized if not prohibited, so the patient's only exposure to people comes through their families and those few staff whose assignment to the patient warrants the time and energy it takes to participate in the strict isolation procedures. Patients come to rely on "their" staff for linkages to the outside world. Current trends away from the rigid procedures of the tents and laminar air flow rooms are easing this, but many patients continue to comment on the importance of staff to ease their loneliness. This request and burden only increases the already close involvement of the staff with these patients (Collins et al. 1989; Holland et al. 1977; Gordon 1975; Graubert and Edmonson 1972).

The predictably close relationship between a bone marrow transplant patient and the staff raises the potential of over-involvement and its emotional cost to the staff. Bone marrow transplant patients experience significant complications and mortality rates, which affect staff. Watching patients in pain and distress is difficult, and increasing the intensity of the relationship only increases this difficulty (Pot-Mees 1987). Over-involved staff may find themselves losing their objectivity and therefore, their professional ability to intervene. However, this problem not only affects patient care, but also affects the staff, draining them of their energy and desire to work with such difficult situations. Such burnout may lead to a staff member's request to transfer out of the bone marrow transplant unit, or to stay but become emotionally and professionally distant. Staff must become vigilant to assess the signs of over-involvement or burn out in themselves and their colleagues.

Trust issues become important when many of the bone marrow transplant patients are from other treatment centers. The specialization of this procedure, as well as the multiple experimental protocols available, sometimes forces patients to travel long distances to receive appropriate treatment. These patients arrive at transplant units with an established history and expectation of treatment procedures from their local hospital, which may not be identical to procedures used at the transplant unit. Patients often have become quite knowledgeable about their disease and treatment by this time and question variations on that treatment. Often this knowledge is limited to how something is done and not why. Transplant nurses spend a great deal of time and energy explaining procedural variations in order to establish and maintain trusting relationships with these scared, concerned patients and families.

Relationships with patients' families can also become intense. Families usually spend a great deal of time with the patient and therefore become quite involved with the staff. These families are often scared, anxious, and are frequently far from home and their normal social support systems and activities. This all contributes to the potential for great closeness and dependency on staff for emotional support. Providing intense support can be rewarding but can also be quite draining, especially if the staff does not think they have adequate time or skills to meet these family demands. Some families may have preexisting struggles that affect the staff as well as the patient. For instance, premorbid marital difficulties or other intrafamily struggles can be exacerbated by the stress of the current illness. Attempting to intervene in these chronic difficulties can be very wearing, especially over the long hospitalizations that transplant patients require. Many times staff realize that the majority of their emotional support and time is being spent with the family, not with the patient. This can be frustrating as well as wearing and can also contribute to staff burnout if there are no other resources to meet family needs.

Aggressive Treatment

Bone marrow transplant patients'treatment acuity can often reach intensive care unit levels. Required care may result in the need for increased staffing ratios, sophisticated monitoring mechanisms, or both. Although patients can be transferred to ICU, some transplant units are designed to keep patients whose care would otherwise require intensive care unit transfer. Providing this level of care requires education and technical skills above and beyond the training and knowledge that typically is offered in a regular oncology unit orientation.

An intensive care emphasis may prove rewarding to some oncology nurses who desire the intellectual and technical challenge, but may be an unwanted burden for oncology nurses who value the psychosocial elements of their work. Critical care staff are continually faced with balancing their patients' intense physical care needs with the great psychosocial needs of the patients or families under their care. Bone marrow transplant regimens are now forcing this dilemma onto oncology nurses. Nurses who strive to be excellent care providers in both realms may face frustration if unable to achieve competence or have adequate resources to reach their goal. An environment that poses continued frustration in reaching treatment goals of staff can lead to burnout (Slaby 1988). Staff can become angry and exhausted, and cope by withdrawing or displaying apathy to the same treatment challenges that originally drew them to bone marrow transplant care. The initial intensive care challenges of bone marrow transplant units may actually become their downfall if resources are not focused on this problem.

Units that specialize in oncology care pride themselves on providing aggressive treatment whether the goal is a cure, palliation, or death with dignity. Patients receiving hospice type care may be located next to patients receiving intensive care level activities. Shifting between patients with such opposing goals can be very difficult. Bone marrow transplant units carry this dichotomy even further, since the cure emphasis may persevere up until only a few hours before a patient's death. There may be little room for a change in care emphasis, let alone a change in the attitudes and hopes of staff when a neutropenic or thrombocytopenic complication can progress so rapidly from being compatible to incompatible with life. This shift in emphasis can be very difficult for staff. Staff that value the goal of cure may feel cheated or defeated when the goal shifts to that of "comfort measures only." They may even lack the skills or desire to feel confident that they can assist a patient in achieving a dignified, comfortable death. On the other hand, staff that value the goal of a caring, dignified death may think that pushing for aggressive treatment until the final hour robs them of the time and environment to properly prepare a patient and family for death.

It is as difficult for patients and family to keep both cure and death at the forefront of their thoughts as it is for staff, so staff are often called upon to assist patients and family to make this transition. However, the suddenness of this switch often catches staff without the time to modify their own goals, let alone help patients and families.

Personal and internalized discord may be played out interpersonally as staff conflict when patient goals are either not clearly defined, or are in the process of change. Staff advocating for continued aggressive treatment clash with staff advocating a peaceful death with dignity. Lack of group cohesiveness, collaboration, and respect becomes apparent at such stressful times. Unfortunately, the morbidity and mortality statistics of bone marrow transplant patients predict that this occurrence is frequent enough to be a common and chronic stressor in a unit devoted to such patients.

Another issue that affects bone marrow transplant nurses is that some of the aggressive treatment of transplant patients requires a great deal of patient participation and compliance. Isolation procedures, hygiene, exercise, and nutrition are but a few of the self-care interventions required of these patients. Much staff time and effort is taken up with educating and motivating patients and families in these activities. Staff emphasize rigid adherence to techniques designed to reduce potential complications that these patients experience from the preparative regimens of high-dose chemotherapy and total body irradiation. Transplant nurses believe in the importance of patient and family participation in the energy draining and time-consuming activities designed to prevent or minimize these complications. However, transplant patients may not be compliant, because of physical debility, fatigue, and pain or due to complex psychological factors that result in regressed, dependent, or acting out behaviors.

Family may not be able to assist staff in motivating patients to be compliant due to lack of knowledge of the problem or due to their fear of the stress on their relationship with the patient that can develop if they play what can seem to the patient to be a "slave driver" role. Patients may resent being asked (or told) to do something that is for "their own good," and families may not tolerate the reactions that this request elicits from the patient. Family members may even interfere with staff who attempt to increase patient compliance. Dealing with compliance issues with the patient as well as with their family can be doubly draining. What complicates this issue even more is the experience staff may have with the noncompliant patient who does well in spite of their refusal to follow staff's advice as compared to the very compliant patient who may do poorly. This individual variation and lack of a perfect correlation between good compliance and low complication rates contributes to staff questioning themselves and each other on the wisdom of expending a lot of time and energy on promoting patient compliance. This questioning can lead to self-doubt and insecurity for individual staff as

well as to interstaff stress on the bone marrow transplant unit.

High Morbidity and Mortality Rates

It is often said that patients are hospitalized in order to receive nursing care. Therefore, nursing care may often seem to be the difference between low and high morbidity rates. However, a treatment such as bone marrow transplant guarantees a high morbidity rate by the very nature of the aggressive antineoplastic and immunosuppressive therapy. In spite of or because of this knowledge, transplant staff strive to perfect their technical skills in order to minimize the predictably high morbidity rates for these patients. This is an admirable but often frustrating goal, since individual patient, environmental, and staff practice variables can affect this goal. Although it may seem logical that the interralated variables would decrease the staff's sense of personal responsibility in affecting these variables, this is not often the case. Staff struggle to devise more and more strategies to reduce the complications and morbidity experienced by bone marrow transplant patients. This is an admirable goal, but one that may be unreachable, or one that may only assist future unknown patients without assisting the initial known sample that inspired the staff to create or vary their interventions. It can be difficult for staff to keep a long-term goal in mind while an individual patient suffers in the short term. This inability to prevent or reduce patient suffering can seem like a nursing failure.

Complications of bone marrow transplants, unlike many other examples of morbidity, are often due to the treatment rather than the disease itself. Patients are brought to transplant in remission, or at most, in early relapse, and morbidity is a direct result of the techniques used to prepare the patient's marrow for the transplant. As such, it is easy to question the reason for the intense suffering experienced by these patients either by complications caused by the preparatory bone marrow ablation or by graft-versus-host disease. (Brack et al. 1988; Pot-Mees 1987; Rappaport 1988). Not only is it stressful to watch such suffering, but staff may even question their role in causing the complication, either by encouraging the patient to have a bone marrow transplant, or by actually administering the preparatory chemotherapy and radiation. This guilt is obviously lessened if a patient has minimal complications and/or survives the transplant with good future quality as well as quantity of life. However, this guilt is heightened if a patient suffers extensive and uncomfortable complications and/or survives the transplant only to have a poor quality of life or dies soon after the transplant due to relapse or a fatal complication. This sense of guilt is dramatized by study results by Brack and colleagues (1988) that showed only 29.4% of a sample of 17 nonphysician members of a bone marrow transplant staff would themselves choose to have a bone marrow transplant. It is difficult for staff not to feel guilty if they themselves would not choose such treatment. This sense of guilt obviously adds to staff stress.

Another complication of bone marrow transplants that may cause staff distress is the treatment of rigors associated with the administration of the broad-spectrum antifungal agent amphotericin B. This agent can cause shaking chills in many patients. This uncomfortable symptom is commonly treated by the use of meperidine (Demerol). Although often effective in treating the rigors, transplant staff may feel uncertain about its use, fearing that although they are treating the distressing symptom of rigors, they may also be contributing to the development of addiction in some of these patients (Fincannon 1988).

Complicating this fear is the lack of consistency of relief obtained by using meperidine, thereby leading to increased dosages in some patients to points where this author as well as Fincannon (1988) have observed patients receiving IV meperidine every two hours, nearly around the clock. It is in this extreme situation where the

staff usually question addiction and worries about their own complicity. This fear produces strong anger and guilt reactions in staff who are in fact well educated about the actual low percentage of addiction caused by narcotics administered in hospitals. This same staff is often well aware of the landmark studies such as the one by Marks and Sachar (1973) that showed gross undertreatment of patients in acute pain due to physician's fear of causing addiction. They are also knowledgeable about the large survey studies that show the risk of developing addiction by using narcotics in hospitalized patients for pain management to be extremely small (Porter and Jick 1980). There is also specific data about the lack of medication abuse or addiction in a sample of 26 bone marrow transplant patients who self-medicated for oral mucositis pain with PCA (patient controlled analgesia) administered morphine (Chapman and Hill 1989). However, the potentially large doses, as well as variable success rate of meperidine in reducing amphoteracin rigors seems to cause this same knowledgeable staff to doubt. Other factors that may increase this staff doubt is the nonanalgesic purpose of the meperidine, as well as the nonterminal nature of the bone marrow transplant patients. Perhaps it is the knowledge that a patient is terminally ill that ordinarily reduces staff fear of addiction. Or, perhaps knowledge of lack of addiction when using narcotics for analgesia does not generalize readily to the use of meperidine for purposes other than analgesia. Finally, the guilt and fear that knowledgeable bone marrow transplant staff feel about the use of meperidine for treating amphotericin-induced rigors may be a repository for, and actually largely symbolic for, the larger fears of causing more morbidity from a bone marrow transplant itself than the patient is currently experiencing from the original disease. If so, this guilt cannot be eliminated by the use of knowledge or observation about narcotic administration.

The closeness of involvement with bone marrow transplant patients leads to staff grief when patients die. Although the hoped for outcome of a transplant is cure of disease, many patients will die either during the transplant of immediate complications of treatment, or afterwards due to chronic complications or relapse of the original disease. The knowledge of the high mortality in these patients can prepare staff intellectually for the inevitable reality, but may do less to prepare staff for the emotional distress. This distress is intensified by the emotional closeness that staff often experience with transplant patients and their families as well as staff ambivalence (Brack et al. 1988) about the worth of the procedure itself. Often, staff may turn from comforting one bereaved family to walking into a pretransplant patient's room and assisting in educating the patient about their upcoming transplant. This leaves little time and emphasis on staff grieving and adjustment. Unresolved staff grief is not only an inevitable negative aspect of transplant nursing, but can be a large factor in the development of staff burnout (Pot-Mees 1987; Rappaport 1988; Brack et al. 1988).

Stresses related to high mortality rates may affect the behavior of the bone marrow transplant staff toward the patient. This behavior has been described as placing the dying patient in a "double bind" situation (Longhofer and Floersch 1980; Brack et al. 1988). A "double bind" situation is one in which there are two contradictory messages coming from the same person. In this case, the staff (or family) say or report positive, hopeful statements about the patient's situation, but clearly show their pessimistic private thoughts and feelings about the situation. This is particularly evident in instances where the transplant patient is deteriorating and death approaches. Patients are torn between their desire to believe the positive, hopeful statements of encouragement that staff and family offer and their own awareness of failing health. In this instance, the reward to the patient in accurately perceiving the true hidden messages of the staff and family is to lose their own hope that they will survive this difficult "last chance" effort. This not only affects their drive and self-care activities designed to decrease

the very same complications that could hasten death, but also results in the patient withdrawing from these difficult interactions (Longhofer and Floersch 1980; Brack et al. 1988). Unfortunately it is often in these situations of patient withdrawal that staff attempts to be more positive, hoping to motivate and provide hope. The cycle continues as the patient reacts by withdrawing even further. This unfortunate situation is most likely to occur when the staff is unable to openly acknowledge the pessimism that is felt about the patient's chance for survival. Not only must the entire team be comfortable with acknowledging their fears as well as hopes, but so must the individual staff member. Coping with the reality of these paradoxes in providing care to bone marrow transplant patients is an important step towards addressing both the staff and patient stress associated with this risky procedure where death can quickly and easily replace success.

Ethical Dilemmas

New technology leads to new ethical dilemmas. The natural lag time between the development of technology and addressing the ethical dilemmas that such technology causes can increase the stress to staff involved in managing the technology. Such is the case with bone marrow transplants. Ethical dilemmas that have been identified include issues around informed consent, concerns about the rights and concerns of donors, and finally, the concern of health care today, allocation of resources.

An acceptable informed consent requires adequate information and comprehension, competence, and voluntariness of the decision. Much debate has occurred over what constitutes adequate information for any informed consent and those for bone marrow transplants are no exception. In a situation where the alternative to the procedure is certain death whereas the procedure offers the chance of survival or the chance of a quicker death, it may be argued that subjects decide solely based on the life or death options. Perhaps for this procedure, lesser issues or values are considered less than in procedures where most outcomes are not life or death issues. In a study by Silberfeld et al. (1988), 70 volunteers (half were law or medical students, half were lay people) were presented with a hypothetical situation in which they were to choose whether or not to have a bone marrow transplant. The investigators provided these volunteers with a videotape of actual patients and staff describing the procedure and real patients' experiences. The overwhelming majority (87%) of the volunteers accepted bone marrow transplant. While there was some exploration of the effect of the individuals' values about courage and logic as well as negative attributional style on their choice, it appeared to the authors that the life or death choice was the biggest motivator in the volunteer's choice (Silberfeld et al. 1988).

Studies of the process of informed consent procedures for bone marrow transplants have explored the patient and staff experience. Lesko and colleagues (1989) questioned 39 adult bone marrow transplant patients, the parents of 61 pediatric BMT patients, and seven oncologists about their informed consent experience. The top three reasons expressed by both adult patients and parents of pediatric patients for choosing the BMT was the "belief that treatment is a cure, fear that the illness will get worse without treatment, and trust in the physician" (Lesko et al. 1989). Most adult patients (95%) and parents (97%) remembered that there was the possibility of complications due to the procedure itself, however, they recalled fewer than half of those complications presented. The complications recalled most often were nausea and graft-versus-host disease/skin reaction. Interestingly, most of the patients and parents thought the content presented was adequate and not too technical, but the physicians involved thought it contained too much information and was too technical in nature. Although patients and parents thought they had freely expressed their doubts or concerns to the physician, they still withheld some questions. Physicians, on the other hand, thought most of them withheld their doubts and concerns. Almost all of the patients and parents ultimately thought the physician wanted them to receive the bone marrow transplant and relied on this advice to make their decision. The physicians underestimated this reliance on their advice although they did think that about half of the patients and parents wanted the physician to make the decision. These findings complement the Silberfeld et al. (1988) study, which also showed the overwhelming weight of the life or death decision, or importance of outcome, in the informed consent procedure for BMT. Although the patients knew there were potential serious complications, the specificity and concern about them was less important in the decision-making.

Carney (1987) explored the experience of informed consent from the staff's perspective. The striking finding in interviews of BMT nurses (N=16) and physicians (N=5) was that the nurses most valued information being told to the patient about potential short- and long-term complications or the process of the procedure, whereas the physicians most valued information about the patient's diagnosis and options, or the outcome of treatment. The Silberfeld et al. (1988) and Lesko et al. (1989) studies support the patient's reliance on making the decision for or against a bone marrow transplant based mostly on the life or death (outcome) issue. Carney (1987) also notes this discrepancy and points out that nurses may need to reevaluate their own focus on the process of the treatment and acknowledge that for most patients the outcome of the treatment is most important in making their decision.

It is understandable that nurses, who grapple with first protecting the patient from the complications and then with promoting the recovery from those complications, would be very concerned with patients' awareness of these problems. Perhaps this is an attempt on the nurses' parts to deal with their own guilt in feeling a part of the process that induces such pain and suffering in these patients. It is logical that one could feel less guilty if the patient were aware of these risks and yet still chose such risky and uncomfortable treatment. However, the intensity of the life or death choice may preclude the ability or interest of a patient in dwelling on the process of getting to that end. Carney (1987) therefore poses the challenge that nurses should "work at tailoring the information we disclose to the needs of the patient and not feel that one has failed as a professional because the patient is not completely informed." This advice may assist individual staff to reconcile their own frustrations at the informed consent procedure and also decrease interstaff accusations of providing inadequate information. Otherwise, nurses will remain frustrated at the physician's and patient's emphasis on outcome because they view the process of treatment as most important.

Concerns have also been expressed about the experience of being a donor of healthy marrow. Issues addressed include confidentiality as well as the psychological adjustment of donors. A case discussed by Caplan et al. (1983) explores the dilemma presented when knowledge was acquired by a potential bone marrow transplant recipient of the existence of a possible matching donor. The dilemma arose because the donor had been tested only because of a family member's need and was not listed on a public, easily accessible list. The donor was contacted, informed of a general request to donate and refused to participate. The potential recipient remained unaware of the identity of the donor, but requested that she be contacted again and informed of the specific request, hoping it would persuade her to help him. Obviously, the confidentiality of the donor was at odds with the principle of beneficence, or promoting good, to the potential recipient. The merits, pro or con, of disclosure revolve around the ability of an unrelated transplant to succeed (benefit of the procedure to the recipient versus harm from donating marrow to the donor), coercion of the donor, autonomy of the donor to refuse to donate marrow, as well as the confidentiality of the donor.

Donating marrow may seem like a small risk relative to the issues facing the recipients of this marrow, but donors should not be ignored. The risky nature of the transplant for the recipient should, in fact, increase our interest and concern for the welfare of the donor. If the donor's experience is negative, it is difficult to promote such a risky procedure as BMT. Risk to the donor has been viewed as mainly psychological since the physical harms are minimal. Most concern has focused on the adverse psychological situation a donor may be in if the recipient experiences serious complications which cause suffering or even death. The ultimate concern is with graft-versus-host disease in which the donor's marrow actually rejects the patient and can cause intense discomfort and even death (Rappaport 1988; Wolcott et al. 1986). In a bizarre sense, the donor could actually perceive his "gift of life" to paradoxically become the instrument of death.

Staff become involved if the donor is a member of the patient's family who is present during the patient's hospitalization. Staff may feel a special need to reward and support the donor, whose psychological health may vary according to the patient's physical status. Concern may also be felt about the potential for coercion involving the donor's choice, especially if the patient's outcome is poor. Wolcott and colleagues (1986) explored this issue in a questionnaire study of 18 donors. Basically, they found few reports of ambivalence about donating, and all said they would donate again if asked. There was little emotional distress associated with the donation but there was an outcome of the study that suggested negative consequences if the recipient deteriorated. However, this study looked only at donors of marrow to surviving recipients. Therefore, although staff probably does not need to be overly concerned about coercion in this group, the issue of the donor suffering if the recipient deteriorates is another potential stressor. It has already been acknowledged that supporting family is difficult for the busy, involved BMT staff. It could be even more difficult if the family includes the donor who stands by helplessly watching his loved one deteriorate as a result of receiving his marrow.

The ethical dilemma of allocation of resources arises with procedures such as bone marrow transplantation that represent current high-cost technology. Staff are faced with specific issues of resource allocation each time a potential transplant patient is turned away due to lack of funds. Durbin (1988) reports the hospital bills for the transplant hospitalization itself to be more than $120,000. Obviously, few patients can pay for this without insurance. However, prepaid insurances such as health maintenance organizations and state public insurances such as Medicaid are evaluating the benefits versus the financial costs of such procedures and many are denying funding (Durbin 1988; Robinson, 1989). Alabama, Arizona, Oregon, Texas, Virginia, and parts of California have already limited the expenditure of public health funds for bone marrow transplants (Robinson 1989). It may be difficult for staff who become close to specific potential recipients to accept these decisions about resource allocation. However, these decisions may become more common as health care dollars become more scarce. It is difficult to justify large expenditures of scarce health care dollars for a procedure that has a high risk of morbidity and mortality (Durbin 1988). Most transplant unit staff have now experienced the pain of this principle of justice as they watch a leukemia patient well known to them not be eligible for transplant because of lack of funds. This grief is much more poignant than the grief of experiencing the death of a leukemia patient who chooses not to have a transplant for non-financial reasons. It remains important to evaluate the costs of this treatment as well as the outcomes in order to more fully address this issue at the health policy and funding levels. Staff should become involved in policy making committees at the local, state, and national level in order to become informed as well as to portray accurately the experience of bone marrow transplantation for these layperson committees. Issues of justice will grow to have larger

and larger importance in ethical decision making as it relates to bone marrow transplantation.

Staff Conflict

The staff stresses previously identified are bound to cause interpersonal conflicts with staff. Disagreements over care goals and interventions, closeness as well as tensions with families and patients, staff guilt and concern over morbidity and mortality, and ethical dilemmas all pose potential areas of discord between staff. These will be addressed further in two ways, conflict between and among nurses, and conflict with other disciplines.

Bone marrow transplant nurses experience conflict with other nurses in a variety of ways. The complexity of physical and psychological care needs of transplant patients and their families requires careful nursing care planning. However, because most of care planning falls to the nursing staff, there is room for disagreement. The very independence of nursing judgement for transplant care that promotes nurse satisfaction also has the potential to increase the nurse-nurse conflict. Each nurse may have his/her own methods or ideas about optimal treatment for physical complications associated with bone marrow transplants. Individual knowledge bases, experiences, and personal biases all affect choices of nursing interventions. This applies as well to the psychosocial needs of patients and families. Nurses must accept accountability for their decisions and resolve conflicts with other nurses so that interventions are optimal and carried through by all shifts. There are few things more frustrating or self-defeating than planning an intricate intervention only to see the next shift reject or ignore it. Not only is patient care compromised by such lack of continuity, but so is the nurse's motivation and confidence in repeating the experience.

Nursing staff also experience conflict with other disciplines. The complex care of bone marrow transplant patients requires teamwork and collaboration among all team members. Energy spent attempting to secure support from the pharmacy or dietary detracts from direct care activities with the patient or family. Territorial feuds over which discipline is to provide psychosocial care to these patients and families can result in nursing staff frustration and lack of care to the patient. Inability to collaborate with physicians about long-term goals or immediate decisions such as the need to address code status with a patient result in staff dissatisfaction, patient suffering, and potentially, nurse burnout (Baggs and Schmitt 1988). Teamwork and collaboration with all disciplines cannot be emphasized enough in the care of bone marrow transplant patients. The necessity for respect and smooth working relationships must be emphasized in such a complicated, morbidity laden, and mortality risky procedure. Recent studies of intensive care unit mortality rates have shown that successful outcomes are significantly affected by nurse-physician interactions and communication (Knaus et al. 1986; Baggs and Schmitt 1988).

There are many skills required for nursing staff to feel adequate to meet the challenge of conflict. Initially, there must be adequate and current scientific knowledge and technological skills for the nurse to be confident in problem solving or decision making. Then, skills such as assertiveness, conflict resolution, and problem solving are important for resolving interpersonal conflicts. This expertise is met best by experienced nurses who can then increase their skills and specialization to meet the challenges and needs of the bone marrow transplant patient. Specific resources to assist nurses in this development will be mentioned later, but conflict resolution and development of teamwork can only occur if the transplant unit environment supports its development with the proper values, supervision, and resource support.

Support Needs for Nurses

The previous sections have identified the many stressors that exist for staff working on a bone marrow transplant unit. The support needs and the services that fulfill those needs are varied as well. It is important to view this programmatically, and not as a single issue or event. In this way, support can be proactive and preventative, rather than constantly crisis oriented. This section will address a variety of support services that a unit could incorporate into a program designed to meet the particular needs of their staff and unit.

Education is a key support service for BMT staff. It is easy to forget that knowledge itself is empowering. Accurately understanding the goals of treatment helps the staff realistically prepare themselves for the types of complications and untoward outcomes that can occur with BMT patients. Predicting and anticipating patient problems allows the staff to intervene promptly and effectively, thus decreasing patient and staff crisis situations. A firm scientific knowledge base is essential in conflict resolution with other staff.

The development of interpersonal skills is also an important component of staff educational programs. Communication skills, as well as negotiation and conflict resolution techniques are but a few of the useful topics for this focus of staff education. The unit and individual staff member's educational needs should be assessed and this then can form the basis for planning orientation, inservice, and continuing education programs that best meet the unit's needs. One such plan was outlined by Ford (1983) for the Fred Hutchinson BMT unit. She points out the importance of scheduling to allow staff to attend inservices and other educational programming. Providing a lecture to staff who are unable to attend, or are so distracted by unit needs that they are unable to fully participate is frustrating and stress producing. However, planning schedules and educational activities to support staff attendance is a frustration as well. What works for one unit may not work for another but there are some techniques that one may generalize. Sometimes it is easier to free up some staff to attend an all day series of educational offerings than it is to support staff to attend a one-, two-, or three-hour program within their regular work day. Organizing short programs at staff meal times is sometimes helpful to stimulate attendance. Repeating a short (15–20 minute) presentation throughout the shifts can eventually reach larger numbers of staff than a single presentation. Videotaping programs can allow staff to choose the time of attendance that is most convenient to them. These are only a few of the ideas that have been shown to assist staff to attend educational programming. Clearly, a combination of well thought out topics and creative scheduling is necessary for the success of an educational program. However, these efforts are worthwhile and essential to meet the educational needs of staff in such specialty units as bone marrow transplant units.

Support groups can be another effective mechanism to help BMT staff cope with their particular unit stresses (Pot-Mees 1987; Sarantos 1988). These groups can address both the complex psychosocial care planning that BMT patients require as well as the staff's reactions to and issues with these patients. Such groups may focus on a particularly trying patient or family situation that affects the staff and come up with useful ideas to modify the situation. Group feedback, support, and ideas can be very helpful in decreasing the frustration for individual staff members who are assigned to the patient. Objectivity and fresh ideas can be obtained by analyzing these difficult situations away from the actual interaction and with peer support. Sometimes the benefit occurs simply by realizing that other staff would also find the situation difficult and frustrating. Staff can also learn techniques or ideas for future difficult situations by assisting their colleague in exploring a current problem. The staff's own issues can also be effectively dealt with in support groups. Issues of control, conflict, and grief can be shared and explored as they affect individuals or groups of staff. Teamwork can be enhanced by discussing and exploring these common themes. Support groups may meet episodically as issues arise, or be scheduled on a routine basis. Leadership varies by the resources available to the BMT unit, but most effective is someone with skill in group dynamics as well as some fa-

miliarity with the issues of the BMT staff and patients.

Support groups should not be confused with psychotherapy groups, however, and leaders must be careful to maintain the focus on the patient's situation and the staff's reaction to that situation. Interstaff conflict may appropriately be addressed in a group format, but unit leaders should be cautious of attempts to scapegoat staff who are not present or the desire of staff to address employment concerns that should appropriately be handled by management. Identifying and maintaining a focus on psychosocial issues of particular patients will assist effective functioning of a staff support group.

Another key stress reduction strategy is adequate peer support. It is easy to become isolated caring for bone marrow transplant patients. This isolation is increased by the rigorous cleansing precautions required to enter these patients' rooms. It is not a simple procedure for a colleague to enter a laminar air flow room to join you to observe a concerning symptom or assist in problem solving. The high level of care needed by these patients often reduces the numbers of patients that any one nurse interacts with. This also promotes staff isolation, making it easy to lose objectivity. Because of this, it is even more important to promote peer support and collaboration. Since this is hampered by the isolation precautions required by BMT patients, staff must actively work on facilitating such interactions. Sharing doubts and indecisions as well as triumphs can decrease individual stress levels and promote the teamwork that is essential in providing BMT patients with the high level of care that their physical states require. However, staff must appreciate this as a benefit and therefore promote collaboration and sharing of ideas. This is not possible in a unit where competition is valued over collaboration. It is important for such staff to confront their own competitiveness and work towards collaboration through peer support. Staff can utilize their already developed patient support skills with each other to promote this cooperative care planning and care provision. The same interpersonal skills the oncology nurses are known for in assisting patients with their stresses can assist them to support each other.

Support from nursing management is essential for any staff support program to be effective. This support includes tangible items such as: equipment; time to plan, provide and evaluate patient care; time to attend educational programs; human resources as well as the intangible items such as supporting and promoting staff achievements; collaboration; peer review; and discussion of both patient and unit problems. Styles and values of unit leaders will obviously set the tone for the unit staff.

Peer support and support by management should not be confused with formal counseling or therapy, however. Staff who are having personal crises or problems with issues outside of work should be encouraged to seek counseling. Ideally, an employee assistance program (EAP) should exist for all staff. This would provide free or low-cost, confidential counseling services. Stresses outside of work obviously affect the individual staff as well as their co-workers. We should be as open about addressing our own problems as we encourage our patients to be. We should be a sign of strength for a staff member to seek counseling and not feel it is a sign of weakness or personal flaw. The presence of an affordable, accessible, and sanctioned counseling service can help staff and management separate work performance issues from personal problems. Issues related to work performance then can be appropriately addressed through peer review and support as well as through leadership supervision and evaluation.

There are a variety of resource people available to BMT staff to assist with care planning, interventions, and evaluation. Both oncology/hematology and psychiatric liaison clinical nurse specialists can be invaluable supports to BMT staff who are dealing with a frustrating patient situation or with their own emotional reactions to this difficult work. These specialists blend the specialty knowledge that the staff needs with a clear understanding and appreciation of the nursing framework upon which staff operate. Non-nurses can also help, specifically with the patient or with staff. These non-nurse resources include chaplains, social workers, psychologists, and psychiatrists (Patenaude and Rappeport 1985; Rappaport 1988). A survey of 52 bone marrow transplant units (Rappaport 1988) indicated that 37 (71%) had some psychosocial/psychiatric support services. Most of these services (78.4%) were provided by nonpsychiatrists, namely nurses, social workers, or psychologists. The large number of BMT units with such support services is proof of the recognition of the stresses inherent in such work.

Finally, BMT staff can receive support and benefit from participation in their professional or charitable organizations. Peer support and education are available in activities provided by the American Cancer Society, the American Nurses' Association, and most specifically, the Oncology Nurses' Society. These organizations provide opportunities for BMT nurses to join a network with other BMT nurses across the country and to benefit from their experiences and expertise. Objectivity and support thus can be obtained for stresses facing BMT patients as well as staff. Opportunities are available for participating in planning and implementing clinical as well as unit and hospital organizational changes that can ultimately modify and decrease the stress felt by BMT staff.

References

Artinian, B.M. 1983. Personal involvement with critically ill patients. *California Nurse 78* (7): 4–5.

Baggs, J.G., and Schmitt, M.H. 1988. Collaboration between nurses and physicians. *IMAGE 20* (3): 145–149.

Brack, G.; LaClave, L.; and Blix, S. 1988. The psychological aspects of bone marrow transplant: A staff's perspective. *Cancer Nursing 11* (4): 221–229.

Caplan, A. et al. 1983. Mrs. X and the bone marrow transplant. *Hastings Center Report 13* (3): 17–19.

Carney, B. 1987. Bone marrow transplantation: Nurses' and physicians' perceptions of informed consent. *Cancer Nursing 10* (5): 252–259.

Chapman, C.R., and Hill, H.F. 1989. Prolonged morphine self-administration and addiction liability: Evaluation of two theories in a bone marrow transplant unit. *Cancer 63*: 1636–1644.

Collins, C., Upright, C., and Aleksich, J. 1989. Reverse isolation: What patients perceive. *O.N.F. 16* (5): 675–679.

Durbin, M. 1988. Bone marrow transplantation: Economic, ethical, and social issues. *Pediatrics 82* (5): 774–783.

Fincannon, J. 1988. Meperidine addiction associated with amphoteracin treatment in leukemia: Case study and staff reaction. *Archives of Psychiatric Nursing 11* (5): 302–306.

Ford, R. 1983. Reducing nursing-staff stress through scheduling, orientation, and continuing education. *Nurs. Clin. North Am. 18* (3): 597–601.

Gordon, A.M. 1975. Psychological adaptation to isolator therapy in acute leukaemia. *Psychotherapy & Psychosomatics 26* (3): 132–139.

Graubert, D.M., and Edmonson, J.H. 1972. Psychologic adaptation of patients isolated in protected environments. *New York State Journal of Medicine 72* (1): 227–228.

Holland, J. et al. 1977. Psychological response of patients with acute leukemia to germ-free environments. *Cancer 40* (2): 871–879.

Knaus, W.A. 1986. An evaluation of outcome from intensive care in major medical centers. *Ann. Intern. Med. 104* (3): 410–418.

Lesko, L.M. et al. 1989. Patients', parents', and oncologists' perceptions of informed consent for bone marrow transplantation. *Medical and Pediatric Oncology 17*: 181–187.

Longhofer, J., and Floersch, J.E. 1980. Dying or living?: The double bind. *Culture, Medicine and Psychiatry 4* (2): 119–136.

Marks, E.M., and Sachar, E.J. 1973. Under treatment of medical inpatients with narcotic analgesics. *Ann. Intern. Med. 78* (2): 173–181.

Patenaude, A.F., and Rappeport, J.M. 1985. Collaboration between hematologists and mental health professionals on a bone marrow transplant team. *Journal of Psychosocial Oncology 2* (3/4): 81–92.

Porter, J., and Jick, H. 1980. Addiction rare in patients treated with narcotics. *N. Engl. J. Med. 302* (2): 123.

Pot-Mees, C. 1987. Beating the burn-out. *Nursing Times 83* (30): 33–35.

Rappaport, B.S. 1988. Evolution of consultation-liaison services in bone marrow transplantation. *General Hospital Psychiatry 10*: 346–351.

Robinson, D. 1989. Who should receive medical aid? *Parade Magazine* May 28, 1989: 4–5.

Sarantos, S. 1988. Innovations in psychosocial staff support: A model program for the marrow transplant nurse. *Seminars in Oncology Nursing 4* (1): 69–73.

Silberfeld, M. et al. 1988. Choosing a risky treatment. *The Psychiatric Journal of the University of Ottawa 13* (1): 9–11.

Slaby, A.E. 1988. Cancer's impact on caregivers. *Advances in Psychosomatic Medicine 18*: 135–153.

Wolcott, D.L. et al. 1986. Psychological adjustment of adult bone marrow transplant donors whose recipient survives. *Transplantation 41* (4): 484–488.

Chapter 17

Procedure Costs and Reimbursement Issues

Marilyn K. Bedell

In this chapter, financial considerations related to bone marrow transplantation will be addressed. Often many of the expenses associated with transplantation are not apparent to the nurse manager confronted with planning and implementing a bone marrow transplant program. A transplant program will require support from all levels of the organization. The program will have an impact on many departments and the people who work in those departments.

The patients served by this program will also feel a financial impact. In the past, health care providers believed that an unlimited amount of health care dollars was available. Third-party payors and the government asked only three questions: Is it safe?; Is it effective?; and Does it have wide acceptance in the medical community? Cost was not a consideration. As we entered the 1980s, health care costs escalated and accounted for 12% of the nation's Gross National Product (GNP). Budget cuts led to a scarce supply of health care

dollars. Due to this shortage of funding a new question is now asked by the government and third-party payors: Is the procedure cost-effective and is there a cost benefit to the patient? As health care providers we cannot assume that the cost of bone marrow transplantation will be covered for all eligible BMT candidates, even if the patient is insured. If the third-party payors will not pay, who will pay?

Nurses can no longer ignore the financial implications associated with providing health care. In order to provide high-quality care we must be aware of costs. The following financial topics will be covered to enable the nurse manager to be better prepared to participate in the development of a bone marrow transplant program:

- Program planning costs
- Nursing costs
- Costs of the procedure
- Costs to the patient
- Reimbursement issues

Program Planning Costs

As with all organ transplant programs there are many financial considerations that must be addressed.

A bone marrow transplant program cannot be developed in isolation. It is a program that will require high-technology resources and skilled labor. As stated in Chapter 18, developing a bone marrow transplant program will require decisions and actions that involve financial, legal, medical, and human resource considerations. Almost every department in a hospital will feel the impact of the program. Early in the design of a program a multidisciplinary team should be identified that will take responsibility for defining the scope of the program. Physicians, nurses, administrators, and representatives from ancillary departments that will be affected by the program should be included in the planning process. A financial liaison needs to be identified early to help identify costs to the institution. By encouraging the team to develop a systematic plan, the nurse manager can help assure that there is a forum to address all issues generated during program development (Mook 1987).

A program manager who will be responsible for managing and coordinating the overall activities of the program should be identified. The manager should be given authority to facilitate program planning, implementation, and evaluation. The program manager can help assure that information is presented in a way that allows management to assess the plan fairly, thoroughly, and in the context of the overall mission of the organization. It is important to demonstrate how the program furthers the organization's goals.

A business plan should be developed to clearly identify the financial risks to the institution. A detailed analysis of potential revenues and expenses should be completed. The projections made during the development stage then can be used as one means to evaluate the program. It is important to try and make patient volume projections as realistic as possible so a fair evaluation can be made.

Cross-organizational implications must be thoroughly explored. Information must be gathered and presented to allow the appropriate managers to make an informed decision about the potential impact of the program on their department. In order to do this analysis, it will be important for the team to define the scope of the program, which should include information on the patient population, types of transplants to be offered, the intensity of service that will be provided, and a prediction of the number of patients to be treated over the next three to five years.

As stated earlier most ancillary departments will be affected by the bone marrow transplant program. For example, the laboratory will most likely see an increase in specialized hematology procedures, cultures, and drug level monitoring. The blood bank will be requested to provide more specialized blood products such as irradiated blood products and HLA-matched platelets. The pharmacy may see an increase in the number and type of antibiotics used by patients who experience such a serious degree of immunosuppression. New drugs may need to be added to the formulary. A clinical pharmacist may be needed to support physicians in making pharmacokinetic decisions. Immunosuppressive medications, which are currently very expensive, will be required with allogeneic transplantation. The radiation therapy department may be requested to do total body irradiation, which may require the purchase of special equipment and generally requires extra staff. All managers need to define which resources will be required. They should consider demands on current available resources including personnel, capital and noncapital equipment, space requirements, and staff educational implications.

Nursing Costs

The nurse manager will be required to analyze the impact of the BMT program on the nursing unit. One of the first issues that needs to be addressed is the environment. Can patients undergoing transplantation be accommodated in the current nursing unit? Room design must be discussed with the bone marrow transplant physicians. It is also helpful to involve an infectious disease physician and the engineering department. The goal should be to make the environment clinically acceptable. The final decision may be limited by economic considerations.

Patients undergoing transplantation will require a private room with attached bathroom including shower. Besides standard furnishings and call-bell systems, it is important to decide if additional oxygen, air, suction, and electrical outlets will be required. Decisions should be made about the amount and type of monitoring equipment. If it is determined that the patients will receive an intensive care unit level of service on the bone marrow transplant unit, different equipment will be required to provide this level of care. Adequate lighting will be necessary to do physical assessments and procedures. Containers for biohazards should be provided.

There are many infection control issues to be addressed. What type of air handling system will be required? How often do air exchanges occur? Is this adequate? Is HEPA filtering or laminar air flow required? Will construction be required to create the appropriate environment? The bone marrow transplant team will need to make the decision about how protected an environment the patient will require. Environmental standards should be established with input from the housekeeping department to help minimize the infection risk to this severely immunocompromised group of patients.

Adequate storage space is required for frequently used supplies. It should be accessible to the nurse and easily cleaned. Again, is any construction required or does any equipment need to be purchased?

The transplant team will require meeting and charting space. Is the space conducive to promoting interdisciplinary communication? Space tends to be a major problem in many hospitals.

If space is inadequate it may hinder confidentiality of communications and thus the delivery of patient care.

It is important to consider other equipment needs such as intravenous pumps, patient scales, exercise cycles, pulse oximeters, automatic blood pressure monitors, cardiac chairs, and other specialized monitoring equipment. Many of these decisions will be based on the number of patients that are predicted to be treated over the next three to five years as well as the level of care that will be provided on the unit. All of the above issues have budget implications, and these anticipated costs need to be included in the program plan.

Once environmental issues have been identified, the nurse manager will need to decide if additional personnel will be required. The impact on the personnel budget will depend on the number of patients expected to undergo transplant and the level of care that will be provided on the unit. The team will need to determine if a patient will ever require a transfer to a critical care unit or if all levels of care will be provided on the bone marrow transplant unit. It is expensive to prepare an entire staff to manage patients requiring all levels of critical care, especially if the patients are few and far between. A decision will need to be made as to whether or not the number of expected critical care patient days will be large enough to keep all staff proficient in critical care skills. If it is decided that some patients may be transferred to a critical care unit, a plan will need to be developed with the nurse manager in that unit to assure that the staff in critical care is prepared to care for this group of severely immunocompromised patients. Once decisions are made about the patients' nursing care requirements, a staffing plan can be developed for the unit.

In order to develop a staffing plan, the nurse manager may want to consult with several other hospitals that are currently doing bone marrow transplantation to determine predicted patient care hours per bone marrow transplant patient day. A review of the proposed bone marrow transplant protocol(s) will also help determine potential nursing care requirements. Predictions regarding **length of stay** (L.O.S.) also need to be made. Once this data is gathered, a **predictive staffing methodology** can be used to estimate the number of staff needed to care for this population of patients. This methodology is a set of mathematical equations for predicting the **variable staffing requirements** for a 12-month period, based on variables of predicted **patient days** (Pt. Day), average **patient care hours** (P.C.H.), a factor for sick vacation and holiday time (S.V.H.), and expected productivity level (Button and Bedell 1988) (Table 17.1). Once the variable staffing requirement number is determined, fixed nursing functions (management staff, secretarial support, and other staff needed to assist nursing roles) should be determined. It is also wise to determine a factor for staff nurse fixed functions, such as time for staff education, orientation, committee time, evaluations, and counselling. The variable staffing requirements plus the **fixed staffing** requirements will provide the nurse manager with an estimate of the **full-time equivalents** (F.T.E.) required to deliver patient care. This methodology is only one consideration in making decisions about staffing levels. Skill level of the nurses also must be considered. The unit design may affect productivity and thus require different staffing levels. It is often helpful to do a mock schedule to verify the predictive methodology and to determine if the staffing level predicted will provide adequate coverage. The nurse manager must also use professional judgement in making a final decision about staffing levels. There may be other variables that only the nurse manager can know. No mathematical model can provide this degree of insight.

Although personnel and environmental issues often become the focal point in bone marrow transplant program planning, there are other costs that should not be overlooked. Often these costs will be ongoing and should be taken into account during the planning stage. For example, the nurse manager should plan on educational expenses to prepare staff to care for this group of patients. Will all staff require a special orientation class on the care of bone marrow transplant patients? Will there be a need to educate non-nursing personnel (interns, residents, housekeepers, pharmacists, social service workers, laboratory personnel, dietary, volunteers and administrators)? This will not be a one time expense, as ongoing orientation will need to be provided for all new personnel.

There can be costs related to equipment and plant maintenance. The nurse manager should review all equipment and determine what periodic service will be required. A capital replacement program should be determined.

Another area of additional expense can be disposable supplies. The disposable supply needs of these patients tend to be higher than the disposable supply needs of general oncology patients. For example, in one setting an autologous bone marrow transplant patient required approximately $35.00 of disposable equipment per day compared to $4.25 for a general oncology patient. Again the financial liaison can help determine variations in supply usage.

Finally, even though the nurse manager will not have to budget for other departments, he/she may be in the best position to help other departments identify other potential expenses associated with bone marrow transplantation. As the nurse manager assesses the environment, he/she should remember to include other managers in the planning process. Concerns and ideas should be shared freely with all team members.

In summary, by doing a thorough assessment of costs, the nurse manager can be assured that appropriate information will be included in the program plan. This information can then be used to help determine whether the bone marrow transplant program should be implemented.

Costs of the Procedure

Another important part of program planning and ongoing monitoring is to estimate the potential revenues and expenses associated with bone mar-

Table 17.1. Predictive Staffing Methodology

Steps		Example	
Step 1:			
Number of transplant patients predicted per year		40	patients
Multiplied by (×) the predicted length of stay (L.O.S.)	×	40	day L.O.S.
Equals (=) the transplant patient days per year	=	1600	patient days per year
Step 2:			
Transplant patient days per year		1600	patient days per year
Multiplied by (×) the average patient care hours (P.C.H.) per patient	×	10	P.C.H. per patient
Equals (=) the P.C.H. for all transplant patients	=	16000	P.C.H. for all transplant patients
Step 3:			
Hours a full-time equivalent (F.T.E.) works annually		40	hrs/week for 1.0 F.T.E.
Multiplied by (×) 52 weeks per year	×	52	weeks per year
Equals (=) hours per F.T.E. per year	=	2080	hours per year
Minus (−) a factor for sick, vacation, and holiday time (nonproductive time)	−	248	hours
Equals the average productive hours per F.T.E.	=	1832	productive hours per F.T.E.
Step 4:			
P.C.H. for all transplant patients		16000	P.C.H. for all transplant patients
Divided by (÷) the average productive hours per F.T.E.	÷	1832	productive hours per F.T.E.
Equals (=) the F.T.E.'s required to meet the workload	=	8.7	F.T.E.'s to meet workload
Step 5:			
F.T.E.'s required to meet workload		8.7	F.T.E.'s
Divided by (÷) an expected productivity level (usually set between 90% and 110%)	÷	98%	(.98)
Equals (=) the F.T.E.'s required to meet the workload at an expected productivity	=	8.9	F.T.E.'s to meet the workload at an expected productivity
Step 6:			
F.T.E.'s required to meet the workload at an expected productivity		8.9	F.T.E.'s to meet the workload at an expected productivity
Plus (+) fixed nursing positions (management staff, secretarial support, and other assistant to nursing roles)	+	3.0	fixed F.T.E. positions
Equals (=) the total number of nursing staff required	=	11.9	F.T.E.'s

row transplantation. The financial liaison will be needed to help predict income and expenses. This person will be able to use their cost-accounting skills to determine direct and indirect costs (see Table 17.2). The financial liaison can also help determine costs by procedure and provide a profile of ancillary and routine services that will be used by patients. He/she can also provide information on payor mix (**third-party payor** utilized by patient). Most hospitals have three or more types of payment systems, such as diagnostic-related groups, negotiated bids, and specific service charges by procedure. Each system can have an impact on the hospital's revenue flow.

Table 17.2. Direct and Indirect Costs

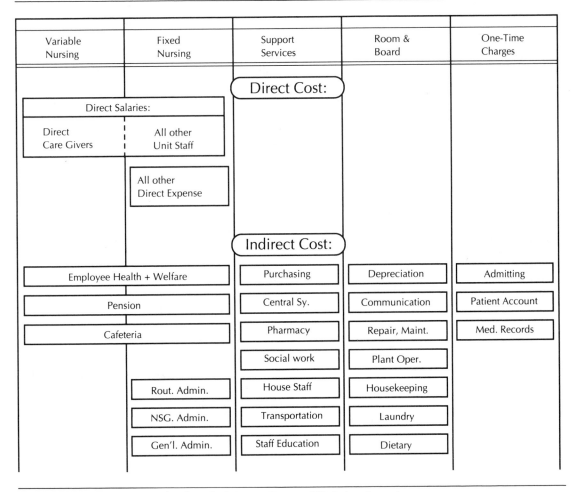

Variable Nursing	Fixed Nursing	Support Services	Room & Board	One-Time Charges

Direct Cost:

Direct Salaries:

| Direct Care Givers | All other Unit Staff |

| All other Direct Expense |

Indirect Cost:

Employee Health + Welfare		Purchasing	Depreciation	Admitting
Pension		Central Sy.	Communication	Patient Account
Cafeteria		Pharmacy	Repair, Maint.	Med. Records
		Social work	Plant Oper.	
	Rout. Admin.	House Staff	Housekeeping	
	NSG. Admin.	Transportation	Laundry	
	Gen'l. Admin.	Staff Education	Dietary	

Source: Henry, S. Dartmouth-Hitchcock Medical Center, Hanover, NH. Patient Acounting.

Thus, it is important to have an understanding of what the hospital can expect from each payor (Cleverley 1986).

Most hospitals also predict that a certain amount of care will be considered free-care and that they will incur a certain amount of bad debt. Again the financial liaison can make predictions about the amount of bad debt and free-care that will result from the bone marrow transplant program. This information will be crucial to predicting revenue flow.

Costs to the Patient

The literature evaluating the cost of bone marrow transplantation (Welch and Larson 1989; Vaughan et al. 1986; Kay et al. 1980) shows that costs range from $75,000 to $200,000 per transplant. Table 17.3 gives a cost estimate for an autologous bone marrow transplant, an expensive procedure that requires a prolonged hospitalization and a continued need for intensive outpatient services. Table 17.4 shows a breakout of costs for

Table 17.3. Summary of Autologous Bone Marrow Transplant Charges Expected for Transplantation Admission (Expected Length of Stay = 40 Days)

Medications	$50,914
Transfusion/Blood products	$30,598
Routine days	$18,792
Laboratory	$18,390
Med. surg. supplies	$6,466
Intensive care	$5,343
Radiology	$2,309
Intravenous therapy	$2,360
Respiratory therapy	$886
Operating room	$857
Radiation therapy	$720
Anesthesia	$208
Recovery room	$205
Physical therapy	$196
Nuclear medicine	$141
Ultrasound	$101
ECG/Stress/Holter	$78
Echocardiography	$71
Cardiopulmonary	$46
Same day services	$17
Total:	$138,698

laboratory tests, medications, and transfusions. Many cost ranges will be similar for allogeneic transplant patients. Recipients of unrelated donor transplants can also expect to pay all of the costs associated with locating a donor as well as marrow acquisition costs from the volunteer donor. The latter charge may be around $10,000.

Besides the hospitalization and professional physician fees for the bone marrow transplant procedure, there are costs associated with pre-transplant evaluation and post-transplant follow-up. For example, bone marrow will need to be harvested from the patient or donor. The cost of bone marrow harvesting varies, based on whether the bone marrow is treated or purged as in a T cell-depleted or autologous transplant (see Table 17.5). Allogeneic bone marrow transplantation requires intensive laboratory tests to determine histocompatibility of potential donors. The cost of these tests are assumed by the patient, and are considerable. The patient will also require an extensive prehospitalization evaluation. Multiple tests may be required to determine whether the patient is eligible for transplantation. The following is a list of possible procedures: baseline complete blood count, renal and liver functions, pulmonary function studies, gated blood pool scan, bone marrow aspirate and biopsy, viral screening, chest x-ray, electrocardiogram, panorex film of the teeth, and a lumbar puncture. A multiple lumen right atrial catheter will need to be placed if the patient does not already have one. After discharge, the patient will require frequent follow-up visits until they are no longer immunocompromised and transfusion dependent. At a minimum, patients will require weekly follow-up visits for the first month, with weekly complete blood counts, electrolyte screening, and renal and liver functions. Most patients will also require periodic blood transfusions.

In addition to the expenses associated with pre- and post-transplant testing and evaluation, there can be other hidden costs. Since most bone marrow transplant procedures are only offered in tertiary referral centers, many patients may have travel expenses (mileage, airfare, lodging). If the patient does not have sick time accrued or disability insurance, income may not be available to help support the family's living expenses.

Family members will have to make decisions concerning whether they can stay with the patient or need to return home. If they stay, they may lose time from work and their salary. Issues such as child care and home maintenance needs may add to expenses. If they return home, phone bills may be significant.

After the transplant, there will be medication bills, right atrial catheter supplies, more time lost from work and more travel expenses. Costs add up quickly.

Bone marrow transplantation will require the patient to make a major investment of money. Patients eligible for bone marrow transplantation

Table 17.4. Average Laboratory Utilization and Patient Charges for Autologous Bone Marrow Transplant Patient

Laboratory Section	Test Description	Average Count	Average Pt. Charges
Microbiology	Fungus blood culture	58	$1,757
Microbiology	Blood culture	62	$1,748
Blood Bank	Compatability test, first unit	12	$1,414
Chemistry	Magnesium, serum	48	$778
Hematology	Blood count complete (no diffs.)	51	$724
Hematology	Differential smearscan, blood	51	$715
Blood Bank	Compatability test, additional UNI	13	$618
Microbiology	Urine culture complete	29	$584
General	Venipuncture	95	$575
Chemistry	Creatinine, serum	52	$570
Chemistry	Blood gases, complete, arterial	18	$481
Chemistry	Urea nitrogen, serum	52	$466
Chemistry	Glucose, random plasma	51	$461
Other Lab	HLA antibodies	6	$443
Microbiology	Fungus culture	14	$387
Hematology	Urinalysis routine	23	$347
Chemistry	Vancomycin	14	$345
Flow cytometry	Reticulocyte count, blood	18	$332
Chemistry	Potassium, serum	51	$305
Chemistry	Sodium, serum	49	$296
Microbiology	*Candida* antigen test	7	$272
Chemistry	Tobramycin level, serum	11	$270
Bone Marrow Processing	Bone marrow transplant	1	$266
Bone Marrow Processing	Marrow processing	0	$262
Chemistry	Chloride, serum	49	$248
Chemistry	Bicarbonate CO_2, content	49	$248
Chemistry	Phosphorus, serum	18	$240
Blood Bank	Autologous bone marrow processing	0	$211
Hematology	Platelet count	21	$171
Laboratory	All other tests	241	$2,869
Total		1,167	$18,390

Medications: Average Utilization of Medications for Autologous Bone Marrow Transplant Patient

Medication	Average Count	Average Pt. Charges
Acyclovir 500mg vial	130	$15,857
Miconazole inj 10mg/ml 200mg/20ml	58	$5,868
TPN solution, adult	30	$3,884
Etoposide 100mg vial	8	$2,255
Mezlocillin 4gm adv vial	59	$2,006
Thio-tepa 15mg vial	17	$1,980
Vancomycin 1gm adv vial	45	$1,809
Lorazepam 2mg/ml 1ml syringe	52	$1,464

(continued)

Table 17.4. *Continued*

Medication	Average Count	Average Pt. Charges
Ceftazidime 1gm adv vial	28	$1,199
Aztreonam inj 1gm vial	25	$880
Cyclophosphamide 2gm vial	6	$805
Carmustine 100mg (BCNU) vial	3	$555
Vancomycin 750mg minibag	9	$519
Vancomycin inj vial 500mg	23	$448
Tobramycin 200mg minibag	8	$424
Tobramycin 160mg minibag	11	$422
Amphotericin 50mg syringe	6	$415
Other drugs	1,183	$10,123
Total	1,302	$50,914

Average Utilization of Blood Products for Autologous Bone Marrow Transplant Patient

Blood Product Type	Average Count	Average Pt. Charges
Platelet pack apheresis, PL100	18	$15,223
Platelet pack apheresis, HLA PL10	10	$9,473
Leukpoor red blood cell, RC100	23	$5,278
Plasma	2	$205
5% albumin, 250ml	2	$88
Cryoprecipitate	2	$68
Platelet pack, apheresis	1	$66
Packed red blood cells	1	$66
Packed red blood cells, PEDI	1	$35
25% albumin, 50ml	1	$32
RH immune globulin, standard dose	1	$24
Platelet concentrate	1	$23
Hespan	1	$17
Total		$30,598

often are not aware of the costs associated with the procedure and are even less prepared for the pre- and post-hospitalization expenses. As much as 30% to 40% of a family's income may be allocated for nonreimbursible expenses (Durbin 1988). Thus, developing a plan to prepare patients and their families for the economic impact of bone marrow transplantation is an important part of any program. Costs can be significant and may require the family to make major changes in life-style.

Initial discussions about bone marrow transplantation should include information about potential financial risks. No testing or other preparations for transplant should be made until the patient has a clear understanding of their financial obligations. If a patient does not have insurance or has limited coverage they may be asked to make

Table 17.5. Cost of Autologous Bone Marrow Harvest

Treated Bone Marrow		Untreated Bone Marrow
$ 9,000	Laboratory	$4,000
2,000	Operating room	1,000
400	Anesthesia	400
550	Routine	1,200
500+/−	Other	1,000+/−
$12,450+/−	Total cost	$7,600+/−

an advanced payment to cover the expense of transplant. Lind (1984) states that information about the financial risks and financial obligations should be included in the informed consent. It can be devastating for a patient to undergo a thorough workup for bone marrow transplantation and then discover they cannot proceed due to lack of funds.

Reimbursement Issues

Insurance Coverage

It can no longer be assumed that procedures such as bone marrow transplantation will be paid for by insurers. Until recently, insurance providers had given implicit support to cover charges. However, skyrocketing health care costs have made third-party payors more reluctant to cover costs of new therapies. Experts say that insurance coverage for transplants can vary from no coverage to full payment (Stiller 1989; Yasko 1988; Fackelmann 1985; Kahn 1984; Evans 1983). Despite the explosion in biotechnology there has been a gradual decline in the funding of biomedical research. In 1970, 3.9% of all health care dollars where devoted to research and development, but by 1982 this number had declined to 2.9% (Boykin 1983). Most insurance contracts exclude investigational treatments from reimbursement. Until recently, exclusion of investigational therapy

had not been rigorously enforced, probably because it is often difficult to determine if a treatment is investigational or not, based on the information provided on the claim form at discharge. Now many insurers are requiring preadmission approval for certain kinds of hospitalization. Requests that include costly interventions such as high-dose chemotherapy with bone marrow transplant are often denied (Wittes 1987). This denial may prevent many patients from participating in bone marrow transplant programs.

There are also many bone marrow transplant candidates who have already incurred significant expenses during the initial treatment of their disease. The adequacy of insurance coverage can be a major problem for many cancer patients. A typical lifetime hospitalization benefit for most comprehensive insurance is $500,000 (Scown 1989). The patient may have already used a significant portion of this benefit.

Why are third-party payors reluctant to pay for bone marrow transplantation? According to Evans (1986), one reason is that there are greater health care priorities that must be met. The goal of health care should be prevention. Critics believe that bone marrow transplantation does not represent a cost-effective use of limited health care dollars. There is increasing pressure to show that all organ transplant procedures are cost-effective and that there is a reasonable cost-benefit ratio (Knox 1980; Evans 1986; Friedlander and Tatterstall 1982; Hicks 1985; Finkler 1982). Cost-benefit analysis provides systematic information about the consequences, both positive and negative, of allocating resources to perform a specific therapy. An attempt is made to assign a monetary value to an outcome. Cost-effectiveness, on the other hand, requires that the outcome be expressed in commensurate units (for example, quality adjusted life years, days of work lost, life span extended) (Hicks 1985). Research to evaluate cost-effectiveness and the cost-benefit ratio has been attempted (Welch and Larson 1989; Kay et al. 1980). Both investigators analyzed costs of treating nonlymphocytic leukemia with and without bone marrow transplantation. Both studies demonstrated that transplantation compared favorably to conventional therapy in terms of cost-benefit but this could not be generalized to all other types of bone marrow transplantation. More research will need to be done to demonstrate that bone marrow transplantation is a reasonable alternative to conventional therapy.

Method of Payment

Health insurance often is not well understood by patients and their care providers. A basic understanding of the types of health insurance (see Table 17.6) and insurance terminology (see Table 17.7) will help nurses care for patients in a more responsible and holistic manner (Brucker and MacMullen 1984).

Historically, third-party payors paid hospitals retrospectively for services provided. A charging structure was set by the hospital. These charges were often reviewed by a regulatory commission for appropriateness. No preauthorization was required prior to admission. A bill for services was only submitted to the insurer after the hospitalization. As long as the bill agreed with the pre-approved charging structure a payment was made. **Retrospective cost reimbursement** systems still exist, but many third party payors are moving to prospective charging systems such as diagnostic-related groups (DRG) and **negotiated bids. Prospective reimbursement systems** establish the rate to be paid prior to the delivery of the service. Even if it costs the provider more money to provide the service, they will only receive a fixed rate (Hoffman 1984).

Medicare began to make payments by DRG in 1983. In the Medicare DRG payment system, diagnostic categories are defined and specific prices are established for each category. Prices by categories are fixed and cannot be negotiated (Cleverley 1986). A new DRG, number 481, has been established for bone marrow transplanta-

tion. Its relative weight is high, and sets an average L.O.S. of 36.6 days.

A new type of prospective payment system is a negotiated bid. A specific contractual agreement is made between the hospital and the third-party payor for services provided. This payment system is frequently used by health maintenance organizations and preferred provider organizations (Cleverley 1986). Health care organizations are asked to submit bids for services and usually the lowest bid receives the contract. State Medicaid programs have also begun to negotiate prices for their patients. For example, the state of Arizona Health Care Cost Containment System Administration has issued a Request for Proposal (RFP) for autologous bone marrow transplantation. Information was sent to hospitals requesting them to bid to provide autologous bone marrow transplantation on both children and adults in a Medicare certified hospital equipped with appropriate professional and environmental support (Veit 1989). Bids are evaluated based on technical aspects, qualifications of the personnel, and the cost. If the technical merits and personnel are evaluated to be equal, the low bidder will get the contract.

Even if the type of insurance and the payment system used by the third-party payor is known, payment for bone marrow transplant cannot be guaranteed. Certain bone marrow transplants are likely to be covered more often than others. Some bone marrow transplants are considered standard therapy, some state-of-the-art, and others investigational. A bone marrow transplant that is seen as a conventional therapy is more likely to be covered than that seen as investigational (see Table 17.8).

Insurance coverage varies from state to state, procedure to procedure, case to case. To ensure that every possible strategy has been explored, it is important to develop a systematic plan and a team approach to help assure that funding will be available. For example, assuring that prior approval is obtained from the third-party payor in writing, and not accepting an immediate "no"

Table 17.6. Types of General Health Insurance Plans

Insurance Type	Advantages	Disadvantages	Comments
Health maintenance organization (HMO)	No out-of-pocket expenses for services covered by HMO providers Ambulatory care is covered Emphasis is on preventive care	Limited number of providers No coverage for outside providers except through referral Expectations may include short in-hospital stay for a procedure (compared with other types of insurance)	Premiums depend on overall health of subscribers. Thus, they may rise if a small HMO has several expensive, catastrophic illnesses in a short period Emphasis on health is attractive to employers In order to meet a wide variety of needs, HMOs tend to be multidisciplinary, multispecialized, and often include nurse-practitioners and midwives
Individual practice association (IPA)	No out-of-pocket expenses for services covered by IPA providers Ambulatory care may be covered Larger number of providers than with HMO because the providers are not exclusive to IPA	No coverage for non-IPA providers except through referral Providers may have limited office hours for IPA clients	System is similar
Preferred provider organization (PPO)	No out-of-pocket expenses for services covered by PPO providers Ambulatory care may be covered Larger number of providers than with HMO because providers are not exclusive to PPO Expenses are limited to cost difference, deductible, or co-payment for care by non-PPO provider	Providers may have limited office hours for PPO clients Limited number of "preferred" providers	System is similar to IPA Since care may be given by a non-PPO provider, the number of "preferred" providers may not be widely multidisciplinary or multispecialized

(continued)

Table 17.6.   *Continued*

Insurance Type	Advantages	Disadvantages	Comments
Medicare	Expenses are limited to co-payment and/or deductible for care by Medicare-approved providers Preventive care is not emphasized Large number of approved providers	Eligibility requirements generally depend upon age Procedure costs are often disputed or subject to usual and customary standards	Funded by public money May be coordinated with Medicaid, thus eliminating the out-of-pocket expense of co-payment or deductible for medically indigent clients
Medicaid	No out-of-pocket costs to medically indigent clients	Some patients are assessed as deductible or "spend-down" amount before they are eligible for program Some providers and institutions refuse to participate because of their low level of reimbursement from program	State and federal funding: eligibility and reimbursement vary from state to state
Civilian health and medical program of the uniformed services (CHAMPUS)	No out-of-pocket costs to subscribers	Eligibility restrictions: in areas of military institutions patients may be limited to those institutions for care	
Unions and commercial insurance (e.g., Blue Cross, John Hancock)	No limitation of providers Preventive care is usually not emphasized Ambulatory care is rarely covered	Out-of-pocket expenses depend upon policy's designation of coverage and deductible	Wide variation among policies even within the same insurance company

Source: Brucker, M.C. and MacMullen, N.J. Health insurance: A summary of basic types. *Home Healthcare Nurse* 4: 8–10, 1984, reprinted by permission of Appleton & Lange, Inc.

answer (denying payment) are but a few good strategies to ensure payment (see Table 17.9). Also other strategies like enlisting the help of the billing office, hospital-based utilization review staff, and the physician to assure that appropriate information has been shared with the third-party payor can do much to ensure the likelihood of payment. It may be helpful to identify a specific person, a case facilitator, to handle the insurance verification process. This person will be able to develop expertise in helping patients move through the financial screening process. This person can participate in a network with other transplant centers to develop strategies to facilitate the verification process. They can assure that verifications are received in writing and can clarify what will and will not be covered. In some cases, if reimbursement is denied, it may be appropriate to seek legal counsel to help with the approval process.

Developing a system to deal with reimbursement issues may be a key factor in determining

Table 17.7. Common Insurance Terms

Fee for service
A method of payment in which a charge is imposed for each service provided.

Usual and customary
A phrase designating the reasonableness of service charges. If the provider's fees do not exceed his usual fees, or fees for similar services in the same geographical area, they will be paid by the insurance company.

Coordination of benefits
If an individual has more than one insurance policy, the companies arrange a payment that does not exceed 100% coverage.

Deductible
Amount to be paid by the subscriber. Once paid, additional costs are covered by the insurance company. Deductibles often need to be paid on a regular (usually annual) basis.

Limitations
Conditions under which the insurance company will not reimburse for services. These conditions frequently include preexisting diseases and fees that exceed usual and customary charges.

Preexisting diseases
Conditions that have been diagnosed and/or treated before the individual obtained the current insurance policy (for example, pregnancy).

Assignment of benefits
The subscriber's designation that the insurance payment may be made directly to someone else, usually the health care provider.

Out-of-pocket expenses
Health care costs that are assumed directly by the subscriber (or patient) and are not reimbursed by the insurance company.

Disease-specific policy
Insurance that is limited to a stated condition (for example, cancer-specific insurance).

Catastrophic illness
A long-term condition requiring costly hospitalization and care.

Basic versus major coverage
A situation in which the basic insurance costs are covered under a specific insurance policy, with usual and customary restraints. After the deductible limitations have been met, additional costs may be paid by a one-time pool of money (deemed major coverage) to decrease out-of-pocket expenses.

Source: Brucker, M.C. and MacMullen, N.J. Health Insurance: A summary of basic types. *Home Healthcare Nurse* 4: 8–10, 1984, reprinted by permission of Appleton & Lange, Inc.

whether the bone marrow transplantation program will be successful. Patients cannot be expected to handle reimbursement issues independently. They will need the help of an organized health care team.

Reimbursement Policy

Health care providers need to become more active in developing long-range strategies to assure reimbursement. Mortenson (1989) states that one of

the most difficult aspects of the reimbursement problem is to figure out who needs to be convinced that something needs to change. Policy makers at the local, state, and national level must be involved in discussions about reimbursement for bone marrow transplantation.

Yasko (1988) has proposed a framework for educating and influencing reimbursement policy makers. She encourages the use of a team approach that includes physicians, nurses, administrators, and pharmacists, who become reim-

Table 17.8. Perspective on Payment for Bone Marrow Transplantation

Examples	Treatment Rating	Payment Potential
Matched sibling donor allogeneic AML childhood	Conventional or standard	Very likely
Unrelated matched	State of the art	Partial
Autologous solid tumor	Investigational	Less likely

bursement experts. The team should also include informed patients and families. Cancer-related professional organizations, cancer research cooperative groups, and appropriate pharmaceutical companies can also be important allies. Yasko (1988) stresses the need to become informed about the success rates of different methods of obtaining reimbursement.

Mobilization of public support is vital. A strategy should be developed to inform and educate the public. Members of the team should look for opportunities to lecture in various public forums, write articles for the lay press, and provide programs that educate the public about the value of new treatment modalities such as bone marrow transplantation. It is important to be clear on how and why you want the public to communicate with policy makers. Keep issues as simple as possible, and put the request in writing. These meas-

Table 17.9. Reimbursement Rules

Call for prior approval
Get names, dates, documentation
Don't accept an immediate "No"
Enlist billing office support
Involve and educate the team
Consider legal counsel

ures will help assure that the policy makers are hearing the message you want them to hear.

Another way to influence policy makers is to work to control costs in your program. Try to keep costs to a minimum. Because the hospital bill for these patients is large ($75,000 to $200,000), they will be audited and scrutinized by the third-party payor. Everyone on the transplant team must be committed to controlling the utilization of resources. Complete and accurate documentation of services provided will help in this process. Economic quality assessments and indications of improvement activities should be evident. This will help demonstrate that there is a commitment to control program costs.

Conclusion

As was stated in the preface, transplant technology is changing daily. The nurse manager will have the challenge of responding to these changes and will be expected to provide leadership in evaluating the financial impact to both the health care organization and the patient. It is hoped that the information in this chapter will guide the nurse manager through the maze of cost and reimbursement issues.

References

Boykin, W.L. (ed.). 1983. NIH Data Book. Washington, DC: Publication #83-1261.

Brucker, M.C., and MacMullen, N.J. 1984. Health insurance: A summary of basic types. *Home Healthcare Nurse 4* (6): 8–10.

Button, P., and Bedell, M.K. 1988. Implementation through staffing practice. In *Proceedings of the Eighth Annual GRASP Conference*. Long Beach, CA: FCG, Inc.

Cleverley, W.O. 1986. *Essentials of Health Care Finance*. Rockville, MD: Aspen Publishers, Inc.

Durbin, M. 1988. Bone marrow transplantation: Economic, ethical and social issues. *Pediatrics 82* (5): 774–783.

Evans, R.W. 1983. Health care technology and the inevitability of resource allocation. *JAMA 249* (15): 2047–2053.

Evans, R.W. 1986. Cost-effectiveness analysis of transplantation. *Surg. Clin. North Am. 66* (3): 603–616.

Fackelmann, K.A. 1985. Organ transplants raise concerns about reimbursement, competition and charges. *Modern Health Care 15* (19): 66–70.

Finkler, S.A. 1982. The distinction between costs and charges. *Ann. Intern. Med. 96* (1): 102–109.

Friedlander, M.L., and Tatterstall, H.N. 1982. Counting the costs of cancer therapy. *J. Clin. Oncology 18* (12): 1237–1241.

Hicks, L.L. 1985. Using benefit-cost and cost-effectiveness analysis in health care resource allocation. *Nursing Economics 3* (2): 78–84.

Hoffman, F.M. 1984. Financial management for nurse managers. Norwalk, CT: Appleton-Century-Crofts.

Kahn, C.R. 1984. A proposed new role for the insurance industry in biomedical research funding. *N. Engl. J. Med. 310* (4): 257–258.

Kay, H.E. et al. 1980. Cost of bone marrow transplants in acute myeloid leukemia. *Lancet 1* (1): 1067–1069.

Knox, R.A. 1980. Heart transplants: to pay or not to pay. *Science 209* (1): 570–573.

Lind, S.E. 1984. Can patients be asked to pay for experimental treatment? *Clinical Research 32* (4): 393–398.

Mook, K. 1987. *Project Life Cycle User Manual*, Unpublished manuscript. Hanover, NH: Management Services, Dartmouth Hitchcock Medical Center.

Mortenson, L.E. 1989. The cancer care reimbursement crisis: Rallying public support. *Oncology Issues 4* (3): 8–10, 15.

Scown, S. 1989. Health insurance and the cancer patient. In J. O'Donnell (ed.). *Oncology for the House Officer.* Baltimore, MD: Williams and Wilkins in press.

Stiller, C.R. 1989. High-tech medicine and the control of health care costs. *Can. Med. Assoc. J. 140* (8): 905–908.

Vaughan, W.P. et al. 1986. Ethical and financial issues in autologous transplantation: A symposium sponsored by the University of Nebraska Medical Center. *Ann. Intern. Med. 105:* 134–135.

Veit, M. 1989. *Notice of Request for Proposal: Autologous Bone Marrow Transplantation #YHO-0009.* Phoenix, AZ: Health Care Cost Containment System.

Welch, H.G., and Larson, E.B. 1989. Cost-effectiveness of bone marrow transplantation in acute nonlymphoctic leukemia. *N. Engl. J. Med. 321* (12): 807–812.

Wittes, R.E. 1987. Paying for patient care in treatment research—Who is responsible? *Cancer Treatment Reports, 71* (2): 107–113.

Yasko, J.M. 1988. Biological response modifiers treatment reimbursement: Present status and future strategies. *O.N.F.* (suppl.) *15* (6): 28–34.

Chapter 18

Developing a Bone Marrow Transplant Program: Planning, Environmental, and Personnel Challenges

Joleen Kelleher

Within the last two decades, bone marrow transplantation (BMT) has successfully expanded the treatment options for both hematologic and malignant diseases. This has created both turbulence and opportunity within hospital organizations considering the expansion of services to include a BMT specialty. As indicated in previous chapters, this specialty can achieve positive patient outcomes and also be financially viable. The treatment however, is lengthy and complex, requiring continuous intensive planning and formidable utilization of the organization's environmental and personnel resources. Organizing a BMT program along traditional hospital departmental and functional lines can often handicap the organization's ability to deliver the appropriate services in relation to the complicated demands. It is the goal of this chapter to provide direction for those individuals who will be developing new BMT programs or modifying existing ones. Table 18.1 out-

Table 18.1. Successful BMT Program Development

- Identify multidisciplinary planning team
- Complete strategic planning process
- Design patient care environment
- Mobilize interdisciplinary resources
- Designate specific unit management

lines the components of successful program development.

Strategic Planning

BMT treatment is usually initiated as a result of an oncologist who wishes to fulfill a therapeutic need in the institution that he/she serves. However, the task of management, in collaboration with medicine, is to make sure of the institution's capacity for survival as well as its capacity to avail

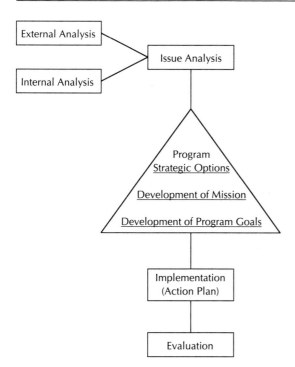

Figure 18.1. Elements of Strategic Planning Process

Table 18.2. Planning Team Composition

BMT medical director
Medical hematology/oncology physician
   representative
Hospital administrator/financial liaison
Nurse manager (inpatient and ambulatory care)
Facility planner
Engineer
Infection control specialist
Laboratory services representative
Pharmacy representative
Blood bank supervisor
Social work representative
Dietary representative
Housekeeping representative
Ad hoc members (optional–as appropriate):
   Staff nurse
   Representatives from various labs/rehab.
      services
   Former BMT patient
   Hospital board member

itself of this new opportunity. Long before a BMT program can be undertaken, certain fundamental factors must be explored. The planning strategies cannot just start with what happened yesterday and project that into the future. Not only success, but survival itself mandates that an organization adopt the view that by careful strategic planning, advantage can be taken of the opportunity presented by the advancement in BMT (Hardy and Lummers 1986).

Strategic planning (see Figure 18.1) requires considerable management skill, both in the planning and implementation of the approved course of action. It almost invariably conserves both time and money (Rowland and Rowland 1985). The competence of the planning team will determine the quality and suitability of the final BMT program design more than any other single factor. The team should be multidisciplinary (see Table 18.2) to assure appropriate resource allocation and utilization, and to eliminate the common interdepartmental power struggles that occur when only one or two people attempt to plan a program with interrelated services. The team may want to include, when appropriate, a patient who has undergone a successful transplant. There is an increasing trend towards more knowledgeable health care consumers who demand greater participation in their own care (Carpman et al. 1986), and this level of input will only enhance the quality of services to be provided.

External Analysis

The full range of external forces that may affect the transplant program need to be identified (see Table 18.3). This tracing of the external environment sets the territorial boundaries for the program. Presently, in the United States, there are well over 150 BMT programs ranging from a two-bed program to a sixty-bed program (BMT SIG 1990). This fact alone should not deter an organization from examining the possibility of de-

Table 18.3. Key Elements of External Analysis

- Demographic forecast
  population characteristics
  area of services
- Consumer demand/preference
- Assessment of competitive programs
  strengths, weaknesses, future plans
  potential for mutual areas of sharing
- BMT program trends (regional, national)
  current research results
  technology changes
- Regulatory environment mapping
  impact of laws/regulations
  insurance trends
- Labor market

veloping their own program, as it may be found that community need and financial feasibility are there. Without this assessment, the team could develop unrealistic planning goals.

Internal Analysis

As painful as it may seem, an internal assessment can develop a balanced framework of the organization's limitations, strengths, and opportunities (see Table 18.4). When evaluating institutional data, it is important to have the perspective of a comparative external benchmark. It is extremely helpful during this phase to visit stable, existing programs in like institutions, as well as

Table 18.4. Elements of Internal Analysis

- Utilization of hospital services
- Diagnosis treated
- Admitting patterns
- Physician characteristics
- Financial performance
- Facility inventory
  technology resources
- Organizational assessment
  evaluate structure
  assess how well structure works
- Present research trends

programs that are newly formed. The BMT Special Interest Group (SIG) of the Oncology Nursing Society (ONS) has compiled a BMT Nursing Resource Directory, which includes information on each BMT program: number of BMT beds, location of BTMU within hospital, type of BMT, nursing research, type of patient education, and isolation practices (BMT SIG 1990). Phoning colleagues across the country in like institutions, and arranging site visits can aid in the critique of one's own institution. Trends and patterns should be examined at this point, without worrying about the financial impact (Rowland and Rowland 1985).

Program Strategy Options

From the external and internal examination should come the identification of the crucial issues. "What kind of program can we afford, support, and need." ASCO/ASH (1990) has approved certain minimum criteria necessary for carrying out a safe and successful BMT program. The criteria (see Table 18.5) have been endorsed by the Executive Committee of the American Society of Hematology and the Governing Board of the American Society of Clinical Oncology. Table 18.6 outlines examples of program options an institution may consider. Several alternatives should be scrutinized with a careful eye for fiscal, environmental, and personnel impact. This analysis sets the course for realistic development of the program's mission. A BMT program should arise from a preexisting cancer program, which includes an active cancer committee, tumor board, tumor registry, multidisciplinary consultation resources, and educational programs related to cancer. To ensure continuity in managing BMT patients, most BMT programs utilize protocols defining the nature of treatment programs that often are research-focused. The planning phase of the BMT program would be the time to examine these protocols in relationship to resources that may be needed or are already available. If an autologous program alone is being considered, the

Table 18.5. Minimal Criteria for Performance of BMT

Area of Focus	Minimal Criteria
Patient volume	Sufficient number per year to allow a designated transplant unit with experienced full-time nursing team (at least 10–20 per year)
	If combination allogeneic/autologous, at least ten transplants each should be performed per year.
	New units should be in compliance within two years of operation.
Facilities	Designated transplant unit with two or more designated beds
	Equipment, experience, and protocols for special handling of marrow after collection (i.e., cryopreservation, ABO incompatibility)
	For allogeneic transplants, certified histocompatibility lab
	Protocol and equiment for required isolation (high-pressure, filtered air, laminar air flow)
	24-hour support from laboratories and radiology
Personnel	Trained BMT physicians
	Consulting physicians with broad range of subspecialties
	Full-time committed nursing staff
	Full-time BMT coordinators
	Adequate support servies (i.e., social work, dietary)
Treatment outcome	Sufficient patient numbers in specific disease groups to be able to compare results with published data from other centers
	Maintenance of patient registry comparing outcomes with other centers
	Policy for identifying deficiencies and improving results
Data reporting	Mechanism for reporting data to available registries (i.e., International BMT Registry)
	Commitment to publish important observations

Adapted from: ASCO/ASH Special Announcement. *Blood* 75 (5): 1209.

degree of intensity of patient's care is similar to that when caring for leukemic patients undergoing induction therapy. The difference being the extent and duration of immunosuppresion for autologous patients, which can be up to 45 days.

Development of Mission

The mission should define the program's responsibility and establish its direction and purpose. It also can be used later to evaluate the program's success. The mission of the BMT program should be compared to, and compatible with, the overall mission of the organization. This part of the process requires the balancing of the following questions:

What do we want to do?
What is our business?

What are we allowed to do?
What does the community need?

Development of Goals/Objectives

The program configuration is further shaped by well-defined goals and objectives. These are action statements that set priorities and describe program strategies. The program goals focus the team on appropriate development of personnel, space, equipment, supplies, and specialty resources and are the foundation for high-quality management by the team. Important in this step is the inclusion of a goal that delineates the relationship of research results to clinical activities and practice (Porter-O'Grady 1986). In many BMT programs, research programs actually *drive* clinical care program development.

Table 18.6. Examples of BMT Program Options

	Autologous BMT Program Characteristics	Allogeneic/Autologous BMT Program Characteristics
Diseases T$_x$	AML 1st Remission Breast Cancer	Leukemias Aplastic anemia Lymphoma
Population	Adult (16–55 yrs)	Adult (18–45 yrs)
Donor Pool	Patient Storage 6–8 mos before treatment	Patient Family members Unrelated donor
Conditioning regimen	High-dose chemotherapy	High-dose chemotherapy Total body radiation
Number of beds/location	Six beds on oncology unit Maintaining critically ill patient on unit	Ten beds near ICU Critically ill moved to ICU
Environment	Five private rooms with HEPA-filter system One isolation room	Two laminar air flow rooms Seven private HEPA-filtered rooms One isolation room
Research	Marrow manipulation GM-CSF studies	Graft-versus-host disease CMV prophylaxis Immunoglobulin

Implementation Plan

The ultimate responsibility for actualizing the BMT plan often rests with the medical director. This is the stage when planning priorities are established and the phasing of the project is completed. Appropriate departments are charged with budgeting, hiring, and training of the additional personnel. Capital expenditures are identified and facility construction or renovation is begun.

Environmental Design

For patients and family members, the time spent in a bone marrow transplant unit (BMTU) is likely to be one of the most physiologically and emotionally stressful periods of their lives. For all those involved, admission to a BMTU means the patient is experiencing a life-threatening illness that necessitates the use of specialized medical technology and treatment. It represents a place where outcome is uncertain and death is a potential. The design of the unit can act together with medical technology, health care staff, and hospital policy, to create an aesthetically pleasing, physically comfortable, and stress-reducing environment, where privacy for patients, family, and staff can be maintained. This can contribute to the patient's well-being and reinforces the caring attitudes shown by the staff (Carpman et al. 1986).

Final design of the environment will depend largely on the number of beds planned, the size and type of patient rooms (i.e., private, laminar air flow, ICU), isolation practices, equipment storage needs, number of unit personnel, anticipated patient-related activities, and support services needed. Special consideration must be given to communication patterns. To function effectively, the work space of the team must be designed to encourage easy and spontaneous interaction. This includes the need to accommodate not only technology, but space for informal consultation and conferencing as well as for interaction with family members. Table 18.7 outlines recommendations for general and specific design requirements (Kel-

Table 18.7.   Recommendations for BMT Unit Design Comments

Environment	Recommend	Optional	Comments
I. General Floor Plan			
• Distinct Unit	X		May be combined with oncology or critical care units on same floor though separation made by double doors to enter unit
• No through traffic	X		Improves infection control practices
• Controlled access			
• Adjacent to:			Supply/professional traffic should be separate from
Elevators		X	public/visitor traffic
Critical care unit		X	If critically ill BMT patients not kept on unit, close proximity to critical care unit may be recommended
• Radiology		X	Frequent use of this service with STAT x-rays, especially CXRs
• Unit size variable			Approximate total floor = 600–800sq. ft. planned/ patient room Units > 12 beds should be on own floor
• Audible/Visible alarms and manual shut-off valve for O$_2$/air	X		Centrally located and identified in both engineering area and BMT unit to permit interruption of supply in case of fire, excessive pressure, or repair purposes
• Special air filter system	X		HEPA-filter air system with negative pressure hallways, positive pressure patient rooms. Air system separate from rest of hospital, 100% fresh air
• Plumbing separate service	X		Water from certified source, especially if dialysis is performed, zone valves must be installed on pipes entering unit to allow service to be turned off should breaks occur
• Emergency power	X		Majority of patient care outlets connected to emergency power source that will supply power with 10 sec. of power interruption
• Windows	X		Take into consideration natural illumination/view, cannot be opened, well-sealed from outside air Drapes easily cleanable between patient use
II. Patient Rooms			
• Double-size room	X		Accommodate multiple infusion pumps (average 4), portable supply storage units, exercise bike, walker, commode, nurse work center, family member sitting area, possible dialysis/critical care equipment, and area for storage and easy access to universal precaution supplies
• Sink	X		Elbow, knee, or foot-operated faucets located *near door* for ease of use
With dialysis hook-ups		X	
• Patient bathroom with shower	X		Severely immunosuppressed patients require daily bathing area: area for disposal of all patient secretion/ waste
• Nurses' work-station	X		Area for storing IV supplies, mixing medications, Sharps disposal and flow sheet charting Night-light for illumination

(continued)

Table 18.7. *Continued*

Environment	Recommend	Optional	Comments
• Services			
—Grounded electrical outlets	X		
12 110-volt outlets	X		Standard electrical equipment: 4–5 infusion pumps, patient bed, patient thermometer, patient light
18 110-volt outlets		X	Anticipating any critical care monitoring equipment
Nurse call system	X		Located at bedside and in bathroom, including emergency call system
—Power panel:			Next to patient bed
2-oxygen outlets	X		Connection to outlets made with keyed plugs to prevent interchange of gases
1-compressed air	X		O_2 and compressed air provided at 50–55psi
2-vacuum outlets	X		Vacuum level of 200mm Hg at each outlet must be provided
• Lighting			
—Low-level 35fc night lighting	X		Allows for patient observation and nurse safety when moving around room
—20 to > 100fc overhead lighting	X		> 100fc for emergency lighting with option for 150fc (high intensity lighting for procedures)
—Patient reading light	X		Mounted approximately 7 feet above floor, may be recessed in power panel with 35fc
• Humidity 30–60%	X		Prevents hazards from static electricity
• Air system	X		Special HEPA-filter
			Minimum six total air exchanges/hour
• Supply storage	X		Mobile storage units, facilitates fluctuating supply demands and daily inventory and restocking
Special Needs			
A. Critical Care monitoring equipment			Depending on policy, if critical care patients to stay on unit: option for specifically equipped critical care room(s) and centralized monitoring or portable monitoring used in any patient room
3- simultaneous display capability	X		
Visible/audible alarms	X		
Trending capabilities		X	
Standard vendor throughout hospital		X	
Cardiac output	X		
Hemodynamic monitoring	X		
Central monitoring		X	Depending on the configuration of ICU specific rooms

Table 18.7. *Continued*

Environment	Recommend	Optional	Comments
B. Laminar air flow units		X	Depending on the infection control practices, diseases transplanted and support services available
• Air system	X		HEPA-filter wall with 120 air exchanges/hour behind patient bed
• Patient zone	X		Minimum 8ft wide × 12ft long
• Anteroom	X		Wide enough to accommodate bathroom/sink facilities, nurse work center, IV pump access, family sitting area
• Special monitoring	X		Weekly cultures of environment/patient: daily cleaning of environment, including walls/floors
C. Isolation room with anteroom	X		Utilized for specific infectious diseases (i.e., disseminated herpes zoster)
			Reverse air flow capabilities located on the periphery of other patient rooms
			Anteroom large enough to accommodate washing and storage
D. Special procedure room		X	Utilize for bronchoscopies, bone marrow aspiration, exam room for new admits

III. Information/Communication Center

• House telephones	X		
• Emergency phone Central nurse call system		X	
• Secretarial area	X		Accessible to all, area for filing
• Charting area	X		Isolated, but central, facilitates concentration
			Space for patient charts
			Large enough to include multidisciplinary team
• Computer space	X		Readily accessible
• Conference area	X		Allows for nursing report, patient/family/staff conferences and multidisciplinary meeting
• Specimen collection/ dissemination space	X		Separate from communication center, easy access to all personnel, adheres to universal precautions policies
• Staff lounge with toilet	X		Separate from central area, includes emergency code alarm signal, locker space, telephone
• Office space	X		Physician director, nurse manager, clinical specialist, social worker

IV. Storage

• Crash cart alcove with electrical outlet	X		On unit
• Equipment storage with electrical outlet	X		Separate room near unit for stretchers, scales, IV pumps, and poles: storage of dialysis and critical care equipment

V. Utility Room

• Clean/Med. room	X		Area for medication preparation, close to pharmacy and includes sink
• Dirty utility	X		Clinical sink, hopper, designated area for infectious/ hazardous waste, dirty equipment

(continued)

Table 18.7. *Continued*

Environment	Recommend	Optional	Comments
VI. Support Services Areas			
• Nourishment preparation	X		Sink, refrigerator, microwave, food preparation area—space for food cart, access 24 hours/day
• Satellite pharmacy		X	Optional, but recommended for large BMT units to avoid errors and delays in pharmacologic therapy Should accommodate 24-hour preparation and admixture services
• On call physician sleep room		X	Depending on location and size of unit, though 24-hour physician coverage is required; need can be shared with critical care areas
• Housekeeping facilities	X		Separate room providing storage shelves, wall hooks, clean hot/cold water supply and disposal sink for dirty/contaminated liquids. Never use interchangeably with public areas because of possibility of cross-contamination
• Family room	X		On peripheral area of unit for families to have privacy and area for children to play
• Outpatient Care	X		Outpatient facilities for care of immediate post-transplant patients, long-term follow-up patients can be part of unit (special procedure room) or in close proximity (with the oncology OPD)

leher and Jennings 1988; Krasinski et al. 1985; Lidwell and Noble 1975; Rotstein et al. 1985; Lingren 1983; Buckner et al. 1978; Streifel et al. 1983). New structures must easily accommodate new techonology and enable rapid and low-cost reprogrammed usage.

Personnel: Organization of Services

Multidisciplinary Services

There are few specialities as complex as BMT with the potential for taxing normal hospital services. Patients are treated for a life-threatening illness; their average length of hospital stay is 35 to 40 days; their acuity can fluctuate from stable to critical in a matter of days, sometimes hours, requiring rapid mobilization of personnel and equipment for support; the family is intimately

involved with day-to-day care; and research results frequently alter standard therapies. The proper balance between the BMT patient's unpredictability, the transplant program research demands, and institutional services and limitations, can only be reached if there is integrated delivery of service (Summers et al. 1988).

As an example, a new protocol may be approved for study, comparing the effects of standard continuous intravenous analgesic infusion with a patient-controlled analgesic (PCA) system in controlling pain from oral mucositis. Successful protocol implementation involves the coordination and collaboration of medicine, nursing, pharmacy, central, and material service. The purchase/lease of new devices and supplies, the development of new medication delivery systems, the allocation of additional storage space, the effective distribution of new devices, and the education of personnel and patients needs to be completed before the protocol is activated. If any one of these services is not involved, the quality of care suffers, space and manpower allocation is ineffective, and expenditures increase (Statland 1989).

Mobilization and cost-effective integration challenges the institution to examine carefully and evaluate each hospital service's capabilities and responsibilities. Table 18.8 delineates the major responsibilities of each department in order to support the BMT program. Service overlaps and/or omissions in services need to be eliminated (Kelleher and Jennings 1988; Statland 1989; Moseley and Brown 1986). Despite an understanding of the need, volume of service will fluctuate. Table 18.9 describes the actual patient utilization of hospital services for an isolated day during the treatment process. The *quality* of services delivered will be dependent on effective communication established between the departments and the BMTU. An integrated "multidisciplinary team approach" can balance each discipline's contribution and vested interest in the shared outcome of efficient and effective service to patients. (Bassett and Metzger 1986). Regular rounds or meetings with the whole team can be useful for both identifying individual patient problems and planning of short- and long-term care interventions and conducting team business.

Nursing Service

Nursing is the most costly and most necessary of the multidisciplinary services, combining a unique complexity of oncology and critical care skills. Capable nursing leadership is paramount to the success of recruiting and maintaining an expert nursing staff. This position is a pivotal cog in the organization (Bassett and Metzger 1986) (see Figure 18.2). If properly encouraged the nursing manager is in a position to make rapid strides in developing a cadre of highly skilled expert nurses. Because of the rapidly changing treatment modality, to be optimally effective the nursing team must be viewed as a group that will challenge the institution's values and standards.

Rapid change can create more tension than previously experienced by the institution. The challenge for the nurse manager is to develop an interactive style of management capable of managing change, being action-oriented, building a sense of shared values, and interfacing with the other programs effectively. Achieving this involves consideration of the underlying rhythm/sequence of events in the transplant process, the unpredictability in individual patient response to treatment, the changing therapies that evolve out of positive research results, and the organization's support for nursing. The place to start is defining the nursing unit structure as briefly reviewed in Table 18.10 and writing unit standards that define the scope of unit function (Marker 1987).

Projecting fiscal, educational, and management needs, requires inclusion of a few critical features (see Table 18.11). The level of patient acuity requires a high RN staff ratio and a staffing approach that is sensitive to the intricacies and unpredictable response of the BMT patient (Kelleher and Jennings 1988). As treatment for BMT patients is constantly changing, education is paramount to maintain the level of nursing expertise and skill (Ford 1983; Orsolits 1984; Stuckey 1983). A strong, well-organized orientation program must be developed and include content as outlined in Table 18.12. A preceptor-based program allows the "novice" nurse to work alongside a "master" or expert, learning not only the procedures but also gaining the experience of doing. The acquisition of those skills is neither easy nor automatic. The average length of orientation is six to eight weeks. Centers starting BMT programs may find it difficult to provide appropriate training for the entire complement of newly hired nurses. Working with an already established center to develop orientation on-site or at the support institution can add the necessary depth and continuity to the education program. Continuing education, both internal and external, is essential as nursing practice can change with each new patient, new protocol, and/or complication. A published monthly calendar of inservices with a focus on

Table 18.8. Multidisciplinary Support Services

Services	*Primary Support	*Secondary Support	Major Responsibilities
Medicine:			
Medical Director	X		Provide medical overview of BMT program
Primary physician	X		Provide 24-hr medical care to BMT patients
Consult medical staff		X	Consultant support for various BMT complications
Infectious disease			
Nephrology			
Critical Care			
Cardiology			
Neurology			
Radiology			
Dental			
BMT Nurse Coordinator	X		Coordinate admissions to unit, work with referring physicians to plan for BMT treatment
Nursing Specialists		X	
Oncology/ Hematology			Consult for clinical care problem-solving
Critical Care			Design orientation programs
Dialysis			Evaluate individual and unit clinical practice learning needs
Psychosocial			Present inservices, provide resource material, provide emotional support, support the nurse managers in planning and change, implementation
Pharmacy	X		Maintain patient profile, monitor drug incompatibilities, allergic reactions; evaluate and monitor protocol compliance; monitor usage of investigational drugs; monitor daily electrolyte, chemistry, and drug levels, and make recommendations for dosage or drug changes; provide drug and compatibility information to physicians and nurses
Nutrition	X		Evaluate patient's nutritional status upon admission and develop appropriate nutritional plan; monitor daily caloric and nutritional intakes, starches, minerals; identify nutritional deficits and make recommendations for maintaining an adequate nutritional balance; provide specialized food selections; maintain special knowledge to meet specific needs of BMT patients, i.e., alteration in taste, inability to eat, and effect of complications, e.g., GVHD; provide education to the health care team, patient, and family regarding nutrition and food preparation

Table 18.8. *Continued*

Services	*Primary Support	*Secondary Support	Major Responsibilities
Social Work	X		Complete psychosocial assessment on each patient/family upon admission; collaborate with patient/family in planning for financial support, living arrangements, psychosocial support, coping and cultural needs; provide counseling and psychosocial interventions, e.g., relaxation, imagery, as appropriate to patients/families; provide 24-hour coverage for emergencies or crisis intervention, e.g., emotional crisis, inability to cope, intrafamily relationship problems, depression, etc.; provide follow-through and continuity of services needed upon discharge, i.e., financial, psychosocial, bereavement, or counseling
Chaplain	X		Provide spiritual and emotional counseling and support to patients and families; resource for referral of other chaplains in the community to specific patients or families, act as a liaison to community churches
Infection control		X	Monitor, control and prevent nosocomial infections; keep statistics to identify changes in infection rates or new occurrences; develop and monitor cleaning policies/practices; establish policies and procedures for the following: Specific isolation practices (herpes zosters, AIDS); Infectious waste handling; Employees' and family members' illnesses and communicable diseases; Educate health care professionals in epidemiology and infection control
Housekeeping	X		Specifically trained in cleaning procedures to reduce risk of infection to BMT patients in protective isolation or laminar air flow units; knowledgeable of infection risks and report repair needs to appropriate supervisor, i.e., cracks in wall, floor, or moldings; coordinate cleaning procedures; develop knowledge and skill in using disinfectants and handling of toxic wastes
Material service (central service)	X		Provide 24-hour service to the unit for equipment and supplies: Daily restocking of patients' supplies; Cleaning, storing, and maintaining patient care/unit equipment; Sterilize supplies and linens for sterile environments; establish standards for sterilization; coordinate new product and equipment evaluations with nursing and other appropriate disciplines

(continued)

Table 18.8. *Continued*

Services	*Primary Support	*Secondary Support	Major Responsibilities
Operating Room		X	Provide surgical support for donors or patients undergoing marrow harvesting, placement of central venous access and special procedures, e.g., open lung biopsy, bronchoscopies, endoscopies; knowledge of BMT patients' special needs with diagnosing and treating acute complications or surgical interventions
Outpatient Clinic	X		Provide clinical support pretransplant for patients and donors; provide follow-up clinical care for post-transplant patients after discharge from hospital
Physical Therapy	X		Evaluate patients upon admission; implement daily exercise program (active and passive)
Blood Bank		X	Provide 24-hour service; maintain special procedures for HLA typing, CMV/HIV screening, irradiation of blood products, pheresis and marrow storage; provide volume and blood product types as needed
Radiology		X	Provide 24-hour service for chest x-rays, abdominal x-rays, CT scanning and MRI
Laboratory Services • STAT • Chemistry • Hematology • Microbiology • Pathology • Genetic assays		X	Provide accurate/timely evaluation of lab values and cultures; prepare for fluctuating volumes of service; establish procedures/policies for culturing BMT patients; assist in training nursing staff in appropriate specimen acquisition and handling
Respiratory Therapy		X	Evaluate and maintain pulmonary care of symptomatic airway obstruction or pulmonary deficits in coordination with the medical plan; maintain respiratory equipment and supplies (cleaning and repair)
Recreational Therapy		X	Plan learning and diversional activities for patients and siblings
Volunteers		X	Provide social activities, friendship, support, and interpretation services

*Primary support: Services having daily *direct* patient care interaction.
*Secondary support: Critical services supporting overall care to patient.

new equipment, procedure changes and updates, assessment skills training, updates on research results, and communication techniques, or inter-personal skills is helpful. Educational time for evening (3–11), night (11–7), and part-time or weekend staff needs to be scheduled on the calendar.

Finally, there are extraordinary demands placed on nursing personnel. These are related to the nature of direct patient care, high morbidity and mortality rates, staff/patient educational needs, increased interpersonal interactions and collaborations, and exposure to new technology (Sinclair 1988; Cox and Andrews 1981; Vincent

Table 18.9.   Example: Patient Utilization of Support Services

History:
- 38 y.o. female with AML, first remission
- Received HLA-matched marrow from sister
- Conditioning therapy:
  Cyclophosphamide 60mg/kg × 2
  Total body irradiation × 7 days
- Lab results:
  WBC–100   BUN–90
  ANC–0   Creat–2.0
  Plts–9,000 Bili–4.0
  Hct–26

Day 12 post-transplant

Clinicial Assessment	Intervention	Service Utilization
1. T–39.4, FUO × 5 days with triple antibiotic coverage	Start antifungal Tx Panculture Cooling blanket	Pharmacy Micro lab; infectious disease consult Central service
2. Severe mucositis with mucosal ulcerations	Morphine drip Saline mouth rinses	Pharmacy Pain consult Dental consult
3. Epistaxis	Transfuse 2 units PRBC; transfuse 8 units platelets Pack nose Repeat Hct and Plt count	Blood Bank ENT consult Hematology lab
4. RR–40 O₂ Sat—89% Rales	Oximeter reading every 6 hours 4L of O₂ Lasix 20mg × 1 STAT CXR	Respiratory therapy Critical Care consult Pharmacy Radiology
5. Elevated BUN/Creat ↑ weight–2kg Hepatic tenderness Elevated LFT	Monitor BUN/Creat Obtain urine/lytes Start Aldactone PO Restrict fluids, change TPN composition	Nephrology consult Clinical lab Pharmacy Dietary/Nutrition support team

and Billings 1988) (see also Chapter 16 on staff stress). As job stress is inherent, research suggests a very strong relationship between the degree of stress perceived by the staff nurse and the nurse manager's leadership style (Jennings 1987). A participatory style of management has been noted to have direct impact on decreasing burnout and increasing job satisfaction among staff nurses (Jennings 1987; Katz 1974; Ulz 1989). This style can generate excitement and commitment to the BMT program as the wise manager taps into knowledge and experience of the individual nurses. The participatory leader can easily support the notion of mentorship, which can enhance staff nurses' professional development. The function of mentoring includes teaching, sponsoring, encouraging, counseling, and befriending. This has benefit for both participants. The relationship is dynamic, noncompetetive, and nuturing, promoting independence, autonomy, and

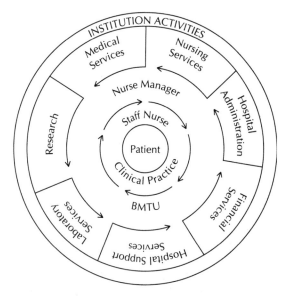

Figure 18.2. Nurse Manager's Relationship to BMTU and Institutional Activities

self-actualization in the protégé, while fostering a sense of pride and fulfillment, support, and continuity in the mentor. The BMT nursing team must have this type of support as they embrace new ideas, challenge old ones, and live with paradox—while providing care to a complex patient population.

Conclusion

Bone marrow transplantation is rapidly becoming a state-of-the-art treatment choice for many hematological and malignant diseases. BMT needs to be viewed as a specialty program and not as an isolated treatment modality. Hospital support for this treatment modality should never be entered into indiscriminately as there are considerable implications to all hospital services. There is no panacea for an effective program. It requires institutionally supported, multidisciplinary commitment and intensive planning with special analysis of the impact of fiscal, environmental, and personnel resources. Once developed, the day-to-day challenges rest with the medical director and nurse manager to develop and maintain a skilled team who, in partnership with other disciplines, deliver holistic and competent care to a very complex patient population.

Table 18.10. Nursing Unit Structure

Elements	Subcomponents
Description	• Location/Size
	• Patient/Unit type
Purpose	• Reason for unit
	• Philosophical ideas and contribution to overall nursing system
Objectives	Delivery of care; data collection
Administration	Organizational chart; narrative; power base of nursing, medical, and administrative decision making
Use of Nursing Unit	Admission mode/criteria; length of stay; discharge preparation/criteria
Governing rules	Safety; infection control; supplies/equipment; confidentiality; services and therapies

Table 18.11. Budgeting Components for BMT Nursing Care

Primary Components	Prerequisites	Comments
1. Development of patient classification system	Identified patient acuity system	Patient acuity can range from modified intensive to life support in a matter of hours during any phase of BMT process
	Clear delineation of nursing tasks	Differentiate between patient assessment, medication administration, nursing interventions, patient activities and critical care management; outlines ''service level,'' which acknowledges fluctuation in care
	Indicate nursing time for each task	Range of hours of care per patient day = 9–20 hours (reflecting direct and indirect patient care activities)
	System coordinated through an information system that integrates clinical and financial data	Computerize system
2. Identification of delivery of care model	The model must: • Maximize productivity • Provide for continuity • Increase autonomy • Enhance collaborative practice with physicians	Patient length of stay ranges 35–45 days; readmission rate can be up to 50%; most usable model is primary nursing, provides for autonomy and accountability for practice; nursing is central to the coordination of ancillary services
3. RN/patient ratio	Ratio should take into account: unit size, patient acuity, type of nursing (primary or other), staff responsibilities (i.e., total care including IVs and chemotherapy)	Usual direct nursing care ratios are: Days: 1:2 Evenings: 1:2–3 Nights: 1:3–4 12-hour shifts may even out staffing ratios (i.e., 1:2–3 q shift)
4a. Recruitment	Be open to varied clinical nursing backgrounds: Oncology, Critical Care, Med./Surg., Pediatrics, and Psychosocial	New graduates can perform well with intensive orientation and strong preceptorship Orientation program 6–8 weeks
4b. Retention	Program directed at: • Promote job satisfaction; involvement in decision making • Adequate staffing • Recognition program • Collaborative relationship with physicians • Professional development • Competitive salaries/benefits • Orientation/continuing education programs • Leadership training	Tailor program to unique needs of unit in relationship to institution; critical to BMTU as it takes 6 months to 1 year for new staff to be fully oriented

Table 18.12.   Orientation Needs of BMT Nursing Staff

Didactic	Preceptor-Supported Experience
Pathophysiology for disease process	Review disease course from diagnosis to transplantation
Introduction to clinical research	Overview of patient's treatment protocols
Revew basic principles of immunology/hemopoietic system	Care for immunosuppressed patient and patients receiving biologic response modifier treatment (i.e., CSF, a monoclonal)
Overview donor selection and types of transplants	Observe marrow aspiration
	Care for patient undergoing autologous, allogeneic (family/unrelated/mismatch) BMT
Review implication of use of right atrial catheters (RAC)	Care for patient undergoing insertion of RAC
Review principles of chemotherapy related to conditioning regimens	Care for patient receiving high-dose chemotherapy
Overview of radiation management and safety	Care for patient receiving total body irradiation (TBI)
Introduction to BMT drug therapy	Care for patient using: prophylaxis for GVHD multiple antibiotics research drugs multiple IV pump manipulations
Review of blood component therapy	Care for patient receiving unirradiated bone marrow, irradiated PRBCs, platelets; signs and symptoms of transfusion reaction
Develop understanding of lab value clinical significance	Review and respond to daily lab value variations
Understanding of unique nutritional needs	Care for patient receiving total parenteral nutrition (TPN) and/or GVHD diet
Introduction to BMT complication, treatment prophylaxis, and pain management	Care for patients experiencing: fluid/electrolyte problems infections/FUO veno-occlusive disease (VOD) hemorrhage multiorgan failure
Overview psychosocial support: coping strategies concept of loss/grief/dying	Participate in family conference Initiate care conferences Relaxation techniques
Introduction to "team"	Participate in rounds
Introduction to infection control: hand washing environmental cleaning patient/room culturing aseptic technique	Care of patient in: private room sterile environment
Principles of self-care for nurses	Participate in stress reduction programs and learn stress reducing techniques

References

ASCO/ASH. 1990. Recommended criteria for the performance of bone marrow transplantation. *Blood 75* (5): 1209.

Arenth, L.M. 1985. The development and validation of an oncology patient classification system. *O.N.F. 12* (6): 17–22.

Bassett, L., and Metzger, N. 1986. *Achieving Excellence: A Prescription for Health Care Managers.* Rockville, MD: Aspen.

Bone marrow transplant nursing resource directory. 1990. BMT Special Interest Group of The Oncology Nursing Society. Pittsburgh, PA.

Bortin, M., and Rimm, A.A. 1986. Increasing utilization of bone marrow transplantation. *Transplantation 43:* 229–234.

Buckner, C.K. et al. 1978. Protective environment for marrow transplant recipients: A prospective study. *Ann. Intern. Med. 89:* 893–901.

Carpman, J.R., Grant, M.A., and Simmon, D.A. 1986. *Design That Cares: Planning Health Facilities for Patients and Visitors.* American Hospital Publishing, Inc.

Cox, A., and Andrews, P. 1981. The development of support systems on oncology units. *O.N.F. 8:* 31–35.

Evans, S.K., Laundon, T., and Yamamoto, W.G. 1980. Projecting staffing requirements for intensive care units. *J. Nurs. Adm. 7:* 34–42.

Ford, R. 1983. Reducing nursing staff stress through scheduling, orientation, and continuing education. *Nurs. Clin. North Am. 18:* 597–601.

Hardy, O.B., and Lummers, L.P. 1986. *Hospitals: The Planning and Design Process,* 2nd ed. Rockville, MD: Aspen Publications, Inc.

Jennings, B. 1987. Social support: A way to a climate of caring. *Nursing Administration Quarterly 11:* 63–71.

Katz, R. 1974. Skills of an effective administrator. *Harvard Business Review 5:* 90–102.

Kelleher, J., and Jennings, M. 1988. Nursing management of marrow transplant units: A framework for practice. *Seminars in Oncology Nursing 4* (1): 60–68.

Krasinski, K. et al. 1985. Nosocomial fungal infection during hospital renovation. *Infection Control 6:* 278–282.

Lidwell, O.M., and Noble, W.C. 1975. Fungi and clostridia in hospital air: The effect of air-conditioning. *Journal of Applied Bacteriology 39:* 251–261.

Lingren, P. 1983. The laminar air flow room: Nursing practice and procedures. *Nurs. Clin. North Am. 18:* 553–561.

Marker, C.G.S. 1987. The Marker Model: A hierarchy for nursing standards. *J. Nurs Qual. Assay 1* (2): 7–20

Mills, D., and Pennoni, M. 1986. A nurturing work environment in philosophy and practice. *Cancer Nursing 9:* 117–124.

Mortenson, L.E. 1984. Are oncology nurses too expensive? *O.N.F. 11:* 14–15.

Moseley, J.R., and Brown, J.S. 1986. The organization and operation of oncology units. *O.N.F. 12:* 17–24.

Orsolits, M. 1984. Effects of organizational characteristics on the turnover in cancer nursing. *O.N.F. 11:* 59–63.

Porter-O'Grady, T. 1986. *Creative Nursing Administration.* Rockville, MD: Aspen.

Rogers, J.M. 1985. You're leaving when? Looking at recruitment and retention in today's economy. *O.N.F. 12:* 72–77.

Rotstein, C. et al. 1985. An outbreak of invasive aspergillosis among allogeneic bone marrow transplants: A case-control study. *Infection Control 6:* 347–355.

Rowland, N., and Rowland, B. 1985. *Nursing administration handbook,* 2nd ed. Rockville, MD: Aspen.

Sinclair, V. 1988. High technology in critical care: Implications for nursing's role and practice. *Focus on Critical Care 15* (4): 36–41.

Skydell, B., and Arndt, M. 1988. The price of nursing care. *Nurs. Clin. North Am. 23*(3): 493–501.

Statland, B. 1989. Quality management: Watch word for the 90's. *MLD July:* 33–40.

Streifel, A.J. et al. 1983. Aspergillus fumigatus and other thermotolerant fungi generated by hospital building demolition. *Applied and Environmental Microbiology 46:* 375–378.

Stuckey, P.A. 1983. Orientation to an oncology unit. *O.N.F. 10* (4): 26–29.

Summers, P.M., and Naderman, W. et al. 1988. Quarterly management: Program design and interdisciplinary approach. *Nurs. Clin. North Am. 23* (3): 665–670.

Tillman, M.C. 1984. A comparison of nursing care requirements of patients on general medical-surgical units and on an oncology unit in a community hospital. *O.N.F. 11:* 42–45.

Ulz, L. 1989. Leadership via participatory management. *Nursing Connections 2* (2): 62–65.

Vincent, P., and Billings, C. 1988. Unit management as a factor in stress among intensive care nursing personnel. *Focus on Critical Care 15* (3): 45–49.

Walker, D.D. 1983. The cost of nursing care in hospitals. *J. Nurs. Adm. 3:* 13–18.

Chapter 19

Patient Perspectives

Dana Grossman

The physiological and pathological facts about bone marrow transplantation are complex and constantly changing. To try to comprehend every medical aspect of the procedure's many variations is a considerable task. Yet even that is not enough for the BMT nurse to gain a full appreciation of the effect of this procedure on the patient. Comprehension of the effects of this disease and the procedure from the patients' point of view is essential to achieving a crucial final measure of understanding and clinical effectiveness. Accordingly, this last chapter consists of the insights and observations of four bone marrow transplant patients.

Their stories have been adapted from a variety of sources—a narrative written especially for this book, the transcript of a taped discussion, a published article, and letters written to family members; the accounts have all been condensed and edited slightly. But regardless of the form in which they set down their thoughts, all four patients were eager to share their experiences in the hope of helping future transplant patients. Much appreciation is extended to each of them and to

their families for their willingness to share so freely of themselves.

* * *

Garreth Gobel, an engineer from Underhill, Vermont, was diagnosed with acute myelogenous leukemia in May 1982. He was 43 years old. After three chemotherapy-induced remissions, he received an autologous BMT at Dartmouth-Hitchcock Medical Center in January 1984.

My goal in life is now simple—to regard each and every day as a gift and live life to the fullest. That sounds like just another cliche, but under the duress of life-threatening illness it takes on great meaning. My decision to undergo the rigorous autologous bone marrow transplant was made somewhat easier because my life has become more meaningful and precious throughout the course of my disease—for the alternative is so very final.

AML is a real roller-coaster type of disease, with many emotional and physical ups and downs. Unfortunately, one of the most difficult aspects of this disease is coping with your own feelings.

When I was first diagnosed with AML, I would lie in my hospital bed and ask myself "Why? What had I done wrong? What had I been exposed to at work, in the Army, or in my travels that could have brought this on? What had I possibly done in the past that I was now to be punished so severely for?" My memory failed to uncover any contributing causes.

This feeling of guilt stayed with me until I convinced myself that I was not being punished. In this imperfect world most things are random, and I just happened to have a breakdown in my immune system. Once I accepted the fact that I had the disease and that I could not change that fact, then it was time to do something about it. From that moment on, I was not going to feel sorry for myself, but with all the determination that I could muster I was going to beat this rap, get well, and live a normal life once again.

The reactions of friends, neighbors, and relatives to my disease varied. Some people felt if they didn't keep in touch the whole thing would just go away; some displayed pity; some were afraid of "catching it." Some very close friends finally admitted almost a year later that they did not stay in close contact with me initially because they didn't know what to say, and the longer they stayed away the more difficult it became for them to approach me. At first, I felt very isolated because of this kind of reaction. Gradually, as people began to realize that I was still the same person they once knew and that it was all right to speak openly about my disease, they began to come around. In the end, many became a real support mechanism. It was such a comfort to know that so many people cared, and this fact has been an additional incentive in my determination to live.

For anyone entering treatment, the important thing to remember is that *you* are the one with the disease and it is *your* body, so *ask questions!* Find out everything you can about the disease, the treatment that is being prescribed, and the other alternatives that are available. Take part in every aspect of your disease. Your doctors and nurses are doing everything possible in your best interests and are more than willing to answer any questions you may have. It will help you tremendously to know what is going on, since this will alleviate at least some of the apprehension and fear that you will surely feel.

My wife and daughter and I have always been very close, and communication among us is and has always been open and honest. The feeling of helplessness on their part was, at times, just too much to bear, and we have had numerous crying sessions together. My wife was hit especially hard, since 15 years before she had lost her first husband to lymphosarcoma. "How could this happen twice, and what did *I* do wrong?" was her biggest question. Again, that ever-present feeling of guilt. A good friend gave me a book entitled *When Bad Things Happen to Good People*, written by Harold S. Kushner. The author and I have remarkably similar beliefs—the most important of which is that guilt is an exhausting, unproductive force and has no positive effect on coping. My wife read this book, and the change in her thinking was significant. Our 13-year-old daughter has managed to cope quite well. She has expressed a strong desire to always be cognizant of everything—good and bad. We have lived up to that promise to her, and she has been a great help to us in keeping our friends abreast of all the latest health bulletins during the times that we were too preoccupied to do so. This gave her a very specific purpose, since everyone needs to be needed at such a time.

Having reached the age of 43, after many years of hard work and planning, I thought that I had complete control of my life. I had a loving family, a comfortable home, job security, financial investments, retirement plans, good health—everything was under control. WRONG! Suddenly, out of the blue, I was told that I had AML—and I had seen my physician with a mere pulled muscle. In one swift moment, it was pointed out to me how little control I suddenly had over my future.

Although I only attend church a few times a year, I am in my own way very religious. It was this strong bond with God that helped give me the extra strength I needed to undergo these treatments. I knew that God did not "give" me this disease but that with His help I would find the strength and determination to cope. I never prayed to be made well but asked Him many times to give me the mental and physical strength to go on. I would never try to convert others to my way of religious thinking, but I would urge others in my situation not to turn their backs on religion.

After exhausting every other means of treatment for my disease and subsequently losing remission, I was told that the best course of action was a bone marrow transplant. Only a small number of people had gone through bone marrow transplantation, and no one so far had gone through the particular treatment used on me. There was no one from whose experience I could benefit.

My decision to undergo this rigorous treatment was made somewhat easier because I was determined to give myself every possible chance to continue my life. On January 16, 1984, I checked into Dartmouth-Hitchcock Medical Center and began my fight for life. This was an especially difficult time for my wife and daughter, for at this point they lost control of the situation to some extent.

I was placed in a specially prepared private room. Reverse isolation procedures were necessary to prevent contamination, since infection is the major fear in the treatment of this disease. This transformed everyone I saw into "blue-masked robots" who came and went to perform their specific duties as swiftly as possible. Physical contact couldn't even be considered, but fortunately my nurses did manage to find ways to circumvent some of the rigid rules and regulations. They will always remain my wonderful friends.

The day of harvesting was relatively uneventful for me. I was given medications to help me relax and was anesthetized during the entire procedure in the operating room. It was the doctors who had a difficult day, dealing with the strenuous task of removing the bone marrow a little at a time and then processing it in the laboratory. During the following week, however, I was tender and sore where the bone marrow had been harvested. But no one should have any anxiety about this part of the procedure.

The next step was high-dose chemotherapy and whole-body radiation. Cytoxan was used in the chemotherapy. I felt much anxiety as I watched them inject it into my Hickman catheter, knowing there was no turning back from that point on but not knowing how sick I might get from it. That was, to say the least, a very scary moment. However, I was fortunate in that my body always tolerated chemotherapy very well. The catheter they inserted into my bladder was uncomfortable, but it was soon removed.

The total body radiation was mentally trying and very scary. There was a feeling of isolation and loneliness in being in the treatment room all alone with that awesome piece of machinery. The television and intercom were some consolation, but there was still the problem of having to hold the tight sitting position for 18 to 20 minutes at a time in order for my entire body to fit into the radiation field. Towards the end of each time period, my entire body would shake with weakness and I would feel that there was no way I could possibly hold the position one second longer—but I did hang in there for the duration of each treatment. For me, this was one of the most trying aspects of the entire treatment. After the third treatment, I experienced the anticipated nausea and vomiting and a complete loss of appetite.

The day I received my treated bone marrow back into my Hickman catheter was a day of excitement and tremendous hopefulness. The only event more exciting for me was that first day when the blood counts started to rise. Until that point, the highlight of each day was learning the result of the day's blood work. There was absolutely nothing anyone could do to alleviate the painful hours of anticipation. What a joy and relief it was when the blood tests finally showed positive signs! That meant the bone marrow had taken and was ready to do its job. From that moment on, our family felt a new sense of being—we had indeed been handed the miracle of a new chance at life!

Following my release from the hospital, while I was recuperating at home, the doctors treated my spinal column with more chemotherapy (methotrexate). This was done to remove any possible leukemic cells from that part of the body, which is resistant to the other methods of treatment. I experienced severe headaches at this time, and they remained for approximately a week following the last treatment.

Another feeling I experienced besides the expected muscular weakness resulting from so many weeks in bed was that I could not tolerate cold temperatures. I found myself shivering while sitting in a warm room where others were comfortable.

But all these symptoms gradually subsided as I gained back my strength and resumed my daily routines.

Many people have asked me where I get my determination to keep on fighting this disease. The truth is that I just plain do not want to be cheated out of life! Details are a newly acquired passion in my life—the sky is so much bluer and the clouds so much whiter and more beautiful than ever before. I now take the time to "smell the flowers" and, above all, I appreciate the most important aspect of my life—LIFE itself! I am more determined than ever to enjoy it to its fullest.

Above all, I am so grateful to have been the first person to go through the Dartmouth transplant program. No matter what the long-term outcome may be, at least I feel that there has been a real meaning to my life and that I have had a chance to bring encouragement and strength to others who are afflicted with leukemia. Doctors have worked for many years trying to find a cure for AML; now perhaps I have been instrumental in the realization of their dream. All the nurses who have gone through the treatments and suffered with me now also see hope for future patients.

Death is a natural part of life. We all know it must happen at some point in time. The only variable is when. When we face cancer and its treatments, we do have a choice; it is our decision and ours alone. I'm a fighter at heart and am determined to go on. That is my decision.

Garreth Gobel died in April of 1984. He finished the account from which these thoughts were excerpted after he had lost his post-BMT remission. Though he knew that the transplant had represented his last chance for a cure, he purposely did not mention that he had relapsed in his account. According to a letter his wife wrote after his death, "He wanted to leave subsequent patients with optimism and hope. I sincerely hope his paper serves that purpose."

* * *

Andrew Baumer, a 37-year-old Operations Manager from Oakland, California, was diagnosed as having multiple myeloma in 1988. He had an allogeneic BMT in Seattle in July 1989. The following comments were adapted from the transcript of a discussion he had in April 1990 with his wife, Lisa Hanauer.

Andrew: The question of whether to die within three years or undergo a bone marrow transplant wasn't one I wasted a lot of time and effort on trying to answer. The only question was when and if the transplant process could begin, which I began asking the night I was diagnosed with multiple myeloma and I was informed that a transplant might be able to save me. The ensuing 18 months were essentially a countdown during which I kept checking off preliminary steps which needed to be completed—starting with getting out of the hospital alive, through getting into remission and finding a donor, to trying not to accidentally die during the transplant procedure itself. So far I've completed the preliminary steps and can now get down to the serious work of trying to stay alive for a long time to come.

Lisa: It is the nightmare of anyone who is in love to be faced with losing that person to a horrible death. While I don't want to minimize what it is to be the patient who's been diagnosed with a disease, I often think that it's just as difficult—and sometimes perhaps more so—to be the one who isn't sick. When we learned that Andrew had multiple myeloma, everything I believed about my future was threatened. I was terrified by the idea that not only might I be a widow by the time I was 30 but I might also be cursed with good health so I would be alone and miserable for the next 60 years. I thought if he were to die it would be over for him, but I would be left behind to remember the pain.

On the night of the diagnosis we were told about the possibility of a cure through a bone marrow transplant. I was determined that Andrew would get into remission and become healthy enough to have a transplant. When Andrew's three siblings were found not to be compatible donors, I was confident that we would find an unrelated donor for him. Against enormous odds, we were fortunate to do so within a relatively short time. Yet with the realization that we would be going to transplant came a whole new set of fears. I was well aware of the fact that a bone marrow transplant is one of the riskiest and most arduous medical procedures there is.

Leaving our home in Oakland to go to Seattle was a trauma for which I wasn't at all prepared. I cried all the way to Seattle and became completely hysterical as we were renting second-rate furniture to put into our rented apartment, after we had taken such care to build all our own to put in the house we loved. Standing at the beginning and not knowing what would lie ahead of us was the most difficult thing of all.

While Andrew was in the hospital during the first phase of the transplant, I felt a tremendous amount of pressure from the nurses to make sure that he was a compliant patient. While I realized how important it was that he get enough exercise, take his oral meds, and apply the antifungal/antibacterial powders and ointments, I felt that I needed more backup from the nurses. I resented being put in the position of "bad guy," and I was afraid of what might happen to Andrew if I failed. But when I expressed this concern to the nurses, not only did I receive increased support but I discovered that Andrew's resistance to compliance was not unusual. There were times when he simply needed to exercise some autonomy in a situation where he felt that he had very little.

Andrew: It's astounding the preposterous things—like this blood-vomiting stuff—to which you can become accustomed when you have nothing better to do. And it's strange the way you can forget just how horrible an ordeal it was. I remember very little that was horrible. I remember a lot that was unpleasant. And I remember everything that was very, very boring. If there is a hell, may the architect of those tiny LAF rooms be condemned to spend eternity stuck inside one. They do what they're supposed to, but those rooms are really very small.

I know I'm obsessed with trivia, but for the duration of my illness and treatment it was exactly those little items of personal trivia that assumed monumental dimensions. Being able to eat or take a shower or use a real toilet behind a door you can shut become Homeric in importance. When your universe contracts to the limits of your own body and the tiny, sterile cubicle in which it's confined, any small triumphs you can achieve in stretching those limits begin to take on the aspect of Achilles's defiance of Agamemnon. What I mean is that when your perception becomes sufficiently distorted, tiny annoyances can become excruciating tortures and excruciating tortures after a while can become boring ordeals.

Lisa: It's true that Andrew doesn't remember the big picture in all of its horrifying clarity as I do. He had drugs designed to serve that purpose. I didn't. And therein lies a great injustice.

Andrew did have a very difficult time dealing with the LAF room. After his counts came in he decided, after much agonizing, that he wanted to "break" LAF. He wanted a bath and a walk. He was becoming extremely depressed and, I felt, his focus had narrowed to the confines of the room to a point where he didn't even seem to notice people on the other side of the plastic curtain. He feared that he might have a nervous breakdown if the curtain remained, and I believed him. A seemingly endless parade of hospital staff spent days trying to convince us that breaking LAF would mean certain danger or worse, even though half the patients had been randomized to non-LAF rooms. They pleaded with him to reconsider. While I was worried about the consequences of breaking LAF, I was equally worried about what might happen to Andrew if he didn't do it. Ultimately we chose to trust what we believed to be the right choice, and on day 25 Andrew broke LAF. His counts continued to flourish, and his spirits rose along with them. The next day, every person who had tried to talk him out of breaking LAF came in to shake his hand. It became apparent that what Andrew had done was more detrimental to the research than to the patient.

After Andrew was released to our apartment in Seattle, he was readmitted on three occasions—twice with HSV and once with a gram-negative septicemia. We had questioned why, with our own house in Oakland being very close to another transplant center, we had to stay in Seattle until 100 days post-transplant. But in the post-transplant days we were glad we did. To know that 24 hours a day we had access to someone with Andrew's chart in front of him or her and whose life work it was to field every possible complication arising from bone marrow transplant turned out to be very confidence-inspiring and on at least one occasion to have saved Andrew's life.

By the time we left Seattle we felt we were truly ready to leave. I had wondered if day 100 would bring with it a magical end to post-transplant complications. In Andrew's case, it did. We are now nine months post-transplant and Andrew is well over the procedure. He still takes a little cyclosporine for a touch of GVH, but even that will soon be tapered down to nothing. He feels stronger and healthier than he has since the diagnosis. We have the date scheduled for his one-

year check-up and I am finding myself increasingly anxious about that. As long as I had the transplant to focus on, I wasn't worried about the cancer. But now it will take time to prove what I believe to be true: that we've accomplished what we set out to do on that bleak night just over two years ago—that Andrew is cured.

Andrew: I know I'm not even supposed to think this, but if I've learned one thing it's that I can think whatever I want: As far as I'm concerned I am cured, and, privately at least, to hell with waiting five years before I can even think the word. Of course my disease could come back tomorrow, but at least it—or enough of it not to worry about—was gone when it was supposed to be. And my transplant worked, or at least as well as they ever do. And if I've learned another thing, it's that I have enough to worry about today without worrying about tomorrow. "One day at a time" may once have been a cliche, but now the concept has sunk so far into my brain that I feel free to use it as justification for breaking any rules that cause me grief.

I started out thinking of this mess as a series of steps I had to get through, one at a time. I set goals for myself, and I've managed to achieve all of them, one at a time. The last step, which is living a long and valuable life that lasts as long as I want it to, is really no different from any of my previous, more immediately achievable goals. It will simply take me much, much longer to find out if I've achieved it. I hope, in fact, that it takes me at least another 40 or 50 or 60 years to find out.

As of October 1990, Andrew Baumer showed no signs of a relapse.

* * *

Paul Cowan of New York City, a staff writer for the Village Voice, *was diagnosed with AML in September 1987, 10 days before his 47th birthday. After several chemotherapy regimens, he was accepted for transplantation at Dartmouth-Hitchcock Medical Center. This account of his treatment is condensed from a feature he wrote for the* Voice *that was published in the May 17, 1988, issue.*

Until the day I was diagnosed with leukemia, I had assumed that health and sickness were separate, distinct terrains. I've since learned that those boundaries don't really exist. Instead, the world is composed of the sick and the not-yet-sick—and, as I hope for myself, the sick and the not-yet-well. They are part of the same continuum. Now I occupy a different place on the continuum than I did when I thought I was in prime physical condition, as recently as early last summer.

During the past five months, I've learned there *is* a land of the sick. When you receive a passport—an unwelcome diagnosis—you learn that the land has its own language (medical terminology), its own geography (hospitals, outpatient clinics, blood-testing labs, doctors' offices), its own citizens (other sick people), its own pantheon of heroes and authority figures (doctors, medical researchers, hospital administrators), its own calendar (dictated by the changes in one's body or by the results of medical tests), and—most of all—its own emotional demands.

In retrospect, I realize that I denied the first manifestations of leukemia. In early August, I noticed several bruises on my legs, friends told me I looked tired and pale, and I felt weak—but I didn't admit this to even my wife, Rachel.

On September 9, in a meeting with editors and publicists about an upcoming publicity tour for a book Rachel and I had written, I felt so tired it was an effort to maintain just a semblance of concentration. On September 11, I called my internist for an appointment. When Dr. Esserman saw me later that day he told me that I had a very low hematocrit and sent me right over to New York University Hospital to see Dr. Julia Smith, a hematologist-oncologist. She said I had "a blood disorder." Clinging to the hope that might mean anemia, I lay on a cot while she did a bone marrow biopsy. I was so frantic, so full of questions, that I barely felt the pain.

Rachel arrived a few minutes after the biopsy. We sat for two hours, clutching each other's hands, unable to talk much, waiting for the biopsy results. At about 5:30, Julia summoned us into a cubicle and waved everyone else away. She said I had leukemia, although there would have to be more tests before she knew what kind. I didn't care much about that distinction, though I felt surprisingly clearheaded. I asked Julia if I would die. There was a reasonable chance I would survive, she said, but the struggle would be long and difficult.

On the night of September 11—only a few hours after I had walked into Dr. Esserman's office—I began a round of blood transfusions to bring my hematocrit and platelets back to a level that would guarantee immediate survival. A resident brought an IV pole and a bag of red blood cells and placed a needle in my vein. It was painless, but I was restricted to a wheelchair. My world had shrunk to my immediate surroundings.

Right then, the question that was at the forefront of my mind was "What should I tell my children?" Lisa had just started her second year at Wesleyan, and Matt was in his senior year of high school. Should I gloss over the truth or present it to them in an unvarnished form? Dr. Esserman was helpful on that point. He said, simply, that when a family member is sick, no one is helped by a lie. I knew he was right, but I felt a surge of guilt about the fact that I was sick at all. Now the people I loved most in the world would feel my illness as a constant weight. But soon my guilt seemed self-indulgent. I didn't blame myself for my leukemia. I knew that if I disguised my sickness or the depths of my fears, the trust that had always held our family together would begin to fray.

On September 14, Julia told me I had AML, and on the 16th I began chemotherapy. Julia said I would receive a high dose of chemotherapy for five days. It had to destroy as much of the marrow as possible in order to destroy the leukemic cells. It would take about three weeks until my marrow regenerated enough blood cells for her to take the crucial biopsy—the one that would show whether or not I was in remission. But I shouldn't think of remission as a cure, she added. It was a plateau that would enable us to choose between various long-term treatments—none guaranteed to work. I had to learn to take this disease one day at a time.

Soon after I entered the hospital I decided to stop asking my doctors the questions about my prognosis that had tumbled out of my mouth when I was first diagnosed. Now that I *was* sick, I didn't want to think of myself as a statistic. I needed all my psychological strength to remember that I was Paul Cowan, a unique person, who had to fight the battle at hand.

During my first weekend in the hospital, I began to learn how important it was for me to retain my ties to the land of the well—to see myself as an exile who would return one day. During those days I was in a four-person ward. One patient moaned through the night; two resolutely cheerful men spent their days comparing symptoms and gossiping about nurses. I didn't want to be part of this hospital culture. I wanted to retain a sense of myself. Luckily, a few days later, it was decided that I needed a private room to protect me from infection. Over time, I would be able to use the room to create my own little island in the midst of the hospital. Gradually, Rachel decorated my room and made it into a haven. She brought in bright posters, a calendar, and snapshots. We arranged my books into a makeshift library. I put my *tefillin* where I could look out over the East River as I said my morning prayers.

During my first days in the hospital I read Norman Cousins's *Anatomy of an Illness* and *The Healing Heart*. I read scores of other books by holistic healers who persuaded me to change my diet, to take up yoga, to visualize my healthy cells conquering leukemic ones. But I balked at the underlying assumption that many of these writers seemed to share—that there is a psychological cause for sickness. Furthermore, these writers argue, there is a correct psychological pathway back to health.

As someone who is seriously sick, I have to struggle to maintain a positive attitude and zest for life. Sometimes it's hard—morbid thoughts are always flickering through my mind. Sometimes I worry that bleak moods undermine my health. Then I remind myself that I'd be unrealistic if I repressed them. I try to maintain hope—or at least the memory of hope—when I am consumed with fear or despair. But I also have to confront the awesome, mysterious power of my disease. Otherwise, if the leukemic cells reenter my bone marrow, I run the risk of blaming myself for relapsing and, if I continue to weaken, of raging at my psyche instead of fighting back.

As I lay on my hospital bed, brooding about the holistic books, I realized I couldn't accept the idea that there was a single set of guidelines to the kind of behavior that enables patients to cope with illness or prolong their lives. Each patient—each person—is unique. They can't change their personalities when they get sick. They can only try to strengthen the strongest part of themselves. That was what I had to do.

When my first round of chemotherapy began, I assumed I'd become nauseated, run high fevers, have incoherent hours. My regimen lasted five days. Each day I expected the nausea to begin. But each day when I awoke I realized that I wasn't running a fever and that I still had an appetite. I was able to hope that I might not get sick from the chemotherapy at all.

About a week after the first infusion of chemotherapy, gray hairs began to shed over my pillows, clothes, and sometimes my food. I didn't mind balding as much as I had expected to. I was worried about my remission, not my hair. But one afternoon as Rachel sat on my bed and stroked my head, tufts of hair came out in her hands. Her pale, bruised husband, who'd been attached to an IV for more than two weeks, was rapidly decomposing. She began to cry as she looked at the clumps of my hair.

I still felt like a foreigner in the land of the sick, and, like most foreigners, I had no context in which to place the information I learned. Once, a young resident felt my abdomen and told me my spleen might have to be removed; I spent a terrified night until Julia told me he was wrong. For my own peace of mind, I had to distinguish between information I wanted to know and information that would depress me. I *did* want to know my blood counts, but I refrained from asking broader questions. I never asked the percentage of AML patients who reach remission. I quit probing for a prognosis. I didn't ask about the choices that awaited me if I reached remission. I didn't want to face frightening decisions I couldn't yet make.

The chemotherapy ended right before Rosh Hashanah. My blood counts started dropping, but two days before Yom Kippur it was clear that they had bottomed out at 1.1. I was terrified that I'd never reach remission. A bone marrow biopsy confirmed my fears—I'd need another round of chemo. In those bleak days, my children became my emotional parents. They couldn't do much for me medically. No one could. One of the most difficult lessons that those who love a sick person must learn is that they can't bring about survival. But they can do a great deal to affect the will to survive. Lisa and Matt showed me how to look inside myself and remember how important it was to be loved. It was the greatest emotional gift they could have offered.

After the second round of chemotherapy, my blood readings fell rapidly. My white blood counts hovered between 0.9 and 0.4 for five days. I was also in pain. My most recent bone marrow biopsy had gotten so badly infected that I could barely stand and I had to receive antibiotics to stave off a fever. I wasn't able to see any visitors except Rachel. But my appetite was still good.

By October 23, my blood counts were skyrocketing, meaning that my immune system was returning. I got permission to walk outdoors, the first time I'd been out of my room in six weeks. I felt as if I'd never walked or tasted fresh air before. When Julia gave me the news that I was in remission this time, I asked her when I could go home. Whenever I wanted to, she said.

I had expected to be very weak when I got out of the hospital, but I was full of energy. I walked three to five miles a day. I was starved to see friends. I felt a childlike pleasure in my strength and stamina.

But no matter how much energy I had, Julia warned me, remission was not a cure. Now that I'd reached remission, my real task was to decide on the next phase of treatment as quickly as possible. There were three possibilities. One choice was to continue with regimen after regimen of chemotherapy and hope that the drugs produced a remission that would last. The second was having a bone marrow transplant; since none of my siblings had marrows that matched mine, my doctors would have to extract my own marrow and treat it to cleanse it of leukemia before transfusing it back into my system. The third alternative was to harvest some of my marrow now, after I'd had some additional chemotherapy to consolidate my remission; but instead of beginning a transplant right away, I could store the marrow and wait to see if I relapsed.

The transplant sounded so arduous that I wanted to talk to as many doctors as possible before I decided to go ahead with it. In November and early December, Rachel and I met with five hematologists and oncologists. I ended up leaning towards having my marrow harvested and stored. But Julia was pushing for an immediate transplant. She reminded me that leukemia is such an aggressive disease you have to fight it as aggressively as possible. And she argued that since I have a strong constitution and an optimistic, cooperative personality I had a good chance of doing well with a transplant. I realized that she knew my body and my cells—and my temperament—better than any of the other doctors I'd consulted. I was a theory as far as they were concerned. I was a human being to her. That made her arguments especially persuasive. I decided to have the transplant as soon as possible.

Besides, I like to be active. I would rather take control of events than have events take control of me. Under the circumstances, the decision to have the transplant—which was as medically sound as the decision to stick with chemo—represented a way of taking action.

Only a few hospitals were equipped to do the kind of transplant I needed: Sloan-Kettering in New York, Johns Hopkins in Baltimore, and Dartmouth-Hitchcock Medical Center in Hanover, N H. Julia thought I should go to Sloan-Kettering, since it would allow Rachel and me to be close to our families and friends.

After I'd had my marrow harvested twice, I learned that the transplant couldn't be done at Sloan-Kettering after all. When my harvested marrow was treated with chemicals to destroy the leukemia, it didn't have enough "progenitor cells"—the cells that would spawn a new marrow.

But Julia had another suggestion. The program at Dartmouth-Hitchcock Medical Center, she said, treated the marrow with genetically cloned antibodies; the antibodies were proteins, not chemicals, so they wouldn't destroy my progenitor cells. I didn't feel like a passive patient. I might be very sick, but I was also part of a team that was at the outermost frontiers of medicine, trying to answer questions that could save me and thousands of people like me.

Early on the morning of March 16, Rachel and I drove from Boston to Hanover. I felt so robust it was hard to remember I was sick. In Hanover, we met Dr. Ted Ball, the chief of transplants, and I had some blood drawn and a routine biopsy done of my bone marrow. My blood counts were perfect, but—shockingly—the biopsy showed that there were leukemic cells in my marrow; I had relapsed. Rachel began to cry. I asked Ted Ball to tell me I was having a nightmare. When I'd arrived in Hanover I'd felt so healthy that I wasn't even sure whether or not I would have a transplant. When I left, I hoped with all the fervor I possessed that I'd return to remission quickly and begin the transplant as soon as possible. I'd worried about my medical decision for months. In the end, it was made for me.

Back in New York on March 23, I started the chemotherapy that might bring me back into re-

mission. I was in the hospital this time for 19 days. My blood count remained at 0.2 for about 12 of them. That meant the chemo was probably working. But I was very weak. Some days I'd sweat and shiver in bed. Words would form in my mind, but I was too weak to say much at all. For the first time, I felt like a patient, not a person. My fever broke on April 9, and on April 12 I had enough white cells that Julia let me go home. On April 18, I finally had enough cells in my bone marrow to allow the biopsy that would determine whether I was in remission or not. I was pacing her office when she came in breathless with the news that I was in remission.

On April 22, I returned to Hanover. After some routine tests, I would be harvested on April 25 and the transplant would begin on May 1. As soon as I got that news, I felt the hope, the energy that had been suppressed since I relapsed.

The bone marrow harvest was bountiful. They got twice as many cells as necessary, and I was set to begin the transplant a few days later. Then I got the word that a spinal tap had revealed leukemic cells in my spinal fluid. That meant returning to New York's University Hospital for spinal taps containing chemotherapy every four days and for another round of chemo to keep my bone marrow in remission. Once again, I felt depressed and fearful. But I believed—I had to believe—that I was on the road to a transplant and a cure.

I came to realize that such frightening setbacks are a routine feature of life in the land of the sick. The truth is that we live with uncertainties. We can't control our bodies, as we did when we were well. They may betray us, our families, our plans, at any time. We can't control our treatments. As I'd seen when the transplants at Sloan-Kettering and at Dartmouth were cancelled, a doctor's well-wrought plan can go askew at the last minute. We don't even possess the minimal security of knowing that we'll be in or out of the hospital on a certain date. There is only one thing over which we can exercise some control—our mood. Our ability to work and love and hope. And our ability to fight.

Over the past five months, I've learned that work is one of the best forms of therapy. I felt compelled to write this article because it channeled my fears—of the transplant when I began, of my relapse when I finished—into an effort to articulate some of what I've been feeling for the past eight months. It has already helped me communicate my feelings to Lisa and Matt. When they read drafts of this article they understood (more clearly than my spoken words had conveyed) just what I have been going through.

I've discovered that love and friendship are therapies too. I've stayed in touch with most of the friends who returned to my life when I was in the hospital. And I've made a new set of friends—other afflicted people. Sometimes these relationships are depressing. It is hard for afflicted people to bear the weight of one another's illnesses. But that doesn't matter. The inhabitants of the land of the sick speak a common language. We can discuss fears we barely admit to others. We can indulge ourselves in bleak jokes we don't dare tell people we love. We're there for one another.

Some of my friends talk about their illness as a precious experience—a threshhold to a new life. I don't agree. I have learned some very important lessons in the past eight months, but not one of them is worth a moment of the hardship my leukemia has inflicted on me and on the people who love me.

I've always wondered how strong I'd be if I were tested. I still don't know. There may be many difficult tests ahead. But I have discovered that I'm stronger than I realized. I've discovered that I can need love and be self-reliant at the same time. I've learned that I can keep loving and laughing and working in the face of relentless fear. I've learned a more important lesson—one I hope stays with me. Dreading death, I've discovered, can still affirm life.

Paul Cowan left the BMT hospitalization, but his

leukemia returned. He died of complications from leukemia on September 26, 1988.

* * *

Peter Zylstra, a nursing home administrator from Statesboro, Georgia, was diagnosed with multiple myeloma in December 1986 at the age of 47. He had an autologous bone marrow transplant at Houston's M.D. Anderson Hospital and Tumor Institute in May 1987. His reflections here were drawn partly from letters he wrote to his wife while he was in Houston and partly from an account he wrote in early 1990 reflecting back on his transplant.

When my doctor told me that what was making me feel exhausted and breathless was not anemia but multiple myeloma, I recall feeling numb and reaching for my wife, Esther's, hand. I had an impulse to either laugh or cry—I wasn't sure which. I couldn't think beyond that moment, as Esther and I held on to each other. It seemed as though I could feel my body drain as I was changed to something different.

I wonder about moments like that. I was present when my father received similar news. I remark to this day on the utter strength I had at that moment. Little did I know at the time that I was to proceed into what would be a special gift for life. Indeed, my life has been changed and every moment since then has been special.

I was sent right away to Houston's M.D. Anderson Hospital, where I was first given a regimen of chemotherapy that put me into remission. The next step was more chemo and then radiation therapy, followed by a bone marrow transplant.

On being told I was a candidate for a bone marrow transplant, I felt both euphoria and fear. My doctor was very honest about the procedure; he held out no false hope but gave me his utter support in making the decision. He reviewed with me what the procedure involves and the mortality of multiple myeloma patients who have this form of treatment (the data coming from circumstances where the patients were far more advanced than I was and not in remission). He went into how my case was different in that I am in better condition than the usual patient. And he explained that I would be the first patient to use this particular bone marrow transplant protocol and that this could mean a very long remission if not a cure!

Having made the decision, I had to prepare for a long separation from my family and for an extended period of confinement in a germ-free "bubble." The informed consent document told me that "one out of ten may not make it," and I made sure my affairs were in order before I traveled to Houston. The hospital had sent me a brochure that made life in the bubble sound easy. My fantasy was that it would be like a retreat—a time to reflect on life, God, and myself, on where I'd been and where I was going, a time to read, write, and listen to music. I tried to prepare for the confinement both psychologically and spiritually. Many family members and friends offered love, support, and hope as I readied myself for the ordeal.

After traveling to Houston and checking into the hospital, I was led to a "protective environment." I would spend the next 48 hours in a preparation room prior to entering the bubble. I received instructions for self-care such as applying antibacterial ointment to my ears, nose, mouth, and perineal area. I learned to take a sterile sponge bath with germicidal soaps and *cold* (!) water and to make my bed with sterile linens. I was introduced to sterile foods prepared by a special process. A nurse helped me sort through my personal things, and anything I wanted to bring in with me was sterilized.

When it came time to actually enter the bubble, I had to take a sterile sponge bath and dress in sterile attire—gown, slippers, robe, hat, and mask. I felt like I was getting ready for a trip into space. When I was ready, I was led through the nurses' station; my entrance was announced, alerting all the staff to put on their masks and remain still. It reminded me of a military maneuver. Then I entered "apartment 1225," an eight-foot by eight-foot cubicle, and the doors clapped shut behind me. I could barely hear the nurse through the barren, stark, cold loneliness tell me to take another sterile bath and change into a new set of sterile clothes. I recall wanting to cry out. I immediately checked out the room and tried to call my wife, only to find the phone out of order. I sat on the bed, feeling physically and emotionally immobile. I tried desperately to stay in touch with myself; however, that ability, which had always been a part of me, seemed to slip away with my loss of independence.

I truly lost it emotionally for a while. A throat is capable of growing a very big lump indeed! Learning of this, a local doctor gave Esther a plane ticket so she could come to see me. I needed that badly and afterwards was able to get hold of myself, establish an attitude change, and grasp the system and protocol under which I would be living for the next six weeks.

On Monday of the second week I received my bone marrow transplant. At this time, a nurse in a "space suit" entered my room to take my vital signs. This was the only time for a four-week period that another human entered my room.

Through all of this, God's goodness abounded. We had a good talk, as I knew we had to proceed through this ordeal together. Each night, as part of devotion time, I would list the blessings of that day. Blessings were mostly those things now taken for granted, such as "my diarrhea was less today," or "I had enough strength to take my sterile sponge bath and do the other self-care chores I needed to accomplish," or "I slept last night," or "I got through five magnum doses of total body radiation and only got sick once."

With the help of God and everyone's prayers, I knew I would make it fine! The phone calls and letters from family and friends were a constant source of support. The doctors and nurses were always encouraging—almost like cheerleaders. I was provided with an "adopt-a-friend" who also helped a lot. I lobbied to get an exercise bike and finally did get one (which had to be sterilized piece by piece before being brought into my bubble). When I rode it, I would visualize myself riding around the Astrodome, which I could see at an angle from my small window.

Getting the lab results was the highlight of every day. I would do the calculations without a calculator in order to prolong the anticipation and pass the time. This was always the day's major event. It was a fabulous experience to learn finally that my new bone marrow had kicked into gear.

When it came time to leave my bubble, I found it to be nearly as hard as entering it had been. I was fearful of leaving the small, safe space; it was like the POW syndrome of a conditioned response to confinement. But with support from the nurses, I was able to leave and join a regular cancer inpatient unit. Here, for the first time, I came to grips with the reality that I belonged to a special fraternity—people with cancer. It was wonderful to see God's spirit evident in each patient I visited with. They all had an attitude about life that was inspiring to me. I could go on and on about this. Bonding with the other patients helped me forge my new life. We understood each other, we could be totally honest, each understood the reality of what life was like for the other.

But this was a painful time too. I felt guilty for having survived. Why did I make it? What was different for me than for the others whom I saw die? How would I handle this new beginning? I was a different person—I'd never be the same Peter again. Would others understand that?

I have learned a lot. One is that God is the center of my life. I feel He always has been, but in a rainy-day sort of way. Now, I find glorifying Him for me must be consistent. I take nothing for granted. I must express gratitude through personal and meaningful prayer for the constant blessings he gives to me and my entire family.

As my checkups over the years have resulted in continued good reports, I realize that cancer truly changed my life. It affected my self-esteem, the mosaic of my relationships with family and friends—the pieces of my life. It truly has been a new beginning!

Peter Zylstra continues to receive a clean bill of health at his checkups.

Appendix A

Nursing Care Plans for the Hospitalized Bone Marrow Transplant Patient

The following nursing care plans reflect the most common problems that develop in the bone marrow transplant patient in the acute care setting. The nursing diagnoses used to describe a patient/family problem are based on the taxonomy developed by the North American Nursing Diagnosis Association. The development of nursing diagnosis is still in its infancy and not yet an exact science based on scientifically tested diagnostic characteristics. Because of this, alternate diagnostic categories may be used in other sources to identify the same phenomenon. Problems are identified as "actual" and related to an etiology if they are likely to occur. "Potential" problems and "risk factors" are used if the problem tends to occur in less than half of the patients. This distinction is somewhat subjective and varies based on the type of transplant being performed.

The problems are also generally listed in order of frequency of occurrence. For instance, almost all patients will develop infections, while neurologic complications occur less frequently and are therefore at the end. The psychosocial care plans are grouped together and follow the physiologic phenomenon.

These care plans were developed by the contributors (listed below) of each of the system chapters. When problems were common to more than one system a collaborative plan was developed. It is our hope that this first proposal will have a twofold benefit. First, as a brief, practical, and useful reference for the novice nurse caring for the bone marrow transplant patient. Second, our hope is that our peers will use and further refine, update, and test our framework so that eventually all of our patients can benefit from the collective consultation of the national nursing experts in bone marrow transplant care.

Contributors to these care plans include: Bruce Ballard, Kathryn Ann Caudell, Deborah Meriney, Peggy Shedd, Karen Vanacek, Marie Whedon, and Terri Wikle.

Nursing Diagnosis	PT/Family Outcomes	Nursing Interventions
Infection, potential for: Risk factors: –leukopenia –immunosuppression –graft-vs.-host disease	Patient is free of infection by discharge as evidenced by: –absence of chills and fever (< 38.5°C) –pulse within normal limits –absence of adventitious breath sounds –absence of burning on urination –absence of redness or swelling at CVC site –intact oral mucous membranes –negative surveillance cultures –absolute neutrophil count at acceptable level Patient is aware of signs and symptoms of infection and reports them immediately	1. Assess patient every four hours for infection or impending septic shock: elevated temperature, flushing, chills, malaise, arthralgias, tachycardia, tachypnea, mental status changes, hypotension, pain on urination or cloudy, foul-smelling urine, dry cough, change in character of breath sounds (decreased or absent), erythema with or without discharge from skin lesions (perirectal, vaginal areas, oral cavity, catheter site, old peripheral intravenous line sites, etc.). 2. Monitor WBC count, particularly absolute neutrophil count to determine period of high risk for infection and return of immune function. 3. Implement protective isolation precautions per institution policy (e.g., laminar air flow, sterile environment, or reverse precautions including hand washing, masking, visitor restrictions, etc.). 4. Perform surveillance cultures per institution protocol and/or obtain cultures with febrile episodes. 5. Teach/perform frequent mouth care (including cleansing with antibacterial, antifungal mouth rinses, moisturizing solutions, dental care including brushing and flossing when appropriate). 6. Initiate antimicrobial diet per institution protocol (e.g., restrictions on fresh fruits, vegetables, only well-cooked foods, etc.). 7. Instruct or assist patient with daily hygiene using antimicrobial soap (chlorhexidine, povidone iodine, etc.). 8. Apply antifungal powders, ointments as ordered (under skinfolds, under breasts, axilla, groin area). 9. Avoid trauma or invasive procedures such as: urinary catheterizations, injections, rectal suppositories, enemas, nasogastric tubes. 10. Initiate measures to prevent rectal trauma from hard stools or constipation (bowel program, stool softeners, sitz baths). 11. Initiate measures to prevent respiratory infection: instruct in/encourage frequent deep breathing, coughing, use of incentive spirometer, increase physical activity, encourage cessation of smoking. 12. Instruct in and/or perform central venous catheter site care per institution protocol. 13. Notify physician immediately for signs and symptoms of infection. Anticipate physician orders: —immediate initiation of antibiotic therapy —reevaluation of current antibiotic therapy, addition of other antimicrobials and/or specific drug level monitoring —obtain appropriate blood, throat, urine, stool, skin cultures, and chest

Nursing Diagnosis	Expected Outcomes	Nursing Interventions
Injury, potential for Risk factors: Thrombocytopenia	Patient is aware of and reports signs and symptoms of bleeding Patient demonstrates measures to prevent bleeding Patient demonstrates absence of bleeding	x-ray —administration of acetominophen. 1. Monitor laboratory values that can indicate bleeding risk or actual occult bleeding, i.e., platelet count, coagulation studies (PT,PTT), bleeding time, hemoglobin, hematocrit, hemetest emesis, urine, and stool 2. Monitor for clinical signs indicative of risk for or actual bleeding: petechiae, ecchymosis, epistaxis, joint pain, or swelling, vaginal or rectal bleeding 3. Monitor neurological status for changes which might reflect intracranial bleed: headache, blurred vision, disorientation, seizures, pupilary changes, etc. 4. Instruct patient and implement measures to protect from injury: —use electric razor —avoid hard-bristled toothbrush and dental floss when thrombocytopenic —avoid forceful nose blowing —carefully supervise toe and fingernail cutting —avoid straining at stool —avoid rectal thermometers, suppositories —avoid injections —apply pressure to injection and bone marrow sites until bleeding ceases (at least 5-10 minutes); consider use of sand bag if bleeding is prolonged —administration of medications to suppress menses during thrombocytopenic period —use of high Fowler's position, ice packs, and nasal packing for epistaxis. 5. Comfort and reassure patient during bleeding episodes. 6. Report bleeding episodes to physician and anticipate physician orders for: —platelet transfusions for count < 20 thousand or if patient is bleeding —treatment of coagulopathies if present from liver dysfunction with appropriate blood components or clotting factors, and or cryoprecipitate, or plasma —possible administration of heparin infusion if disseminated intravascular coagulation is source of bleeding —topical methods of controlling bleeding (e.g., thrombin, silver nitrate sticks, Gelfoam) —antiemetics and/or sedatives to control nausea and vomiting.
Breathing patterns, Ineffective related to: —interstitial pneumonitis	Patient will exhibit adequate respiratory function as evidenced by normal rate, rhythm, and depth of	1. Assess/monitor for hypoxia or altered respiratory function regularly including: —shallow, rapid respiratory rate —use of accessory muscles of respiration —abnormal (absent, diminished, or adventitious) breath sounds —dusky or cyanotic skin color

Nursing Diagnosis	PT/Family Outcomes	Nursing Interventions
—respiratory infection —fluid overload —compromised cardiac status (Gas exchange, Impaired—may occur in relation to the above. Treatment of this diagnosis generally requires referral to the physician.)	respirations, absence of dyspnea, abnormal breath sounds, cyanosis, and normal blood gases, pulse oximentry, chest x-ray, and pulmonary function studies	1. —increased sputum production —decreased activity level —changes in neurological/mental status. 2. Monitor results of laboratory and diagnostic testing: —arterial blood gases/pulse oximetry —sputum cultures —pulmonary function tests —chest x-rays —lung scans. 3. Implement measures to improve respiratory status: —place patient in high Fowler's position —maintain oxygen therapy as ordered —instruct/assist patient in regular coughing, deep breathing, and use of incentive spirometry —encourage aerobic exercise to patient tolerance, e.g., walking, stationary bike. 4. Assist with measures to facilitate removal of pulmonary secretions, i.e., chest physiotherapy, positioning, hand-held or nasotracheal suction, airway humidification, increased fluid intake. 5. Teach patient breathing relaxation exercises. 6. Administer mucolytic agents via nebulizer per order. 7. Administer other agents which may assist with easing breathing pattern: —diuretics to decrease pulmonary edema —morphine sulfate to decrease pulmonary vascular congestion and reduce apprehension-associated dyspnea —bronchodilators —anxiolytics.
Fluid volume Excess related to: —high volume of intravenous fluid (medications) infused —blood product transfusions —impaired renal function	Patient will have a normal fluid and electrolyte balance as evidenced by achieving baseline body weight and normal serum chemistries	1. Strict monitoring of intake and output (especially intravenous fluids. Pharmacy consultation to determine absolute minimum volumes to safely mix medications for administration). 2. Weights BID. 3. Pulmonary assessment every four hours for signs and symptoms of fluid overload (i.e., rales, rhonchi, wheezes, moist cough, increased respiratory effort). 4. Cardiovascular assessment for edema (increased BP, gallops, increased pulse pressure). 5. Neurological assessment for headache, decreased level of consciousness, seizures.

—impaired hepatic function (VOD) —impaired cardiac function (congestive heart failure)		6. Serum and urinary lab values including electrolytes, blood urea nitrogen (BUN), creatinine, hematocrit, urine for specific gravity, osmolality. 7. Measure abdominal girths to detect or monitor ascities. 8. Assess for peripheral and/or dependent edema. 9. Report any evidence of fluid overload (2kg increase in body weight in 24 hours, greater than 1000ml fluid excess on intake, 500ml for pediatric patients) to the physician. 10. Anticipate the following MD orders: —administer diuretics —fluid restriction —administer albumin —"renal dose" dopamine.
Fluid volume deficit related to: —diarrhea —vomiting —mucositis —fever	Patient maintains normal fluid volume and electrolyte balance as evidenced by normal blood and urinary lab values, normal skin turgor, absence of thirst, moist mucous membranes, and normal mentation	1. Monitor blood and urinary lab values for signs of dehydration including: electrolytes, hemoglobin and hematocrit, specific gravity, osmolality. Specifically monitor patients for clinical manifestations of electrolyte imbalance: hypokalemia—muscular weakness, irregular pulse, muscle cramps hypomagnesemia—tachycardia, arrhythmias, increased neuromuscular irritation, paresthesias hyponatremia—anorexia, weakness, abdominal cramping, lethargy, confusion. 2. Monitor vital signs for postural changes and instruct patient to call for assistance when changing position until fluid balance achieved. 3. Monitor body weight for sudden loss. 4. Monitor intake and output for excess output (including careful measurement of emesis, diarrhea, etc.). 5. Frequent mouth care, especially if patient is unable to take oral fluids. 6. Notify physician of early signs of dehydration and anticipate physician orders: —increase fluid intake with corresponding electrolyte replacement —administer acetominophen for fever, also cooling blanket or tepid sponge bath for prolonged, severe fever. Also see the following care plans for specific interventions for related etiologies: —Nausea and vomiting (alteration in nutrition) —Diarrhea (bowel elimination, alteration in bowel elimination) —Mucositis (alteration in tissue integrity).
Nutrition, altered: Less than body requirements	Patient maintains adequate nutritional status during periods of decreased	1. Assess past history of nausea and vomiting to determine pattern and measures that cause or relieve symptoms. Tailor specific plan of care based on this history.

Nursing Diagnosis	PT/Family Outcomes	Nursing Interventions
Related to: —nausea and vomiting	oral intake Patient experiences minimal or no nausea and vomiting	2. Assess nutritional intake and monitor serum and urinary laboratory values that reflect fluid and electrolyte and nutritional status (e.g., BUN, creatinine, glucose, total protein, albumin, electrolytes, iron and total iron binding capacity (TIBC), etc.). 3. Provide small, frequent meals with input from the patient about preferences (often low-fat, bland, and dry foods are tolerated best). Maintain antimicrobial restrictions per institution protocol. 4. Determine with patient which foods to avoid (usually spicy, GI irritating foods and fluids are withheld, for example citric juices, caffeine, foods with strong odors or flavors such as fish). 5. Eliminate noxious sights and smells from the environment at meal times. 6. Administer antiemetics prophylactically, in combination, and at frequency that relieves nausea and vomiting. Attempt different drug combinations and schedules in collaboration with physician and per patient response. 7. Relieve pain from concurrent stomatitis/mucositis if present. 8. Consult with dietician and/or physician to supplement if intake inadequate (i.e., with total parenteral nutrition). 9. Consider behavioral medicine intervention for use of relaxation techniques or measures to control anticipatory nausea and vomiting.
Nutrition, altered: Less than body requirements Related to: —Xerostomia —Taste changes	Patient reports/maintains adequate nutritional status during periods of decreased oral intake Patient reports strategies to manage altered taste	1. Assess quality and severity of dryness or altered taste. 2. Assess general nutritional status and other aspects of oral and dental health that might affect xerostomia, e.g., use of dentures, oral infections, etc. 3. Consult with dietician regarding patient food preferences, aversions; encourage choices that have a high liquid content. 4. Consider use of artificial saliva. 5. Maintain mouth moisture by use of other measures like oral rinses, increasing fluid intake. 6. Maintain integrity of lips by use of moisturizing balms. 7. Recommend that patient avoid drying substances like alcohol, tobacco, commercial mouthwashes, lemon glycerin swabs. 8. Provide room humidification unless contraindicated. 9. Offer foods with a variety of flavors and consistencies to determine preferences given altered taste.
Skin integrity, impaired related to: Skin	Patient's skin will remain intact and/or free of infection	1. Monitor for early signs and symptoms of skin GVHD, i.e., maculopapular rash, dryness, scaling, pruritus, redness of palms and soles. 2. Monitor for evolution of bullae and skin desquamation.

Nursing Diagnosis	Patient Outcomes	Nursing Interventions
manifestations of graft-vs.-host disease		3. Avoid use of harsh soaps and hot water. 4. Daily bathing with antibacterial soap (chlorhexidine or povidone iodine if appropriate) to keep skin clean and dry. Consider use of emollients like Keri-oil, Eucerin cream, aloe cream, as appropriate. 5. Keep bed linens free of wrinkles and avoid use of plastic-backed incontinence pads. 6. Trim nails and discourage patient scratching. Consider hand mitts, anti-pruritic medication, soothing baths, etc. 7. If bullae and skin desquamation occur: —consider use of low air loss or silicon bead bed —apply Burow's solution-soaked gauze (Domeboro) on desquamated areas and remove to aid in debridement and cleansing —apply antibiotic ointment-painted hydrogel dressing to desquamated areas. 8. Administer pain medications as indicated.
Tissue integrity, impaired related to: Radiation, drug-, or infection-induced mucositis	Patient performs prescribed prophylactic and/or therapeutic oral regime at appropriate frequency. Patient maintains adequate nutritional state during period of mucositis. Patient reports adequate oral pain relief when mucositis is present. Patient demonstrates healing of disrupted mucous membranes.	1. Assess for preexisting dental problems. 2. Perform daily oral assessment including assessment for dysphagia. 3. Initiate and instruct patient in oral care regime. 4. Culture suspicious oral lesions for bacterial, fungal, and/or viral pathogens. 5. Monitor degree and severity of lesions and/or dysphagia. 6. If dysphagia present: —Provide oral suction to assist patient in clearing oral secretions —Aspiration precautions —Assess the consistency of foods best tolerated by patient (liquids vs. solids). 7. Apply topical anesthetics or parenteral analgesia for control of oral pain as appropriate. 8. Determine with patient tolerable oral diet to assist in maintaining proper nutrition (e.g., soft, bland diet, ice chips, popsicles, etc.) 9. Consult with dietician and physician for alternative nutritional support if patient unable to tolerate adequate oral nutrition (e.g., total parenteral nutrition, enteral feedings through nasogastric tube). 10. Administer and monitor patient's response to therapeutic medications for oral infections.
Bowel elimination, alteration in, related to: Radiation or GVHD-induced diarrhea	Patient fluid and electrolyte status is maintained within normal limits. Patient returns to normal defecation pattern.	1. Modify oral intake to minimize further risk of exacerbating hypermotility: i.e., minimize caffeine, cooked fruits and vegetables, some lactose-containing products. 2. Offer foods that have antidiarrheal effect, e.g., cheeses. 3. Monitor laboratory values that reflect dehydration and other adverse effects of diarrhea, i.e., electrolytes, serum protein, hemoglobin and hematocrit.

Nursing Diagnosis	PT/Family Outcomes	Nursing Interventions
		4. Monitor stool character for additional complications of bleeding and infection. Perform stool cultures or other diagnostic studies as ordered.
		5. Monitor weight and intake and output for adverse effects from diarrhea and administer proper fluid and nutritional supplementation.
		6. Administer antidiarrheal medications as ordered.
		7. Meticulous perineal care including sitz baths after stools, soothing creams and emollients, anti-inflammatory creams or anesthetic agents.
		8. Regular monitoring of perineal area for breakdown and infection.
		9. Anticipate other physician orders to keep patient NPO, to administer specific medications for GVHD, and to treat other effects of chronic, prolonged diarrhea.
Urinary elimination, alteration in, related to: bladder irritation from cyclophosphamide metabolites (acrolein) and/or adenovirus	Patient is free of signs and symptoms of hemorrhagic cystitis	1. Maintain vigorous oral and intravenous hydration during administration of cyclophosphamide.
		2. Maintain bladder irrigation with 500–1000ml of GU irrigation solution prior to, during, and for 8–24 hours after cyclophosphamide per institution protocol. (Intravenous mesna bladder protectant may also be ordered.)
		3. Continue strict measurement of fluid and electrolyte balance throughout period of bladder irrigation.
		4. Monitor appropriate serum and urinary laboratory tests for evidence of urinary bleeding (i.e., heme test urine, serum hemoglobin and hematocrit).
		5. Immediately report any signs and symptoms of hemorrhagic cystitis to the physician. Anticipate physician orders of: —continuous bladder irrigation —diagnostic bladder testing —administration of platelets, and/or red blood cells.
Activity intolerance related to: —fatigue, —debilitation, —weakness, —anemia	Patient will maintain (or have identified plan to achieve) maximal Karnofsky performance status	1. Offer support and encouragement to perform ADLs and other activities.
		2. Aggressive physical therapy program to enhance conditioning.
		3. Aggressive occupational therapy program if indicated from any resulting deficits.
Potential for injury risk factors: —drug or infection-	Patient is maintained in a safe environment during periods of confusion and disorientation	1. Regular assessment of mentation and neurological function.
		2. Monitor serum lab values and anticipate physician order to replace or correct electrolyte imbalances that interfere with neurological function (e.g., magnesium, sodium, potassium, etc.).

Nursing Diagnosis	Expected Outcomes	Interventions
induced neurological impairment, —metabolic encephalopathies	Patient regains maximal independence and function following resolution of temporary neurologic impairments	3. Know hepatically metabolized drugs and discuss with physician ways to decrease doses or minimize administration of these while patient is hepatically impaired (e.g., narcotics, antibiotics, total parenteral nutrition). 4. Provide safe environment when patient is confused, disoriented: —determine appropriateness of raising bedrails —assess for need for constant supervision —assess appropriate restraint use if necessary —call bell within reach —bed in low position. 5. Orient regularly and provide a clock and calendar for concrete reminders of time. 6. Institute seizure precautions if indicated. 7. Assist with all aspects of self-care until patient is able (e.g., feeding, bathing, toileting, etc.). 8. Support patient and family during periods of confusion, somnolence, coma. Reassure them if condition is predicted to be temporary and reversible.
Social isolation related to protective isolation precautions	Patient/Family will determine plan to optimize contact with appropriate social supports during hospitalization Patient will express tolerable level of loneliness while hospitalized	1. Assess with patient and family normal social supports. 2. Assist patient to determine list of friends and family who would be most helpful supports during hospital stay (appropriate visitors). 3. Explore availability of appropriate visitors. Assist patient to formulate a schedule of visits in accordance with isolation precautions, unit visitor policy, and patient's care needs. 4. Discuss alternate ways of communicating with appropriate visitors: phone calls, cards and letters, audio and video tapes, photographs. 5. Offer staff and volunteer visitors as available: social worker, CNS, chaplain, volunteers, Cansurmount (ACS) visitors. 6. Offer BMT patient/family support group if allowed by isolation precautions. 7. Instruct visitors in isolation precautions, emphasizing the importance of interaction with the patient. Specify what contact they are permitted to have with the patient.
Anxiety related to nausea and vomiting or pain	Patient/family will evaluate effectiveness of anti-anxiety component of antiemetic or pain regimen Patient will identify approach to modify anxiety associated with	1. Evaluate patient's previous experience with nausea/vomiting or pain. What made it worse? Individualize care plan accordingly. 2. Explain and teach use of relaxation exercises to patient/family. Encourage patient to practice exercises 2–3X/day as well as when nauseated or in pain. 3. Evaluate and encourage patient's use of relaxation exercises, modify or correct as necessary. 4. Explore with patient the use of other available behavioral techniques: guided imagery, quiet music or television for distraction, biofeedback, hypnosis.

Nursing Diagnosis	PT/Family Outcomes	Nursing Interventions
	N/V or pain Patient verbalizes satisfaction with anxiety level achieved through approach	5. Evaluate patient's current pharmacological program for effective analgesic and antiemetic effect. Modify as necessary for optimal effect. 6. Provide adequate information for patient/family to understand care routines, diagnostic tests, etc.
Alteration in patient/family coping related to powerlessness	Patient/family will determine appropriate coping strategies for hospitalization Patient will report acceptable level of control for him/her as well as for staff/family while hospitalized	1. Explore patient's previous methods of coping with hospitalization and cancer. 2. Identify coping methods by which patient attempted to cope with lack of control or power in past: sleeping, sedation, treatment refusal, demanding behavior, repetitive questions, extensive reading or searching for information, formulating schedules of activities, alliance with care givers for care planning, keeping a journal of activities, blood counts, test results, etc. 3. Allow appropriate expressions, verbalizations of anger, fear, anxiety, loss of independence, role performance. 4. Encourage and reward the use of positive, healthy, past coping strategies—incorporate into routine care. 5. Collaborate with patient in care planning. Allow choices when possible. 6. Explore outcome of any past regressive coping strategies—assist patient to notice negative outcomes. 7. Assess family's understanding of patient's coping strategies. Validate appropriate strategies and encourage family to support these with patient. 8. Offer support group, psychosocial resource staff as available.
Alteration in parenting related to prolonged hospitalization	Patient and spouse are able to identify realistic and appropriate ways for patient to function as parent while hospitalized Patient, family will verbalize acceptance and comfort with patient's role as parent while hospitalized	1. Explore patient's role as parent precancer and how it has changed since diagnosis of cancer. 2. Acknowledge difficulties of maintaining parental role while sick or in hospital. 3. Evaluate patient's strategies to meet parental role obligations while hospitalized. Encourage use of effective and appropriate strategies: phone calls, visits from children, reports of school and other activities, identification of parental activities patient can continue while hospitalized, problem solving disciplinary action as necessary and child care substitutions. 4. Explore spouse's thoughts of patient's current ability to function as parent. Reinforce importance of patient maintaining as much parental activity as able. 5. Offer psychosocial resource staff as available and necessary.
Noncompliance	Patient will perform necessary procedures at minimum level of	1. Assess patient's reasons for noncompliance. A. If related to lack of knowledge—educate patient/family as to reasons for and correct methods of performing procedures.

acceptability while hospitalized	B. If related to pain—explore and modify pain management to provide adequate relief for patient to perform required procedures. C. If related to fatigue—arrange patient's daily schedule to allow rest period before procedure. Assist patient when fatigued. D. If related to lack of belief in care givers and therefore lack of belief in importance of procedure, establish trust by consistency in care givers, respect for patient's autonomy and knowledge, collaboration with patient in care planning. 2. Assess all procedures and rank order by level of necessity. Allow patient as much flexibility in performance as possible. 3. Praise patient for achievements. 4. Assess family's appreciation of necessity of patient's compliance with procedures. Educate as necessary. 5. Enlist family's encouragement of patient's compliance or at least support for nursing interventions to improve compliance.
Grieving, anticipatory Patient/family will openly express their thoughts and feelings regarding potential death during transplant hospitalization Patient/family is able to verbalize comfort with level of preparation for death	1. Explore patient's and family's beliefs and concerns regarding their/patient's mortality. 2. Acknowledge reality of patient's/family's concerns, correct misperceptions. 3. Support patient and family in their ambivalence regarding hope for cure and fear of morbidity/mortality. 4. Evaluate patient's preparation for death: will, living will, durable power of attorney, CPR status, funeral arrangements, child care wishes, etc. at patient's level of tolerance for discussion. 5. Utilize chaplains, social workers, psychosocial resources as appropriate.

Appendix B

Bone Marrow Transplant Resource List

This list was adapted from the list of transplant centers in the *International Bone Marrow Transplant Registry* (except for those centers which are listed as "so" under the **SIG** column). After each center an "x" appears in the **AUTO** or **ALLO** column indicating the type(s) of transplants reported to be performed by each center.

SIG—an "sa" in this column indicates that the center is *also* listed in the 1990 Oncology Nursing Society Special Interest Group *Bone Marrow Transplant Nursing Resource Directory*. An "so" in this column indicates that this center was listed *only* in the SIG directory and not in the international registry. The reader should contact either of these directories for specific physician or nurse names and phone numbers.

NMDP—an "x" in this column indicates that this center is listed as one of the National Marrow Donor Program transplant centers. These centers have applied for and met particular criteria to become NMDP-recognized centers (see Chapter 5 for full details of the definition of this criteria).

International Bone Marrow Transplant Registry (IBMTR)
Statistical Center
Medical College of Wisconsin
P.O. Box 26509
Milwaukee, WI 53226
414-257-8325

Mortimer M. Bortin, M.D.
Scientific Director

Mary M. Horowitz, M.D.
Assistant Scientific Director

The IBMTR, located in the Division of Biostatistics/Clinical Epidemiology at the Medical College of Wisconsin, is a research organization for the collection and analysis of data regarding allogeneic bone marrow transplantation. Most transplant centers worldwide voluntarily report detailed information regarding their consecutive bone marrow transplants on specialized reporting forms. Results of IBMTR analyses are presented at scientific meetings throughout the world and published in scientific journals and medical textbooks.

The International Autologous Bone Marrow Transplant Registry (ABMTR)
c/o Dr. N.C. Gorin
Department of Hematology
Hopital St. Antoine
184 rue du Faubourg St. Antoine
75571 Paris Cedex 12, France

The ABMTR is a voluntary association of North American and European physicians representing centers performing autologous bone marrow transplants. Results reported to the ABMTR are periodically reported in scientific journals and presented at symposia. Currently, there is no central office for the group and officers of the advisory committee will change periodically so that the most accurate address for correspondence will only be available from individual transplant physicians or through publications of the group.

U.S. Transplant Centers	AUTO	ALLO	SIG	NMDP
Baptist Medical Center—Princeton 701 Princeton Avenue, SW Birmingham, AL 35211 205-783-7483	x		so	
Arkansas Children's Hospital 800 Marshall Street Little Rock, AR 72202 501-370-1495	x	x	sa	
Arizona Cancer Center Room 4945 1515 North Campbell Avenue Tucson, AZ 85724 602-626-4196	x	x	sa	
Regional Cancer & Blood Disease Center of Kern San Joaquin Hematology/Oncology Medical Group 3550 Q Street Bakersfield, CA 93301 805-327-5529	x			
Bone Marrow Transplant Program Alta Bates Herrick Hospital 3001 Colby Street Berkeley, CA 94705 415-540-1591	x	x	sa	
Department of Hematology/BMT City of Hope National Medical Center 1500 East Duarte Road Duarte, CA 91010 818-359-8111 x2403	x	x	sa	x
Weingart Center for Bone Marrow Transplantation Scripps Clinic & Research Foundation 10666 North Torrey Pines Road La Jolla, CA 92037 619-455-9100	x	x	sa	

U.S. Transplant Centers	AUTO	ALLO	SIG	NMDP
Kaiser Hospital 4950 Sunset Boulevard Los Angeles, CA 90022 213-667-4011	x	x	sa	
BMT Program Kaiser Permanente Southern California Permanente Medical Group 4700 Sunset Boulevard Los Angeles, CA 90027 213-667-5306	x	x	sa	pend.
Pediatric BMT Program Department of Pediatrics UCLA Medical Center Los Angeles, CA 90024 213-825-3046		x		x
Division of Hematology/Oncology Department of Medicine UCLA—Center for Health Sciences CHS Room 37068 10833 Le Conte Los Angeles, CA 90024-1678 213-825-3046		x	sa	x
BMT Program Norris Cancer Center University of Southern California 1441 Eastlake Avenue Los Angeles, CA 90033 213-224-6443	x	x	sa	
Division of BMT and Research Immunology Children's Hospital of LA 4650 Sunset Boulevard Los Angeles, CA 90027 213-669-2546	x	x	sa	x
Department of Hematology Children's Hospital Medical Center Bone Marrow Transplant Unit Oakland, CA 94609 415-428-3690	x	x		
Children's Hospital of Orange County 455 South Main Orange, CA 92705 714-532-8636	x	x	sa	

U.S. Transplant Centers	AUTO	ALLO	SIG	NMDP
Bone Marrow Transplant Program Stanford University Hospital 300 Pasteur Drive Room H1353 Stanford, CA 94305 415-723-0822	x	x	sa	x
Children's—San Diego 8001 Frost Street San Diego, CA 92123 619-576-5811	x	x	sa	
Department of Pediatrics Pediatric Bone Marrow Transplant Program University of California Moffitt Hospital Room 679 San Francisco, CA 94143 415-476-2188	x	x		x
BMT Program UCSF Medical Center 400 Parnassus Avenue Room A—502 San Francisco, CA 94143 415-476-1220	x	x	sa	
Pacific Presbyterian Medical Center Division of BMT 2351 Clay Street Stanford 414 San Francisco, CA 94115 415-923-3646	x	x	so	
University of Colorado Health Sciences Center 4200 East Ninth Avenue B140 Denver, CO 80262 303-394-8796	x			
Department of Medicine University of Connecticut Health Center Farmington, CT 06032 203-679-2255	x	x	sa	
Bone Marrow Transplant Program Yale University School of Medicine 333 Cedar Street New Haven, CT 06510 203-785-4744	x	x	sa	

U.S. Transplant Centers	AUTO	ALLO	SIG	NMDP
BMT Program Lombardi Cancer Research Center Georgetown University Medical Center 3800 Reservoir Road, NW Washington, DC 20007 202-687-2253	x	x	sa	x
George Washington University 2150 Pennsylvania Avenue, NW Washington, DC 20037 202-994-4200	x	x	sa	
Children's Hospital National Medical Center 11 Michigan Avenue, NW Washington, DC 20010 202-745-2140	x	x	so	
Pediatric Hematology/Oncology Pediatric BMT Unit P.O. Box J296 University of Florida J. Hillis Miller Health Center Gainesville, FL 32610 904-392-4470	x	x		x
Shands Hospital Division of Medical Oncology P.O. Box J277 University of Florida J. Hillis Miller Health Center Gainesville, FL 32610 904-372-0937	x	x	sa	x
Bone Marrow Transplant Program All Children's Hospital 801 Sixth Street South St. Petersburg, FL 33701 813-892-4235		x	sa	x
Bone Marrow Transplant Program Division of Medical Oncology H. Lee Moffitt Cancer Center & Research Institute University of South Florida 12902 Magnolia Drive Tampa, FL 33612-9497 813-979-7202	x	x	sa	x
Henritta Egleston Hospital for Children 1405 Clifton Road, NE Atlanta, GA 30322 404-325-6460	x	x	so	

U.S. Transplant Centers	AUTO	ALLO	SIG	NMDP
Northside Hospital 1000 Johnson Ferry Road Atlanta, GA 30042 404-851-8000	x		so	
Department of Pediatrics Emory University 2040 Ridgewood Drive Atlanta, GA 30322 404-727-4451	x	x		
Emory University—Box AE 718 Woodruff Memorial Building Atlanta, GA 30322 404-727-5830	x	x	sa	
St. Francis Medical Center 2230 Liliha Street Honolulu, HI 96817 808-547-6536	x	x	sa	
Division of Pediatrics Hematology/Oncology University of Chicago Hospitals 5841 South Maryland Avenue Box 97 Chicago, IL 60637 312-702-6808	x	x	sa	
Rush Presbyterian-St. Lukes Medical Center BMT Center 1653 West Congress Parkway Chicago, IL 60612 312-942-3047	x	x	sa	
Loyola University Medical Center Building 54 Room 067H 2160 South First Avenue Maywood, IL 60153 312-531-2056	x	x	sa	
Bone Marrow Transplantation Methodist Hospital 1701 N. Senate Boulevard Indianapolis, IN 46206 317-929-3400	x	x		x
Department of Medicine Indiana University Hospital, W608 926 W. Michigan Avenue Indianapolis, IN 46202-5250 317-274-0843	x	x	sa	x

U.S. Transplant Centers	AUTO	ALLO	SIG	NMDP
Pediatric BMT Department of Pediatrics University of Iowa Hospitals 2524 JCP Iowa City, IA 52242 319-356-1608	x	x	sa	x
Hematology Division University of Kansas 39th and Rainbow Boulevard Kansas City, KS 66103 913-588-6077	x	x	sa	
St. Francis Regional Medical Center 818 Emporia #403 Wichita, KS 67214 316-262-4467	x	x	sa	
BMT University of Kentucky Medical Center Lexington, KY 40536-0084 606-233-5768	x	x	sa	x
Division of Hematology James Graham Brown Cancer Center 529 S. Jackson Street, Room 427 University of Louisville Louisville, KY 40292 502-588-8050	x	x	sa	x
BMT Program Section of Hematology/Oncology Louisiana State University School of Medicine 1542 Tulane Avenue New Orleans, LA 70112-2822 504-568-5843		x	sa	x
Tulane Medical Center 1430 Tulane Avenue New Orleans, LA 70112 504-588-5412	x	x	sa	
Pediatric Hematology/Oncology Children's Hospital Louisiana State University Medical Center 200 Henry Clay Street New Orleans, LA 70118 504-896-9505 504-568-6221	x	x		

U.S. Transplant Centers	AUTO	ALLO	SIG	NMDP
Division of Hematology/Oncology Louisiana State University Medical Center Shreveport, LA 71130 318-674-5970	x			
Johns Hopkins Oncology Center 600 North Wolfe Street Baltimore, MD 21205 301-955-8785	x	x	sa	x
Department Health & Human Services Public Health Service NIAID National Institutes of Health 9000 Rockville Pike Building 10 Room 11B13 Bethesda, MD 20892 301-496-7196	Syngeneic in AIDS only			
Bone Marrow Transplant Program Brigham and Women's Hospital 75 Francis Street Boston, MA 02115 617-732-6782	x	x	sa	x
Dana-Farber Cancer Institute 44 Binney Street Boston, MA 02115 617-732-3465	x	x	sa	
Bone Marrow Transplant Unit Children's Hospital Medical Center 300 Longwood Avenue Boston, MA 02115 617-732-3315	x	x	sa	
Bone Marrow Transplant Program University of Michigan Room F7828 Box 0247 1500 East Medical Center Drive Ann Arbor, MI 48109-0247 313-936-8785	x	x	sa	
Wayne State University School of Medicine 3990 John R. Detroit, MI 48201 313-745-9160	x	x	sa	x
Abbott Northwestern Hospital 800 E. 28th Street Minneapolis, MN 55407 612-863-5383	x		so	

U.S. Transplant Centers	AUTO	ALLO	SIG	NMDP
University of Minnesota P.O. Box 86 University Hospitals Minneapolis, MN 55455 612-625-4659	x	x		x
Adult BMT Program University of Minnesota Hospital and Clinics 420 SE Delaware Street P.O. Box 480 UMHC Minneapolis, MN 55455 612-624-5422	x	x	sa	
Pediatric BMT Program 420 SE Delaware Street P.O. Box 366 UMHC Minneapolis, MN 55455 612-626-2778				
Department of Internal Medicine Division of Hematology Mayo Clinic Rochester, MN 55905 507-284-2511 x4100		x	sa	
Boone Hospital Center 1600 E. Broadway Columbia, MO 65201 314-875-3381	x		so	
Barnes Hospital #1 Barnes Hospital Plaza St. Louis, MO 63110 314-362-5084	x	x	so	
Hematology/Oncology Association 3401 Berrywood Drive Suite 301 Columbia, MO 65201 314-874-7800	x			
Division of Hematology/Oncology Washington University School of Medicine P.O. Box 8125 660 S. Euclid St. Louis, MO 63110 314-362-7589	x	x		
Department of Medicine University of Nebraska Medical Center 42nd and Dewey Avenue Omaha, NE 68105 402-559-7290	x	x	sa	x

U.S. Transplant Centers	AUTO	ALLO	SIG	NMDP
Bone Marrow Transplant Unit Department of Pediatrics University of Nebraska Medical Center 42nd and Dewey Avenue Omaha, NE 68105 402-559-4062	x	x		
Bone Marrow Transplant Unit Department of Internal Medicine University of Nebraska Medical Center 42nd and Dewey Avenue Omaha, NE 68105 402-559-5170	x	x		
Bone Marrow Transplant Program Bishop Clarkson Memorial Hospital Dewey Avenue at 44th Omaha, NE 68105 402-559-3645	x	x	sa	
Department of Medicine Dartmouth Hitchcock Medical Center Hanover, NH 03756 603-646-7671	x	pend.	sa	
Bone Marrow Transplantation St. Joseph's Hospital & Medical Center 703 Main Street Paterson, NJ 07503 201-977-2122	x	x	sa	
Hematologic Oncology Department Roswell Park Memorial Institute 666 Elm Street Buffalo, NY 14263 716-845-3087	x	x		
Adult BMT Unit North Shore University Hospital 300 Community Drive Manhasset, NY 11030 516-562-4160	x	x	sa	
Atran Building P.O. Box 1275 Mt. Sinai Hospital 1 Gustave Levy Plaza New York, NY 10029 212-241-6021	x	x	sa	
Memorial Sloan-Kettering 1275 York Avenue New York, NY 10021 212-639-5957	x	x	sa	x

U.S. Transplant Centers	AUTO	ALLO	SIG	NMDP
Montefiore Medical Center 111 East 210 Street Bronx, NY 10467 212-920-6648	x	x	sa	x
Division of Oncology New York Medical College Valhalla, NY 10595 914-285-8374	x	x	sa	
University of Rochester Medical Center 601 Elmwood Avenue Rochester, NY 14642 716-275-2884	x	x	sa	
Duke University Medical Center 363 Jones Building P.O. Box 2898 Durham, NC 27710 919-684-2922 919-684-6707	x		sa	
Bowman Gray School of Medicine 300 South Hawthorne Road Wicke Forest University Winston-Salem, NC 27103 919-748-2088	x	x		
University of Cincinnati Medical Center Mail Location No. 562 Cincinnati, OH 45267 513-558-4233	x	x	sa	
BMT Program Children's Hospital Medical Center CHRF 1-18 Cincinnati, OH 45229 513-559-4266	x	x	sa	x
Department of Medicine University Hospital of Cleveland 2074 Abington Road Cleveland, OH 44106 216-844-3629	x	x	sa	
Department of Hematology/Oncology Cleveland Clinic 9500 Euclid Avenue Cleveland, OH 44106 216-444-6922	x	x	sa	x

U.S. Transplant Centers	AUTO	ALLO	SIG	NMDP
Case Western Reserve University Hospital Bone Marrow Transplant Program University Circle Cleveland, OH 44106 216-444-3330	x	x		
Ohio State University Bone Marrow Transplant Program 410 W. 10th Avenue Room N1025 DN Columbus, OH 43210 614-293-8939	x	x	sa	x
University of Oklahoma Department of Medicine Section of Oncology P.O. Box 26901 940 Stanton L. Young Oklahoma City, OK 73190 405-271-4022	x	x	sa	x
Division of Immunology/Rheumatology Department of Pediatrics Oregon Health Sciences University 3181 SW Sam Jackson Park Road Portland, OR 97201 503-279-8447		x		
Children's Hospital of Philadelphia 34th and Civic Center Boulevard Philadelphia, PA 19104 215-590-2141	x	x	sa	x
BMT Program Temple University Parkinson Pavilion Room 759 3400 North Broad Street Philadelphia, PA 19140 215-221-2847	x	x	sa	
BMT Program University of Pennsylvania Cancer Center G Penn Tower 3400 Spruce Street Philadelphia, PA 19104-4385 215-662-3402 x6313	x		sa	
Institute for Cancer & Blood Disease Hahnemann University Broad Street and Vine Street Philadelphia, PA 19102 215-448-8026	x	x	sa	x

U.S. Transplant Centers	AUTO	ALLO	SIG	NMDP
Montefiore Hospital 3459 5th Avenue Pittsburgh, PA 15213 412-648-6436	x	x	sa	x
Allegheny General Hospital 320 East North Avenue Pittsburgh, PA 15212 412-359-3131	x		x	
Department of Pediatrics University of Tennessee Medical Center P.O. Box 50642 Knoxville, TN 37950-0642 615-544-9320 615-971-1000	x	x		
St. Jude Hospital Children's Research Hospital 332 North Lauderdale 10 Box 318 Memphis, TN 38101 901-522-0300	x	x		
A2127 Medical Center North Vanderbilt University Nashville, TN 37232 615-322-2829	x	x	sa	x
Baylor University Medical Center 3500 Gaston Avenue Dallas, TX 75246 214-820-2619	x	x	sa	x
Children's Medical Center 801 7th Avenue Fort Worth, TX 76104 817-885-4006	x	x	sa	
Section of BMT Department of Hematology M.D. Anderson Cancer Center University of Texas 1515 Holcombe Boulevard Box 65 Houston, TX 77030 713-792-3611	x	x	sa	x
Baylor College of Medicine 6565 Fannin Mailing Station 902 Houston, TX 77030 713-790-2155	x	x	sa	

U.S. Transplant Centers	AUTO	ALLO	SIG	NMDP
Texas Children's Hospital Pediatric Immunology 6621 Fannin Street Houston, TX 77030 713-798-1319	x	x	sa	
Bone Marrow Transplant Program Department of Medicine/SGHMMH Wilford Hall USAF Medical Center Lackland AFB, TX 78236-5300 512-670-7312 512-670-7311	x	x	sa	
San Antonio Tumor & Blood Clinic Baptist Medical Center 8527 Village Drive Suite 101 San Antonio, TX 78217 512-656-7177	x		sa	
Bone Marrow Transplant Program Department of Medicine University of Texas Health Science Center and Southwest Texas Methodist Hospital 7703 Floyd Curl Street San Antonio, TX 78284 512-567-4848	x	x		x
Audie-Murphy VA Hospital University of Texas HSC 7400 Merton Minter Boulevard San Antonio, TX 78284 512-696-9960	x		so	
Department of Medicine LDS Hospital Eighth Avenue and C Street Salt Lake City, UT 84143 801-268-0303	x	x		
University of Virginia P.O. Box 465 Charlottesville, VA 22901 804-924-1693	x	x	sa	x
Bone Marrow Transplant Program Division of Hematology/Oncology Medical College of Virginia Virginia Commonwealth University P.O. Box 230 Richmond, VA 23298-0001 804-786-9641	x	x	sa	

U.S. Transplant Centers	AUTO	ALLO	SIG	NMDP
BMT Program Fred Hutchinson Cancer Center 1124 Columbia Street Seattle, WA 98104 206-467-5111 206-467-4324	x	x	sa	x
Swedish Hospital Medical Center 747 Summit Avenue Seattle, WA 98104 206-386-6000	x	x	so	
VA Medical Center 1660 South Columbian Way Seattle, WA 98108 206-764-2709	x	x	sa	x
University of Wisconsin Hospital & Clinics K4/434 Clinical Science Center 600 Highland Avenue Madison, WI 53792 608-263-6201	x	x	sa	pend.
Department of Oncology/Marshfield Clinic 1000 North Oak Avenue Marshfield, WI 54449 715-387-5416	x	x	sa	
Bone Marrow Transplant Program Medical College of Wisconsin 8700 West Wisconsin Avenue Milwaukee, WI 53226 414-257-7142	x	x	sa	x

Alphabetical by state

Donor Registries

National Marrow Donor Program
100 South Robert Street
St. Paul, MN 55107
612-291-3871

The National Marrow Donor Program serves as the hub organization within the United States to maintain a centrally organized registry of unrelated potential marrow donors. The NMDP also coordinates activities of donor centers and transplant centers to facilitate unrelated marrow transplants and conducts donor and histocompatibility-related research. (See Chapter 5 for a full explanation of the function of the NMDP.)

LIFE-SAVERS Foundation of America
529 South Second Avenue
Covina, CA 91723
818-967-1500

A charitable, nonprofit corporation dedicated to the education, recruitment, and testing of potential marrow donors. LIFE-SAVERS can provide assistance to families and communities in marrow donor recruitment. They also maintain a "Donor Hotline" at 1-800-999-8822 to provide additional information to prospective donors about the donation process.

Nursing-Related Resources

The Bone Marrow Transplant Special Interest Group of the Oncology Nursing Society
1016 Greentree Road
Pittsburgh, PA 15220-3125
412-921-7373

The BMT SIG, established in 1989, provides a formal structure within ONS to facilitate networking of ONS members who are interested in the specialty of BMT. The primary goals of the SIG are to maintain a Nursing Resource Directory, to develop guidelines for BMT nursing practice, to develop collaborative nursing research projects, and to plan educational offerings. Information on how to become a SIG member or how to access any of the above-mentioned resources is available by contacting the national office of ONS at the above address and phone.

Patient-Related Resources

American Cancer Society
Tower Place
3340 Peachtree Road, NE
Atlanta, GA 30026
404-320-3333

The local state or division office should be contacted first, these phone numbers are located in your local phone book. The ACS provides a variety of cancer-related services and materials to patients and health professionals.

Aplastic Anemia Foundation of America
P.O. Box 22689
Baltimore, MD 21203
301-955-2803

Provides information to patients about coping with their disease.

BMT Newsletter
c/o Susan Stewart
1985 Spruce Avenue
Highland Park, IL 60035
708-831-1913

A newly developed newsletter, written by a former BMT patient, designed for bone marrow transplant patients, their families and friends, and members of the general public who are interested in learning more about bone marrow transplants and related issues.

Candlelighters Childhood Cancer Foundation
Suite 1001
1901 Pennsylvania Avenue
Washington, DC 20006
202-659-5136

Formed in 1970 by parents of young cancer patients at local hospitals in the Washington, DC, area, this group's primary focus is to help parents and other family members share the experience of having a child with cancer and to obtain consistent and adequate federal support for cancer research.

Corporate Angel Network
Westchester County Airport
Building One
White Plains, NY 10604
914-328-1313

A nonprofit organization that arranges free air transportation for cancer patients going to or from recognized treatments, consultations, or checkups. The program uses available seats on corporate aircraft. A person must be in stable condition, able to board unassisted, and have backup reservations available as service is not guaranteed. Available regardless of financial need.

Leukemia Society of America
733 Third Avenue
New York, NY 10017

A national voluntary health agency dedicated to seeking the control and eventual eradication of leukemia and related diseases. The Society is concerned with public and professional education, patient aid, and research. Patient financial aid and informational booklets about the disease and treatment are available. There are 56 chapters in 31 states and the District of Columbia.

National Coalition of Cancer Survivorship
323 Eighth Street, SW
Albuquerque, NM 87102
505-764-9956

An organization of independent groups and individuals interested in issues of cancer survivorship and support of cancer survivors. "The mission of NCCS is to communicate that there can be vibrant, productive life following the diagnosis of cancer." A quarterly newsletter is published.

Ronald McDonald Houses
500 North Michigan Avenue
Chicago, IL 60611
312-863-7100

Ronald McDonald Children's Charities
One McDonald's Plaza
Oak Brook, IL 60521
312-575-7048

First established in 1974, over 100 Ronald McDonald houses have been established worldwide to provide temporary low-cost lodging to families of children who are undergoing treatment at nearby hospitals for cancer, leukemia, and other serious illnesses.

Appendix C

List of Abbreviations

ALL—acute lymphocytic leukemia
AML—acute myelogenous leukemia
ANV—anticipatory nausea and vomiting
ARAC—cytosine arabinoside
ARDS—adult respiratory distress syndrome
ATG—antithymocyte globulin
BID—twice a day
BMT—bone marrow transplant
cGy—centigray
CML—chronic myelogenous leukemia
CTZ—chemoreceptor trigger zone
Cy—cyclophosphamide
CyA—cyclosporine
DHPG—gancyclovir
DIC—disseminated intravascular coagulation
ECG—electrocardiogram
GVHD—graft-versus-host disease
HLA—human leukocyte antigens
IBMTR—International Bone Marrow Transplant
  Registry

IPn—interstitial pneumonitis
MRI—magnetic resonance imaging
NBTE—nonbacterial thrombotic endocarditis
NMDP—National Marrow Donor Program
OLB—open lung biopsy
PBSC—peripheral blood stem cells
QD—daily
SAA—severe aplastic anemia
SCIDS—severe combined immunodeficiency
  syndrome
SIADH—syndrome of inappropriate antidiuretic
  hormone
TBB—transbronchial biopsy
TBI—total body irradiation
TID—three times a day
TLI—total lymphoid irradiation
VC—vomiting center
VOD—veno-occlusive disease

Glossary

Ablation. Removal or destruction, as in to remove or destroy the hematopoietic system with chemoradiotherapy.

Absorption. The active renal tubule process that moves material in the renal filtrate from the lumen of the renal tubule into the capillary surrounding the tubule.

Acute tubular necrosis. The type of renal failure caused by damage to the epithelial cells lining the renal tubules, typically from nephrotoxic or ischemic insult.

Akinetic mutism. A state in which the individual makes no spontaneous movement or sound.

Allogeneic BMT. Bone marrow is derived from another person, usually an HLA-matched sibling.

Alveolar/Capillary block. Impaired ability of gasses to pass through the pulmonary alveolar/capillar membrane.

Aphasia. Defect or loss of the power of expression by speech, writing or signs, or of comprehending spoken or written language, due to injury or disease of brain centers.

Ataxia. Failure of muscular coordination; irregularity of muscular action.

Autologous BMT. Bone marrow is derived from self.

Bronchiectasis. Chronic dilatation of a bronchus or bronchi, with secondary infection that usually involves the lower portion of the lung.

Cardiac ejection fraction. Fraction of the end dyastolic volume that is ejected from the ventricle of the heart at the end of a contraction. It is reported as a percent of normal.

cGy. (centi gray) A dose measurement of radiation therapy. It is sometimes interchangeably used with rad. One centigray equals one rad. One hundred centigrays equals one Gy (Gray).

Chimera. In greek mythology, an animal composed of a lion's head, goat's body, and a serpent's tail. In bone marrow transplantation the term has come to mean the outcome of transplanting a foreign hematopoietic system into a recipient host.

Concomitant infection. An infection taking place at the same time as at least one other organism.

Conditioning. The process of preparing the host to receive bone marrow.

Consolidation. Solidification of the lungs due to pathologic engorgement of lung tissue usually due to an infectious process.

Cor pulmonale. Hypertrophy or failure of the right ventricle resulting from disorders of the lungs, pulmonary vessels, or chest wall.

Dysarthria. Imperfect articulation of speech due to disturbances of muscular control that result from damage to the central or peripheral nervous system.

Dysdiadokokinesis. Decreased ability to perform rapid alternating movements.

Dysesthesia. Impairment of any sense, especially that of touch. A painful and persistent sensation induced by a gentle touch of the skin.

Dysmetria. A condition in which there is improper measuring of distance in muscular acts; decreased ability to gauge distance.

Dysphagia. Difficulty in swallowing.

Engraftment. The process whereby normal hematopoiesis resumes following a bone marrow transplant because bone marrow stem cells have returned to the marrow space and reinstated the production and normal maturation of blood cells.

Excretion. The renal process that passes the product of the renal nephron processes, from the kidney out of the body.

Filtration. The process of moving water and dissolved substances through a permeable membrane from an area of higher pressure to an area of lower pressure. In the renal tubule, this occurs at the glomerulus, and is measured by the glomerular filtration rate (gfr).

Fixed staffing. Nursing staff that provide support services to a nursing unit and are required in the same number no matter how many patients are on the nursing unit (e.g., management staff, secretarial staff, and others assistive to nursing roles).

Full-time equivalent. An employee who works 40 hours per week (i.e., 40 hours = 1 FTE; 32 hours = .8 FTE; 24 hours = .6 FTE, etc.).

Genotype. The entire genetic constitution of an individual.

Glomerular filtration rate. The rate at which filtrate is produced at the glomerulus by the process of filtration and passed on to the renal tubules.

Graft-versus-host disease. A common complication of bone marrow transplantation between recipients other than identical twins and autologous donors. An immunologic response occurs in the recipient whereby immunologically competent T cells from the donor marrow attack the seemingly "foreign" host resulting in varying degrees of damage to three target organs: the skin, gastrointestinal tract, and liver.

Guillain-Barré syndrome. Acute febrile polyneuritis.

Haplotype. A set of alleles of a group of closely linked genes; usually inherited as a set (such as the HLA complex). One set is usually inherited from each parent.

Hemiparesis. Muscular weakness affecting one side of the body.

Hemorrhagic cystitis. A condition of ulcerated bladder mucosal tissue secondary to infection or the toxic effects of acrolein, a metabolite of cyclophosphamide.

Human leukocyte antigens. A series of antigens found on white blood cells and most other cells of the body that are responsible for one of the major histocompatibility systems in man. Often referred to as the human body "fingerprint." HLA typing is performed between the donor and potential recipient to determine the degree of similarity between these individuals' body tissues.

Intention tremor. Tremor that arises, or which is intensified when a voluntary, coordinated movement is attempted.

Interstitial pneumonitis. An inflammatory process involving the intra-alveolar linings of the lung.

Intrarenal failure. The type of renal failure that is characterized by an injured nephron tubule such that the processes of absorption and secretion are impaired.

Length of stay. The number of days each individual patient is hospitalized.

Leukoagglutinin. An antibody that causes the clumping together of white blood cells.

Meningismus. Signs and symptoms of meningeal irritation associated with acute febrile illness or dehydration without actual infection of the meninges.

Meningoencephalitis. Inflammation of the brain and meninges.

Myopathy. Any disease of a muscle.

Negotiated bid. A specific contractual agreement that is made between the hospital and the third-party payor for services to be provided.

Neuralgia. Paroxysmal pain that extends along the course of one or more nerves.

Nuchal rigidity. Extreme stiffness of the back of the neck.

Nystagmus. Involuntary rapid movement of the eyeball, which may be horizontal, vertical, rotary, or mixed.

Obtundation. State of mental dullness or bluntness.

Opportunistic organisms. Organisms that cause an infection due to the opportunity afforded by the altered physiological state of the host.

Ototoxicity. Exerting a deleterious effect upon the eighth cranial nerve or upon the organs of hearing and balance.

Parkinsonism. Group of neurological disorders characterized by hypokinesia, tremor, and muscular rigidity.

Patient care hours. A measurement of time for each individual patient's nursing care requirements.

Patient day. Each individual day a patient is hospitalized.

Phenotype. The unit of inheritence.

Photophobia. Abnormal visual intolerance of light.

Positive end expiratory pressure. A method of holding alveoli open during expiration. The goal is to achieve adequate arterial oxygenation without using toxic levels of oxygen.

Postrenal failure. The type of renal failure that is characterized by an inadequate glomerular filtration rate secondary to impaired delivery of blood to the glomerulus, or inadequate pressure differential across the glomerular capillary wall to allow sufficient filtration to occur.

Predictive staffing methodology. A mathematical method for predicting variable staffing requirements, i.e., the staff that provides direct patient care.

Prospective reimbursement. The rate to be paid for health care services is established with the third-party payor prior to the period over which the rate is to be applied.

Ptosis. Drooping of the upper eyelid from paralysis of the third cranial nerve or from sympathetic innervation.

Pulmonary compliance. The distensibility of the lungs. It is reduced by anything that obstructs the normal flow of air in and out of the lung.

Quadriparesis. Paralysis of the arms and legs.

Retrospective reimbursement. Payments by the third-party payor are made after health care services have been provided.

Secretion. The active renal tubule process that moves material in the capillaries surrounding the renal tubule into the lumen of the tubule.

Spasticity. Increase over the normal tone of a muscle with heightened deep tendon reflexes.

Stupor. Marked reduction in mental and physical activity; marked slowness and reduction in response to commands or stimuli.

Superinfection. A new infection caused by an organism different from that which caused the initial infection. The microbe responsible is usually resistant to the treatment given for the initial infection.

Syngeneic BMT. Bone marrow transplant between identical twins.

Third-party payor. The agency that pays all or part of a patient's hospital and health care bills, usually an insurance company, Medicare, or Medicaid.

Tinnitus. Noise in the ears, such as ringing, buzzing, roaring, clicking, etc.

Tumor lysis syndrome. The syndrome resulting from the rapid destruction of tumor cells with cytotoxic therapy. High serum levels of intracellular materials are common with risk of hyperkalemia, hyperuricemia, hyperphosphatemia, and hypocalcemia.

Variable staffing requirements. The staff that is required to meet patient care requirements. This number will vary based on the number of patients and their individual nursing care requirements.

Veno-occlusive disease (VOD). A disease of the liver induced by toxic effects of high-dose chemotherapy and/or radiation characterized by an occlusion in the venous outflow tract of the liver.

Index

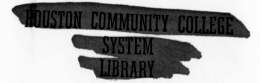